CLINICAL OUTLINE
OF ORAL PATHOLOGY:
Diagnosis and Treatment

CLINICAL OUTLINE
OF ORAL PATHOLOGY:
Diagnosis and Treatment

LEWIS R. EVERSOLE, D.D.S., M.S.D.
Chairman, Department of Pathology and Medicine
Director, Facial Pain Research Center
University of the Pacific
School of Dentistry
San Francisco, California

SECOND EDITION

LEA & FEBIGER   1984 • Philadelphia

Lea & Febiger
600 Washington Square
Philadelphia, PA 19106-4198
U.S.A.
(215) 922-1330

First Edition, 1978
  Reprinted, 1981

Library of Congress Cataloging in Publication Data

Eversole, Lewis R.
  Clinical outline of oral pathology.

  Includes bibliographical references and index.
  1. Mouth—Diseases. 2. Teeth—Diseases. I. Title.
[DNLM: 1. Mouth Diseases—diagnosis—handbooks. 2. Mouth
Diseases—therapy—handbooks. 3. Tooth Diseases—
diagnosis—handbooks. 4. Tooth Diseases—therapy—hand-
books. WU 39 E93c]
RC815.E9 1984   617.6   84-7870
ISBN 0-8121-0929-5

PRINTED IN THE UNITED STATES OF AMERICA

Print No.   4   3   2   1

To Chris and Laura

Preface

This book is written with the full knowledge that many comprehensive texts dealing with the information recorded herein are available to the dental clinician and the student of oral diseases. Indeed, some of these textbooks on oral diseases explore them in such detail that students are inundated with description and may find themselves in a quandary regarding salient features, resulting in a lack of assimilation and retention of the knowledge originally sought. In addition to this dilemma, in the conventional textbook approach, disorders are considered on a pathogenetic or etiologic basis (e.g., developmental, inflammatory, neoplastic diseases, etc.). Unfortunately, patients do not present themselves for diagnosis and treatment in this fashion but, rather, manifest certain signs and symptoms. The pathogenetic approach to the presentation of oral pathologic entities is under no criticism here; indeed, initial confrontation with the basic concepts of oral disease is perhaps dealt with most logically in this fashion. Once these basic concepts have been studied, however, students must filter through this knowledge to construct a differential diagnosis dependent upon the presenting signs and symptoms. Herein lies the value of this clinical outline.

This second edition maintains the general format of the previous edition whereby diseases of the oral cavity have been categorized according to presenting signs and symptoms, with a primary objective being the development of a differential diagnosis. Each chapter outlines diseases according to these features, and the various clinical parameters used to differentiate among lesions manifesting common signs and symptoms are enumerated. An introductory chapter provides guidelines for the development of an approach to the patient. Once the chief complaint and history of the present illness have been obtained along with other aspects of the data base, the sleuthing process begins, thus requiring appropriate sequencing of interrogation, clinical testing, and laboratory data procurement. The introductory chapter provides the student with a protocol for developing a differential diagnosis, evaluating patient responses and clinical signs so as to limit the differential, and ultimately securing a definitive diagnosis so that a treatment plan can be generated. Whereas microscopic characteristics are not featured in detail, for the emphasis is on clinical diagnosis, the vital role of biopsy for the confirmation of a clinical impression must be remembered. As stated, the diseases discussed in this outline are categorized according to their most common presenting features; since, however, exceptions can and do arise, a diagnosis must be considered tentative until confirmed by biopsy or, in some instances, by use of certain laboratory tests.

Preceding each chapter are clinical taxonomic tables followed by diagrams that elucidate the pathogenic basis for collective clinical signs characterizing each chapter heading. The disease entities included in each chapter have been reordered in some instances; the last chapter, which deals with facial pain and neurologic and functional disorders, has been revised and expanded.

Another goal of this book is to rank disorders according to frequency and life-threatening importance. Each chapter considers the most common pertinent entities and emphasizes those diseases with serious prognostic implications. With each entity, references are given for standard texts and publications that pursue more detailed accounts of the subject; in this respect, this outline may be used as an adjunctive text.

Finally, once a definitive diagnosis has been evolved, the matter of treatment becomes paramount. For each entity, the most widely accepted form of treatment—be it surgical, medical, psychologic, or radiotherapeutic—is given. Oral abnormalities may be manifestations of diseases of a systemic nature, and under these circumstances, patient management becomes the responsibility of a physician. Recommendations of this nature are dealt with under the treatment sections.

It is my hope that this text will integrate the precepts of basic oral pathology, oral radiology, and oral medicine into a usable chairside outline, enabling the clinician to construct a differential diagnosis, arrive at a definitive diagnosis, and ultimately provide appropriate management and treatment for the patient.

San Francisco, California   Lewis R. Eversole

Acknowledgments

This book was designed as a practical, useful chairside aid to clinical diagnosis of oral lesions. Its utility depends upon the use of representative illustrative material. In this regard, I am deeply indebted to many people who provided me with clinical photographs from previous publications and from their own personal collections. In particular, I wish to acknowledge the cooperation of Dr. Sheldon Rovin; Dr. Henry Cherrick, Dean, University of Nebraska School of Dentistry; Dr. Alan Leider, Asssociate Professor of Diagnostic Sciences, University of the Pacific, School of Dentistry; Dr. Robert Gorlin, Chairman of Oral Pathology, University of Minnesota; Dr. Carl Witkop, Chairman of Human and Oral Genetics, University of Minnesota, School of Dentistry; Dr. Stefan Levin, Department of Otolaryngology, the Johns Hopkins University, School of Medicine; and Dr. Charles Tomich, Department of Oral Pathology, Indiana University, School of Dentistry.

My appreciation is also warmly extended to Dr. Willard Fee, Department of Otolaryngology, Stanford University, School of Medicine, and to Dr. Roger Bowles, Chairman of Otolaryngology, University of California at San Francisco, School of Medicine, for contributing illustrative materials for the chapter on extraoral soft tissue swellings.

Included in the appendix are listings of prescription drugs employed in the practice of oral medicine. I wish to acknowledge Dr. Peter Jacobsen and Dr. Constance Stone who have compiled a student drug booklet at the University of the Pacific from which much of this material was compiled.

One of the most tedious tasks in the preparation of a textbook is, of course, the typing of the manuscript. I am deeply indebted to my secretaries, Miss Myrna Pantangco and Miss Doris Low, for their patience and diligence in this regard. Mr. Arnold Eilers, Director of Audiovisual Aids, University of the Pacific, School of Dentistry, deserves my gratitude for his preparation of literally hundreds of photographs used to illustrate the various disorders compiled in this text. I am deeply indebted to Mr. George Mundorff, editor for Lea & Febiger, for his constructive comments and assistance during the course of planning and revising the manuscript.

Lastly, I wish to extend appreciation to my family, children, and friends for their encouragement and patience with me during the months of work required to prepare this book.

L.R.E.

Contents

1
The Diagnostic Process

PROCUREMENT OF THE DATA BASE
  Chief Complaint and History of the Present Illness
  Medical and Dental History
  Physical Examination
  Radiographic Examination

ASSESSMENT OF THE FINDINGS

FORMULATING A DIFFERENTIAL DIAGNOSIS

SECURING A DEFINITIVE DIAGNOSIS

FORMULATING A TREATMENT PLAN

The diagnostic process involves four sequential steps: (1) obtainment of a comprehensive overview of the patient's past and current health status, referred to as the historical data base; (2) evaluation of all the findings to correlate the chief sign or symptoms with the current history, other physical findings, and the medical history; (3) formulation of a differential diagnosis to include all disease processes that could conceivably account for the collective findings; and (4) arrival at a definitive diagnosis on the basis of interrogation and specific clinical and laboratory tests that serve to exclude specific diseases and point to a definite disease process. Once the diagnostic process is consummated, a plan for treatment can be generated with establishment of a follow-up assessment program.

Thorough and open communication between doctor and patient is a prerequisite to the diagnostic process. Since the ultimate goal is the definitive diagnosis, the doctor is charged with the duty of sleuth par excellence, meaning he or she must develop the communication skills to become an eminent interrogator. The questioning process is as important as having a large knowledge base regarding disease processes and the skills necessary to recognize tissue changes. The process of interrogation helps to exclude diseases that, on the basis of physical appearance or symptoms alone, would have been included as initial possibilities. What questions does one ask? First, the physician must have a reasonable comprehensive knowledge of the possible disease entities he or she may encounter. Without this knowledge base, the appropriate line of questioning may not be obvious. Alternatively, the examiner who is aware of the various diseases sharing common symptoms or physical signs can ask appropriate questions to begin the process of elimination (i.e., limiting the differential diagnosis). As we proceed through the sequential steps of the diagnostic process, emphasis will be placed on the development of a logical approach to interrogation.

PROCUREMENT OF THE DATA BASE

Chief Complaint and History of the Present Illness

The initial contact with the patient should be met with concern conveying a desire to be of assistance. Patients are often upset, fearful, annoyed, or short-tempered when they feel they are ill or have something wrong with them. This is particularly true when pain is the primary complaint or when they have sought help from other health practitioners who were unable to arrive at a diagnosis. Nonverbal communication such as a hand on the shoulder, a look of kindness, or a comment expressing concern and determination to help will open the doors to trust and communication. Once these subtle gestures have helped

1

to establish rapport, an assessment of the patient's problem or chief complaint can be explored. The chief complaint usually emerges as a symptom, a sign, or both.

Symptoms are subjective, representing a definite problem expressed by the patient. Common symptoms of oral and maxillofacial disease processes include the following.

Discomfort: Pain, ache, numbness (hypesthesia), tingling (paresthesia), itching (pruritus), burning, rawness, tenderness, and clicking/popping of TMJ.

Textural Changes: Roughness, dryness (xerostomia, xerophthalmia), and swelling (growth, enlargement).

Functional Changes: Difficulty with swallowing, opening, or chewing: altered bite, taste, or hearing: difficulty with speech: tooth clenching or grinding: joint sounds; loose teeth and bleeding from mouth, gingiva, or nose.

Once the chief symptom is recorded, questioning helps to define the problem more accurately. Interrogation revolving around the chief complaint should explore the nature of the problem, the duration, the periodicity, the location, and association with factors known to the patient. For example, if a patient complains of pain, the examiner should explore its nature (i.e., sharp, dull, throbbing, etc.). How long has the symptom been a problem? Has it persisted for a few hours, a few days, or for weeks or months? What is the periodicity of the pain? Is it constant, intermittent, only at night, only at mealtime? Where is the pain located? It is localized or does it radiate? Can it be associated with hot liquids, cold liquids, spicy foods, citrus fruits, sugar, pressure, percussion? A similar line of questioning can be pursued for other subjective complaints or symptoms.

Signs are objective changes that can be observed or detected by palpation, percussion, auscultation, or analysis of laboratory data. Common signs of oral and maxillofacial disease processes include the following.

Soft-tissue Changes: White, red, or pigmented spots or patches; ulcerations; blisters; multiple small nodules (papules); nodules; papillary growths; localized swellings; and diffuse swellings.

Hard-tissue Changes (Clinical): Dental changes in number, shape, or structure; localized or diffuse osseous swellings; and facial asymmetry.

Hard-tissue Changes (Radiographic): Dental changes, radiolucent or radiopaque lesions, and mixed radiolucent/radiopaque lesions.

Neuromuscular Functional Changes: Paralysis or flaccidness, muscle spasm or hypertrophy, special sensory deficits, and alteration in salivation.

Not all patients will relate a specific symptom. Often they will observe a change in the tissues. Objective signs can be noticeable tissue changes that the patient observes or changes that may be unknown to the patient but have been detected during the course of the physical examination. Signs should be characterized in more detail by exploring their features and history. When a patient states that he or she discovered a tissue change, the physician should attempt to uncover, through questioning, the nature of the disease from the patient's perspective, the duration, the location, and any associated factors. For example, a patient may state that while looking in the mirror he or she discovered a white patch on the tongue. The examiner will want to know how the patient perceives the change. Is it sore? Can you feel its presence? How long ago did you first notice it? Is that the only place in your mouth you've noticed a change? Do you recall biting your tongue or burning it?

Medical and Dental History

The recording of the problem—be it a symptom, a sign, or both—along with the history of the illness should have allowed the examiner to contemplate a partial list of suspected disease processes. At this point, the chief complaint is put aside until other aspects of the data base are procured. The next step in the diagnostic process is to evaluate the patient's history of illness. The patient's general health status is reviewed by determining how the patient feels. Does he or she feel weak or febrile? Has there been any significant weight loss or loss of appetite? A history of past illness according to the body's organ systems is reviewed; the examiner knows that certain medical problems require dental treatment precautions. Furthermore, many systemic diseases manifest observable oral and facial lesions. Habits and medications can also affect the tissues of the head and neck. Previous hospitalizations and any complications from past medical treatment can have a bearing on the oral and maxillofacial tissues. Finally, the dental history might have some influence with regard to the presenting problem.

Physical Examination

Provided there are no significant medical problems that would militate against proceeding with the physical examination, the examiner should begin a systematic evaluation of the tissues. In medicine, physical diagnosis involves examination of the organ systems. In dentistry, the primary emphasis is examination of the head and neck. Usually, prior to a detailed evaluation of these tissues, the vital signs, including blood pressure, pulse, respiration, and temperature are assessed. Subsequently, physical examination should include the external structures of the scalp, face, exposed skin and hands; the oral, nasal, and laryngeal cavities; the tympanic membrane; the salivary glands and neck; the temporomandibular joint; and the dentition and periodontium. During the physical examination deviations from normal are recorded.

Once the physical examination has been completed, the examiner should recall the chief complaint and focus attention on physical changes associated with the presenting signs and symptoms. Once a lesion has been uncovered and clinically characterized, the examiner should proceed by ordering adjunctive diagnostic tests. Many tests are available in the diagnostic armamentarium, and these tests should be used discriminantly to avoid excessive cost to the patient. In general, a differential diagnosis is established once the data base from the history and physical examination has been completed. However, when signs and symptoms point to a disease process in bone, radiographs are usually obtained prior to formulation of a differential diagnosis.

Radiographic Examination

When the patient's history and physical examination suggest pain of dental or osseous origin, salivary occlusion, asymmetry, or osseous enlargement, appropriate radiographs are obtained in order to characterize dental or intraosseous disease processes. In general, periapical and panoramic films are used initially. The location of the suspected problem will indicate specific radiographs (see table 1.1). New technology is emerging rapidly in radiology; detailed tissue imaging is possible with the use of three-dimensional computerized tomography, radioisotopic scanning, xeroradiography, and nuclear magnetic resonance imaging techniques. Many of these techniques are costly yet may be extremely valuable diagnostically as well as for determining extent of disease.

In most cases, routine radiographs and tomograms are obtained initially and are followed by special films as needed or when indicated.

Radiographic interpretation is rarely diagnostic. The ability of the radiologist or clinician to describe the radiomorphology and list diseases known to exhibit specific patterns is of major importance.

ASSESSMENT OF THE FINDINGS

Once all the preliminary data base including initial radiographs is secured, the physician must return to the chief complaint and physical findings. All this data must now be placed in perspective by focusing on the problems and correlating them with the overall findings. During this process, new lines of interrogation may emerge. The problems and findings represent a mosaic that must achieve the best fit in order to arrive at a diagnosis. Provided the examiner's knowledge base is comprehensive, the pieces of the puzzle will usually fall into place readily. Occasionally, however, some of these puzzles are quite complex and require more sophisticated diagnostic procedures. After all the data have been reviewed, collated, and correlated, the dentist should be able to list possible disease entities that could be responsible for the findings. This list of entities represents the differential diagnosis.

FORMULATING A DIFFERENTIAL DIAGNOSIS

The list of entities subsumed under the designation "differential diagnosis" can be quite staggering, particularly when only the presenting signs or symptoms are taken into account. To the astute clinician, the interrogative process along with the review of all findings should have eliminated many entities from the differential diagnosis list. In this regard the "differential" has already been limited in scope. Perhaps only two or three disease processes remain worthy of consideration.

So far, the discussion has revolved around principles and generalities. A specific example may help to clarify some of these general considerations. Suppose a 40-year-old woman comes to you with a chief complaint of painful sores in her mouth. This is a presenting symptom. If you were to develop a differential diagnosis including all lesions that manifest mouth sores, you would probably use up an entire notebook. This might be a terrific academic exercise, but the patient is waiting for help. At this point you would want to obtain more history. She states that they appeared

TABLE 1.1. Radiographs in Oral and Maxillofacial Medicine

Area of Investigation	Radiographs
Dental caries	Bite-wing
Infections of dental origin	Periapicals
Impactions	Panoramic
Jaw lesions	Panoramic
Salivary stones (submandibular)	Mandibular occlusal
Salivary stones (parotid)	Panoramic
Salivary occlusion, inflammation, tumors	Sialogram
Sinus lesions	Water's sinus, Cauldwell sinus, sinus tomograms
Other paranasal sinuses	Paranasal sinus tomograms, CT scans
Facial deformities	CT scans, Cephalometric survey
Temporomandibular joints	TMJ tomograms, arthrograms, CT scans
Facial fractures	Many different films are available to visualize specific sites.
Jaw and facial tumors	CT scans, radioisotope scans, nuclear magnetic resonance imagery

two weeks ago, she never had anything like this before, and they are getting worse. Despite all this, she does not feel tired or feverish. Review of her medical history is noncontributory, meaning she has a clean bill of health. Furthermore she is not taking any medication. At this point the long list in your differential diagnosis may be somewhat shortened.

Now you conduct the physical examination and find multiple oral lesions that are red, ulcerated, and sloughing. Furthermore, you discover a few large intact blisters. Being a sharp clinician, you conclude that this patient suffers from one of the bullous disorders. You have now considerably shortened the list because less than a dozen bullous diseases affect the oral tissues. Also, during your examination you failed to note any conjunctival, nasal, or skin lesions. What you have is a limited, working differential diagnosis. Furthermore, based on her age, sex, and distribution of the oral lesions, you can eliminate some of the entities in the bullous disease category.

This example, then, helps to clarify the process of limitation of the differential diagnosis. The final step in the diagnostic phase of the approach to the patient involves devising a plan to secure a definitive diagnosis.

SECURING A DEFINITIVE DIAGNOSIS

Once a reasonable limited differential diagnosis is formulated, specific tests are conducted. These tests can further limit the differential by excluding some diseases (i.e., the rule-out process). It is more advisable, however, to rule in probable disease processes. In oral medicine, the most useful diagnostic tool is biopsy. In most, yet not all instances, the pathologist can provide a definitive diagnosis based on histologic evaluation of the diseased tissue. Some diseases exhibit ambiguous or nonspecific histologic changes, and clinical or laboratory findings are more germane to the process of inclusion or exclusion.

Another important concept is the principle of "cause and effect." Just because two factors occur simultaneously (i.e., they are correlated) doesn't mean one causes the other. For example, an ulcer may occur on the tongue adjacent to a fractured tooth cusp. Before concluding a cause-and-effect relationship, the dentist should restore the tooth to normal contour and allow two weeks to pass. If the lesion persists, the initial observation ascribing an irritational causative role can no longer be substantiated. A biopsy should then be performed, and it may reveal an early cancerous lesion. Therefore, a cause should be searched for in all cases, and if found, documentation should be pursued in order to determine whether or not the observation was indeed causative or merely correlative.

In most instances, a definitive diagnosis can be secured on a clinical, histologic, radiologic, and/or laboratory finding basis. Occasionally, a final diagnosis cannot be made because all definitive tests and criteria are ambiguous. Under these circumstances therapeutic trials may be in order. Perhaps the diagnosis is limited to two or three possibilities; if so, the most likely disease is selected and treated accordingly. If the treatment succeeds, then one can usually conclude, on the basis of response to treatment, that the probable diagnosis was correct.

FORMULATING A TREATMENT PLAN

Once a definitive diagnosis is made, the most efficacious treatment must be selected. Depending upon the disease, the following management strategies will be considered: (1) no treatment, (2) surgical removal, (3) pharmacologic agents, (4) palliative treatment, (5) behavioral or functional treatment, and (6) psychiatric therapy. Referral to a medical or dental specialist may be required. One should realize that many diseases cannot be cured, and treatment is aimed at control and alleviation of symptoms. Some diseases resolve of their own accord, some require a single curative treatment, and others require prolonged or indefinite treatment.

After a management strategy has been formulated and implemented, a plan for prevention of recurrence should be devised. For example, a patient with leukoplakia showing microscopic evidence of premalignant change (i.e., dysplasia) may have been successfully treated by surgery. Failure to eliminate important etiologic factors such as continued alcohol and tobacco use could result in a recurrence of the disease in the same site or in a new location. The clinician should advise the patient about these potentially harmful habits and help the patient to curtail them.

The final consideration, and one of paramount importance, is patient follow-up and assessment. Patients with a disease that has a potential for recurrence should be placed on periodic recall. The length and periodicity are determined by the behavior and natural history of the disease process. Some diseases never recur, and initial therapy is conclusive and complete; therefore, short-term follow-up and assessment are adequate. Alternatively, neoplastic diseases and chronic illnesses may require frequent recall assessment and retreatment.

The diagnostic process must be thorough and include history procurement, physical examination, and radiologic examination when indicated. All patient findings are integrated to synthesize a differential diagnosis. The differential diagnosis is pared down with selective interrogation and specific diagnostic procedures such as biopsy and clinical laboratory tests. With establishment of a definitve diagnosis, a management plan can be devised; results of therapy should be evaluated by follow-up assessment, and preventive measures, when applicable, should be instituted.

The remainder of this text is designed to aid the clinician in the attainment of a definitve diagnosis; each disease is described so that the examiner can efficiently evaluate the signs and symptoms in order to arrive at a definitive diagnosis. Most chapters are arranged according to physical findings; the final chapter, dealing with facial pain, being subjective, is outlined according to presenting symptoms. The recommended therapy is mentioned briefly, and the reader may find more detail regarding management by referring to the current references listed for each disease.

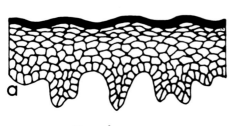

Normal mucosa

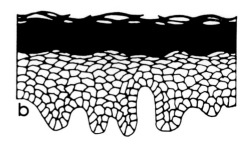

Hyperkeratosis

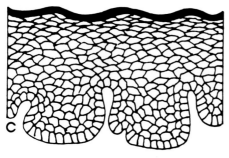

Acanthosis

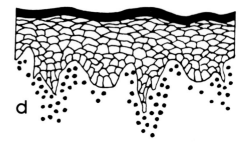

Lymphocytic infiltration

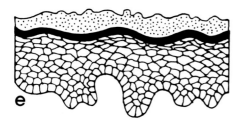

Extrinsic coating

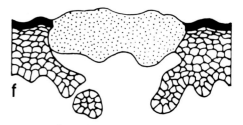

Ulcerative pseudomembrane

White Lesions

2
White Lesions

GENOKERATOSES

　Leukoedema
　White Sponge Nevus
　Hereditary Benign Intraepithelial Dyskeratosis
　Keratosis Follicularis
　Pachyonychia Congenita
　Incontinentia Pigmenti

LEUKOPLAKIAS

　Friction/Trauma Associated Leukoplakia
　Idiopathic/Tobacco Associated Leukoplakia
　　Planar Leukoplakia
　　Verruciform Leukoplakia
　　Speckled Leukoplakia
　　Snuff Leukoplakia
　Actinic Cheilitis
　Dysplasia, Carcinoma in Situ, Squamous Cell
　　Carcinoma, and Verrucous Carcinoma

DERMATOSES

　Lichen Planus
　Lupus Erythematosus

INFLAMMATIONS

　Koplik Spots of Measles
　Mucous Patches of Syphilis
　Chemical Burns
　Candidiasis

MISCELLANEOUS WHITE SPOTS AND PAPULES

　Fordyce's Granules
　Dental Lamina Cysts, Bohn's Nodules, and Epstein's
　　Pearls
　Stomatitis Nicotina

White lesions of oral mucous membranes appear thus because (1) one or more of the epithelial layers is thickened or (2) an extrinsic or intrinsic pseudomembrane is adherent to the surface mucosa. The white lesions encountered in practice may be subdivided into groups on the basis of pathogenesis or etiologic factors. Developmental white lesions are generally bilateral in distribution. Patients will relate that a familial pattern exists, since most of the developmental white lesions are genetically inherited (genokeratosis).

As a gardener's hands become calloused from hours of friction from the hoe, so may the oral epithelium become calloused or thickened in response to chronic trauma. Tobacco in its many forms is also considered a local irritant, and indeed is associated with carcinomatous transformation in white lesions of the oral mucosa. The white lesions associated with physical or tobacco-product irritation are grouped under the heading leukoplakias, as are other white lesions of undetermined origin. Since tobacco-associated and idiopathic white lesions may show microscopic evidence of malignancy, biopsy must be performed when (1) a cause cannot be detected or (2) the suspected traumatic agent is eliminated yet the lesion fails to involute or regress.

White lesions of nonhereditary diseases may coexist with skin lesions. These keratotic dermatoses may, however, occur as oral lesions with skin involvement. As no etiologic agent can be discerned in oral keratotic dermatoses, biopsy must be undertaken to confirm the diagnostic impression when classical clinical features of these disorders are lacking.

Inflammatory lesions that may produce thickened epithelium and/or a surface pseudomembrane will appear white, and in these instances the surface coating may be rubbed away with gauze. The diagnosis of inflammatory white lesions can be secured by obtaining a thorough history, including questions regarding use of drugs, sexual habits or promiscuity, recent contact with persons manifesting similar illness, or contact with injurious chemicals.

The last group of white lesions is characterized by multifocal spots on the mucosa that are generally diagnostic on a clinical basis for the entities in this group.

This chapter illustrates and enumerates the features of white lesions in the aforementioned context. The differential diagnosis for a given white lesion will depend upon obtaining a history, with primary considerations of: (1) a familial pattern, (2) presence or absence of a causative agent with notations on oral habits, particularly tobacco use, (3) presence or absence of associated skin lesions, (4) questions relating to contact with individuals showing similar lesions, (5) presence or absence of fever, and (6) exploration of the nature of the white patch as to tenacity to underlying structures and ease of removal by rubbing. Based upon responses and findings regarding the above considerations, a ranking of entities in the differential diagnosis may ensue and ultimately biopsy, or in certain instances serology and blood count, must be performed to obtain a definitive diagnosis.

The most frequently encountered white lesions are: (1) friction, idiopathic or tobacco associated leukoplakias, (2) lichen planus, (3) candidiasis, (4) leukoedema.

White lesions associated with a potentially lethal outcome include: (1) premalignant leukoplakias and (2) lupus erythematosus.

GENOKERATOSES

Leukoedema

Age: No predilection
Sex: No predilection

Clinical Features: Leukoedema occurs in blacks and dark-skinned Caucasians and is so frequently encountered that it should be considered a normal variation in these individuals. The lesion is bilateral and diffuse, involving the buccal mucosa, and shows a filmy, mother-of-pearl appearance, often with delicate overlapping curtain-like mucosal folds. When the mucosa is stretched the white appearance is diminished.

Microscopic Features: The epithelium displays acanthosis, parakeratosis, and spongiosis.

Differential Diagnosis: The diffuse delicate

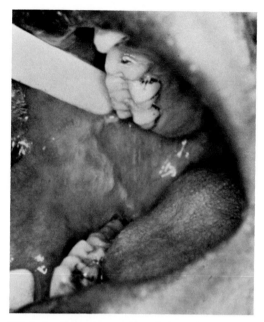

FIG. 2–1.　Pale mucosa with a slight tendency to form curtain-like folds in leukoedema.

mother-of-pearl sheen and the propensity to involve members of the Negro race are characteristics that permit differentiation from other hereditary white lesions of the genokeratosis group. The primary entities in the differential diagnosis include white sponge nevus and hereditary benign intraepithelial dyskeratosis, both of which are thicker, plaque-like, and show specific microscopic features.

Treatment: No treatment is necessary.

References

1. Archard, H. O., Carlson, K. P., and Stanley, H. R.: Leukoedema of the human oral mucosa. Oral Surg. 25:717, 1968.
2. Durocher, R. T., Thalman, R., and Fiore-Donno, G.: Leukoedema of the oral mucosa. J. Am. Dent. Assoc. 85:1105, 1972.
3. Martin, J.L. and Crump, E.P.: Leukoedema of the buccal mucosa in Negro children and youth. Oral Surg. 34:49, 1972.

White Sponge Nevus

Age: Childhood onset
Sex: No predilection

Clinical Features: White sponge nevus, inherited as an autosomal dominant trait, appears from ultrastructural observations to represent a defect in epithelial maturation involving tonofilament formation with impaired normal desquamation of the superficial strata of cells. It is characterized by

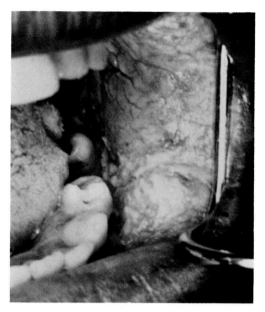

FIG. 2–2. Thickened, diffuse white lesion of buccal mucosa in white sponge nevus.

diffuse and sometime patchy white lesions of the buccal mucosa, bilaterally, with involvement of the tongue and occasionally other oral mucosal sites. The conjunctivas are spared; however, vaginal, esophageal, and anal mucous membranes may harbor white lesions similar to those of the oral tissues.

Microscopic Features: The epithelium shows parakeratosis and acanthosis with spongiosis. Parallel striae of condensed parakeratin traverse the surface layers in oblique planes. Individual cell keratinization may be seen in the spinous cell layer.

Differential Diagnosis: Other white lesions do not tend to be as thick and diffuse as white sponge nevus; however, hereditary benign intraepithelial dyskeratosis, lichen planus, and candidiasis should be considered in the differential diagnosis. Biopsy will disclose characteristic features.

Treatment: No treatment is necessary.

References

1. Cannon, A. B.: White sponge nevus of the mucosa (naevus spongiosus albus mucosae). Arch. Dermatol. Syph. *31:*365, 1935.
2. Cooke, B. E. D.: Oral epithelial nevi. J. Dent. Res. *35:*954, 1956.
3. Witkop, C. J. and Gorlin, R. J.: Four hereditary mucosal syndromes. Arch. Dermatol. *84:*762, 1961.
4. Stiff, R. H. and Ferraro, E.: Hereditary keratosis. Oral Surg. *28:*697, 1969.
5. Whitten, J. B.: The electron microscopic examination of congenital keratosis of the oral mucous membranes. I. White sponge nevus. Oral Surg. *29:*69, 1970.

Hereditary Benign Intraepithelial Dyskeratosis

Age: Childhood onset
Sex: No predilection

Clinical Features: Hereditary benign intraepithelial dyskeratosis (HBID) is inherited as an autosomal dominant trait, and electron microscopic studies have disclosed a defect in keratinization characterized by cytoplasmic accumulation of tonofilaments with loss of cellular interdigitation and desmosomes. As with the other genokeratoses, HBID manifests diffuse white plaques of the buccal mucosa and tongue. In addition to the oral signs are coexistent conjunctival telangiectasias and occasionally thickened plaques of the bulbar conjunctiva, which may eventuate in blindness. The disease was originally described in a racial isolate group in the Carolina states.

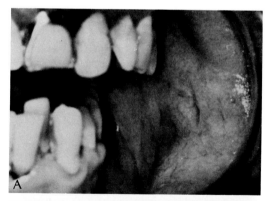

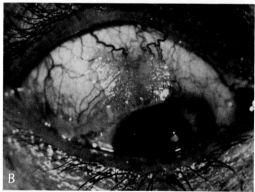

FIG. 2–3. Hereditary benign intraepithelial dyskeratosis. *A:* Buccal mucosal white lesions. *B:* Conjunctival telangiectasia and gelatinous plaque. (Courtesy of Dr. Carl J. Witkop.)

Microscopic Features: Acanthosis with both hyperorthokeratosis and hyperparakeratosis is present within the epithelium. The pathognomonic features seen are benign dyskeratotic changes consisting of the cell-within-a-cell phenomenon and individual cell keratinization, similar to those features encountered in Darier-White's disease; however, no intraepithelial cleavage occurs.

Differential Diagnosis: The oral white lesions must be differentiated from those in white sponge nevus, pachyonychia congenita, and lichen planus. The combination of eye and oral lesions in this disease should not be confused with the muco-oculocutaneous syndromes in which the oral lesions are either ulcerative, bullous, or erythematous.

Treatment: No treatment is necessary. Because of the potential for blindness, genetic counselling may be in order.

References

1. Witkop, C. J., et al.: Hereditary benign intraepithelial dyskeratosis. II. Oral manifestations and hereditary transmission. Arch. Pathol. *70*:696, 1960.
2. Von Sallman, L. and Paton, D.: Hereditary benign intraepithelial dyskeratosis. I. Ocular manifestations. Arch. Ophthalmol. *63*:421, 1960.
3. Witkop, C. J. and Gorlin, R. J.: Four hereditary mucosal syndromes. Arch. Dermatol. *84*:762, 1961.
4. Sadeghi, E. M. and Witkop, C. J., Jr.: Ultrastructural study of hereditary benign intraepithelial dyskeratosis. Oral Surg. *44*:567, 1977.

Keratosis Follicularis (Darier-White's Disease)

Age: Generally adult onset
Sex: No predilection

Clinical Features: Keratosis follicularis is a dermatologic disorder manifesting orange-yellow papular and white keratotic lesions of skin. It is inherited as an autosomal dominant trait. Oral lesions are not universally seen in all patients, yet when present they are papular and usually keratotic in appearance. Buccal mucosa, lips, palate, and tongue are the favored oral locations. Other mucous membranes including vulva, vagina, and anus may be involved.

Microscopic Features: Surface hyperkeratosis is present. Within the spinous cell layer are dyskeratotic changes represented by the cell-within-a-cell phenomenon known as *corps ronds* and pyknotic elongated nuclei termed *grains*. A suprabasilar cleavage is present with acantholysis; formation of wandering rete ridges manifesting cleft-like spaces produces a villous pattern. The micro-

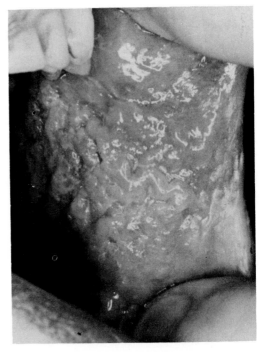

FIG. 2–4. Multiple keratotic papules in keratosis follicularis. (From Weathers, D. R. and Driscoll, R. M.: Darier's disease of the oral mucosa. Oral Surg. *37*:711, 1974.)

scopic appearance may be confused with pemphigus vulgaris and familial pemphigus (Hailey-Hailey disease).

Differential Diagnosis: The multipapular or cobblestone appearance and characteristic skin lesions differentiate Darier-White's disease from the other genokeratoses that generally manifest oral white lesions in a more diffuse or plaque-like pattern. This white papular eruption may be confused with other oral lesions showing multiple polyps or papules, including pyostomatitis vegetans, verrucous carcinoma, oral florid papillomatosis and denture papillomatosis. Biopsy will afford a definitive diagnosis.

Treatment: Retinoids have been employed in high doses, the rationale being an attempt to eliminate the degree of skin keratinization. This treatment is of limited value.

References

1. Gorlin, R. J. and Chaudhry, A. P.: The oral manifestation of keratosis follicularis. Oral Surg. *12*:1468, 1959.
2. Spouge, J. D., et al.: Darier-White's disease: a cause of white lesions of the mucosa. Oral Surg. *21*:441, 1966.

3. Weathers, D. R. and Driscoll, R. M.: Darier's disease of the oral mucosa. Oral Surg. *37*:711, 1974.

Pachyonychia Congenita

Age: Childhood onset
Sex: No predilection
Clinical Features: Pachyonychia congenita is an autosomal dominant inherited disorder manifesting oral white lesions and laminated thickening of the finger- and toenails. The oral white lesions are located bilaterally on the buccal mucosa, tongue, and other sites and are usually limited in terms of the extent of mucosal tissues affected.

Microscopic Features: A nonspecific thickening of the parakeratin and spinous cell layer is seen.

Differential Diagnosis: The bilateral mucosal white lesions of pachyonychia congenita may be confused with white sponge nevus, HBID, and lichen planus; however, the fingernail changes, when considered in conjunction with the oral lesions, provide the diagnostic clinical features of the disease. Candidiasis of the oral mucosa with fingernail involvement should be considered in the differential diagnosis and can be ruled out by obtaining an oral cytologic smear that can be stained for hyphae.

Treatment: No treatment is necessary.

References

1. Gorlin, R. J. and Chaudhry, A. P.: Oral lesions accompanying pachyonychia congenita. Oral Surg. *11*:541, 1958.
2. Joseph, H. L.: Pachyonychia congenita. Arch. Dermatol. *90*:594, 1964.
3. Young, L. L. and Lenox, J. A.: Pachyonychia congenita; a long-term evaluation of associated oral and dermal lesions. Oral Surg. *36*:663, 1973.
4. Maser, E. D.: Oral manifestations of pachyonychia congenita: report of a case. Oral Surg. *43*:373, 1977.

Incontinentia Pigmenti

Age: Begins during infancy
Sex: Females
Clinical Features: Incontinentia pigmenti is inherited as a dominant trait, is lethal in males, and manifests both skin and dental defects. The skin lesions vary from reticulated slate-gray pigmentations to vesicles and verrucous keratoses. Oral mucosal white lesions may occur on the buccal mucosa, yielding a patchy plaque or verrucous appearance. Partial anodontia, strabismus with nystagmus, and epilepsy may also be seen.

Microscopic Features: Skin lesions in the vesicular stage show intraepithelial vesicle formation with numerous eosinophils. Pigmented zones display incontinence of melanin granules from the basal cells with accumulation in dermal or submucosal macrophages. White lesions are characterized by hyperorthokeratosis, hyperparakeratosis, and acanthosis. Individual cell keratinization may be present.

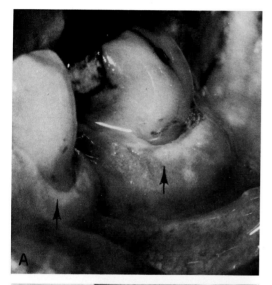

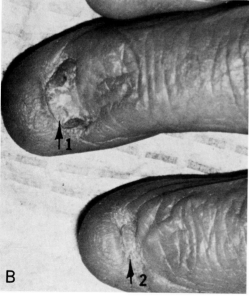

FIG. 2–5. *A:* Gingival white lesions in pachyonychia congenita. *B:* Dystrophic nail changes (arrow #1) and surgically removed fingernail (arrow #2). (From Young, L. L. and Lenox, J. A.: Pachyonychia congenita; long-term evaluation of associated oral and dermal lesions. Oral Surg. *36*:663, 1973.)

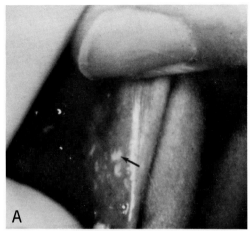

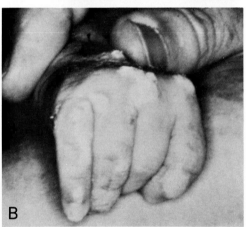

FIG. 2–6. *A:* Oral lesions on buccal mucosa in an infant with incontinentia pigmenti. *B:* Keratoses and focal pigmentations of skin. (Courtesy of Dr. Sheldon Rovin.)

Differential Diagnosis: The white lesions encountered intraorally may resemble those seen in other genokeratoses yet are generally focal and patchy in distribution. The other components of this disorder, including skin discoloration and keratosis as well as partial anodontia, separate this entity from other genetic diseases manifesting oral white lesions.

Treatment: There is no treatment.

References

1. Schulze, C: In *Thoma's Oral Pathology,* 6th Ed., edited by R. J. Gorlin and H. M. Goldman. St. Louis, C. V. Mosby Co., 1970, Vol. 1, p. 130.
2. Shafer, W. G., Hine, M. K., and Levy, B. M.: *A Textbook of Oral Pathology,* 4th Ed. Philadelphia, W. B. Saunders Co., 1983, p. 823.
3. Russell, D. L. and Finn, S. B.: Incontinentia pig-

menti (Bloch-Sulzberger syndrome): a case report with emphasis on dental manifestations. J. Dent. Child. *34:*494, 1967.

LEUKOPLAKIAS

Friction/Trauma Associated Leukoplakia

Age: No predilection

Sex: No predilection

Clinical Features: Frictional keratoses represent callus formation from chronic trauma with resultant thickening of one of the epithelial cell layers. The white lesions are therefore associated with various etiologic agents, including ill-fitting

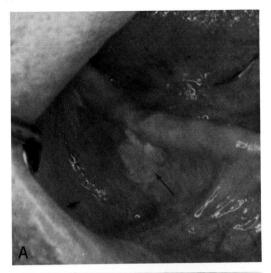

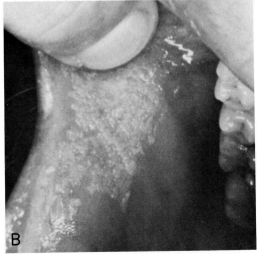

FIG. 2–7. *A:* Hyperkeratosis of mandibular alveolar ridge due to ill-fitting denture. *B:* Cheek-biting keratosis.

dental prostheses, chronic irritational habits such as cheek- or lip-biting, and overzealous tooth brushing. The individual lesions may be smooth or irregular in texture, and their location and configuration will coincide with the corresponding location of the causative agent.

Microscopic Features: Frictional irritation may cause thickening of any layer or combination of layers of the epithelium with hyperorthokeratosis, hyperparakeratosis, and/or acanthosis. Depending upon the degree of irritation, the underlying submucosa may show an inflammatory cell infiltrate, usually chronic in nature.

Differential Diagnosis: White lesions due to chronic irritation may be diagnosed as such when a causative agent presents itself. Providing the cause can be eliminated or markedly reduced (e.g., leaving ill-fitting dentures out of the mouth for two weeks, smoothing down irritating tooth cusps, avoiding habits) and the white lesion regresses or resolves, a cause-and-effect relationship can be substantiated. Failure of a white lesion to regress subsequent to elimination of the causative agent(s) should arouse suspicion with regard to precancerous leukoplakia, and biopsy is then indicated. Additionally, other diseases manifesting white lesions may coincidentally correspond to denture-bearing zones; however, diseases such as lichen planus, moniliasis, or the genokeratoses will generally be located in regions beyond the confines of a potential irritant.

Treatment: Elimination of the causative agent is indicated. White lesions attributed to a chronic irritant probably have a limited tendency to undergo malignant change. However, should the lesions fail to resolve after removal of the irritant, a biopsy should be performed in order to rule out atypical cell changes that occur independently.

References

1. Waldron, C. A.: In *Thoma's Oral Pathology.* 6th Ed., edited by R. J. Gorlin and H. M. Goldman. St. Louis, C. V. Mosby Co., 1970, Vol. II, p. 811.
2. Shafer, W. G., Hine, M. K. and Levy, B. M.: *A Textbook of Oral Pathology,* 4th Ed. Philadelphia, W. B. Saunders Co., 1983, p. 92.
3. Cooke, B. E. D.: Leukoplakia buccalis and oral epithelial naevi. Br. J. Dermatol. 68:151, 1956.
4. Cawson, R. A.: Leukoplakia and Oral Cancer. Proc. Roy. Soc. Med. 62:610, 1969.

Idiopathic/Tobacco Associated Leukoplakia: Planar Type

Age: Middle-aged and elderly adults

Sex: Males predominantly

Clinical Features: White plaques of unknown

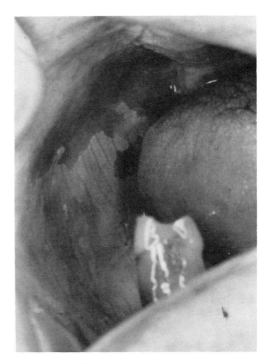

FIG. 2–8. Diffuse planar white lesion with well-demarcated border on buccal mucosa in a chewing-tobacco user.

etiology or those encountered in smokers and tobacco chewers are a common malady that may occur on any oral mucosal surface yet are more often seen on the buccal mucosa, mucobuccal fold, and oral floor. These leukoplakias may be smooth, ridged, rough, delineated, or diffuse. The smooth form or planar type fails to exhibit surface irregularity, being homogeneously white without a verrucous texture. The term leukoplakia is strictly clinical and has no implications with regard to microscopy. These lesions are usually benign yet may show microscopic evidence of premalignant cellular change. Whereas leukoplakias as a collective group display microscopic evidence of dysplasia, carcinoma in situ, or squamous cell carcinoma in approximately 20 percent of the cases, evidence suggests that the atypical cell changes are not as prevalent in the smooth planar form. Leukoplakias of the oral floor manifest the highest incidence of atypical cell change.

Microscopic Features: The clinical extent does not necessarily predict the microscopic features. Idiopathic or tobacco-induced leukoplakias may merely show hyperorthokeratosis, hyperparakeratosis, acanthosis, or a combination. Alternatively, and most important, cellular atypia, dysplasia, carcinoma in situ, or frank superficially invasive squamous cell carcinoma may microscopically be encountered.

Differential Diagnosis: Idiopathic and tobacco-associated leukoplakia must be differentiated from frictional leukoplakia on the basis of history. Lichen planus, lupus erythematosus, the genokeratoses and inflammatory white lesions must also be eliminated from consideration on the bases of history and biopsy.

Treatment: Biopsy should be performed in all instances of idiopathic or tobacco-associated leukoplakia to ascertain whether or not premalignant cell changes exist. Benign cellular features do not preclude future malignant change in the same location or in a new site. For this reason patients should be subjected to periodic follow-up with rebiopsy, particularly when a change in the clinical character of a lesion evolves. Lesions with a microscopic diagnosis of dysplasia or carcinoma in situ should be surgically stripped or removed *in toto* by cryosurgery or laser surgery. Invasive carcinoma is usually managed by combined radiotherapy and surgery.

References

1. Waldron, C. A. and Shafer, W. G.: Leukoplakia revisited. A clinicopathologic study of 3256 oral leukoplakias. Cancer 36:1386, 1975.
2. Silverman, S., Jr. and Rozen, R.: Observations on the clinical characteristics and natural history of oral leukoplakia. J. Am. Dent. Assoc. 76:772, 1968.
3. Bánóczy, J. and Csiba, A.: Comparative study of the clinical picture and histopathologic structure of oral leukoplakia. Cancer 29:1230, 1972.

Idiopathic/Tobacco Associated Leukoplakia: Verruciform Type

Age: Middle-aged and elderly adults
Sex: Males predominantly

Clinical Features: Verruciform leukoplakia is a variant form that is occasionally associated with frictional irritation yet may also be associated with tobacco use. Clinically, the lesions are white with a verrucous or washboard-like corrugated pattern. In the floor of the mouth the corrugations may simulate sand remaining from an ebbing or receding tide. Elsewhere, the leukoplakia may resemble fissured, cracked desert sand. Atypical cell changes are slightly more prevalent among verruciform lesions than the flat smooth planar leukoplakias. Also, oral floor lesions show a greater propensity for harboring atypical cells.

Microscopic Features: Verruciform leukoplakia is characterized by an atrophic to normal

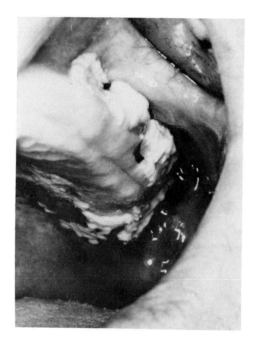

FIG. 2–9. Verruciform leukoplakia of the maxillary alveolar ridge and palate.

spinous cell layer with a thickened keratin layer. The entire epithelium shows a verrucous corrugated pattern with church-spire projections. The individual epithelial cells may fail to exhibit atypical changes or may evince dysplasia, carcinoma in situ or frankly invasive carcinoma.

Differential Diagnosis: This lesion must be differentiated from verruciform xanthoma and from verrucous carcinoma, which is generally more extensive both in lateral spread and overall thickness. Clinically, the other white lesions outlined in this chapter do not manifest a corrugated verrucous pattern.

Treatment: Lesions with a benign histology can be observed and rebiopsied periodically should any notable changes develop. Alternatively, even benign lesions may be stripped, particularly in tobacco users who are recalcitrant with regard to eliminating their habit. Dysplastic or carcinoma-in-situ lesions should be totally excised or removed by other means (e.g., cryosurgery, laser surgery). Invasive carcinoma is usually managed by combined radiotherapy and surgery.

References

1. Hobaek, A.: Leukoplakia oris. Acta Odontol. Scand. 7:61, 1946.
2. Bánóczy, J. and Sugar, L. Longitudinal studies in oral leukoplakias. J. Oral Pathol. 1:265, 1972.

3. Shear, M. and Pindborg, J. J.: Verrucous hyperplasia of the oral mucosa. Cancer 46:1855, 1980.
4. Eversole, L. R. and Shopper, T. P.: Oral leukoplakia: prevalence of dysplastic and carcinomatous change in verruciform and planar patterns. Cal. Dent. Assoc. J. Oct.:45, 1981.

Idiopathic/Tobacco Associated Leukoplakia: Speckled Type

Age: Middle-aged and elderly
Sex: Males predominantly

Clinical Features: Whereas the prevalence of atypical and malignant change in leukoplakia is approximately 20 percent (somewhat less prevalent among planar forms, more prevalent among the verruciform type), speckled leukoplakias are the most ominous in this regard. Clinically, speckled leukoplakia is a white patch with multiple red foci or appears as a red velvet discoloration with superimposed multiple white flecks or plaques. Therefore it represents a combined leukoplakia-erythroplakia. Speckled leukoplakia is usually encountered on the oral floor, lateral tongue, and soft palate.

Microscopic Features: Foci of hyperkeratosis, parakeratosis, and acanthosis alternate with zones of epithelial atrophy devoid of a cornified layer. The atrophied foci correspond to those regions that appear red clinically, and usually the cells occupying the attenuated spinous layer show pleomorphism, hyperchromatism, and increased mitotic activity. The keratinized or parakeratinized regions representing the clinically evident white plaques may also harbor atypical cells.

Differential Diagnosis: Speckled leukoplakia, with its mixed red and white appearance, may be confused clinically with erosive lichen planus and candidiasis. Whereas these two entities are usually multifocal, speckled leukoplakia is usually, yet not invariably, an isolated lesion. Biopsy is required to obtain a definitive diagnosis.

Treatment: Speckled forms of leukoplakia are usually found to harbor atypical cells. Dysplastic or carcinoma-in-situ lesions require surgical stripping, cryosurgery, or laser surgery with liberal margins of normal mucosa. Invasive cancer is managed by surgery and/or radiation therapy.

References:
1. Pindborg, J. J., Renstrup, G., Jolst, O., and Roed-Petersen: Studies in oral leukoplakia: A preliminary report on the period prevalence of malignant transformation in leukoplakia based on a follow-up study of 248 patients. J. Am. Dent. Assoc. 76:767, 1968.
2. Mashberg, A., Morrissey, J. B., and Garfinkel, L.: A study of the appearance of early asymptomatic oral squamous cell carcinoma. Cancer 32:1436, 1973.

Idiopathic/Tobacco Associated Leukoplakia: Snuff Dipper Keratosis

Age: Middle-aged and elderly adults
Sex: No predilection

Clinical Features: White lesions caused by snuff usage are located under the area in which snuff granules are habitually placed; they are therefore encountered in the mucobuccal fold region. The lesion is somewhat rough in texture and may manifest an undulating or wrinkled surface. The white areas are relatively well circumscribed and localized to the area of snuff placement.

Microscopic Features: As with other forms of tobacco-induced leukokeratosis, snuff keratosis may show a thickening of one of the epithelial layers (i.e., hyperorthokeratosis, hyperparakeratosis, acanthosis), yet, importantly, cytologic atypia may be encountered.

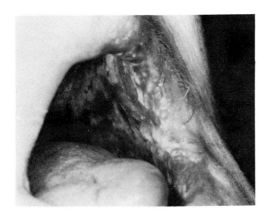

FIG. 2–10.   Speckled leukoplakia, a mixed red and white lesion.

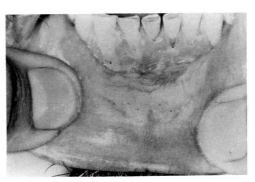

FIG. 2–11.   Snuff dipper's leukoplakia in labial sulcus and on the lip mucosa.

Differential Diagnosis: A white lesion in the mucobuccal fold may represent frictional keratosis or leukoplakia related to tobacco products. A thorough history will indicate whether or not the lesion is snuff related. The "ebbing-tide" effect on the white surface implicates snuff usage.

Treatment: All suspected snuff-associated white lesions must be examined microscopically to rule out premalignancy. If atypical cytologic changes are present, complete excision is recommended. Absence of cellular premalignant changes does not preclude future evolution to cancer; therefore, the snuff habit should be curtailed.

References

1. Rosenfeld, L. and Callaway, J.: Snuff dipper's cancer. Am. J. Surg. *106*:840, 1963.
2. Brown, R. L., et al.: Snuff dipper's intraoral cancer; clinical characteristics and response to therapy. Cancer *18*:2, 1965.
3. Roed-Petersen, B. and Pindborg, J. J.: A study of Danish snuff-induced oral leukoplakia. J. Oral Path. *2*:301, 1973.

Actinic Cheilitis

Age: Middle-aged and elderly adults
Sex: Males predominate

Clinical Features: Solar or ultraviolet light exposure may predispose the vermilion border to keratotic change, and certain individuals whose occupations or hobbies provide continuous sun exposure are most prone to develop actinic cheilitis. The lower lip is more prominent and therefore more prone to actinic change than is the upper. The lesion is white and usually smooth and diffuse.

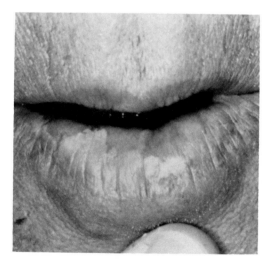

FIG. 2–12.   White lesion of lower lip in an outdoor construction worker representing actinic cheilitis.

The borders may be sharply delineated from uninvolved vermilion, or the transition may be gradual. Ulcerations or focal zones of highly thickened keratin plaque may indicate early carcinomatous transformation.

Microscopic Features: Solar cheilitis reflects a spectrum of microscopic changes similar to leukoplakia. The early limited changes are restricted to the keratin layer, which manifests thickening, and the subjacent connective tissue zones, which characteristically show clumping, fragmentation, and granulation of elastic fibers known as solar or senile elastosis. Progression to cytologic atypia, dysplasia, and frank invasive carcinoma can develop in actinic cheilitis. The earliest premalignant atypicality is represented by atrophy of the spinous cell layer, fragmentation of the basement membrane, and mild hyperchromatism and/or pleomorphism of the basal cells.

Differential Diagnosis: Habitual lip chewing must be differentiated from actinic cheilitis. Tobacco irritants (cigars, pipe stems, and reverse smoking) may induce hyperkeratotic lesions of the lips.

Treatment: A biopsy should be performed to determine whether or not cytologic atypia is present. A lack of premalignant cellular changes in actinic cheilitis does not preclude future evolvement. Protection from the sun with solar protective cream containing para-aminobenzoic acid is recommended. Histologically atypical change should be managed by lip stripping with incontinuity wedge resection if a zone of superficial carcinomatous invasion is coexistent.

If no foci of carcinoma exist, topical application of 1 percent 5-fluorouracil cream twice daily for 2 weeks will remove dysplastic epithelium, allowing for regeneration of normal epithelium.

References

1. Waldron, C. A.: In *Thoma's Oral Pathology*, 6th Ed., edited by R. J. Gorlin and H. M. Goldman. St. Louis, C. V. Mosby Co., 1970, Vol. II, pp. 826–829.
2. Mitchell, D. F., Standish, S. M, and Fast, T. B.: *Oral Diagnosis/Oral Medicine*, 3rd Ed. Philadelphia, Lea & Febiger, 1978, pp. 130, 308.
3. Shafer, W. G., Hine, M. K., and Levy, B. M.: *A Textbook of Oral Pathology*, 4th Ed. Philadelphia, W. B. Saunders Co., 1983, p. 848.
4. Bernier, J. L. and Reynold, M. C.: The relationship of senile elastosis to actinic radiation and to squamous cell carcinoma of the lip. Milit. Med. *117*:209, 1955.
5. Warnock, G. R., Fuller, R. P., Jr., and Pelleu, G. B., Jr.: Evaluation of 5-fluorouracil in the treatment

of actinic keratosis of the lip. Oral Surg. 52:501, 1981.

Dysplasia, Carcinoma in Situ, Squamous Cell Carcinoma, and Verrucous Carcinoma

Age: Elderly adults
Sex: Males predominate

Clinical Features: Early cancerous change within the oral epithelium may initially manifest as a white lesion or may arise in a preexisting leukoplakic area. Depending upon the extent of the tumor, the white lesion may be relatively macular or plaque-like or, in larger lesions, associated with tumefaction and induration. Whereas oral cancer is generally localized, it may on occasion be multifocal with numerous isolated separate white lesions manifesting microscopic evidence of neoplastic transformation. Location is highly significant when considering the possibility of malignancy; while malignant change may be seen on any surface, the most common locations are oral floor, alveolar ridge and vestibule, and lateral posterior tongue.

The most important contributing etiologic factors regarding carcinogenesis of oral epithelium are use of tobacco and a high intake of alcohol. Patients with untreated syphilis and the Plummer-Vinson syndrome are also prone to develop oral or oropharyngeal cancer. As emphasized under the section on leukoplakias associated with tobacco, the apparent clinical innocence of white patches can be misleading; the most innocuous lesion may be cytologically malignant. One ex-

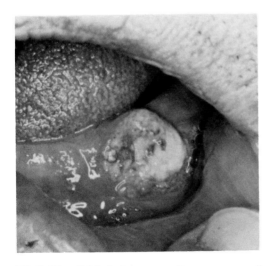

FIG. 2–13.   White lesion representing squamous cell carcinoma.

ception to clinical predictability regarding suspicion of potential malignancy may be encountered in the white lesion associated with zones of erythema, so-called speckled leukoplakia. Isolated mixed red and white lesions should be considered malignant until proven otherwise (i.e., biopsy).

A variant form of oral squamous cell carcinoma that is classically a warty-appearing keratotic white lesion is verrucous carcinoma (see Chapter 6, Intraoral Soft Tissue Swellings, Verrucous Carcinoma).

Microscopic Features: Epithelial dysplasia, carcinoma in situ, and invasive squamous cell carcinoma are, respectively, progressively advanced stages of malignancy. When they are characterized clinically as white lesions, they manifest a thickening of the keratin or parakeratin layer. The earliest changes, termed *dysplasia,* begin in the dividing cells of the basilar and parabasilar layers. Initial changes include nuclear hyperchromatism, pleomorphism, and an increase in mitotic figures. By definition, all layers, top to bottom, must evince atypical cell changes in carcinoma in situ; however, the basement membrane remains intact without evidence of invasion into the subjacent connective tissue. Violations of the basement membrane integrity results in superficially invasive carcinoma, which then progresses to frank squamous cell carcinoma.

Invasive squamous cell carcinoma may contain islands and nests of tumor cells that retain the characteristics of oral epithelium by manufacturing the chief protective products of that organ, albeit disorganized, keratin and parakeratin. These differentiated tissues are often arranged in laminated whorls termed *keratin pearls.* Tumors with this histologic morphology are termed well-differentiated carcinomas and are associated with a slower course, lower metastatic potential, and thus a better prognosis. A lack of or a diminution in keratin formation connotes a more rapidly progressing lesion with a poor prognosis and is termed poorly differentiated carcinoma. A moderately differentiated lesion logically falls between these two extremes both morphologically and behaviorally.

Differential Diagnosis: White lesions associated with tumefaction and induration present no problem in the clinical diagnosis, yet biopsy is indicated to determine the grade of malignancy (i.e., differentiation of tumor cells) prior to planning therapy. Early malignant change manifesting a plaque-like white lesion must be differentiated primarily from frictional leukoplakias, benign leukoplakias, and lichen planus. When a causative agent cannot be identified or eliminated, an adequate history and biopsy are necessary.

Treatment: Dysplasia or carcinoma in situ, if localized, can be managed by wide local excision, obtaining margins free from atypical changes; margins 1 cm away from clinically involved tissue should be adequate, yet microscopic confirmation is mandatory. Diffuse or multifocal dysplasia or carcinoma in situ may be treated by surgery or radiation therapy. Invasive carcinoma requires a complete workup with evaluation of the neck, chest roentgenogram, and the presence of other symptoms. As treatment may employ a variety of therapeutic modalities either alone or in combination, including surgery, radiation, and chemotherapy, invasive squamous cell carcinoma should be evaluated and managed by a physician experienced in oncology.

References

1. Ackerman, L. V.: Verrucous carcinoma of the oral cavity. Surgery 23:670, 1948.
2. Pindborg, J. J., Restrup, G., Poulsen, H. E., and Silverman, S., Jr.: Studies in oral leukoplakias. V. Clinical and histologic signs of malignancy. Acta Odont. Scand. 20:407, 1963.
3. Silverman, S., Jr., and Rozen, R. D.: Observations on the clinical characteristics and natural history of oral leukoplakia. J. Am. Dent. Assoc. 76:772, 1963.
4. Waldron, C. A. and Shafer, W. G.: Leukoplakia revisited. A clinicopathologic study of 3256 oral leukoplakias. Cancer 36:1386, 1975.
5. Bánóczy, J. and Csiba, A.: Occurrence of epithelial dysplasia in oral leukoplakia: Analysis and follow-up study of 12 cases. Oral Surg. 42:766, 1976.

DERMATOSES

Lichen Planus

  Age: Adults
  Sex: Females affected slightly more often

Clinical Features: Lichen planus is a dermatologic disorder, yet oral lesions without skin involvement are a common presentation of the disease. Whereas the etiology is unknown, lichen planus-like lesions are occasionally associated with systemic medications such as thiazides and quinidines. If withdrawal of the drug is accompanied by regression or ablation of lesions, the condition is appropriately designated a lichenoid drug eruption. The classic appearance is one of reticulated interconnected white thread-like lesions, striae of Wickham, located bilaterally on the buccal mucosa. Other areas such as tongue and gingiva may also be involved; indeed, vir-

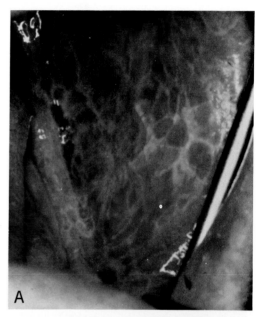

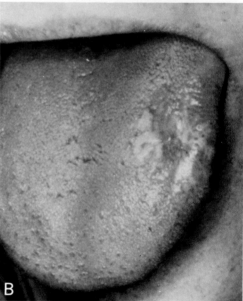

FIG. 2–14. A: Lacy reticulated white striae of lichen planus. B: Plaque form of lichen planus on tongue.

tually any oral mucosal tissue may evince manifestations of lichen planus. Whereas the aforementioned features are most common, oral lichen planus may have protean clinical signs. The plaque form resembles leukoplakia with a multifocal distribution. Plaque-like lichen planus is usually a smooth to slightly irregularly surfaced white lesion found primarily on buccal and glossal mucosae. A circinate variety can be encountered. Circinate, oval, and target-appearing white lesions of lichen planus are seen most often on buccal mucosa.

Skin lesions, when present, are scaly keratoses overlying an erythematous or violaceous base and are most frequently seen on the extensor surfaces of the extremities.

Multifocal white lesions with an erythematous component are seen in the erosive and bullous forms of lichen planus, which are considered elsewhere.

Microscopic Features: Hyperkeratosis or parakeratosis may or may not be present. The basal cell layer is disrupted with loss of polarity; lymphocytes may be interposed between basal cells. If rete ridges are present, they taper off into the underlying connective tissue, imperceptibly blending into a subepithelial lymphocytic infiltrate below yielding a sawtooth pattern. The basement membrane is irregular and thickened. The juxtaposed lymphocytic infiltrate is zonal, localized only in the submucosa without involvement of the deeper connective tissue.

Differential Diagnosis: The reticulated form is easily separated from other oral white lesions. Plaque forms may be confused with leukoplakias or premalignant conditions, moniliasis, or the genokeratoses. Evidence is emerging that a significant number of instances of lichen planus are associated with malignant transformation. Whether or not these cases represent true lichen planus undergoing malignant change or leukoplakias and mucositis with a marked resemblance to oral lichen planus microscopically is presently unknown. Regardless, the plaque form may mimic other oral white lesions, and biopsy is often necessary to render a definitive diagnosis.

Treatment: The nonerosive, nonbullous forms of lichen planus are generally asymptomatic, requiring no treatment. An anxiety component often accompanies the disorder and, if this feature is prominent, counselling by a psychiatrist or psychologist may be recommended. Importantly, a significant number of patients with oral lichen planus are diabetic. For this reason, any patient with oral lichen planus should be subjected to a glucose tolerance test.

References

1. Grinspan, D., et al.: Notre experience sur le lichen *Ruber planus* de le muqueuse buccale. Ann. Dermatol. Syph. 93:531, 1966.
2. Andreason, J.: Oral lichen planus. Oral Surg. 25:31, 1968.
3. Almeyda, J. and Levantine, A.: Lichenoid drug eruptions. Br. J. Derm. 85:604, 1971.
4. Howell, F. V. and Rick, G. M.: Oral lichen planus and diabetes: a potential syndrome. J. Calif. Dent. Assoc. 1:58, July 1973.
5. Silverman, S., Jr., and Griffith, M.: Studies on oral lichen planus. Oral Surg. 37:705, 1974.
6. Krutchkoff, D. J., Cutler, L., and Laskowski, S.: Oral lichen planus: the evidence regarding potential malignant transformation. J. Oral Path. 7:1, 1978.

Lupus Erythematosus

Age: Young adults
Sex: Females

Clinical Features: Lupus erythematosus, the discoid type, is a disorder manifesting erythematous dermatologic scaly lesions of skin. A more serious form, the systemic type, evinces lesions in the kidney and other visceral organs as well as on skin, being one of the collagen-vascular immunopathic diseases. Oral lesions are sometimes seen with lupus erythematosus, particularly the systemic type. The lesions are white and plaque-like, resembling lichen planus, and occasionally an erythematous component accompanies the white lesions. Disc and circinate patterns are common, and lesions often involve the vermilion border. The facial butterfly pattern—a plaque of erythema over the nasal bridge with bilateral flaring

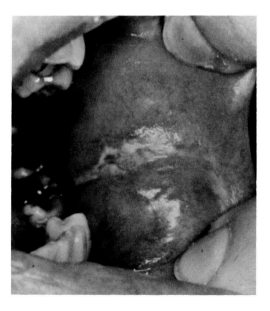

FIG. 2–15. White plaques in a patient with lupus erythematosus. (Courtesy of Dr. S. Silverman.)

on the skin of the malar eminence region—is a classical feature of lupus erythematosus.

Microscopic Features: The microscopic features are most characteristic when a biopsy is obtained from skin. Hyperkeratosis is accompanied by some disruption of the basal cell layer. The basement membrane is thickened with fibrinoid change. A lymphocytic infiltrate prevails, is patchy in distribution, and typically is localized in the vicinity of pilosebaceous structures. Oral lesions manifest microscopic features not unlike those of lichen planus, yet deeper zones of perivascular lymphocytic infiltration can be noted.

Differential Diagnosis: White lesions of lupus erythematosus must be differentiated from lichen planus, the genokeratoses, and leukoplakias. The characteristic skin lesions and butterfly pattern, when present, are important diagnostic signs. Lupus erythematosus may also show erythematous and erosive oral lesions, usually admixed with a white component. Antinuclear factor, anti-DNA antibodies, immunofluorescent microscopic tests, and the L.E. prep are usually positive in lupus, and elevated IgG may be seen.

Treatment: Patients with lupus erythematosus may manifest systemic complications, particularly in the kidney. Prolonged systemic steroids are the treatment of choice, and these patients should be managed by a physician, usually a dermatologist.

References
1. Andreasen, J. O.: Oral manifestations of discoid and systemic lupus erythematosus. 1. Clinical investigations. Acta Odontol. Scand. 22:295, 1964.
2. Edwards, M. B. and Gayford, J. J.: Oral lupus erythematosus. Oral Surg. 31:332, 1971.
3. Nisengard, R. J., et al.: Diagnostic importance of immunofluorescence in oral bullous diseases and lupus erythematosus. Oral Surg. 40:365, 1975.
4. Schiodt, M., Halberg, P., and Hentzer, B.: Clinical study of 32 patients with oral discoid lupus erythematosus. Int. J. Oral Surg. 7:85, 1978.
5. Schiodt, M., et al.: Deposits of immunoglobulins, complement, and fibrinogen in oral lupus erythematosus, lichen planus, and leukoplakia. Oral Surg. 51:603, 1981.

INFLAMMATIONS

Koplik Spots of Measles

Age: Children
Sex: No predilection

Clinical Features: During the prodromal stages of rubeola infection when fever and malaise are waxing, focal white spots less than 1 cm in diameter may be encountered on the buccal mu-

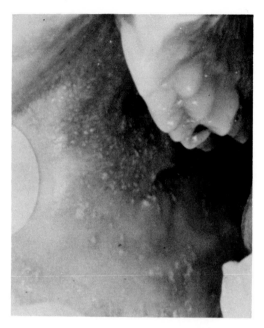

FIG. 2–16. Multiple white spots on buccal mucosa heralding the onset of rubeola infection.

cosa. There may be only one lesion or as many as fifty on each side of the mouth. The lesions are plaque- or dome-like and are oval to round in contour. When the maculopapular skin rash appears, Koplik spots begin to disappear.

Microscopic Features: The epithelium shows superficial necrosis with an avid neutrophilic inflammatory cell infiltrate in the subjacent submucosa.

Differential Diagnosis: Koplik spots are usually not difficult to separate from other white lesions as they are focal and seen most often in children. Large Fordyce's granules and cheek-biting keratosis should be considered in the differential diagnosis. A diagnosis of Koplik spots is confirmed upon appearance of the classic rubeola maculopapular rash.

Treatment: Supportive care, including high fluid intake and the use of salicylates to control fever, with bed rest is recommended treatment. The child's physician should be notified; complications, while uncommon, may occur in measles.

References
1. Hornstein, O. P. and Gorlin, R. J.: In *Thoma's Oral Pathology*, 6th Ed., edited by R. J. Gorlin and H. M. Goldman. St. Louis, C. V. Mosby Co., 1970, Vol. II, p. 756.
2. Mitchell, D. F., Standish, S. M., and Fast, T. B.:

Oral Diagnosis/Oral Medicine, 3rd Ed. Philadelphia, Lea & Febiger, 1978, p. 325.

3. Shafer, W. G., Hine, M. K., and Levy, B. M.: *A Textbook of Oral Pathology,* 4th Ed. Philadelphia, W. B. Saunders Co., 1983, p. 378.

4. Koplik, H.: The diagnosis of the invasion of measles from a study of the exanthem as it appears on the buccal mucous membrane. Arch. Pediatr. *13:*981, 1896.

5. Bhaskar, S. N.: *Synopsis of Oral Pathology.* St. Louis, C.V. Mosby Co., 1969, p. 357.

Mucous Patches of Syphilis

Age: Adults
Sex: No predilection

Clinical Features: Mucous patches are smooth-surfaced plaques that manifest a glistening, opalescent character and are seen 6 to 8 weeks following formation of the chancre. In addition to the mucosal patches, split papules at the commissure and a maculopapular rash may be present. A history of promiscuous sexual activity can usually be obtained, although some patients may deny such activities. The lesions persist for 1 to 3 weeks, after which they resolve. The lesions in this stage are infectious.

Microscopic Features: Parakeratosis and fibrinous exudate over both intact and focally ulcerated epithelium can be seen. The submucosa contains an avid plasma cell infiltrate. The spirochete is not visible on routine staining; a Warthin-Starry silver stain will demonstrate the micro-organism in tissue sections.

Differential Diagnosis: Mucous patches may resemble a variety of white lesions of the oral cavity; because they are highly infectious, the clinician should always be aware of the fact that oral white lesions may be luetic. The primary considerations in the clinical differential diagnosis include moniliasis, plaque-form lichen planus, or leukoplakia of one type or another. An adequate history should elicit suspicion of syphilis, and the diagnosis may be confirmed by FTA (fluorescent treponemal antibody test) or VDRL test. A smear with dark-field microscopy will demonstrate motile spirochetes.

Treatment: Treatment for syphilis is penicillin. The patient can be referred to a dermatologist or general physician for treatment.

References

1. Meyer, I. and Shklar, G.: The oral manifestations of acquired syphilis. Oral Surg. 23:34, 1967.
2. Fiumara, N. J.: Oral lesions of syphilis. Med. Aspects Hum. Sexuality 6:68, 1972.
3. Fiumara, N. J.: Venereal disease of the oral cavity. J. Oral Med. *31:*36, 1976.

Chemical Burns

Age: No predilection
Sex: No predilection

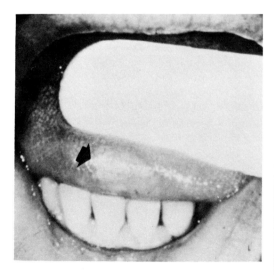

FIG. 2–17.   Filmy white plaque representing a mucous patch in secondary syphilis. (Courtesy of Dr. William Sabes.)

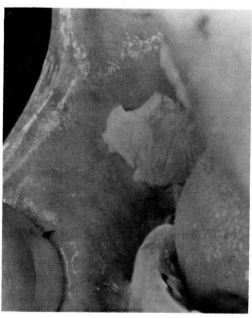

FIG. 2–18.   Aspirin burn causing coagulation necrosis of surface epithelium.

Clinical Features: Burns due to caustic chemical agents will produce coagulation necrosis of the epithelium with subsequent inflammation. The necrotic tissue loses its translucency and appears white. The white areas correspond to the areas of contact with the caustic agent and show a tendency to slough; initially, however, they may be adherent to the mucosa so that scraping with an instrument may not result in desquamation. The chief incriminating agents include aspirin, phenol, acids, and alkalies. The contactants may be introduced on a factitial or iatrogenic basis.

Microscopic Features: Chemical burns cause coagulation necrosis of the epithelium so that microscopically the upper layers show a homogeneous appearance with loss of structure and a failure of nuclei to take stains. Desquamation occurs, and an inflammatory cell infiltrate within the underlying connective tissue can be seen.

Differential Diagnosis: The white necrotic surface is smooth with regional fissuring; this shiny surface, seen clinically, usually differentiates the necrotic surface from the keratotic lesions. Candidiasis should also be included in the differential diagnosis; however, the presence of pain and procurement of an adequate history will provide evidence for a diagnosis of mucosal burn.

Treatment: Treatment is supportive with a consideration of eliminating pain until healing occurs. This may be accomplished by the use of Orabase gel, or palliation may result from the anesthetic effects of an antihistaminic mouth rinse in combination with Kaopectate.

References

1. Greither, A. and Hornstein, O. P.: In *Thoma's Oral Pathology,* 6th Ed., edited by R. J. Gorlin and H. M. Goldman, St. Louis, C. V. Mosby Co., 1970, Vol. II, p. 781.
2. Mitchell, D. F., Standish, S. M., and Fast, T. B.: *Oral Diagnosis/Oral Medicine,* 3rd Ed. Philadelphia, Lea & Febiger, 1978, p. 375.
3. Shafer, W. G., Hine, M. K., and Levy, B. M.: *A Textbook of Oral Pathology,* 4th Ed. Philadelphia, W. B. Saunders Co., 1983, pp. 572–573.
4. Kawashima, Z., Flagg, R. H., and Cox, D. E.: Aspirin-induced oral lesion: report of case. J. Am. Dent. Assoc. *91:*10, 1975.

Candidiasis (Moniliasis, Thrush)

Age: Infants and adults
Sex: No predilection in oral form

Clinical Features: Candida albicans is a superficial fungus that infects the mucous membranes of infants whose mothers display vaginal infestation at the time of parturition and of adults

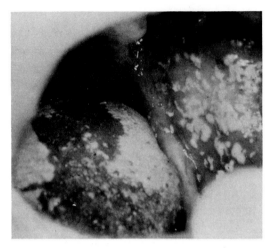

FIG. 2–19.   Diffuse curd-like pseudomembranous patches in moniliasis.

who have experienced an upset in their oral microflora from the use of conventional antibiotics. In addition, oral candidiasis may be associated with other systemic alterations, including diabetes mellitus, hypoparathyroidism, and immunodeficiency diseases. Instances are also commonly seen in the absence of preexisting or intercurrent systemic disease. The oral lesions consist of either multifocal or diffuse white velvety-appearing surfaces resulting from matted mycelia and parakeratotic cells. The lesions may be wiped away with gauze; however, they are often tenacious and resist such treatment. In elderly patients, moniliasis has been found occasionally to coexist with dysplastic or carcinomatous change. A cocarcinogenic effect has been suggested for Candida in these instances, yet no cause-and-effect relationship has been proven. While Candida is generally characterized by white lesions, an erythematous component may accompany the white areas. Deep or systemic and granulomatous infection by Candida may occur in severely debilitated states such as uncontrolled diabetes or severe immunodeficiency diseases. Indeed chronic oral candidiasis is a common finding in the aquired immunodeficiency syndrome (AIDS).

Microscopic Features: Superficial infection is microscopically represented by surface parakeratosis with infiltration of the parakeratin and upper to middle spinous cell layers by PAS-positive mycelia and yeast forms. The submucosa may be free from inflammation or may contain a chronic inflammatory cell infiltrate.

Differential Diagnosis: The velvety surface is unique, yet the lesions of candidiasis may resemble white lesions of plaque-form lichen planus, leukoplakias or even one of the genokeratoses, particularly since familial candidiasis has been described. A complete history, particularly questions relating to the recent use of antibiotics, will significantly limit the differential diagnosis. A cytologic smear with staining for mycelium with periodic acid-Schiff will confirm the diagnosis. Instances of Candida infection without any predisposing factors should arouse suspicion of underlying systemic disease. In these cases appropriate laboratory tests for diabetes, hypoparathyroidism, and immunodeficiency states—fasting blood glucose and glucose tolerance tests, serum calcium, and immunoglobulin complement and lymphocyte blast transformation studies respectively—should be obtained.

Candida infection in the older age groups may coexist with precancerous or carcinomatous change. Biopsy is then indicated.

Treatment: Referral to a physician for control of any systemic derangement is mandatory. Management of the local infection employs the use of nystatin oral suspension 100,000 units/cc, 1 teaspoon of which is mixed with ¼ cup of water and used as an oral rinse, followed by swallowing, 3 times daily. Vaginal suppositories are effective when taken orally as lozenges. This regimen is usually sufficient to eliminate the infection if utilized over a 10-day period.

References

1. Woods, J. W., et al.: Monilial infections complicating the therapeutic use of antibiotics. J. Am. Med. Assoc. *145*:207, 1951.
2. Lehner, T.: Oral thrush, or acute pseudomembranous candidiasis: a clinico-pathologic study of forty-four cases. Oral Surg. *18*:27, 1964.
3. Cawson, R. A.: Chronic oral candidiasis and leukoplakia. Oral Surg. *22*:582, 1966.
4. Eyre, J. and Nally, F. F.: Oral candidosis and carcinoma. Br. J. Dermatol. *85*:73, 1971.
5. Lehner, T., Wilton, J. M., and Ivanyi, L.: Immunodeficiencies in chronic mucocutaneous candidiasis. Immunology *22*:775, 1972.
6. Lozada, F., Silverman, S., Migliorati, C. A., Conant, M. A., and Volderding, P. A.: Oral manifestations of tumor and opportunistic infections in the acquired immunodeficiency syndrome (AIDS): Findings in 53 homosexual men with Kaposi's sarcoma. Oral Surg. *56*: 491, 1983.

MISCELLANEOUS WHITE SPOTS AND PAPULES

Fordyce's Granules

Age: All ages
Sex: No predilection

Clinical Features: Fordyce's granules or ectopic sebaceous glands are present in 90 percent of the population. They are multifocal, less than 2 mm in diameter and actually more yellow than white in appearance. They are located on the mucosal surfaces of the lips and buccal mucosa.

Histologic Features: Submucosal clusters of sebaceous acini are present and communicate with the oral epithelium by way of ducts.

Differential Diagnosis: The small size, multiplicity, and yellow color are characteristic and are unlikely to be confused with other mucosal diseases.

Treatment: No treatment is necessary.

References

1. Gorlin, R. J.: In *Thoma's Oral Pathology,* 6th Ed., edited by R. J. Gorlin and H. M. Goldman, St. Louis, C. V. Mosby Co., 1970, Vol. 1, pp. 24–25.
2. Mitchell, D. F., Standish, S. M., and Fast, T. B.: *Oral Diagnosis/Oral Medicine,* 3rd Ed. Philadelphia, Lea & Febiger, 1978, pp. 374–375.
3. Shafer, W. G., Hine, M. K., and Levy, B. M.: *A Textbook of Oral Pathology,* 4th Ed. Philadelphia, W. B. Saunders Co., 1983, p. 20.
4. Fordyce, J.: A peculiar affection of the mucous membrane of the lip and oral cavity. J. Cutan. Genito-Urin. Dis., *14*:413, 1896.
5. Miles, A. E. W.: Sebaceous glands in the lip and cheek mucosa of man. Br. Dent. J. *105*:235, 1958.

Dental Lamina Cysts, Bohn's Nodules, and Epstein's Pearls

Age: Infants
Sex: No predilection

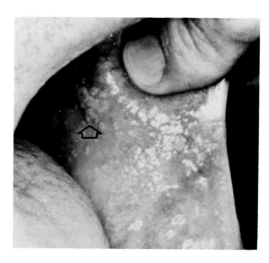

FIG. 2–20. Clusters of submucosal sebaceous glands constituting Fordyce's granules.

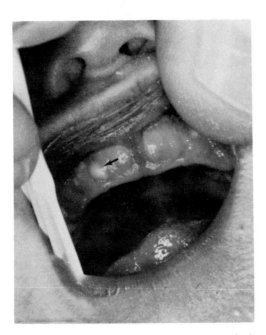

FIG. 2–21. Dental lamina cysts appearing as multiple pearl-like spots on this infant's alveolar ridge.

Clinical Features: Focal white nodules seen on the alveolar ridges, palatal raphe area, or lateral palatal mucosa represent dental lamina cysts, Bohn's nodules, and Epstein's pearls respectively. These nodules are encountered in neonates and represent keratin cysts that are remnants of embryonic processes of dental or minor salivary gland origin or, in the case of midpalatal Bohn's nodules, small cystic remnants of palatal process fusion.

Microscopic Features: Microscopically all three entities are identical. They are characterized by submucosal epithelial cysts that contain no true lumen but, instead, are filled with concentric swirls of keratin.

Differential Diagnosis: Neonatal alveolar ridge nodules may be confused with natal teeth, but closer scrutiny will obviously disclose the true nature of the spots as submucosal nodules and not prematurely erupting teeth.

Treatment: No treatment is necessary as these small cysts spontaneously regress within 1 to 3 months.

References

1. Kreshover, S. J.: The incidence and pathogenesis of gingival cysts. Presented at 35th General Meeting, International Association for Dental Research, March, 1957.
2. Fromm, A.: Epstein's pearls, Bohn's nodules and

inclusion cysts of the oral cavity. J. Dent. Child. *34*:275, 1967.
3. Cataldo, E. and Berkman, M.: Cysts of the oral mucosa in newborns. Am. J. Dis. Child. *116*:44, 1968.
4. Maher, W. P. and Swindle, P. F.: Etiology and vascularization of dental lamina cysts. Oral Surg. *29*:590, 1970.

Stomatitis Nicotina

Age: Middle-aged and elderly adults
Sex: Males predominate

Clinical Features: Inveterate pipe and cigar smokers may manifest multiple focal keratotic papules restricted to the palatal mucosa, generally the posterior hard palate and anterior soft palate. The center of each papule in stomatitis nicotina evidences a pinpoint erythematous depression with an umbilicated appearance.

Microscopic Appearance: The epithelium surrounding the palatal minor salivary gland duct orifice is thickened, with involvement of both keratin and spinous cell layers. The excretory salivary duct is acanthotic and may show mucous cell metaplasia. A periductal inflammatory cell infiltrate composed of lymphocytes and plasma cells accompanies capillary proliferation and dilatation in this zone.

Differential Diagnosis: The restriction of umbilicated papules to the palate in pipe smokers is characteristic for stomatitis nicotina. Oral keratotic papules may also be seen in keratosis follicularis (Darier-White's disease). Stomatitis nicotina differs from papillomatosis (papillary hyperplasia) in that the papules of the former are generally focal with clinically normal-appearing intervening mucous membrane; additionally, papillary hyperpla-

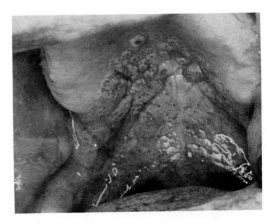

FIG. 2–22. Multifocal umbilicated keratotic papules on posterior hard palate in a pipe smoker.

sia is not keratotic and does not show a centrally depressed area.

Treatment: The presence of stomatitis nicotina is an indication that the patient is utilizing tobacco to a level that is toxic to his mucosa. While malignancy is not associated with this mucosal change, the patient may nevertheless manifest leukoplakia plaques in other mucosal locations. The habit should be eliminated or severely limited.

References

1. Saunders, W. H.: Nicotine stomatitis of the palate. Ann. Otol. Rhinol. Laryngol. 67:618, 1958.
2. Schwartz, D. L.: Stomatitis nicotina of the palate. Oral Surg. 20:306, 1965.
3. Thoma, K. H.: Stomatitis nicotina and its effect on the palate. Am. J. Orthod. Oral Surg. 27:38, 1941.

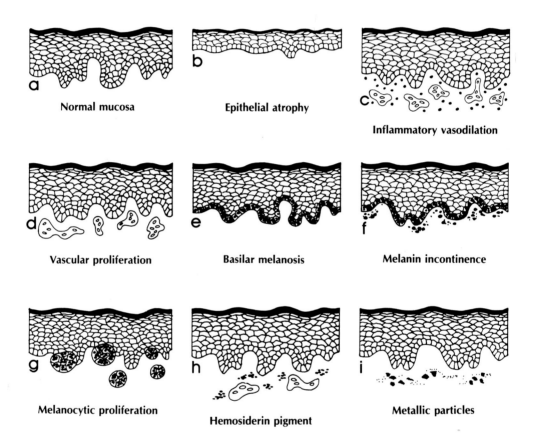

Normal mucosa

Epithelial atrophy

Inflammatory vasodilation

Vascular proliferation

Basilar melanosis

Melanin incontinence

Melanocytic proliferation

Hemosiderin pigment

Metallic particles

Red and Pigmented Lesions

3
Red and Pigmented Lesions

FOCAL ERYTHEMAS

Nonspecific (Irritational) Mucositis
Mucosal Burn
Macular Hemangioma
Erythroplakia (Precancerous)

DIFFUSE AND MULTIFOCAL RED LESIONS

Geographic Tongue
Erythema Migrans
Vitamin Deficient Glossitis
Radiation Mucositis
Xerostomic Mucositis
Lupus Erythematosus
Allergic Mucositis
Erythema Multiforme
Candidiasis
Lymphonodular Pharyngitis
Scarlet Fever
Erosive Lichen Planus
Dermatitis Herpetiformis
Ecchymosis and Clotting Factor Deficiencies
Field Cancerization

PETECHIAE

Suction Petechiae
Infectious Mononucleosis
Thrombocyte Disorders
Hereditary Hemorrhagic Telangiectasia

FOCAL PIGMENTATIONS

Amalgam and Graphite Tattoo
Mucocele
Hematoma
Hemangioma and Varix
Nevus
Ephelis, Oral Melanotic Macule

DIFFUSE AND MULTIFOCAL PIGMENTATIONS

Malignant Melanoma
Kaposi's Sarcoma
Racial Pigmentation
Pigmented Lichen Planus
Peutz-Jeghers Syndrome
Multiple Neurofibromatosis
Addison's Disease
Hemochromatosis
Heavy Metal Ingestion
Hairy Tongue

Redness of the gingiva is the hallmark of plaque-related inflammatory disease, gingivitis and periodontitis. These two entities have been intentionally omitted since they are dealt with extensively in dental practice and need no consideration here. When dental plaque cannot be incriminated as a source of inflammation, the clinician is obliged to pursue other causes. Diffuse gingivitis, often exhibiting pronounced erythema, may be encountered in association with systemic alterations (e.g., diabetes, pregnancy). In these instances, gingival enlargement accompanies the erythema; systemically associated gingivitis is discussed in the chapter dealing with intraoral tumefactions.

Red lesions or erythemas of the oral mucosa, including the gingiva, generally present to the assessing eye of the clinician a promulgation of inflammation. This generality should not, however, be made to the point of excluding other disease processes, particularly malignant neoplasia. Intense erythema represents increased vascularity as an expression of the inflammatory response, yet early oral cancer frequently heralds its own presence by accompanying inflammatory changes that often coexist.

In this section, red lesions are classified according to degree of involvement with regard to surface area and the size of the isolated erythematous zone (i.e., focal erythemas, diffuse and multifocal erythemas, petechiae, and focal telangiectasia). When considering a grouping of disease entities as collective components of the differential diagnosis, one must be constantly cognizant of the fact that ulcerative and vesiculobullous lesions usually manifest a circumlesional erythematous halo. The primary character of the early lesion is of utmost relevance in the development of a differential diagnosis. Lesions that evince an erythematous component yet are primarily ulcerative or vesiculobullous-desquamative in nature are considered in a separate chapter.

A previously mentioned concept warrants reemphasis: Most individual diseases encompassed within the erythematous group are inflammatory idiopathic disorders. Some represent a response to physical and chemical irritants; others are a manifestation of hypersensitivity to various allergens including foods and drugs. Importantly, premalignancy or incipient carcinomatous change may appear red clinically. As with other oral diseases, thorough history procurement relative to both the present illness and past medical history is imperative when one attempts to limit the differential diagnosis. Observation of the distribution, longevity, and temporal relationship of lesions to suspected causative agents will, in conjunction with the case history, lead to a tentative diagnosis. These features are detailed for each disease entity included here.

Pigmentations other than red lesions are considered in this section and may be black, brown, or blue. The discolorations may be due to the accumulation of either intrinsic or extrinsic chemicals in the mucosal tissues. The primary intrinsic pigmentations of the oral mucosa include the melanins and hemoglobin or hemosiderin. Extrinsic pigments responsible for discolorations are usually heavy metal particles introduced either locally or systemically. Pigmented areas that blanch when pressed represent vascular lesions. The differential diagnosis is based on extent; multiple pigmentations are associated with certain disorders whereas focal, isolated pigmentations encompass a different group of diseases.

Common focal erythemas are nonspecific mucositis and erythroplakia (premalignant and malignant). Erythroplakia is potentially lethal.

The most common multifocal red lesions are geographic tongue, erosive lichen planus, and moniliasis. Multifocal red lesions associated with a potential lethal outcome include field cancerization, lupus erythematosus, and ecchymosis from clotting factor deficiencies.

The most common petechial lesions usually found on the palate are suction petechiae and infectious mononucleosis. Petechiae connoting a potentially lethal course include leukemia and primary thrombocyte disorders.

The most common focal pigmentations are amalgam or graphite tattoo and mucocele. Melanoma is a potentially lethal, pigmented lesion that may be focal during the incipient phase, yet usually appears diffuse. All diffuse pigmentations, with the exception of racial melanosis, are rare.

FOCAL ERYTHEMAS

Nonspecific (Irritational) Mucositis

Age: No predilection
Sex: No predilection

Clinical Features: Localized zones of redness are often related to a physical agent that has irritated the mucosa. Ill-fitting dental prostheses or factitial injuries from chronic habitual irritation are the chief contributing factors. The zone of erythema will correspond to the source of irritation.

Microscopic Features: The epithelium may be atrophic with regions bordering on ulceration. The submucosa displays capillary proliferation with dilation and a mixed inflammatory cell infiltrate.

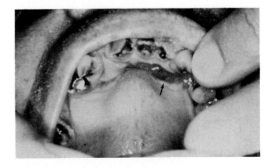

FIG. 3–1. Linear focal erythema corresponding to a partial denture gold connector that had mechanically irritated the palatal mucosa.

Differential Diagnosis: In older individuals, precancerous erythroplakia must be ruled out, particularly when an immediate cause is indeterminate or when removal of the suspected causative agent fails to mitigate or limit the extent of the lesion.

Treatment: Elimination of the irritating agent is necessary. If the area is painful, Orabase gel or an oral bandage may alleviate or palliate the symptoms until healing takes place.

References

1. Greither, A.: In *Thoma's Oral Pathology*, 6th Ed., edited by R. J. Gorlin and H. M. Goldman. St. Louis, C. V. Mosby Co., 1970, Vol. II, pp. 780–781.
2. Mitchell, D. F., Standish, S. M., and Fast, T.B.: *Oral Diagnosis/Oral Medicine*, 3rd Ed. Philadelphia, Lea & Febiger, 1978, p. 381.

Mucosal Burn

Age: No predilection
Sex: No predilection

Clinical Features: Chemical agents that are caustic or irritational often cause coagulation of the epithelium with the appearance of a white lesion. If these same chemicals are dilute or contact mucosa for a short period of time, they will induce intense inflammation and redness without producing superficial necrosis. Thermal burns display the same features. A common oral mucosal burn due to thermal injury from contact by hot foods, such as pizza cheese, results in palatal erythema. The lesions will logically correspond to the region of contact, and the red mucosa is usually painful. Incriminating chemical agents include acids, alkalies, caustic organic compounds, and volatile oils.

Microscopic Features: The epithelium may be intact, eroded, or show microvesicles. The sub-mucosa is diffusely infiltrated with inflammatory cells that are usually subacute in nature.

Differential Diagnosis: The history of contact with a chemical irritant is, of course, the primary differentiating event. Contact with chemicals known to be devoid of caustic or irritational qualities may point to a hypersensitivity reaction. Lack of an identifiable contact irritant necessitates biopsy to eliminate the possibility of cytologic atypia.

Treatment: Refraining from use of the irritant and applying Orabase are recommended. Spicy foods and vegetables should be avoided until healing has occurred.

References

1. Greither, A.: In *Thoma's Oral Pathology*, 6th Ed., edited by R. J. Gorlin and H. M. Goldman. St. Louis, C. V. Mosby Co., 1970, Vol. II, p. 781.
2. Mitchell, D. F., Standish, S. M., and Fast, T. B.: *Oral Diagnosis/Oral Medicine*, 3rd Ed. Philadelphia, Lea & Febiger, 1978, pp. 375, 381.
3. Shafer, W. G., Hine, M. K., and Levy, B. M.: *A Textbook of Oral Pathology*, 4th Ed. Philadelphia, W.B. Saunders Co., 1983, pp. 572–573.

Macular Hemangioma (Port-wine Stain)

Age: Congenital or childhood onset
Sex: Female predilection

Clinical Features: Macular hemangiomas of the facial skin have been termed port-wine stains or nevus flammeus. They tend to follow the vascular components of neurovascular tracts of the trigeminal nerve pathways. The Sturge-Weber syndrome, encephalotrigeminal angiomatosis, manifests nevus flammeus of the facial skin with accompanying vascular hamartomas of the cerebrum and radiographically demonstrable serpentine calcifications. Ocular involvement may be present. Patients with this syndrome will often suffer from epilepsy, contralateral hemiplegia, and visual disturbances. The angiomatous component

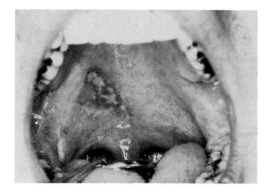

FIG. 3–2. Focal red lesion with surface pseudomembrane caused by contact of the mucosa with phenol.

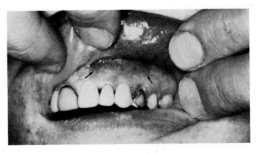

FIG. 3–3. Macular hemangioma limited to the mucosal surface of the upper lip and maxillary gingiva.

may extend as a macular or tumorous lesion of the oral mucosa. Focal macular hemangiomas without evidence of skin involvement or central nervous system manifestations are also encountered in the oral cavity, although they are somewhat rare. The tumorous palpable type is more common.

Microscopic Features: The submucosal or dermal connective tissue underlying the surface epithelium displays randomly dispersed small-caliber vessels, which are usually engorged with erythrocytes.

Differential Diagnosis: Nevus flammeus of the facial skin, when considered in conjunction with a history of long duration, poses no problem in the differential diagnosis. A diagnosis of Sturge-Weber syndrome requires radiographic demonstration of intracranial calcifications and onset of the characteristic symptomatology. Focal mucosal hemangiomas may be confused with erythroplakia, mucositis, or chemical burns; however, history of onset and duration provides helpful clues as to the nature of the red lesion. Blanching on pressure may be evoked, and biopsy will confirm the diagnosis.

Treatment: Patients with Sturge-Weber syndrome should be managed by a physician for control of epilepsy. Cosmetic surgery and tattooing may be indicated for the concerned patient with nevus flammeus. Oral macular hemangiomas may spontaneously regress after puberty. Once the diagnosis is established, no treatment is necessary for focal mucosa macular hemangiomas.

References

1. Gorlin, R. J. and Pindborg, J. J.: *Syndromes of the Head and Neck.* New York, Blakiston Division, McGraw-Hill Book Co., 1964.
2. Watson, W. L. and McCarthy, W. D.: Blood and lymph vessel tumors; a report of 1,056 cases. Surg. Gynecol. Obstet. *71*:569, 1940.
3. Yukua, R. A., Cassingham, R. J., and Carr, R. F.: Periodontal manifestations and treatment in a case of Sturge-Weber syndrome. Oral Surg. *47*:408, 1979.
4. Royle, H. E., Lapp, R., and Ferrara, E. D.: The Sturge-Weber syndrome. Oral Surg. *22*:490, 1966.

Erythroplakia (Precancerous)

Age: Middle-aged and elderly adults
Sex: Male predilection

Clinical Features: Erythroplakia is the red counterpart to leukoplakia and should be used strictly in the clinical sense meaning, simply, red patch. Erythroplakia may therefore be represented by any of the focal erythemas listed in this chapter.

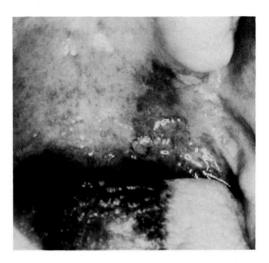

FIG. 3–4.   Focal red lesion of soft palate representing carcinoma in situ. This type of red lesion is referred to as erythroplakia. The patient also has a hairy tongue.

Premalignant or malignant erythroplakia was originally described as a penile cancerous lesion termed *erythroplasia.* The oral mucosal counterpart is clinically similar in that a focal zone of redness may exist alone or accompanied by leukoplakic zones. When multifocal keratotic white patches are superimposed upon an erythematous base, the lesion is descriptively termed *speckled leukoplakia* or erythroplakia. Importantly, a focal red lesion with no identifiable cause is a prime suspect for premalignant erythroplakia. Precancerous erythroplakia is most prevalent in the oral floor, on the soft palate, buccal mucosa, and ventral tongue.

Microscopic Features: The epithelium may or may not possess a cornified layer. The spinous cell layer is atrophic, and rete ridge formation is either absent or shows bulbous projections. The spinous layer contains cells displaying atypia, hyperchromatism, pleomorphism, and increased numbers of mitotic figures. The underlying connective tissue is generally infiltrated by mononuclear inflammatory cells.

Differential Diagnosis: Focal erythemas representing precancerous erythroplakia can be clinically confused with irritational mucositis, macular hemangioma, or chemical burn. Absence of any identifiable irritants warrants biopsy.

Treatment: Wide local excision of focal lesions, including 1 cm of clinically normal tissue, is recommended. The specimen should be evaluated microscopically for dysplastic free margins.

References

1. Shear, M.: Erythroplakia of the mouth. Int. Dent. J. 22:460, 1972.
2. Shafer, W. G., and Waldron, C. A.: Erythroplakia of the oral cavity. Cancer 36:1021, 1975.
3. Mashberg, A.: Erythroplasia: the earliest sign of asymptomatic oral cancer. J. Am. Dent. Assoc. 96:615, 1978.
4. Mashberg, A. and Morrissey, J. B.: A study of the appearance of early asymptomatic oral squamous cell carcinomas. Cancer 37:2149, 1976.

DIFFUSE AND MULTIFOCAL RED LESIONS

Geographic Tongue (Migratory Glossitis)

Age: Onset in childhood or early adult life

Sex: Slight female predilection

Clinical Features: Multifocal circinate and irregular zones of surface erosion characterized by loss of the filiform papillae are seen on the dorsum and lateral margins of the tongue. The fungiform papillae remain intact and may show mild swelling with variable degrees of erythema. The eroded zones are rimmed by keratotic white circumlesional hypertrophic filiform papillae. Whereas most cases are asymptomatic, some patients will complain of glossodynia. The disease has been stated to occur in 1 to 2 percent of the population. The term *geographic tongue* is descriptive in that the foci of desquamation appear as islands and continents in a sea of normal-appearing glossal mucosa. The lesions wax and wane with periods of remissiion. During recurrent episodes, lesions appear in a different location.

Microscopic Features: The epithelium evinces loss of filiform papillae with spongiotic abscesses similar to those encountered in psoriasis with migration of neutrophils into the spinous cell layer.

The submucosa generally displays a mild chronic inflammatory cell infiltrate with variable degrees of capillary proliferation.

Differential Diagnosis: The clinical features, age, and history of chronicity with a tendency of the lesions to migrate are characteristic. Other diffuse erythemas that may mimic geographic tongue include moniliasis and erosive lichen planus, both of which manifest lesions in extraglossal mucosa. Geographic tongue may accompany other dermatologic conditions; therefore, the exposed skin should be examined for accompanying lesions.

Treatment: No treatment is necessary. The patient should be reassured as to the benignity of the condition.

References

1. Redman, R. S.: Prevalence of geographic tongue, fissured tongue, median rhomboid glossitis, and hairy tongue among 3,611 Minnesota school children. Oral Surg. 30:390, 1970.
2. Weathers, D. R., Baker, G., Archard, H. O., and Burkes, E. F., Jr.: Psoriasiform lesions of the oral mucosa (with emphasis on "ectopic geographic tongue"). Oral Surg. 37:872, 1974.
3. Kullaa-Mikkonen, A, Mikkonen, M., and Kotilainen, R.: Prevalence of different morphologic forms of the human tongue in young Finns. Oral Surg. 53:152, 1982.
4. Eidelman, E., Chosack, A., and Cohen, T.: Scrotal tongue and geographic tongue: Polygenic and associated traits. Oral Surg. 42:591, 1976.

Erythema Migrans (Migratory Stomatitis)

Age: Young adults

Sex: No predilection

Clinical Features: Erythema migrans is probably the extraglossal counterpart to geographic tongue. The lesions may actually accompany those of geographic tongue, or they may be in-

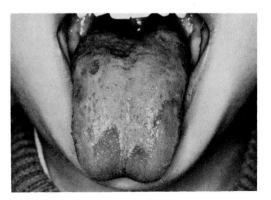

FIG. 3–5. Multifocal zones of denuded tongue with mild erythema alternating with normal tongue mucosa, representing geographic tongue.

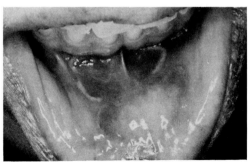

FIG. 3–6. Erythematous macules with circinate keratotic borders that migrate from one site to another, representing erythema migrans.

dependent. They are found on the buccal mucosa, lips, soft palate, oral floor, and ventral tongue mucosa. Multifocal erythematous patches are rimmed by a keratotic white margin and have a circinate pattern. As with geographic tongue, a history of migration is elicited. The erythematous regions are usually asymptomatic; however, stomatodynia may be a complaint in rare instances.

Microscopic Features: The epithelium displays psoriasiform patterns; spongiosis with neutrophilic infiltration is seen in the spinous cell layer. The epithelium may be atrophic or may manifest elongated rete ridges with superficially oriented submucosal papillae.

Differential Diagnosis: A history of migration, lack of pain, and a circinate appearance are characteristic. Erythematous moniliasis, erosive lichen planus, lupus erythematosus, and field cancerization should be considered in the clinical diagnosis; biopsy should be performed to rule out these diseases.

Treatment: The cause is unknown and no treatment is necessary. Assurance as to the benignity of the condition is indicated, particularly if the patient is cancerophobic.

References

1. Weathers, D. R., et al.: Psoriasiform lesions of the oral mucosa (with emphasis on "ectopic geographic tongue"). Oral Surg. 37:872, 1974.
2. Burkes, E. J.: Ectopic geographic tongue. J. N. C. Dent. Soc. 57:22, 1974.
3. Saprio, S. M. and Shklar, G.: Stomatitis areata migrans. Oral Surg. 36:28, 1973.

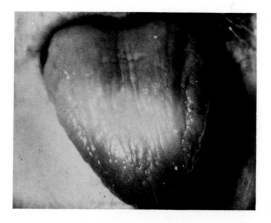

FIG. 3–7. Bald tongue generally reddened in pernicious anemia or B-complex deficiency.

Vitamin Deficient Glossitis

Age: Children and elderly adults
Sex: No predilection

Clinical Features: Vitamin deficiencies are endemic in some regions of the world; in western populations they are usually restricted to alcoholics suffering from malnutrition. Deficiency of the B vitamins such as riboflavin, niacin, and cyanocobalamine (B_{12}) with pernicious anemia, as well as folic acid deficiency and sprue resulting from an intolerance to gluten, may be accompanied by atrophic glossitis. Atrophic glossitis accompanying pernicious anemia has been termed Hunter's or Moeller's glossitis. The tongue is smooth, devoid of papillae, and shows diffuse erythema. The condition is reversible with adequate therapy.

Microscopic Features: Tongue papillae are absent; there is a flattened epithelial layer. The submucosa shows mild chronic inflammatory cell infiltration.

Differential Diagnosis: Atrophic erythematous glossitis, when diffuse, is usually indicative of vitamin B complex, or B_{12}, deficiency. Luetic glossitis should be considered in the differential diagnosis, yet usually lacks an erythematous component. Hematogram, bone marrow aspiration, and gastric analysis will disclose the presence of pernicious anemia. Similar blood studies and stool analysis for steatorrhea are necessary when sprue is suspected.

Treatment: The nutritional deficiency should be rectified by proper diet and multiple vitamin tablets. Pernicious anemia should be managed by a physician and can be treated by vitamin B_{12} injections. Tropical sprue is managed by a nutritional diet, whereas nontropical sprue may be controlled by a gluten-free diet.

References

1. Cagnone, L. D.: In *Thoma's Oral Pathology,* 6th Ed., edited by R. J. Gorlin and H. M. Goldman. St. Louis, C. V. Mosby Co., 1970, Vol. II, pp. 612–614.
2. Shafer, W. G., Hine, M. K. and Levy, B. M.: *A Textbook of Oral Pathology,* 4th Ed. Philadelphia, W. B. Saunders Co., 1983, pp. 649–653.
3. Adlersberg, D.: Newer advances in sprue. Oral Surg. 1:1109, 1948.
4. Dreizen, S., et al.: Oral manifestations of nutritional disorders. Dent. Clin. North Am. July: 429–440, 1958.

Radiation Mucositis

Age: Middle-aged and elderly adults
Sex: Male predilection

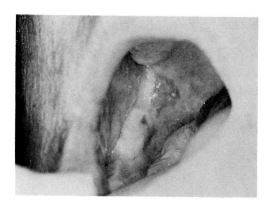

FIG. 3–8. A pale red lesion on soft palate with similar lesions in the oropharynx in patient who received radiation for a carcinoma of the tongue.

Clinical Features: Patients who have received external radiation therapy to the oral mucosa in excess of 3500 to 4000 rads for the treatment of oral, pharyngeal, or salivary malignant neoplasms will often evince a diffuse erythema with telangiectasia of the mucosa. The red zones may initially be associated with a white pseudomembrane and are located in the zone of maximal radiation.

Microscopic Features: The surface epithelium may show ulceration or atrophy; depending upon whether the area examined was involved with neoplastic change, residual cytologic atypia can be observed. Later changes show an inflammatory cell infiltrate in the submucosa with an attenuated spinous cell layer. Telangiectasia with nuclear pleomorphism of endothelial cells is often encountered; intimal thickening and even thrombosis may be observed. Atypical cytologic features are no longer observed six weeks after radiation unless recurrence has developed.

Differential Diagnosis: A history of radiation therapy to the head and neck area points to a diagnosis of radiation mucositis. Persistence of the red lesion or increase in size should arouse suspicion that an erythroplakia connoting recurrence of carcinoma is evolving.

Treatment: Radiation mucositis regresses with time. Persistence or an increase in topographic extent may herald recurrence of carcinoma. Cytologic smears are the method of choice for monitoring postradiation mucositis. Unnecessary tissue breakdown, often evoked by surgical biopsy, can be avoided by this procedure. A bland dentifrice is recommended along with a soft diet. A soothing mouth rinse such as an antihistaminic with Kaopectate will offer pain relief.

References

1. Chase, L. P., et al.: Radiation-induced changes in the epithelium of the buccal mucosa. J. Dent. Res. 40:929, 1961.
2. Mouriquand, J., et al.: Radiation cell changes from the oral cavity. Acta Cytol. 3:451, 1960.
3. Greenspan, D. and Silverman,S., Jr.: Study of bland dentifrice for persons with radiation-induced mucositis and vesiculo-erosive disease. J. Am. Dent. Assoc. 99:203, 1979.
4. Blozis, G. G. and Robinson, J. E.: Oral tissue changes caused by radiation therapy and their management. Dent. Clin. North Amer. 643: Nov., 1968.

Xerostomic Mucositis

Age: Adults

Sex: Female predilection

Clinical Features: Diffuse erythema from lack of salivary secretion is painful, with dry mucous membranes, and is severe on the gingiva. The diagnosis of xerostomic mucositis is realized upon manual palpation of the major salivary glands with resultant failure to elicit flow from Wharton's and Stensen's ducts. Xerostomic mucositis may be due to: (1) radiation fields in the region of the major salivary glands, (2) immunopathologic sialadenitis as seen with collagen diseases, Sjögren's syndrome or Mikulicz's disease or (3) prolonged use of antihistamines or antisialogogues. Rampant dental caries may accompany xerostomia, particularly when associated with radiation injury or long-standing Sjögren's syndrome. Notably, xerostomia may occur in the absence of any mucosal alterations.

Microscopic Features: Xerostomic mucositis

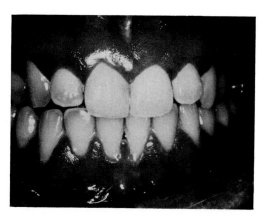

FIG. 3–9. Generalized erythema of the gingiva and other oral mucous membranes occurring in severe xerostomia associated with Sjögren's syndrome.

shows a nonspecific chronic inflammatory cell infiltrate with capillary dilation in the submucosa.

Differential Diagnosis: Diffuse erythema of xerostomic mucositis must be differentiated from primary mucosal damage by direct irradiation (radiation mucositis). Failure to elicit salivary flow on palpation, symptoms of dry mouth, history of radiation to salivary gland regions, and bilateral parotid enlargement are all indicative of oral erythema due to xerostomia. A definitive diagnosis can be made only by uncovering the cause of the condition.

Treatment: Management of xerostomic mucositis due to antisialogogues requires elimination or limitation of the drug. Treatment of dry mouth and mucositis due to compromised salivary function as a result of organic disease is problematic. Frequent rinsing with water or a saliva substitute and use of soft-line denture bases with Orabase may afford some degree of comfort. Use of sialogogues is of limited benefit and may cause gastrointestinal irritability because of their cholinergic properties. Daily fluoride application and meticulous oral hygiene will diminish the caries incidence.

References

1. Bertram, U.: Xerostomia. Acta Odontol. Scand. 25:Suppl. 4, 1967.
2. Nakamoto, R. Y.: Use of a saliva substitute in post-radiation xerostomia. J. Prosthet. Dent. 42:539, 1979.
3. Dreizen, S., Brown, L. R., Daly, T. E., et al.: Prevention of xerostomia-related dental caries in irradiated cancer patients. J. Dent. Res. 56:99, 1977.

Lupus Erythematosus

Age: Young and middle-aged adults

Sex: Female predilection

Clinical Features: The oral lesions seen in lupus erythematosus may be red, white, or bullous. Often, red and white zones are present bilaterally on buccal mucosa with diffuse or multifocal involvement. The dermatologic features are invariably present, and the "butterfly rash" over the nasal bridge and malar eminence region bilaterally is diagnostic when other skin lesions coexist. The systemic form more frequently manifests oral lesions. Antinuclear antibodies are present in most cases, being demonstrated more often in the systemic than in the discoid form of the disease. The presence of circulating antibodies to DNA is of more diagnostic significance.

Microscopic Features: The oral mucosal changes in lupus erythematosus may resemble

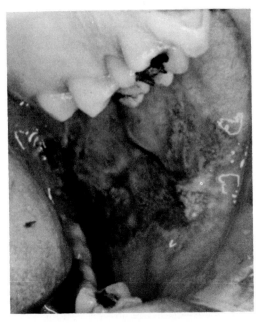

FIG. 3–10. Diffuse red lesions of the buccal mucosa in lupus erythematosus. (Courtesy of Dr. T. Daniels.)

those in lichen planus. The basal lamina is thickened with subepithelial and perivascular lymphocytic infiltrates. Immunofluorescent microscopy reveals the presence of granular in vitro tissue-bound immunoglobulins in the basal lamina and epithelial nuclei.

Differential Diagnosis: The red and mixed red and white lesions of lupus erythematosus resemble those seen in erosive lichen planus. Candidiasis, allergic mucositis, erythema migrans, and multifocal precancerous erythroplakia must also be considered in the differential diagnosis. Antinuclear antibody, anti-DNA antibody, L.E. Prep, and renal function tests, with a consideration of the dermatologic condition, will limit the differential diagnosis.

Treatment: Lupus erythematosus is treated by systemic immunosuppressant therapy and should be managed by a physician.

References

1. Andreasen, J. O.: Oral manifestations in discoid and systemic lupus erythematosus. 1. Clinical investigation. Acta Odontol. Scand. 22:295, 1964.
2. Archard, H. P., et al.: Oral manifestations of chronic discoid lupus erythematosus. Oral Surg. 16;696, 1963.
3. Schiodt, M., Halberg, P., and Hentzer, B.: A clinical study of 32 patients with oral discoid lupus erythematosus. Int. J. Oral Surg. 7:85, 1978.
4. Schiodt, M. and Pindborg, J. J.: Histologic differ-

ential diagnostic problems for oral discoid lupus erythematosus. Int. J. Oral Surg. 5:250, 1976.

Allergic Mucositis

Age: No predilection
Sex: No predilection

Clinical Features: Inflammatory oral red lesions from immediate systemic hypersensitivity to drugs (stomatitis medicamentosa) or contact allergy (stomatitis venenata) may occur at any site on oral mucosa. Immediate antibody-mediated hypersensitivity may be seen with any parenteral medication, but is most commonly associated with antibiotics, sulfa drugs, iodine and barbiturates. Diffuse and multifocal red lesions are usually accompanied by a pseudomembrane, desquamation or occasionally bullae. Contact allergy can be seen in the region in direct continuity with the incriminating allergen, which may be any dental material including heavy metals, topical medications, or dental preparations such as toothpastes and mouth rinses. The lips and face may show erythematous lesions when cosmetics are the cause of allergy. A specific form of contact mucositis due to an allergen in chewing gum has been observed and is characterized by severe diffuse gingival erythema with ulceration of the lips and commissure. This has been termed *plasmacytosis gingivae,* so named because of the profuse infiltration of plasma cells into the submucosa of the gingiva. In both immediate and contact allergic reactions, pruritus or burning may be a primary symptom.

Microscopic Features: The submucosa in immediate hypersensitivity evinces capillary dilation and nonspecific infiltration of the inflammatory

cells. Eosinophils are present in variable numbers yet are not usually a prominent feature. In plasmacytosis gingivae an avid plasma cell infiltrate prevails, producing myeloma-like features microscopically. Delayed reactiions are T-cell mediated and exhibit a lymphocytic submucosal infiltrate with scattered plasma cells and chronic epidermitis; the histologic features may be similar to lichen planus.

Differential Diagnosis: Hypersensitivity-related oral red lesions may clinically mimic erosive lichen planus, lupus erythematosus, erythema migrans, or any of the other diffuse red lesions outlined in this section. The differential diagnosis may be limited by procuring a history of drug ingestion or occurrence of lesions following use of a suspected allergenic substance. Biopsy shows nonspecific features. Epimucous patch testing may be accomplished by applying the suspected allergen on dried mucosa overlaid with an oral bandage. Provided the material is not naturally caustic, a zone of erythema 24 to 48 hours later generally denotes allergy if the procedure can be reduplicated. Alternatively, most allergens causing mucositis will evoke a positive cutaneous patch test which is easier to perform. Patch testing is reserved for delayed contact reactions. If immediate hypersensitivity is suspected, scratch tests with suspected allergens can be performed or *in vitro* radioallergosorbant assays can be diagnostically employed.

Treatment: Elimination of the allergen is necessary to provide cure. Acute reactions and symptoms can be minimized by prescribing antihistamines for systemic reactions or topical triamcinolone in Orabase for contact allergy.

References

1. Tillman, H. H.: Problems of allergy encountered in dentistry. Oral Surg. *11*:1372, 1958.
2. Crissey, J. T.: Stomatitis, dermatitis and denture materials. Arch. Dermatol. *92*:45, 1965.
3. Kerr, D. A., McClatchey, K. D., and Regezi, J. A.: Allergic gingivostomatitis (due to gum chewing). J. Periodontol. *42*:709, 1971.
4. Eversole, L. R.: Allergic stomatitides. J. Oral Med. *34(4),* 1979.
5. Rickles, N. H.: Allergy in surface lesions of the oral mucosa. Oral Surg. *33*:744, 1972.

Erythema Multiforme

Age: Young adults
Sex: Male predilection

Clinical Features: Erythema multiforme shows protean clinical manifestations and is included with both red and bullous lesions. When erythem-

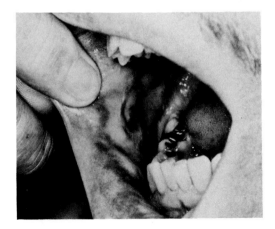

FIG. 3–11. Allergy to mouthwash showing diffuse erythema of the buccal mucosa.

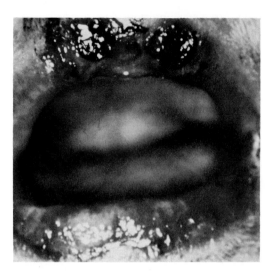

FIG. 3–12. Erythematous and hemorrhagic crusts of the lips in erythema multiforme. Diffuse red lesions were encountered on the oral mucous membranes as well.

atous zones are present, areas of bulla formation and ulceration with hemorrhage may coexist. No site is favored; lesions occur on virtually any oral surface. As opposed to other diffuse red lesions, the lips are invariably affected, including the vermilion surface. The red, eroded mucosa is painful, and the patient may be mildly febrile. Erythema multiforme may occur spontaneously but is often precipitated by parenterally administered medications, particularly sulfa drugs and sulfur-containing hypoglycemic agents, implying an atypical allergic reaction. Onset subsequent to viral infection, predominantly herpetic, is also common. Skin lesions are usually encountered and classically manifest an iris or target pattern, a focal macule with a clear zone enveloped by an erythematous halo. The muco-oculocutaneous syndromes, including Stevens-Johnson and Reiter's syndromes, are diseases similar to erythema multiforme. In the Stevens-Johnson syndrome, oral, conjunctival, and genital erythematous and bullous lesions are accompanied by pain, fever, and malaise. Reiter's syndrome shows a myriad of mucosal and cutaneous lesions including urethritis, conjunctivitis, and arthritis. These diseases are discussed in more detail in the section on vesiculobullous-ulcerative diseases.

Microscopic Features: The histopathologic appearance of erythema multiforme lacks any characteristic or pathognomonic features. The parakeratin layer may show excessive accumulation

of hyalinized eosinophilic globules, so-called mucopolysaccharide keratin dystrophy. Intraepithelial abscesses can be seen, and subbasilar separation may be encountered. A submucosal subacute inflammatory cell infiltrate prevails.

Differential Diagnosis: When bullous lesions accompany oral diffuse erythematous zones, the bullous dermatoses must be considered in the differential diagnosis. When erythematous lesions predominate, other diseases encompassed within the diffuse and multifocal red lesion groupings must be considered—chiefly erythema migrans, allergic mucositis, erythematous candidiasis, erosive lichen planus, and premalignant diffuse erythroplakia. As opposed to erythema multiforme, most of these diseases manifest only minimal pain and, in addition, the external labial mucosa and vermilion border are usually not involved.

Treatment: A topical palliative rinse of an antihistaminic elixir mixed 50:50 with Kaopectate should be employed in conjunction with short-term, low-dose systemic steroids.

References

1. Shklar, G.: Oral lesions of erythema multiforme: Histologic and histochemical observations. Arch. Dermatol. *92*:495, 1965.
2. Shelley, W. B.: Herpes simplex virus as a cause of erythema multiforme. J. Am. Med. Assoc. *201*:153, 1967.
3. Wooten, J. W., et al.: Development of oral lesions in erythema multiforme exudativum. Oral Surg. *24*:808, 1967.
4. Lozada, F. and Silverman S., Jr.: Erythema multiforme; clinical characteristics and natural history in fifty patients. Oral Surg. *46*:628, 1978.
5. Nazif, M. M. and Ranalli, D. N.: Stevens-Johnson syndrome; A report of fourteen pediatric cases. Oral Surg. *53*:263, 1982.

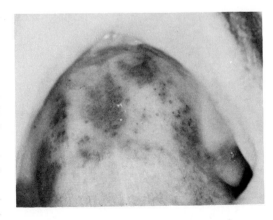

FIG. 3–13. Multifocal red lesions of candidiasis underlying an ill-fitting maxillary dental prosthesis.

Candidiasis

Age: Infants and adults

Sex: No predilection

Clinical Features: The classic pseudomembranous white lesions of Candida albicans infection may occasionally be supplanted or obscured by diffuse and multifocal red patches. A common clinical manifestation of erythematous candidiasis has been termed *denture sore mouth.* The red lesions are confined to denture-bearing mucosa, usually on the palate, and exhibit a patchy distribution often associated with speckled curd-like white lesions, which are generally easily displaced by rubbing. Angular cheilitis often accompanies such changes. In addition to candidal-induced red lesions under dentures, erythematous candidiasis occasionally involves mucous membranes devoid of any overlying dental prosthesis. The red patches may be strictly erythematous or speckled as seen in denture sore mouth. The erythematous component in this form of candidiasis is a reflection of inflammation and may represent hypersensitivity to the organism. Although rare, this mycosis may become systemic with a granulomatous response, is potentially lethal, and usually heralds the presence of an immunodeficiency disorder.

Microscopic Features: The epithelium is attenuated, and PAS staining exhibits superficially oriented mycelia. The underlying submucosa evinces a mild to avid chronic or subacute inflammatory cell infiltrate.

Differential Diagnosis: Denture sore mouth candidiais must be distinguished from a true allergic reaction to denture-base resin (an extremely rare condition). Nondenture-related erythematous candidiasis may be confused with erythema migrans, radiation change, lupus erythematosus, erosive lichen planus, dermatitis herpetiformis, or malignancy. Indeed, candidial infection may coexist with carcinoma. A cytologic smear with periodic acid-Schiff stain will disclose mycelia, or culture may be performed. Failure to respond to antifungal therapy should be followed by biopsy and consideration of other possible diseases in the differential diagnosis.

Treatment: Nystatin cream may be applied to the denture base for rapid resolution of erythema followed by reconstrucion or relining. Erythematous candidiasis not related to ill-fitting dentures can be managed by nystatin oral suspension used 3 times per day as a mouth rinse for 7 to 10 days or nystatin vaginal tablets dispensed as an oral troche to be used 4 times daily. Alternatively, clo-trimazole vaginal tablets may be employed in similar fashion.

References

1. Cawson, R. A.: Denture sore mouth and angular cheilitis. Br. Dent. J. *115*:441, 1963.
2. Davenport, J. C.: Incidence of immediate and delayed hypersensitivity to Candida albicans in denture stomatitis. J. Dent. Res. *50*:892, 1971.
3. Roed-Peterson, B., Renstrup, G., and Pindborg, J. J.: Candida in oral leukoplakia. Scand. J. Dent. Res. *78*:323, 1970.
4. Lehner, T.: Oral candidosis. Dent. Pract. *17*:209, 1967.

Lymphonodular Pharyngitis

Age: Children and young adults

Sex: No predilection

Clinical Features: Multifocal nodules with a pronounced erythematous base localized primarily to the soft palate and oropharynx are seen in lymphonodular pharyngitis, a Coxsackie virus type A infection. Patients complain of sore throat and general malaise, are febrile, and manifest regional nodal lymphadenitis. The nodules are multifocal and measure approximately 0.5 cm in diameter with a wide erythematous base. Similar lesions may occasionally be seen anterior to the oropharynx. The disease resolves spontaneously in 5 to 7 days.

Microscopic Features: The epithelium displays both intracytoplasmic and intranuclear inclusions with transmigration of neutrophils. The submucosa is infiltrated with nodular accumulations of lymphocytes that distend the overlying epithelium.

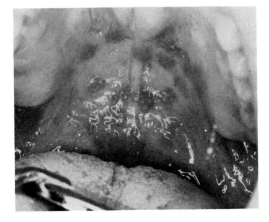

FIG. 3–14. Multiple red papules of the soft palate and oropharynx characteristic of lymphonodular pharyngitis, a Coxsackie virus infection.

Differential Diagnosis: The lesions differ from those of other oral viral infections in that they are erythematous and nodular rather than vesicular. The coexistence of palatal and oropharyngeal lesions with fever allows segregation from other elements in the differential diagnosis, yet allergic mucositis and erythema multiforme should be considered. In these diseases, temperature is not elevated over 100°, whereas in lymphonodular pharyngitis it usually exceeds 101°. Definitive diagnosis can be achieved by procuring a stool culture for isolation of Coxsackie virus.

Treatment: Treatment of lymphonodular pharyngitis is palliative. The symptoms may be mitigated by prescribing a soothing oral rinse such as an antihistaminic expectorant mixed with equal parts of Kaopectate, with subsequent swallowing for sedative affects.

References

1. Steigman, A. J., Lipton, M. M., and Braspennickx, H.: Acute lymphonodular pharyngitis: A newly described condition due to Coxsackie A virus. J. Pediatr. *61*:331, 1963.
2. Lennette, E. H. and Magoffin, R. L.: Virologic and immunologic aspects of major oral ulcerations. J. Am. Dent. Assoc. *87*:1055, 1973.

Scarlet Fever

Age: Children
Sex: No predilection

Clinical Features: Scarlet fever is caused by beta-hemolytic streptococci, which generate an erythrogenic toxin. The toxin induces vascular dilation and damage with an erythematous macular rash on the skin. A fiery red pharyngitis is accompanied by cervical lymphadenopathy. The tongue similarly becomes overtly erythematous with hypertrophy of the fungiform papillae, termed *straw-*

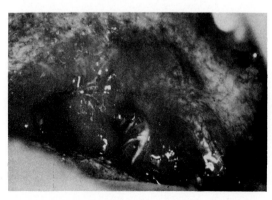

FIG. 3–15. Acute erythematous pharyngitis, a feature of streptococcal sore throat seen in scarlet fever.

berry tongue. Constitutional signs of infectious disease are epitomized by fever and malaise. Potential complications include rheumatic fever, otitis media, and pharyngeal abscess. The disease was often fatal before antibiotic treatment became available.

Microscopic Features: The pharyngeal mucosa may display superficial necrosis, a pseudomembranous exudate and microbial colonies. The submucosa will evince an acute or subacute inflammatory cell infiltrate. The tongue is generally devoid of ulceration yet shows vasodilation with inflammatory cell infiltration, being a nonspecific mucositis.

Differential Diagnosis: The clinical tetrad of erythematous macules, pharyngitis, lymphadenopathy, and so-called strawberry tongue constitutes the hallmark of the disease. The tongue lesion may simulate a chemical burn. Atrophic glossitis seen in vitamin deficiency and pernicious anemia is usually mild and not nearly as bright red in appearance. Swab cultures of the oropharynx disclose the presence of hemolytic streptococci, and antistreptolysin-O titers are elevated.

Treatment: Penicillin is preferred if no allergy to the drug exists. Intramuscular injection of 1,000,000 units is followed by oral penicillin daily. As dangerous complications occasionally occur, the patient should be referred to his or her physician.

References

1. Shafer, W. G., Hine, M. K., and Levy, B. M.: *A Textbook of Oral Pathology,* 4th Ed. Philadelphia, W. B. Saunders Co., 1983, pp. 340–341.
2. Krugman, S. and Ward, R.: *Infectious Diseases of Children,* 4th Ed. St. Louis, C. V. Mosby Co., 1968, Chapter 25.
3. Schwentker, F. F., Janney, J. H., and Gordon, J. E.: The epidemiology of scarlet fever. Am. J. Hyg. *38*:27, 1943.
4. Wesselhoeft, C. and Weinstein, L.: Scarlet fever. N. Engl. J. Med. *232*:500, 531, 1945.

Erosive Lichen Planus

Age: Middle-aged adults
Sex: Predilection for females

Clinical Features: The conventional form of lichen planus is discussed in the section on white lesions. When erythema, superficial ulceration, and desquamation accompany the white component, the term *erosive lichen planus* is used. The buccal mucosa and mucobuccal fold are favored locations, yet other sites are generally involved as well. Reticulated white lines or striae are often, but not invariably, present and are su-

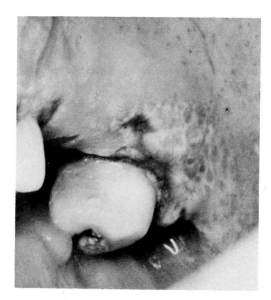

FIG. 3–16. Erosive lichen planus showing multifocal erythematous erosions with associated white lacy striae of Wickham.

perimposed over a red base. The lesions are patchy in distribution with or without an overt slough. Bullae may sometimes be seen with a predominantly erosive form of lichen planus. Pain and burning are frequently encountered. Skin lesions are infrequently associated with oral erosive lichen planus. Most patients are tense or anxiety prone, and the lesions wax and wane corresponding to periods of emotional stress. The erosive form of lichen planus has been associated in rare instances with oral carcinoma.

Microscopic Features: The epithelium is generally attenuated and the basal cell layer is disorganized, with diffuse zones of degeneration. Transmigration of lymphocytes into the basal and parabasilar cell regions is a prominent feature, and the basement membrane is eosinophilic and thickened. A junctional separation at the level of the basement membrane is generally noted in multiple areas to the extent that the epithelial layer may be completely detached or missing. The immediate subjacent connective tissue evinces a zonal lymphocytic band. Immunofluorescent staining fails to demonstrate precipitation of immunoglobulins. Rather, fibrinogen globular deposits are demonstrated along the epidermal-submucosal interface corresponding to the zones of desquamation and basal lamina thickening.

Differential Diagnosis: When a white component with reticulated striae accompanies the red lesions, a clinical diagnosis of erosive lichen planus should be the foremost consideration. Radiation mucositis, allergic mucositis, lupus erythematosus, and erythroplakic precancerous lesions show similar clinical features. If bullous lesions accompany the red lesions, other bullous dermatoses should be considered in the differential diagnosis. Biopsy is indicated to secure a definitive diagnosis.

Treatment: Topical steroid application (triamcinolone in Orabase or .05 percent fluocinonide ointment 50/50 with Orabase) is generally the treatment of choice and results in a clearing of the painful erythematous component. As erosive lichen planus is a paroxysmal chronic disease, this medication can be used periodically during the more severe episodes. Because of the occasional occurrence of carcinoma in this form of lichen planus, patients should be subjected to periodic follow-up. Biopsy of areas that are refractory to treatment should be performed.

References

1. Shklar, G.: Erosive and bullous oral lesions of lichen planus: Histologic studies. Arch. Dermatol. 97:411, 1968.
2. Silverman, S., Jr., and Griffith, M. Studies on oral lichen planus. Oral Surg. 37:705, 1974.
3. Laskaris, G., Slavounou, A., and Angelopoulos, A.: Direct immunofluorescence in oral lichen planus. Oral Surg. 53:483, 1982.
4. Shklar, G.: Lichen planus as an oral ulcerative disease. Oral Surg. 33:376, 1972.

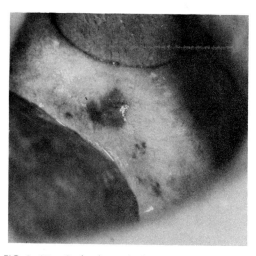

FIG. 3–17. Oral red macular lesions in dermatitis herpetiformis. (From Fraser, N. G., et al.: Oral lesions in dermatitis herpetiformis. Br. J. Dermatol. 89:439, 1973.)

Dermatitis Herpetiformis

Age: Adults
Sex: Male predilection

Clinical Features: Dermatitis herpetiformis is a rare dermatologic disease, which is essentially a vesiculobullous dermatosis. Whereas bullae may occur orally, the predominant oral manifestation is one of multifocal erythematous macular patches. The skin bullae and erythematous papules are pruritic and cluster in groups located primarily on the extremities, with minimal involvement of other skin areas. The oral erythematous macules may show surface ulceration. A protracted course with periodic remissions is most often encountered.

Microscopic Features: The predominant finding is a cluster of inflammatory cells, chiefly eosinophils and neutrophils, localized in the dermal or submucosal papillae interposed between adjacent rete ridges. A subbasilar or junctional separation with bulla formation occurs on the skin yet may not be obvious in the oral mucosal lesions.

Differential Diagnosis: The oral red lesions may mimic a variety of diseases including erythema multiforme, allergic and radiation mucositis, candidiasis, and erosive lichen planus. In conjunction with pruritic vesiculobullous eruptions, other bullous dermatoses should be considered. Biopsy discloses characteristic findings, particularly when obtained from the skin lesions. Immunofluorescent microscopy shows bound IgA deposits of a granular nature in the dermal papillary regions adjacent to, yet not within, bullae.

Treatment: Dermatitis herpetiformis classically responds to sulfapyridine. Indeed, this drug has been used to confirm the diagnosis. As the disease is primarily a dermatologic disorder, management rests with a skin specialist.

References

1. Shafer, W. G., Hine, M. K., and Levy, B. M.: *A Textbook of Oral Pathology,* 4th Ed. Philadelphia, W. B. Saunders Co., 1983, pp. 840–841.
2. Mitchell, D. F., Standish, S.M., and Fast, T. B.: *Oral Diagnosis/Oral Medicine,* 3rd Ed. Philadelphia, Lea & Febiger, 1978, pp. 386–387.
3. Rusotto, S. B. and Ship, I. I.: Oral manifestations of dermatitis herpetiformis. Oral Surg. *31:*42, 1971.
4. Fraser, N. G., Kerr, N. W., and Donald, D.: Oral lesions in dermatitis herpetiformis. Br. J. Dermatol. *89:*439, 1973.

Ecchymosis and Clotting Factor Deficiencies

Age: No predilection
Sex: No predilection

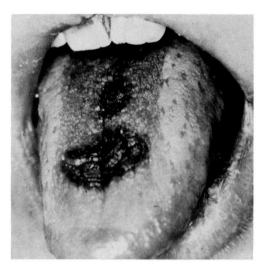

FIG. 3–18. Multiple reddish-brown ecchymotic pigmentations observed in hemorrhagic diatheses due to clotting factor deficiencies. (Courtesy of Dr. Sheldon Rovin.)

Clinical Features: Red lesions caused by extravasation of blood will appear clinically as a submucosal erythema or a diffuse slightly elevated smooth surfaced bruise. The color will range from red to brown to bluish-black, depending upon the duration. Ecchymosis from trauma is common, yet when no traumatic incident can be recalled or when the presence of ecchymosis far outweighs the degree of trauma experienced by the patient a defective clotting mechanism should be suspected. Without exhaustive explanation, the following causes should be considered in the pathogenesis: (1) hereditary clotting factor deficiencies (e.g., hemophilia, Christmas disease), (2) use of medications with anticoagulant activity (e.g., coumarin), and (3) primary liver disease. Gingival hemorrhage and uncontrolled bleeding are also features associated with clotting factor deficiencies. Purpura is encountered in various platelet disorders and leukemia as well.

Microscopic Features: Ecchymosis is characterized by submucosal extravasation of erythrocytes with varying amounts of hemosiderin pigment and organization by fibrovascular and inflammatory cell elements.

Differential Diagnosis: Ecchymosis of the oral mucosa associated with clotting factor disorders will in general be complicated by cutaneous manifestations or hemarthrosis. The oral lesions often appear as blood filled diffuse bullae and therefore are not readily confused with other diffuse or multifocal red lesions. Defective thrombocyte deficiencies are generally heralded by petechial rather than ecchymotic hemorrhages; nevertheless, severe platelet anomalies will manifest ecchymotic lesions. Patients with ecchymosis with no history of undue trauma should be initially subjected to a coagulation panel evaluation, including partial thromboplastin time, prothrombin time, thrombocyte count, thrombocyte aggregation assay, bleeding and clotting time, and a tourniquet test.

Treatment: Detection of an abnormal value in any of these tests warrants referral to an internist or hematologist. Oral surgical procedures should be deferred until the coagulation defect has been corrected.

References

1. Curtis, A. B.: Childhood leukemias: initial oral manifestations. J. Am. Dent. Assoc. *83*:159, 1971.
2. Rettberg, W. A. H.: Symptoms and signs referable to the oral cavity in blood dyscrasias. Oral Surg. *6*:614, 1953.
3. Archer, W. H.: *Oral and Maxillofacial Surgery,* 5th Ed. Philadelphia, W. B. Saunders Co., 1975, pp. 1558–1560.

Field Cancerization

Age: Middle-aged and elderly adults
Sex: Male predilection

Clinical Features: Multifocal erythroplakias will show the same features as focal precancerous erythroplakia, being velvety-red macules often accompanied by a patchy or speckled leukoplakia component. As with leukoplakia, most patients use tobacco and are heavy consumers of alcoholic beverages. Importantly, patients with a history of oral cancer in the past are at risk for developing not merely a recurrence in the previous site of involvement but multifocal oral carcinomas. The larynx may also be the site for other primary carcinomas.

Microscopic Features: The epithelium is invariably attenuated, with foci of hyperorthokeratosis or parakeratosis. The individual epithelial cells may evince changes ranging from atypia to frank invasive carcinoma. The submucosa is traversed by dilated capillaries with an accompanying dense diffuse inflammatory cell infiltrate.

Differential Diagnosis: Multifocal red lesions in eldery patients, particularly those with tobacco and alcohol habits, should arouse suspicion of malignancy. Biopsy is indicated immediately if no cause is discernible, even when other diseases are considered likely components of the differential diagnosis. Field cancerization made manifest by multifocal erythroplasia may mimic erythema migrans, radiation mucositis, lupus erythematosus, allergic mucositis, erythema multiforme, erythematous candidiasis, or erosive lichen planus.

Treatment: Field cancerization is an extremely difficult management problem and is particularly enigmatic when a preexisting carcinoma was present and was managed by radiation therapy. Surgical stripping of carcinoma in situ and radiation therapy remain the treatment modalities of choice. Complete examination with workup for other primary lesions in the oropharynx and larynx is indicated, with management by an experienced oncologist.

References

1. Waldron, C. A.: In *Thoma's Oral Pathology,* 6th Ed., edited by R. J. Gorlin and H. M. Goldman. St. Louis, C. V. Mosby Co., 1970, Vol. II, pp. 824, 826.
2. Shafer, W. G., Hine, M. K. and Levy, B. M.: *A Textbook of Oral Pathology,* 4th Ed. Philadelphia, W. B. Saunders Co., 1983, p. 115.
3. Slaughter, D. P., et al.: "Field cancerization" in oral stratified squamous epithelium; clinical implications of multicentric origin. Cancer 6:963, 1953.
4. Meyer, I. and Shklar, G.: Multiple malignant tumors involving the oral mucosa and the gastrointestinal tract. Oral Surg. *13*:295, 1960.
5. Moertel, C. G., et al.: Multiple primary malignant neoplasms III. Tumors of multicentric origin. Cancer *14*:238, 1961.

PETECHIAE

Suction Petechiae

Age No predilection
Sex No predilection

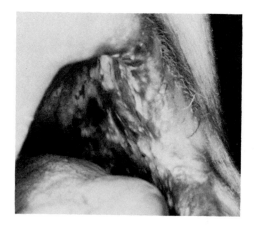

FIG. 3–19. Hyperkeratotic white lesions admixed with red zones (the darkened regions in this clinical photograph) representative of widespread carcinoma in situ.

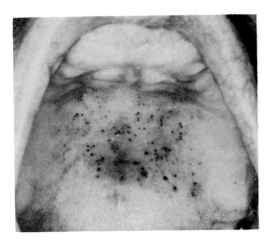

FIG. 3–20.   Petechial hemorrhages evolving as the result of negative pressure on the oral tissues. This patient wore a maxillary denture with a relief area corresponding to the region occupied by petechiae.

Clinical Features: Petechiae are characterized by pinpoint-sized red spots 1 to 3 mm in diameter, are multifocal, and may show confluency. Suction petechiae are located either beneath a denture with a relief zone or on the soft palate in patients complaining of pruritus in that region. They may begin as a prodromal sign for sore throat, influenza, or the common cold. Onset of "itchiness" in the soft palate may induce the patient to suck or click the area for relief, with resultant microvascular rupture. Soft palate petechiae are also the result of orogenital sexual activity.

Microscopic Features: Damaged vascular walls of small vessels in the submucosa manifest a juxtaposed zone of erythrocyte extravasation.

Differential Diagnosis: Infectious mononucleosis may be present with palatal petechiae, yet other clinical and laboratory features provide data that will eliminate consideration in the differential diagnosis. If the patient does not recall clicking his or her soft palate and if other mucocutaneous petechiae are observed, thrombocyte deficiencies or leukemia should be ruled out by instituting appropriate laboratory studies. Hereditary hemorrhagic telangiectasia shows other characteristics essential for the diagnosis. Scurvy may include petechiae as a component of vitamin C deficiency, but this disease is encountered with extreme rarity in this day and age.

Treatment: No treatment is necessary for non-denture-related suction petechiae. Those lesions related to a denture relief zone will resolve following relining or rebasing the prosthesis.

References

1. Giansanti, J. S., Cramer, J. R., and Weathers, D. R.: Palatal erythema: Another etiologic factor. Oral Surg. 40:379, 1975.
2. Schlesinger, S. L., Borbotsina, J., and O'Neill, L.: Petechial hemorrhages of the soft palate secondary to fellatio. Oral Surg. 40:376, 1975.
3. Damm, D. D., White, D. K., and Brinker, C. M.: Variations of palatal erythema secondary to fellatio. Oral Surg. 52:417, 1981.

Infectious Mononucleosis

Age: Young adults
Sex: No predilection

Clinical Features: Palatal petechiae are commonly seen in infectious mononucleosis, located on the soft palate. The petechiae are probably engendered by suction on a pruritic soft palate by the tongue as outlined for suction petechiae; however, other hemorrhagic manifestations such as epistaxis have been reported. A generalized stomatitis with erythema and ulceration may also be evident. Other clinical features implicating onset of infectious mononucleosis, a herpes virus infection (Epstein-Barr virus), include extreme malaise with lethargy, lymphadenopathy, hepatosplenomegaly, sore throat, and fever.

Microscopic Features: Damaged vascular walls of small vessels in the submucosa manifest a juxtaposed zone of erythrocyte extravasation.

Differential Diagnosis: Palatal petechiae are seen in sore throat independent from infectious mononucleosis, in platelet disorders, and in hereditary hemorrhagic telangiectasia. The diagnosis

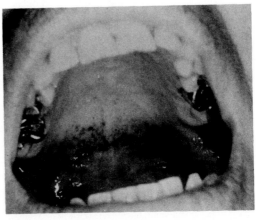

FIG. 3–21.   Soft-palate petechiae in infectious mononucleosis.

of infectious mononucleosis may be confirmed when the heterophil antibody titer exceeds 1:28. The monospot screening serologic test, while not as accurate as the heterophil antibody titration, is rapidly performed and is usually adequate diagnostically. The appearance of atypical lymphocytes (Downey cells) on the differential blood count is also a diagnostic finding.

Treatment: Treatment for infectious mononucleosis is supportive, with bed rest and high liquid intake. A mild analgesic and antipyretic are recommended.

References

1. Shafer, W. G., Hine, M. K., and Levy, B. M.: *A Textbook of Oral Pathology,* 4th Ed. Philadelphia, W. B. Saunders Co., 1983, pp. 736–740.

2. Dunnett, W. N.: Infectious mononucleosis. Br. Med. J. *1:*1187, 1963.

3. Holzel, A.: An early clinical sign of infectious mononucleosis. Oral Surg. *12:*685, 1959.

4. Shiver, C. B., Berg, P., and Frenkel, E. P.: Palatine petechiae: An early sign in infectious mononucleosis. J. Am. Med. Assoc. *161:*592, 1956.

5. Cassingham, R. J.: Infectious mononucleosis: A review of the literature, including recent findings on etiology. Oral Surg. *31:*610, 1971.

Thrombocyte Disorders

Age: Children and young adults
Sex: No predilection

Clinical Features: Petechiae due to platelet deficiency or malfunction may be present on oral mucosa, yet lesions will be encountered on skin surfaces as well. Various diseases may inhibit platelet formation. Myelophthisic anemia with thrombocytopenia can occur with leukemia, lymphoma, metastatic carcinoma to bone, and marble bone disease. Primary thrombocytopenic purpura, pancytopenia, and bone marrow depression from cytotoxic drugs result in lack of platelets. Malfunctioning platelets may be responsible for petechial hemorrhages in thrombocytopathic purpura, thrombasthenia or secondary to overuse of salicylates. In addition to these bleeding disorders, a variety of nonthrombocytopenic purpuras exist, including anaphylactoid purpura, snake venom purpura, and certain infectious diseases. In all thrombocyte disorders, petechiae may be accompanied by gingival hemorrhage or prolonged bleeding after extraction.

Microscopic Features: Damaged vascular walls of small vessels in the submucosa manifest a juxtaposed zone of erythrocyte extravasation.

Differential Diagnosis: Thrombocyte disorders may be differentiated clinically from other petechial-producing diseases in that the lesions are not confined to the palate, yet may be ubiquitous with lesions on the skin of the extremities and trunk. The tourinquet test is positive. A workup for the underlying cause includes complete blood count and platelet count and other clinical and laboratory tests specific for the diseases enumerated under clinical features. A history of drug use is of utmost significance when considering causes of petechiae. Because evaluation of disease entities producing petechiae involves manifold considerations and complex relationships, the patient should be referred to a hematologist for definitive diagnosis and treatment.

Treatment: Management of platelet disorders is governed by the underlying cause. Definitive diagnosis and treatment should be determined by a physician.

References

1. Williamson, J. J.: In *Thoma's Oral Pathology,* 6th Ed. edited by R. J. Gorlin and H. M. Goldman. St. Louis, C. V. Mosby Co., 1970, Vol. II, pp. 925–927.

2. Wintrobe, M. M.: *Clinical Hematology,* 7th Ed. Philadelphia, Lea & Febiger, 1974.

3. Linenberg, W. B.: Idiopathic thrombocytopenic purpura. Oral Surg. *17:*22, 1964.

4. Lynch, M. A. and Ship, I. I.: Oral manifestations of leukemia; a post-diagnostic study. J. Am. Dent. Assoc. *75:*1139, 1967.

5. Stafford, R., Sonis, S., Lockhart, P., and Sonis, A.: Oral pathoses as diagnostic indicators in leukemia. Oral Surg. *50:*134, 1980.

Hereditary Hemorrhagic Telangiectasia

Age: Begins in infancy
Sex: No predilection

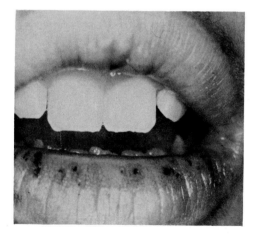

FIG. 3–22. Petechial hemorrhages in a leukemic patient with secondary thrombocytopenia. (Courtesy of Dr. A. Leider.)

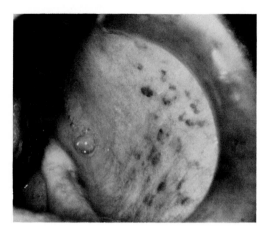

FIG. 3–23. Red papules in hereditary hemorrhagic telangiectasia. (Courtesy of Dr. A. Leider.)

Clinical Features: Hereditary hemorrhagic telangiectasia is inherited as a dominant trait and is characterized by the appearance of spider telangiectasias of skin, primarily on the face and neck with petechia-like lesions of the oral mucosa. Epistaxis is a prominent clinical sign. Bleeding from the gingiva is also a feature. Platelet and clotting factor functions are normal. Perivascular supportive tissue appears to be defective.

Microscopic Features: Submucosal dilated vessels are present and evince leakage of the vascular contents with fibrin deposition in the perivascular region.

Differential Diagnosis: The resemblance to petechial disease is striking; however, close scrutiny of the skin lesions discloses the spider-like angiomas rather than true petechial macules, and a hereditary history will generally lead to a diagnosis of hereditary hemorrhagic telangiectasia. Bleeding and clotting times are normal. Platelets and clotting factors are within normal limits unless profuse hemorrhage has resulted in a blood-loss anemia with thrombocytopenia.

Treatment: Genetic counselling is recommended. A normal life span can be expected; however, death from epistaxis may occur. Hemorrhage can generally be controlled by placement of pressure packs.

References
1. Shafer, W. G., Hine, M. K., and Levy, B. M.: A Textbook of Oral Pathology, 4th Ed. Philadelphia, W. B. Saunders Co., 1983, p. 157.
2. Scopp, I. W. and Quart, A.: Hereditary hemorrhagic telangiectasia involving the oral cavity. Oral Surg. 11:1138, 1958.
3. Gorlin, R. J. and Pindborg, J. J.: Syndromes of the Head and Neck. New York, Blakiston Division, McGraw-hill Book Co., 1964.
4. Everett, F. G. and Hahn, C. R.: Hereditary hemorrhagic telangiectasia with gingival lesions: Review and case reports. J. Periodontol. 47:295, 1976.
5. Austin, G. B., Quart, A. M., and Novak, B.: Hereditary hemorrhagic telangiectasias with oral manifestations: Report of periodontal treatment in two cases. Oral Surg. 51:245, 1981.

FOCAL PIGMENTATIONS

Amalgam and Graphite Tattoo

Age: No predilection
Sex: No predilection

Clinical Features: Tattoos caused either by traumatic implantation of dental amalgam or by graphite from a lead pencil will produce a grey to black pigment in the mucosa. The borders are generally somewhat diffuse, and the pigment will not blanch on pressure. Amalgam tattoos are usually located on the gingiva, alveolar ridge, or buccal mucosa, whereas graphite tattoos are more often seen on the palate where a pencil wound was self-inflicted. Large amalgam tattoos can be demonstrated radiographically. Amalgam tattoos are usually solitary but occasionally may be multiple.

Microscopic Features: Brown or black foreign material is present yet fails to elicit a giant cell response. Stippling of collagen, reticulin, and perivascular connective tissues with particulate granules is a prominent feature, and inflammatory cells are present in limited number.

Differential Diagnosis: Amalgam tattoos must be differentiated from nevi and superficial mela-

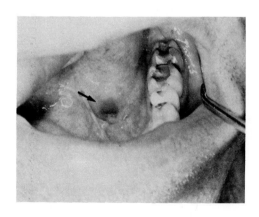

FIG. 3–24. Dark area in floor of mouth representing an amalgam tattoo.

noma. Pressure without blanching will differentiate amalgam tattoos from vascular lesions.

Treatment: Failure to demonstrate radiopaque particles on roentgenogram for suspected amalgam tattoo necessitates biopsy to rule out nevus or melanoma. No treatment is necessary for those lesions that are radiographically demonstrable.

References

1. Orban, B.: Discoloration of the oral mucous membrane by metallic foreign bodies. J. Periodontol. 17:55, 1946.
2. Weathers, D. R. and Fine, R. M.: Amalgam tattoo of oral mucosa. Arch. Dermatol. 110:727, 1974.
3. Buchner, A. and Hansen, L. S.: Amalgam pigmentation (amalgam tattoo) of the oral mucosa. A clinicopathologic study of 268 cases. Oral Surg. 49:139, 1980.
4. Harrison, J., Rowley, P., and Peters, P.: Amalgam tattoos. Light and electron microscopy and electron-probe micro-analysis. J. Pathol. 121:83, 1977.

Mucocele

Age: No predilection
Sex: No predilection

Clinical Features: Mucoceles may appear as focal reddish-blue elevations if hemorrhage has occurred. As with the conventionally appearing fluid-filled mucous retention phenomena, hemorrhagic mucoceles follow trauma with rupture or severance of a minor salivary duct with pooling of mucus within the submucosa; they are most frequently encountered on the lips, buccal mucosa, and ventral tongue.

Microscopic Features: The epithelium is distended by an underlying zone of pooled mucin encompassed by a granulation tissue pseudocystic membrane. Extravasated erythrocytes and fibrin are admixed with mucin and inflammatory cells.

Differential Diagnosis: Hemorrhagic muco-celes may be indistinguishable clinically from hemangioma, varix, hematoma, nevus, or even melanoma. A history of antecedent trauma can usually be elicited.

Treatment: Local excision with extirpation of the underlying minor salivary lobules is recommended. Failure to remove the glandular tissue may contribute to recurrence.

References

1. Robinson, L. and Hjorting-Hansen, E.: Pathologic changes associated with mucous retention cysts of minor salivary glands. Oral Surg. 18:191, 1964.
2. Cataldo, E. and Mosadomi, A.: Mucoceles of the oral mucous membrane. Arch. Otolaryngol. 91:360, 1970.
3. Harrison J. D.: Salivary mucoceles. Oral Surg. 39:268, 1975.

Hematoma

Age: No predilection
Sex: No predilection

Clinical Features: Mucosal hematomas or bruises result from vascular severance due to trauma. They are brown or blue in color and may be macular or swollen. Since the blood is not intraluminal but extravasated, hematomas will not blanch on pressure.

Microscopic Features: The submucosa evinces profuse erythrocyte extravasation with fibrin deposition. Variable degrees of fibrovascular organization with inflammation are present.

Differential Diagnosis: Hematomas are the result of trauma yet may be confused clinically with hemorrhagic mucocele, tattoo, hemangioma or varix, nevus, and melanoma. Ecchymosis is identical, yet in blood dyscrasias trauma is minor and the lesions are usually multifocal.

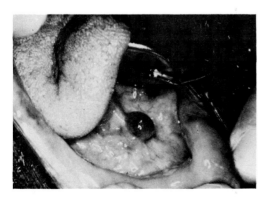

FIG. 3–25. Mucocele containing extravasated blood and appearing as a brown pigmented cystic nodule.

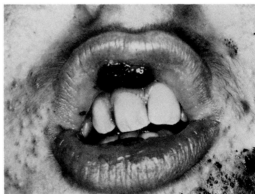

FIG. 3–26. Hematoma of the upper lip. (Courtesy of Dr. Sheldon Rovin.)

Treatment: A suspected hematoma should be observed over a 2-week period. Failure to resolve indicates the clinical impression was incorrect and biopsy should be performed. Any hematoma observed without significant provocation or trauma should arouse suspicion of purpura secondary to a blood dyscrasia.

References

1. Mitchell, D. F., Standish, S. M., and Fast, T. B.: *Oral Diagnosis/Oral Medicine*, 3rd Ed. Philadelphia, Lea & Febiger, 1978, p. 407.
2. Archer, W. H.: *Oral and Maxillofacial Surgery*, 5th Ed. Philadelphia, W. B. Saunders Co., 1975, pp. 1554–1556.

Hemangioma and Varix

Age: No predilection
Sex: Female predilection

Clinical Features: Hemangiomas begin in childhood, while focal venous dilations (varices) are found in adults and the aged. Trauma may play a role in the induction of a varix. Both lesions are frequently seen on the lips and buccal mucosa, where they appear as tumefactions with blue pigmentation. Digital pressure will produce blanching, provided a thrombus is not present within the vascular lumen.

Microscopic Features: Both hemangiomas and focal varices show large dilated erythrocyte-engorged blood channels. Thrombus formation is not uncommon.

Differential Diagnosis: Differentiation from other focal pigmentations such as tattoos, nevi, melanoma, and hematoma may be accomplished provided that blanching can be induced, as only vascular lesions behave in this manner.

Treatment: Treatment of choice is excisional biopsy; excessive hemorrhage from lesions less than 2 cm is generally not encountered. Large hemangiomas may be reduced with sclerosing solutions or cryosurgery. Radiation is contraindicated, as the risk for development of sarcoma in adjacent exposed bone is a distinct possibility.

References

1. Shklar, G. and Meyer, I.: Vascular tumors of the mouth and jaws. Oral Surg. *19*:335, 1965.
2. Weathers, D. R. and Fine, R. M.: Thrombosed varix of the oral cavity. Arch. Dermatol. *104*:427, 1971.
3. Minkow, B., Laufer, D. and Gutman, D.: Treatment of oral hemangiomas with local sclerosing agents. Int. J. Oral Surg. *8*:18, 1979.

Nevus

Age: No predilection
Sex: Female predilection

Clinical Features: Oral nevi are rare and are characterized by a plaque- or dome-shaped sessile nodule with blue or black pigmentation. Occasionally nonpigmented forms occur intraorally. They may be seen at any age, but are likely to have been present since childhood. Pigmented nevi do not blanch on pressure and are most frequently encountered on the palate, gingiva, buccal mucosa, and lips. They generally reach a given size and the growth becomes static. Various types exist, including junctional, compound, intramucosal, blue nevus, and spindle cell nevus.

Microscopic Features: The histology of nevi is variable. Nevocellular nevi are composed of oval epithelioid cells arranged in clumps or theques, junctional nevi maintain continuity with the epithelium, whereas intramucosal types are confined to the underlying connective tissue. Spindle cell nevi contain elongated spindle cells with a junctional (intraepithelial) component. Melanocytic or blue nevi are confined to the submucosa and are composed of fibroblast-like spindle cells with fas-

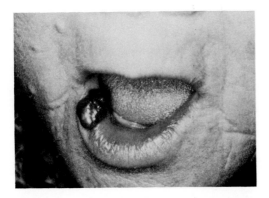

FIG. 3–27. A varix appearing as a reddish-brown tumefaction.

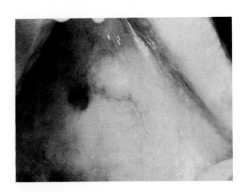

FIG. 3–28. Pigmented nevi appear brown, black, or blue and may be papular or macular.

ciculation. Melanin granules may be seen in all forms and may be sparse or pervasive.

Differential Diagnosis: Nevi do not blanch under pressure and may clinically be indistinguishable from a tattoo, hematoma, or superficial melanoma. An ephelis is flat, lacking any tumefaction, yet is often indistiguishable clinically from junctional nevi and tattoos

Treatment: Junctional nevi in adults may evolve into malignant melanoma. For this reason, all pigmented lesions in the mouth in which nevus is a consideration in the differential diagnosis should be excised and submitted for microscopic examination.

References

1. Weathers, D. R.: Benign nevi of the oral mucosa. Arch. Dermatol. *99*:688, 1969.
2. Trodahl, J. N. and Sprague, W. G.: Benign and malignant melanocytic lesions of the oral mucosa: An analysis of 135 cases. Cancer *25*:812, 1970.
3. Giansanti, J. S., Drummond, J. F., and Sabes, W. R.: Intraoral melanocytic cellular nevi. Oral Surg. *44*:267, 1977.
4. Bhaskar, S. N. and Jacoway, J. R.: Blue nevus of the oral mucosa. Oral Surg. *19*:678, 1965.
5. Buchner, A. and Hansen, L. S.: Pigmented nevi of the oral mucosa: a clinicopathologic study of 32 new cases and review of 75 cases from the literature. Oral Surg. *48*:131, 1979.

Ephelis, Oral Melanotic Macule

Age: No predilection

Sex: Female predilection

Clinical Features: Ephelis, or freckle, occurs on sun-exposed skin and is common on the face, yet unusual on the vermilion border. The lesion is brown or brownish-black and macular; in most cases it is less than half of 1 cm. The melanotic macule occurs on oral mucosa and therefore is not related to actinic radiation. Oral melanotic macules are focal brown, blue, or black spots that are most frequently observed on the gingiva and buccal mucosa.

Microscopic Features: Melanotic macules do not evolve from proliferation of melanocytes; rather, the epithelium is unremarkable, and the basal cells exhibit diffuse deposition of melanin pigment. Occasionally, melanin incontinence is observed with pigment granules identifiable in subepithelial melanophages.

Differential Diagnosis: The focal macular appearance of ephelis of the lip or melanotic macule of oral mucosa may be identical to amalgam tattoo, junctional nevus, or early superficial spreading melanoma. Pigmented lesions of this nature

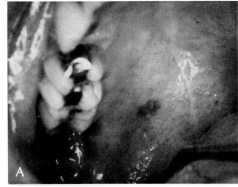

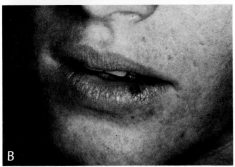

FIG. 3–29. A. Oral melanotic macule. B. Ephelis of the lower lip.

cannot be diagnosed without microscopic evaluation.

Treatment: Excision is the treatment of choice.

References

1. Shapiro, L. and Zegarelli, D. J.: The solitary labial lentigo; a clinicopathologic study of 20 cases. Oral Surg. *31*:87, 1971.
2. Weathers, D. R., Corio, R. L., Crawford, B. E., Giansanti, J. S., and Page, L. R.: The labial melanotic macule. Oral Surg. *42*:196, 1976.
3. Page, L. R., Corio, R. L., Crawford, B. E., Giansanti, J. S., and Weathers, D. R.: The oral melanotic macule. Oral Surg. *44*:219, 1977.
4. Buchner, A. and Hansen, L. S.: Melanotic macule of the oral mucosa; A clinicopathologic study of 105 cases. Oral Surg. *48*:244, 1979.

DIFFUSE AND MULTIFOCAL PIGMENTATIONS

Malignant Melanoma

Age: Middle age and above

Sex: Male predilection

Clinical Features: Oral melanomas exhibit a striking predilection for the palatal mucosa, chiefly anterior palate and maxillary alveolar ridge or gingiva. Most are markedly pigmented, being either

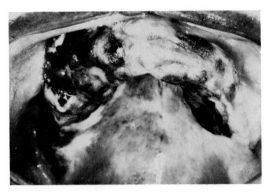

FIG. 3–30. Malignant melanoma of the oral cavity, usually seen on the anterior maxillary or palatal mucosa. It begins as a brown-black or blue pigmentation with irregular borders and becomes progressively more diffuse. (Courtesy of Drs. L. Hansen and P. Merrill.)

bluish-black or dark brown. They begin as macular focal lesions but may rapidly grow to fungating diffuse tumefactions. Ulceration is a common finding. As proliferation ensues, satellite lesions or streaking of pigment can be noted at the lateral margins. The tumor may or may not be indurated. Survival rates for oral and cutaneous melanomas are extremely low; less than 5 percent live for five years. Widespread dissemination to both nodes and distant sites is common. A superficial form known as malignant freckle of Hutchinson has a more favorable prognosis; while usually located on facial skin, oral cases have been reported. Malignant freckle is macular with minimal tumefaction. Nonpigmented varieties of melanoma occur and may be confused clinically with inflammatory and other neoplastic swellings.

Microscopic Features: Three specific microscopic patterns are observed in melanoma. The Hutchinson's freckle variety is a slowly growing lesion usually seen on the malar skin and is characterized by proliferation of pleomorphic, palisaded melanocytes distributed along the epidermal/dermal junction with a horizontal or lateral direction of proliferation. These atypical cells fail to invade the upper epithelial layers. The second variety also proliferates along the epidermal/dermal junction and is termed superficial spreading type. This type exhibits a pagetoid appearance with ovoid tumor cell nests showing a propensity for invasion of the upper epithelial layers. The third variety is invasive melanoma. This form may arise de novo or evolve from either of the aforementioned lesions. The invasive type is usually nodular and exhibits a vertical growth pattern

which invades the underlying connective tissues. The cells are spindle, ovoid, or polygonal and are pleomorphic with variable amounts of melanin pigment. Invasive melanomas are graded 1 to 5, depending upon their depth of growth: Grade 1 is confined to epithelium, grade 2 invades papillary dermis, grade 3 invades to the level of reticular dermis, grade 4 invades the reticular dermis, and grade 5 extends into the subcutaneous fat.

Differential Diagnosis: Early oral melanoma may be confused with other focal pigmentations. As melanin will not blanch, differentiation from a vascular lesion can be made clinically. Since melanoma must be detected at its earliest stage to achieve cure, it is recommended that biopsies be performed with all oral focal pigmentations.

Treatment: Radical surgery is indicated and should be managed by a cancer surgeon. Prophylactic neck dissection in the absence of clinically palpable nodes probably does not improve the prognosis.

References

1. Chaudhry, A. P., et al.: Primary malignant melanoma of the oral cavity; a review of 105 cases. Cancer 11:923, 1958.
2. Trodahl, J. N. and Sprague, W. G.: Benign and malignant melanotic lesions of the oral mucosa; an analysis of 135 cases. Cancer 25:812, 1970.
3. Eneroth, C. M.: Malignant melanoma of the oral cavity. Int. J. Oral Surg. 4:191, 1975.
4. Jackson, D. and Simpson, H. E.: Primary malignant melanoma of the oral cavity. Oral Surg. 39:553, 1975.
5. Regezi, J. A., Hayward, J. R., and Pickens, T. N.: Superficial melanomas of oral mucous membranes. Oral Surg. 45:730, 1978.

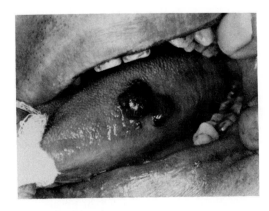

FIG. 3–31. Pigmented vascular lesions in Kaposi's sarcoma.

Kaposi's Sarcoma

Age: Young and elderly adults
Sex: Male predilection
Clinical Features: Kaposi's sarcoma is a rare type of angiosarcoma that is usually mucocutaneous in presentation and yet may also involve lymph nodes, particularly among Africans. Until recently, the disease was encountered primarily on skin of the lower extremities and in the oral cavity of elderly males. Within the past few years, numerous cases have been reported to occur in young homosexual males as a component of acquired immunodeficiency syndrome. In this syndrome, which occurs predominantly in promiscuous gay males with a drug abuse history, one encounters infectious diseases including herpes simplex, candidiasis and/or a parasitic pulmonary infection by Pneumocystis carinii, elevated antibody titers to cytomegalovirus, immunodeficiency, and appearance of otherwise rare neoplastic diseases, primarily Kaposi's sarcoma. The lesions appear blue or dark brown and are usually raised and plaque-like or appear as blebs. In most instances, multiple oral lesions are observed. Cutaneous lesions of a similar nature may be observed on the lower extremities. The disease is probably caused by T–cell leukemia virus type III.
Microscopic Features: The early stages of the disease are characterized by endothelial enlargement such that the vessel linings exhibit a hobnail appearance. The proliferative phase is represented by multinodular foci of spindle-shaped endothelial cells with a fasciculated pattern oriented about slit-like vascular spaces. Pleomorphism is observed, and hemosiderin pigment deposition is a prominent feature.
Differential Diagnosis: The clinical findings are rather unique; however, one must consider multiple foci of ecchymosis and multiple hemangiomas in the differential diagnosis. A biopsy will disclose the pathognomonic microscopic features.
Treatment: Patients suffering from the acquired immunodeficiency syndrome show an extremely poor prognosis, with most instances being fatal. Oral lesions may be excised. Referral to a physician for overall management is recommended.
References
1. Braner, M. K., Gates, P. E., and Doyle, J. L.: Visceral Kaposi's sarcoma presenting with gingival lesions. Oral Surg. 50:151, 1980.
2. Alper, R. A. and Wiggins, H. E.: Hemorrhagic palatal lesion. J. Oral Pathol. 4:222, 1975.
3. Dterak, D.: Opportunistic infections and Kaposi's sarcoma in homosexual men. N. Eng. J. Med. 305:1465, 1981.
4. Eversole, L. R., Leider, A. S., Jacobsen, P. L., and Shaber, E. P.: Oral Kaposi's sarcoma associated with acquired immunodeficiency syndrome among homosexual males. J.A.D.A. 107:248, 1983.

Racial Pigmentation

Age: Present at birth
Sex: No predilection
Clinical Features: The oral mucosa of Negroes and many dark-skinned Caucasians is often stippled with multifocal and diffuse macular pigmentations generally dark brown in color. These zones may occur anywhere in the mouth and are more often encountered on the gingiva. They are innocuous manifestations of racial or ethnic origin and have no premalignant potential.
Microscopic Features: Melanin granules are densely accumulated in the basal cell layer.
Differential Diagnosis: When the patient's skin is heavily pigmented, oral pigmentation can be considered normal. In Caucasians, other diseases must be considered, e.g., Addison's disease, neurofibromatosis, or heavy metal ingestion.
Treatment: No treatment is necessary.
References
1. Mescon, H., Grots, I. A., and Gorlin, R. J.: In *Thoma's Oral Pathology*, 6th Ed., edited by R. J. Gorlin and H. M. Goldman. St. Louis, C. V. Mosby Co., 1970, Vol. II, p. 672.
2. Mitchell, D. F., Standish, S. M., and Fast, T. B.: *Oral Diagnosis/Oral Medicine*, 3rd Ed. Philadelphia, Lea & Febiger, 1978, p. 382.
3. Dummett, C. O.: Physiologic pigmentation of the oral and cutaneous tissues in the Negro. J. Dent. Res. 25:421, 1946.
4. Dummett, C. O.: Oral pigmentation—physiologic and pathologic. N. Y. State Dent. J. 25:407, 1959.

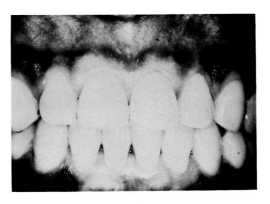

FIG. 3–32. Racial melanosis. Can be seen anywhere in the mouth but is more commonly identified on the gingiva of Negroes or dark-skinned Caucasians.

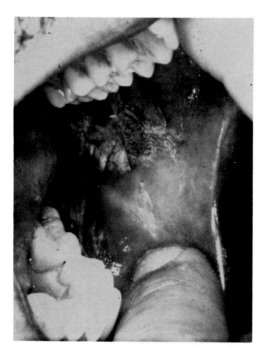

FIG. 3–33.   Gray melanin deposition associated with white stria in pigmented lichen planus.

Pigmented Lichen Planus

Age: Adults
Sex: Females more often affected

Clinical Features: Whereas lichen planus is usually characterized by either white striated lesions or mixed red and white lesions in the erosive form, a pigmented variety is occasionally encountered. The pigmented zones are macular with a black, brown, or slate-gray appearance and are most prevalent on the buccal mucosa. Invariably, the pigmented mucosa is surrounded by a zone of white, and reticulated striae can be discerned.

Microscopic Features: The surface keratin is thickened, and transmigration of lymphocytes into the basilar and parabasilar zones occurs. The basal cell layer contains melanin granules, and this layer is disrupted with melanin incontinence. The submucosa is occupied by a band-like lymphocytic infiltrate with interposed free melanin granules and melanophages.

Differential Diagnosis: The pigmented zones of this form of lichen planus may be confused with other diffuse pigmented lesions included here; however, one is usually able to detect the presence of accompanying white striae. A biopsy will confirm the diagnosis.

Treatment: Provided an erosive component is lacking, no treatment is necessary.

Reference

1. Murti, P. R., Bhousle, R.B., Daftary, D. K., and Mehta, F. S.: Oral lichen planus associated with pigmentation. J. Oral Med. *34*:23, 1979.

Peutz-Jeghers Syndrome

Age: Childhood onset
Sex: No predilection

Clinical Features: Peutz-Jeghers syndrome is inherited as an autosomal dominant trait and is characterized by multifocal macular melanin pigmentation in perioral locations. These macules or freckles stipple the vermilion and may extend into the facial skin as well as the oral mucosa. Intestinal polyposis with no tendency for malignant change may contribute to colic pain in affected individuals. In addition to perioral lesions, the extremities may show dermal foci of pigmentation.

Microscopic Features: The basal cell layer contains a profusion of melanin granules.

Differential Diagnosis: The perioral location is unique and diagnostic. Intestinal radiographic studies will disclose the presence of polyps located primarily in the small intestine.

Treatment: Provided an erosive component is lacking, no treatment is necessary. Patients can be

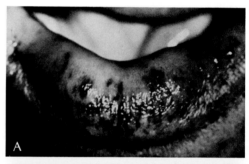

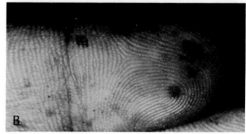

FIG. 3–34.   Peutz-Jeghers syndrome. *A:* Melanotic macules of the lips. *B.* Melanotic macules of the fingers. (Courtesy of Dr. T. K. O'Brien.)

advised of the genetic character of the disease. Referral to a gastroenterologist is recommended.

References

1. Bartholomew, L. G., et al.: Intestinal polyposis associated with mucocutaneous pigmentation. Surg. Gynecol. Obstet. *115*:1, 1962.
2. Dummett, C. O. and Barens, G.: Oromucosal pigmentation: an updated literary review. J. Periodontol. *42*:726, 1971.
3. Wesley, R. K., Delaney, J.R., and Pensler, L.: Mucocutaneous melanosis and gastrointestinal polyposis (Peutz-Jeghers syndrome): clinical considerations and report of case. J. Dent. Child. *44*:131, 1977.
4. Jeghers, H., McKusick, V. A., and Katz, K. H.: Generalized intestinal polyposis and melanin spots of the oral mucosa, lips and digits. N. Engl. J. Med. *241*:993, 1031, 1949.

Multiple Neurofibromatosis

Age: Childhood onset

Sex: No predilection

Clinical Features: An inheritable disease characterized by multiple neurofibromatous nodules, von Recklinghausen's disease of skin also manifests pigmented macules of skin termed *cafe-au-lait spots*. The pigment is light brown and the macules vary considerably in size, displaying smooth demarcated borders. The neurofibromas exist in two forms: nodular, with a putty-like feel on palpation, or flabby pendulous folds. The neurofi-

bromas and macular pigmentations may involve the oral mucous membranes as well as the skin.

Microscopic Features: Cafe-au-lait pigmentation is represented by diffuse deposition of melanin granules within the basal cell layer.

Differential Diagnosis: Oral pigmentations of neurofibromatosis are similar to those of Peutz-Jeghers syndrome, racial pigmentation, and Addison's disease. The accompanying neurofibromatous tumefactions on skin differentiate von Recklinghausen's disease from the aforementioned entities.

Treatment: When function is compromised the neurofibromas can be excised. The pigmented areas have no malignant potential; however, sarcomatous change in preexisting benign neurofibromas of von Recklinghausen's disease has been reported to occur in as many as 5 percent of the population with the disease.

References

1. Shafer, W. G., Hine, M. K., and Levy, B. M.: *A Textbook of Oral Pathology*, 4th Ed. Philadelphia, W. B. Saunders Co., 1983, pp. 206–208.
2. Kragh, L. V., et al.: Neurofibromatosis (von Recklinghausen's disease) of the head and neck; cosmetic and reconstructive aspects. Plast. Reconstr. Surg. *25*:565, 1960.
3. O'Driscoll, P. M.: The oral manifestations of multiple neurofibromatosis. Br. J. Oral Surg. *3*:22, 1965.
4. Crowe, R. W. and Schull, W. J.: Diagnostic importance of café-au-lait spots in neurofibromatosis. Arch. Intern. Med. *91*:758, 1953.

Addison's Disease

Age: Middle-aged adults

Sex: Slight female predilection

Clinical Features: Addison's disease is caused

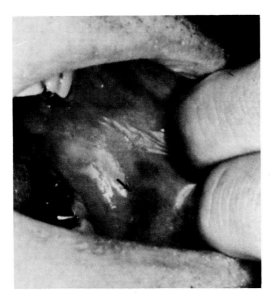

FIG. 3–35. Cafe-au-lait pigmentations of buccal mucosa in neurofibromatosis.

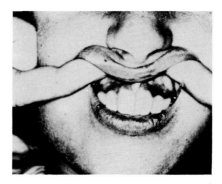

FIG. 3–36. Progressive diffuse pigmentation of the mucosa in regions previously devoid of such change is suggestive of Addison's disease. (Courtesy of Dr. Sheldon Rovin.)

by adrenal cortical insufficiency of idiopathic origin or by cortical replacement as seen in granulomatous infection by tuberculosis or the deep mycoses. Decreased steroid levels stimulate pituitary ACTH output with increased levels of a melanocyte-stimulating factor. The skin becomes bronzed or shows brown pigmentation in skin folds or over joints. Oral pigmentation is multifocal or diffuse and macular. Other symptoms of the disease include weakness, hypotension, and cold intolerance. Anorexia, vomiting, and diarrhea are also commonly encountered symptoms. Cushing's syndrome associated with pituitary hyperfunction may also be associated with pigmentation on mucocutaneous surfaces.

Microscopic Features: Pigmentation in Addison's disease is a manifestation of increased melanin production represented by diffuse melanin granule deposition in the basal cell layer.

Differential Diagnosis: Addisonian pigmentation in the mouth simulates that of racial pigmentation, Peutz-Jeghers disease, and von Recklinghausen's disease. The skin coloration particularly in pressure areas, lack of lesions seen in other diseases with oral pigmentations, history of recent onset with progressive deepening of the pigment, and the other clinical manifestations require workup for adrenal cortical insufficiency.

Treatment: Addison's disease is managed by the physician. Any underlying cause must be treated, and maintenance levels of steroid therapy are required.

References

1. Wilkins, L.: *The Diagnosis and Treatment of Endocrine Disorders of Childhood and Adolescence,* 3rd Ed. Springfield, Charles C Thomas, 1965, pp. 342–423.
2. Wood, N. K. and Goaz, P. W.: *Differential Diagnosis of Oral Lesions,* 2nd Ed. St. Louis, C. V. Mosby Co., 1980, pp. 201–202.

Hemochromatosis

Age: Adults
Sex: Male predilection

Clinical Features: Characterized by excessive deposition of iron pigment within tissues, hemochromatosis represents a primary heritable disease with a pronounced male predilection or evolves as a secondary aquired defect accompanying cirrhosis, chronic anemia, porphyria, excessive dietary iron intake, or a postcaval shunt for portal hypertension. Classic clinical signs include hepatomegaly, diabetes, and bronze skin. Pigmentation of the palate and, less frequently, the gingiva

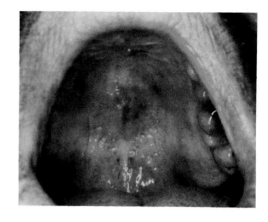

FIG. 3–37.   Palatal blood pigment deposition in hemochromatosis.

is encountered. The pigmentation is slate-gray to brown with diffuse macular appearance. Oral and skin pigmentations are attributable to iron deposition as well as melanosis, probably secondary to adrenal cortical insufficiency due to pathologic deposition of iron in the adrenal cortex with subsequent elevations in melanogenic ACTH secretion.

Microscopic Features: A biopsy of oral mucosa may disclose basilar melanosis with deposition of brown granular hemosiderin or ferritin pigment within connective tissue and underlying salivary acini. A Prussian blue iron stain is especially useful for demonstrating the nature of the pigment. An inflammatory reaction is usually not present.

Differential Diagnosis: The macular diffuse slate-gray pigmentation observed in hemochromatosis may resemble early laterally spreading melanoma, diffuse tattoo, Addisonian pigmentation, and heavy metal ingestion. A history or documentation of cirrhosis with concomitant diabetes and bronzing of the skin should arouse suspicion of hemochromatosis. A biopsy with demonstration of diffuse iron deposition, in conjunction with the clinical findings, along with elevated serum iron will allow for a definitive diagnosis.

Treatment: Hemochromatosis is a metabolic medical problem with many causes and should be managed by a physician.

References

1. Powell, L. W.: Changing concepts in haemochromatosis. Postgrad. Med. J. 46:200, 1970.
2. Frantzis, T. G., Sheridan, P. J., Reeve, C. M., and Young, L. L.: Oral manifestations of hemochromatosis. Report of a case. Oral Surg. 33:186, 1972.

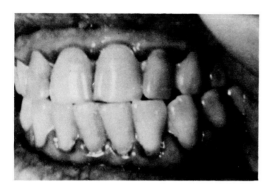

FIG. 3–38. Heavy metal deposits in the marginal gingiva. (Courtesy of Dr. J. Hasler.)

Heavy Metal Ingestion

Age: Adults

Sex: No predilection

Clinical Features: Various heavy metals including lead, mercury, and bismuth may be ingested for medicinal reasons or as an occupational hazard. (Bismuth, lead, and mercury are the more common metals causing oral pigmentation.) The metal becomes deposited diffusely along the free gingival margin that scallops around the cervix of the teeth. The metallic line is gray. Occasionally, other mucosal sites show macular pigmentation. Systemic symptoms are often encountered, particularly in lead poisoning. These include abdominal pain, vomiting, anorexia, tremor, headaches, and mania.

Microscopic Features: Metallic crystals are located within the submucosal fibrous connective tissue immediately subjacent to the oral epithelium.

Differential Diagnosis: The limitation of pigment to the gingival margin is characteristic of heavy metal pigmentation. History of metal ingestion confirms the visual clinical impression.

Treatment: No treatment is necessary for the pigmented lesions. Once a metallic line has formed, the patient should be considered to be in a state of metal poisoning and exposure should be immediately terminated. Advanced periodontal disease may accompany mercury poisoning.

References

1. Dreeson, W. C.: Health of lead-exposed storage battery workers. J. Invest. Hyg. Toxicol. 25:60, 1943.
2. Robinson, H. M.: An evaluation of the bismuth blue line. J. Invest. Dermatol. 18:341,1952.
3. Bruggenkate, C. M., Cordozo, E. L., Maaskant, P., and van der Waal, I: Lead poisoning with pigmentation of the oral mucosa. Oral Surg. 39:747, 1975.
4. Gordon, N. C., Brown, S., Khosla, V. M., and Hansen, L. S.: Lead poisoning; A comprehensive review and report of a case. Oral Surg. 47:500, 1979.

Hairy Tongue

Age: Middle-aged adults

Sex: More common in males

Clinical Features: Diffuse brown or black pigment of the dorsal surface of the tongue accompanied by elongate hair-like projections of the filiform papillae is termed hairy tongue. The pigment is extensive and probably represents a combination of food products, tobacco stain, and chromogenic bacteria. A host of causative agents have been considered; however, the etiology remains obscure.

Microscopic Features: The filiform papillae are markedly elongated, with voluminous amounts of stratified parakeratin. Food and microbial debris are impacted between papillae.

Differential Diagnosis: Pigmentation localized to the dorsum of the tongue accompanied by elongated papillae is pathognomonic.

Treatment: Podophyllum resin has been used successfully, painted over the affected area as 1 percent solution. After application, the tongue should be rinsed thoroughly and the rinse expectorated, as ingested podophyllum can produce dangerous side effects. Three to five daily treatments are satisfactory. Many patients respond to brushing of the tongue with a hard-bristle toothbrush. This treatment is preferable initially, with

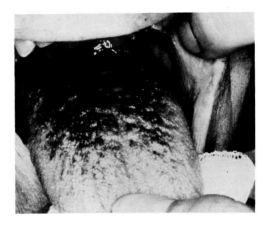

FIG. 3–39. Hairy tongue characterized by elongation of the filiform papillae, which appear matted and pigmented, brown or black coloration being most common.

podophyllum reserved for cases that fail to resolve
with mechanical abrasion.

References

1. Winer, L. H.: Black hairy tongue. Arch. Dermatol.
   77:97, 1958.
2. Standish, S. M. and Moorman, W. C.: Treatment of
   hairy tongue with podophyllin resin. J. Am. Dent.
   Assoc. 68:535, 1964.
3. Farman, A. G.: Hairy tongue (lingua villosa). J. Oral
   Med. 32:85, 1977.
4. Svejda, J., Skach, M., and Plackova, A.: Hairlike
   variations of filiform papillae in the human tongue.
   Oral Surg. 43:97, 1977.

PLATE I

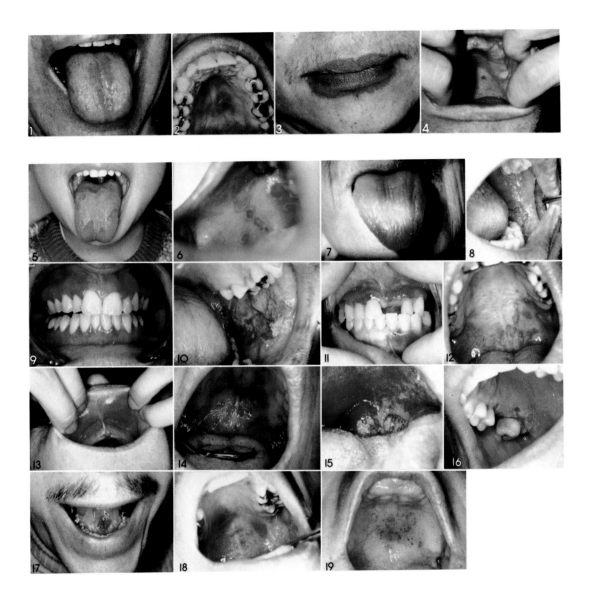

Red Lesions

Focal Erythemas. 1. Nonspecific mucositis of tongue. 2. Thermal burn of the palate. 3. Hemangioma, macular type, of lower lip. 4. Focal erythroplakia of palate.

Diffuse and Multifocal Erythemas. 5. Migratory glossitis. 6. Erythema migrans. 7. Atrophic glossitis in pernicious anemia. 8. Radiation mucositis of buccal mucosa. 9. Diffuse erythema associated with xerostomia. 10. Lupus erythematosus. (Courtesy of Dr. Troy Daniels.) 11. Allergic (plasma cell) gingivitis. 12. Erythema multiforme. 13. Atrophic candidiasis. 14. Erythematous papules in acute lymphonodular pharnygitis. 15. Pharyngitis in scarlet fever. 16. Erosive lichen planus. 17. Ecchymosis in floor of mouth. 18. Multifocal erythroplakias in field cancerization. 19. Palatal petechiae.

PLATE II

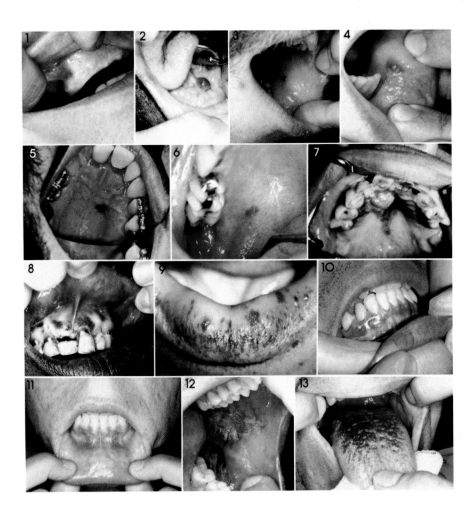

Pigmented Lesions

Focal Pigmentations. 1. Amalgam tattoo. 2. Hemorrhagic mucocele. 3. Focal hematoma. 4. Varix of buccal mucosa. 5. Nevus. 6. Oral melanotic macule. 7. Malignant melanoma.

Diffuse Pigmentations. 8. Physiologic (racial) pigmentation of the gingiva. 9. Labial melanotic macules in the Peutz-Jeger syndrome. 10. Gingival melanosis in Addison's disease. 11. Hemosiderin pigmentation of gingiva in hemochromatosis. 12. Pigmented lichen planus. 13. Black hairy tongue.

4
Oral Ulcerations and Fistulae

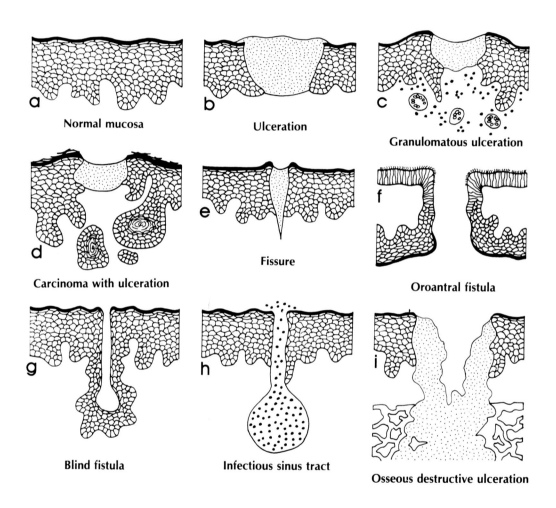

a Normal mucosa

b Ulceration

c Granulomatous ulceration

d Carcinoma with ulceration

e Fissure

f Oroantral fistula

g Blind fistula

h Infectious sinus tract

i Osseous destructive ulceration

Ulcers, Fistulae, and Sinuses

4
Oral Ulcerations and Fistulae

RECURRENT AND MULTIPLE ULCERATIONS

Aphthous Stomatitis
Major Scarring Aphthous Stomatitis
Behcet's Syndrome
Agranulocytosis
Cyclic Neutropenia
Uremic Stomatitis
Viral Vesicular Stomatitis
Acute Necrotizing Ulcerative Gingivitis
Acute Streptococcal Stomatitis
Gonococcal Stomatitis

FOCAL ULCERATIONS

Traumatic Ulcer
Necrotizing Sialometaplasia
Specific Granulomatous Ulcer
Chancre
Squamous Cell Carcinoma

PERIORAL AND COMMISSURAL ULCERATIONS AND FISTULAE

Commissural Pits
Congenital Lip Pits
Angular Cheilitis
Carcinoma

ORAL FISTULAE

Periapical Abscess and Osteomyelitis
Periodontal Abscess
Actinomycosis
Oroantral Fistula
Soft Tissue Abscess
Developmental Oral Sinuses
Cutaneous Fistulae

NECROTIC AND OSSEOUS DESTRUCTIVE LESIONS

Factitial Injury and Trauma
Midline Lethal Granuloma and Wegener's
 Granulomatosis
Tertiary Syphilis
Osteoradionecrosis
Mucormycosis
Antral Carcinoma

Ulcerative lesions of the oral cavity are common. Assessment of the nature of oral ulcers requires a thorough history of the present illness. Certain ulcerations occur in multiples, and many of these are recurrent. Signs and symptoms relative to general health with review of organ systems will point to a diagnosis of certain systemic problems that can manifest oral ulceration. The nature of the ulcer itself is vitally important when a definitive diagnosis is pursued. One should always remember that oral vesiculobullous diseases are subject to trauma, with loss of the characteristic vesicular nature of the lesions clinically. For this reason the patient should be questioned concerning the nature of the lesions at their outset, and attempts should be made to search for an intact vesicle. If the ulcerations prove to be or to have been vesiculobullous, refer to the next chapter for discussion of vesiculobullous diseases. In this section, only diseases that begin as ulcers will be considered.

Draining tracts or fistulae are included in this chapter since clinically they may appear as areas of ulceration. By definition, a fistula represents an epithelial lined tract connecting two body cavities, whereas a sinus is a drainage tract associated with an infection. Many clinicians do not make this distinction and refer to all tracts as fistulae. This is the context in which the term fistula is used here. Palpation of the underlying tissues will usually elicit flow of purulent exudate from an area of tissue breakdown suspected to represent a fistula. Insertion of a probe or gutta-percha point will also aid in detecting a tract. The exudate may be subjected to culture and sensitivity tests to determine the specific infectious agents responsible for infection.

The most common recurring oral ulcerations are aphthae, whereas the most frequently encountered nonrecurring multifocal ulcerative disease is acute necrotizing ulcerative gingivitis. Potentially lethal diseases with multifocal ulcerations are agranulocytosis and uremia.

The traumatic ulcer from biting or denture irritation is the most common focal oral ulceration. Carcinoma, tuberculous, and mycotic ulcers are potentially lethal diseases.

Common perioral ulcerations include angular cheilitis and cancer, the latter being most serious.

Parulis of pulpal or periodontal origin is the most common form of oral fistula. All necrotic and osseous destructive lesions with drainage are serious disorders.

RECURRENT AND MULTIPLE ULCERATIONS

Aphthous Stomatitis

Age: Teenagers and young adults
Sex: No predilection

Clinical Features: Aphthous ulcers may occur singly or in crops. The lesions are shallow and flat

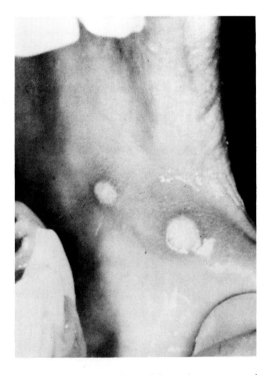

FIG. 4–1. Aphthous ulcers of the oral mucosa—oval, shallow, and displaying an erythematous halo.

with a central white fibrinous pseudomembrane surrounded by an erythematous halo. Commonly known as canker sore, these lesions are prone to appear during times of stress; frequency of recurrence and multiplicity are extremely varied. They are quite painful, remain for 10 to 14 days, and then spontaneously regress. They occur most often on the oral soft tissues that are not bound to bone, yet occasionally the gingiva is involved. Aphthae can be small, punctate, and present in great numbers; lesions of this nature have been referred to as herpetiform ulcers, despite the fact that they are not caused by herpesvirus. Aphthous ulcers are occasionally a concomitant of chronic inflammatory bowel disease. L-form streptococci have been isolated from the lesions, and cell-mediated immune responses to oral epithelium have been demonstrated. While a specific etiology has not been definitively identified, there is some evidence that food allergens may be responsible in some instances.

Microscopic Features: The epithelium is ulcerated, with an eosinophilic fibrinous coagulum on the surface. The connective tissue is infiltrated with mononuclear cells, chiefly lymphocytes, and the reaction is superficial.

Differential Diagnosis: Recurrent aphthous stomatitis must be differentiated from cyclic neutropenia by obtaining periodic blood counts when the recurrence of lesions is periodic and regular. Behcet's syndrome should be investigated since oral lesions in that disease are indistinguishable from aphthae.

Viral infection can be ruled out if no history of vesicle formation can be obtained. With the exception of palatal secondary herpesvirus infection, herpes of the oral soft tissues does not occur on a recurrent basis as do aphthae.

Treatment: Single lesions or instances in which only a few ulcers appear can be treated by applying a wet applicator impregnated with silver nitrate for a few seconds, cauterizing the central core of the ulcer. Tetracycline oral suspension may invoke early involution. Selective elimination of suspected foods can be attempted.

References

1. Graykowski, E.A., et al.: Recurrent aphthous stomatitis; clinical, therapeutic, histopathologic and hypersensitivity aspects. J. Am. Med. Assoc. 196:637, 1966.
2. Lehner, T.: Pathology of recurrent oral ulceration and oral ulceration in Behcet's syndrome. Light, electron and fluorescence microscopy. J. Pathol. 97:548, 1969.

3. Ship, I. I.: Epidemiologic aspects of recurrent aphthous ulcerations. Oral Surg. *33*:400, 1972.
4. Cohen, L.: Etiology, pathogenesis and classification of aphthous stomatitis and Behcet's syndrome. J. Oral Pathol. *7*:347, 1978.
5. Antoon, J. W. and Miller, R. L.: Aphthous ulcers— A review of the literature on etiology, pathogenesis, diagnosis and treatment. J. Am. Dent. Assoc. *101*:803, 1980.

Major Scarring Aphthous Stomatitis

Age: Young adults

Sex: No predilection

Clinical Features: Major aphthae, also known as periadenitis mucosae necrotica recurrens or Sutton's disease, are similar in appearance to minor aphthae. However, the ulcers are more deep-seated, exceed 0.5 cm in size (indeed, they may be several centimeters in diameter), and, like minor aphthae, soft tissues not bound to bone are predisposed to them. The faucial pillars and oropharynx are often the initial sites of ulceration. After resolution, which may require 1 to 4 weeks, healing with scar formation is seen. Remissions are short, with a new crop of ulcers appearing shortly after the older lesions resolve. Most patients are tense and anxious, and the lesions are extremely painful. The cause is unknown, but mounting evidence points to an immune defect. Both immunoglobulin and cell-mediated responses to oral epithelium have been demonstrated.

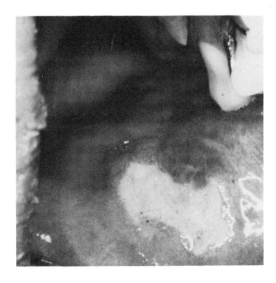

FIG. 4–2. Major aphthous ulcers—extensive, often showing irregular margins and with inflamed surrounding mucosa. They leave depressed scars after healing.

Microscopic Features: The epithelium is ulcerated with an eosinophilic fibrin surface. A mononuclear inflammatory cell infiltrate composed predominantly of lymphocytes extends deeply into the submucosa.

Differential Diagnosis: Major aphthae are differentiated from minor aphthous stomatitis on the basis of size and tendency to heal with scarring. Cyclic neutropenia and agranulocytosis may be ruled out by obtaining a leukocyte and differential count.

Treatment: Initial attempts to control the severity and distress of major aphthae include the use of gauze compresses soaked in tetracycline oral suspension and applied three times daily. A palliative mouth rinse such as an antihistamine oral suspension mixed with equal parts of Kaopectate often minimizes pain. If tetracycline is ineffective, prednisone, 20 mg daily in divided doses for 10 days, usually induces regression of ulcerations. These treatment regimens must be repeated when new lesions periodically appear. Psychiatric consultation is also recommended.

References

1. Hjørting-Hansen, E. and Siemssen, S. O.: Stomatitis aphthosa recurrens cicatricians. Odontol. Tidskr. 69:294,1961.
2. Monoteleone, L.: Periadenitis mucosa necrotica recurrens. Oral Surg. 23:586, 1967.
3. Lehner, T.: Pathology of recurrent oral ulceration and oral ulceration in Behcet's syndrome. Light, electron and fluorescence microscopy. J. Pathol. 97: 548, 1969.
4. Stanley, H. R.: Management of patients with persistent recurrent aphthous stomatitis and Sutton's disease. Oral Surg. 35:174, 1973.

Behcet's Syndrome

Age: Young and middle-aged adults

Sex: Significant male predilection

Clinical Features: One of the muco-oculocutaneous syndromes, Behcet's disease represents an immunopathic disorder characterized by oral aphthous ulcerations, uveoconjunctivitis, and genital ulceration. L-form bacteria have been implicated in the pathogenesis of the disease. Not all components of the syndrome triad are present at any given time. The oral ulcerations are small with a white pseudomembrane and erythematous halo, indistinguishable from ordinary aphthae. The eye lesions consist of recurrent conjunctivitis, ulceration, uveitis and hypopyon, with visual damage being a common sequela. In males, the genital lesions are located on the penis and scrotum; in females, the vulva is frequently affected.

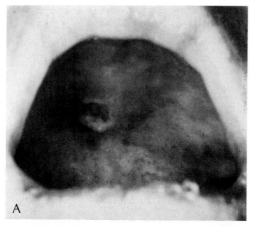

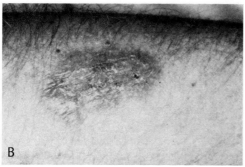

FIG. 4–3. *A:* Oral ulcerations in Behcet's syndrome, resembling aphthae. *B:* Skin lesions appearing as erythematous plaques with a keratotic scale.

References

1. Steinmetz, P. R. and Green, J. P.: Reiter's syndrome. U. S. Armed Forces Med. J. *10*:1185, 1959.
2. Mason, R. M. and Barns, C. G.: Behcet's syndrome with arthritis. Ann. Rheum. Dis. *28*:95, 1969.
3. Lehner, T.: Pathology of recurrent oral ulceration and oral ulceration in Behcet's syndrome: Light, electron and fluorescence microscopy. J. Pathol. *97*:481, 1969.
4. Chajek, T. and Fainaru, M.: Behcet's disease. Report of 41 cases and a review of the literature. Medicine *54*:179, 1975.
5. Rapidis, A. D., Langdon, J. D., and Patel, M. F.: Recurrent oral and oculogenital ulcerations (Behcet's syndrome). Oral Surg. *41*:457, 1976.

Agranulocytosis

Age: No predilection
Sex: No predilection

Clinical Features: A deficiency in circulating blood granulocytes may represent a primary idiopathic disorder or may be secondary to bone marrow suppression by certain drugs that are cytotoxic for hematopoietic tissue. Cancer patients receiving antitumor chemotherapy are most often affected. Since the granulocytic series are vital to defense against infection, patients with agranulocytosis are extremely prone to develop infections, pulmonary bacterial infections in particular. Death from uncontrollable infection is common. The leukocyte count is usually under 2500 per cu mm, and the differential count shows severely depressed numbers of neutrophilic granulocytes. The oral ulcers

Gastrointestinal complaints in the form of diarrhea and pain are frequently encountered, as are joint pain and discomfort.

Microscopic Features: The epithelium shows ulceration, being replaced by an eosinophilic coagulum. The connective tissue is infiltrated with mononuclear cells, chiefly lymphocytes.

Differential Diagnosis: The extraoral signs are sufficient to differentiate Behcet's syndrome from simple aphthae. When the dominant features are arthritis, dermatitis of the palms and soles, conjunctivitis, and genital ulceration, then the disease is more correctly termed Reiter's syndrome. Both Behcet's and Reiter's syndromes are probably variants of the same immunopathologic process.

Treatment: Systemic steroids are required for control. Because of the multiplicity of defects, these patients should be managed by a general physician or dermatologist.

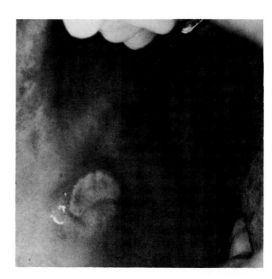

FIG. 4–4. Agranulocytic ulcers, flat with a necrotic center.

are oval in shape and variable in size. In addition, gingivitis or periodontitis is a frequent finding with ulcerations located on the attached gingivae. Pain is a feature.

Microscopic Features: The microscopic changes are pathognomonic. The epithelium is lacking and there is an eosinophilic fibrin surface. Underlying the pseudomembrane and imperceptibly merging with it is a zone of amorphous necrotic tissue, which is strikingly devoid of neutrophils. Indeed, other inflammatory cells, including round cells, are present in only limited numbers, probably because the lesions are detected and taken for biopsy early in their course.

Differential Diagnosis: Agranulocytic ulcers may appear identical to aphthae, major aphthae, and cyclic neutropenia. Differentiation from these entities requires biopsy and a complete blood count.

Treatment: Oral ulceration in agranulocytosis is an ominous sign denoting severe depression of cellular defense mechanisms. If drug induced, it is a sign of dangerous toxicity levels and the dose of medication should be decreased immediately; otherwise the patient is open to rapidly progressive infection. If no cause can be determined, the disease is of the idiopathic primary type, and referral to a hematologist is essential.

References

1. Andrews, R. G., et al.: Chronic benign neutropenia of childhood with associated oral manifestations. Oral Surg. 20:719, 1965.
2. Swenson, H. M., et al.: Agranulocytosis. J. Periodontol. 35:466, 1965.
3. Kander, R. and Mauer, A. M.: Neutropenias of childhood. J. Pediatr. 69:147, 1966.
4. Awbrey, J. J. and Hibbard, E. D.: Congenital agranulocytosis. Oral Surg. 35:526, 1973.
5. Mishkin, D. J., Akers, J. O., and Darby, C. P.: Congenital neutropenia. Report of a case and a biorationale for dental management. Oral Surg. 42:738, 1976.

Cyclic Neutropenia

Age: Childhood onset
Sex: No predilection

Clinical Features: Oral ulcerations that are multifocal, are located primarily on movable mucosa, appear every 20 to 25 days, persist for 5 to 8 days, and reappear on a periodic basis probably represent oral manifestations of cyclic neutropenia. The ulcers are shallow, may show an erythematous halo, and vary in size. Coexistent severe premature periodontal lesions are common. The gingival papillae are erythematous and edem-

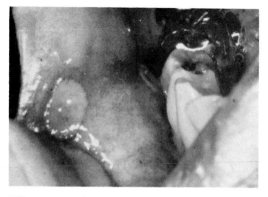

FIG. 4–5. Cyclic neutropenia, characterized by premature periodontitis and focal ulcerations that appear every 20 or 25 days.

atous, and may be ulcerated. Vertical alveolar bone loss with pocket formation is encountered in many regions throughout both dental arches. Otitis media, joint pain, and headache are often present during the neutropenic phase. The leukocyte count is depressed, as are the neutrophilic granulocytes during the period of ulceration. Throughout the course of the 20-day remission, the hemogram is within normal limits. During the agranulocytic phase, susceptibility to infection is a complication. The cause of this mysterious paroxysmal hematologic disorder is unknown, but is related to a maturation arrest in the bone marrow.

Microscopic Features: The ulcers are typically agranulocytic. The epithelium is lacking, and there is an eosinophilic necrotic zone. The submucosa is characterized by a paucity of inflammatory cells in general and a complete lack of neutrophils.

Differential Diagnosis: The ulcers of cyclic neutropenia are indistinguishable from aphthae, major aphthae, agranulocytosis, and Behcet's syndrome. The consistent cyclic nature of the lesions is highly suggestive of cyclic neutropenia; however, recurrent aphthae often show this pattern in the absence of an altered hemogram. The presence of premature periodontal lesions is another factor in favor of a diagnosis of cyclic neutropenia. The diagnosis can be established by obtaining leukocyte and differential blood counts every three days during periods of affliction and regression.

Treatment: Patients with cyclic neutropenia require management by a hematologist. While the periodontal prognosis is poor, periodontal therapy is required for its own sake as well as to eliminate a focus of infection.

References

1. Gorlin, R. J. and Chandhry, A. P.: The oral manifestations of cyclic (periodic) neutropenia. Arch. Dermatol. *82*:344, 1960.
2. Wade, A. B. and Stafford, J. L.: Cyclical neutropenia. Oral Surg. *16*:1443, 1963.
3. Cohen, L.: Recurrent oral ulceration and cutaneous infections associated with cyclical neutropenia. Dental Pract. *16*:97, 1966.
4. Degnan, E. and Perlow, A.: Infected oral lesions of cyclic neutropenia. J. Oral Med. *28*:29, 1973.

Uremic Stomatitis

Age: Young and middle-aged adults
Sex: No predilection

Clinical Features: Patients suffering end-stage renal disease with elevated creatinine or blood urea nitrogen and electrolyte derangements will occasionally develop oral ulcerations. Uremic oral ulcers vary in size, are irregular in shape, and are usually shallow. They connote a poor prognosis, with death being imminent unless renal dialysis or kidney transplant is performed. The cause for ulceration is unknown, yet has been suggested to be the consequence of strongly alkaline saliva due to ammonia formation from retained urea secreted in the saliva. In other cases the use of orally administered alkaline solutions used to alleviate metabolic acidosis may cause ulceration.

Microscopic Features: The epithelium is lacking, having been replaced by an eosinophilic coagulum with a subjacent inflammatory cell infiltrate.

Differential Diagnosis: Patients with uremic ulcers will manifest the clinical signs of the uremic syndrome: an ammonia odor on the breath, weight loss, anemia, cardiac arrhythmias, and, in many instances, secondary hyperparathyroidism. The oral ulcers are chronic rather than recurrent and may clinically simulate agranulocytic ulcers.

Treatment: Uremia may be secondary to pyelonephritis, glomerulonephritis, diabetic glomerulosclerosis, or lupus erythematosus. Management lies with a physician.

The oral ulcers, if painful, may be treated by prescribing a palliative oral rinse such as an antihistaminic oral suspension 50:50 with Kaopectate.

References

1. Halazonetis, J. and Harley, A.: Uremic stomatitis. Oral Surg. *23*:572, 1967.
2. Newell, G. B. and Stone, O. J.: Irritant contact stomatitis in chronic renal failure. Arch. Dermatol. *109*:53, 1974.
3. Tyldesley, W. R., Rotter, E., and Sells, R. A.: Oral lesions in renal transplant patients. J. Oral Pathol. *8*:53, 1979.

Viral Vesicular Stomatitis

Age: Children and young adults
Sex: No predilection

Clinical Features: Viral infections that manifest oral ulcerations do so secondarily, in that the early lesion is vesicular and, under masticatory trauma, the vesicles rupture and yield areas of ulceration. Herpes virus, varicella-zoster virus, and Coxsackie viruses are the common infectious agents. The specific features encountered in oral viral infections are enumerated in the section on vesiculo-

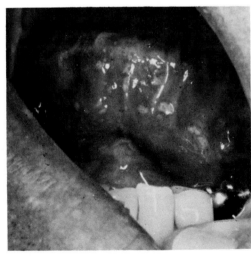

FIG. 4–7.   Viral stomatitides. Vesicles form and rupture within 24 hours, yielding shallow ulcers as seen in this example of primary herpetic gingivostomatitis.

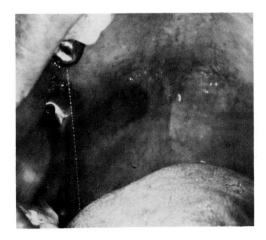

FIG. 4–6.   Diffuse stomatitis with zones of ulceration manifested in renal failure.

bullous and desquamative lesions. In general terms, oral ulcers that develop from viral infection are shallow, small, multifocal, and painful. A constant finding is elevation in temperature during primary infection.

Microscopic Features: The classic cytologic changes unique to oral vesicular eruptions are usually not apparent after the vesicles rupture to leave ulcers. The ulcerated zones may show ballooning degeneration of spinous cells in the marginal epithelium. Usually only an area of ulceration with a subacute inflammatory cell infiltrate is seen, with evidence of regenerating epithelium on the surface.

Differential Diagnosis: Viral ulcerations are most frequently confused with aphthous stomatitis. If the oral ulcers are of a recurrent nature, then viral ulceration can be eliminated as a possibility; the viruses causing oral infection do so only as a primary disease and do not manifest intraoral recurrent infections.

Exceptions to this are recurrent herpes labialis, which is not intraoral, and recurrent palatal herpes, which is unilaterally localized to the palatal gingiva as microvesicles that ulcerate, leaving tiny pinpoint ulcerative foci.

Treatment: Treatment for primary viral stomatitis is palliative. Soft diet, liquids, analgesic/antipyretic drugs, and a soothing oral rinse consisting of an antihistaminic oral suspension with equal parts of Kaopectate are recommended.

References

1. Ship, I. I.: Virus and viral-like diseases of the mouth. Postgrad. Med. *38*:499, 1965.
2. Weathers, D. R. and Griffin, J. W.: Intraoral ulcerations of recurrent herpes simplex and recurrent aphthae: two distinct clinical entities. J. Am. Dent. Assoc. *81*:81, 1970.
3. Cawson, R. R.: Oral ulceration—clinical aspects. Oral Surg. *33*:912, 1972.
4. Lennette, E. H. and Magoffin, R. L.: Virologic and immunologic aspects of major oral ulcerations. J. Am. Dent. Assoc. *87*:1055, 1973.

Acute Necrotizing Ulcerative Gingivitis

Age: Teenagers and young adults
Sex: Male predilection

Clinical Features: Acute necrotizing ulcerative gingivitis (ANUG), Vincent's disease, manifests multifocal pseudomembranous ulcerations localized primarily to the gingival interdental papillae. The papillae are blunted, with necrotic craters showing a marginal zone of erythema. Pain is a chief complaint, and halitosis is a constant feature. Uncommonly, ulcerations extend beyond the gin-

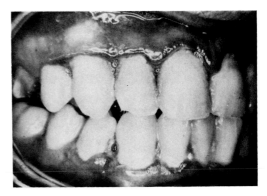

FIG. 4–8. Gingivitis accompanied by crateriform ulcers with blunting of the papillae. The multifocal ulcers of ANUG are generally confined to the interdental papillae.

giva to include the palate and mucobuccal fold, where they may be extensive. The infectious microorganisms associated with acute necrotizing ulcerative gingivitis are anaerobic fusiform and spirochetal bacteria that are saprophytic members of normal oral flora. They proliferate and may be considered pathogenic when the patient is under undue stress. In this context it is not surprising that the disease often occurs among college students during final examination periods.

Microscopic Features: Smears and dark-field scrapings disclose the presence of fusiform and mobile spirochete bacterial forms. Tissue sections show nonspecific ulceration with superficial necrosis and a subacute inflammatory cell infiltrate. Bacterial colonies populate the necrotic surface.

Differential Diagnosis: Localization to gingival papillae and presence of a foul odor are essentially diagnostic of acute necrotizing ulcerative gingivitis. These features differentiate this disease from the other ulcerative disorders outlined in this section.

Treatment: In severe cases systemic antibiotics (e.g., penicillin 250 mg 4 times daily for 1 week) are recommended. Less severe forms can be managed by 3 percent hydrogen peroxide rinses. Two to three days after therapy is instituted, dental prophylaxis should be performed.

References

1. Schluger, S.: Necrotizing ulcerative gingivitis in the Army. J. Am. Dent. Assoc. *38*:174, 1949.
2. Carter, W. J. and Ball, D. M.: Results of a three year study of Vincent's infection at the Great Lakes Naval Dental Department. J. Periodontol. *24*:187, 1953.
3. Coslet, R. S.: The psychological factor in the etiol-

ogy of acute necrotizing gingivitis. Dent. Hyg. 53:257, 1979.

Acute Streptococcal Stomatitis

Age: Young adults
Sex: No predilection

Clinical Features: Acute streptococcal stomatitis is a rare disease that is characterized by gingival, oral mucosal, and tonsillar inflammation associated with cervical lymphadenopathy. It is conceivable that the disease could represent a secondary bacterial infection following primary herpetic gingivostomatitis. The lesions are ulcerative with an erythematous base and involve both fixed and movable mucosa. The gingiva is boggy with diffuse erythema; the ulcers do not confine themselves to the intradental papilla, nor are they restricted only to marginal gingiva. Fetid odor is not a feature. Beta-hemolytic streptococci can be cultured, and antistreptolysin O titers are elevated during the convalescent period. The white blood cell count is elevated with a neutrophilic leukocytosis.

Microscopic Features: The mucosa is ulcerated with a pseudomembranous fibrin surface. The ulcer bed is represented by granulation tissue exhibiting a nonspecific subacute inflammatory cell infiltrate.

Differential Diagnosis: Viral vesicular stomatitis, particularly primary herpetic gingivostomatitis, exhibits almost identical clinical features. Whereas primary herpes typically manifests a marginal gingivitis in addition to oral ulcers, streptococcal gingivitis fails to show this feature. Most of the other ulcerative diseases are not accompanied by fever and lymphadenopathy. A definitive diagnosis rests with a positive culture for beta-hemolytic streptococci with elevated antistreptolysin O titers in the convalescent period.

Treatment: Acute streptococcal stomatitis is managed by prescribing penicillin or synthetic penicillin analogs 250 mg every 6 hours for 2 weeks. A palliative oral mouth rinse or tetracycline oral suspension is also recommended.

References

1. Blake, G. C. and Trott, J.R.: Acute streptococcal gingivitis. Dent. Pract. *10*:43, 1959.
2. Tyldesley, W. R.: Infections of the oral mucosa. Br. Dent. J. *20*:449, 1973.
3. Littner, M. M., et al.: Acute streptococcal gingivostomatitis: Report of five cases and review of the literature. Oral Surg. *53*:144, 1982.

Gonococcal Stomatitis

Age: Young adults
Sex: No predilection

Clinical Features: Whereas gonorrhea is a common urethral infection, localization in the oral cavity and oropharynx is rare. When the oral mucosa is infected, irregular ulcerations ranging from 0.5 to 2.0 cm are observed and are accompanied by a perilesional zone of erythema. Tonsilar and pharyngeal involvement is characterized by a pseudomembranous reaction with tonsilar enlargement accompanied by an erythematous pharyngitis. Lymphadenopathy and fever are also observed.

Microscopic Features: The mucosa may be intact or ulcerated with a fibrinous pseudomembrane. The submucosa displays a nonspecific subacute inflammatory cell infiltrate. Cytologic smears prepared with a gram stain disclose free and intraepithelial gram-negative diplococci.

Differential Diagnosis: The ulcerations of gon-

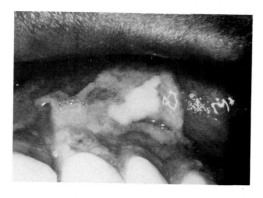

FIG. 4–9. Child with diffuse ulcer and pseudomembrane in acute streptococcal stomatitis. (Courtesy of Dr. D. Adams.)

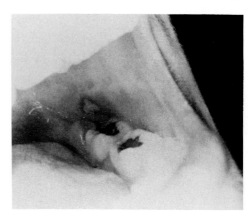

FIG. 4–10. Irregularly outlined ulcer in gonococcal stomatitis.

ococcal stomatitis may simulate other diseases included here as ulcerative diseases. The variation in size and configuration and elevated temperature should arouse suspicion of gonorrhea along with a history of contact with a known carrier of the disease. A smear will often, yet not invariably, disclose the presence of gram-negative diplococci. A culture is required in order to secure a definitive diagnosis.

Treatment: Penicillin is the treatment of choice. One gram of probenecid followed 30 minutes later by 4.8 million units of intramuscular procaine penicillin is recommended therapy. Alternatively, 500 mg oral penicillin every 6 hours for 10 days will generally eliminate the infection. Penicillin resistant cases should be evaluated by culture and sensitivity testing.

References

1. Kohn, S. R., Shaffer, J. F., and Chomenko, A. G.: Primary gonococcal stomatitis. J. Am. Med. Assoc. *219*:86, 1972.
2. Chue, P.W. Y.: Gonorrhea—Its natural history, oral manifestations, diagnosis, treatment, and prevention. J. Am. Dent. Assoc. *90*:1297, 1975.
3. Merchant, H. W. and Schuster, G. S.: Oral gonococcal infection. J. Am. Dent. Assoc. *95*:807, 1977.
4. Jamsky, R. J. and Christen, A. G.: Oral gonococcal infections; report of two cases. Oral Surg. *53*:358, 1982.

FOCAL ULCERATIONS

Traumatic Ulcer

Age: No predilection
Sex: No predilection

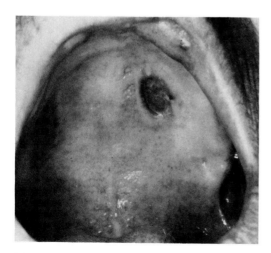

FIG. 4–11. Traumatic ulcer evolving in response to an ill-fitting, recently fabricated maxillary denture. Size of ulcer depends on etiology.

Clinical Features: The traumatic ulcer is by far the most common type of focal ulceration. It may occur in response to a variety of traumatic insults including denture irritation, cheek- or tongue-biting, pizza burn, or other forms of self-inflicted trauma or iatrogenic injury occurring in the dental office. The cause is usually readily determined by examining for flange overextension on dentures using pressure-indicating paste, or by checking for jagged or malposed cusps and restorations. The ulcer is generally shallow, yet may show rolled borders as a result of granulation tissue response. Marginal erythema is usually, yet not invariably, present. Traumatic ulcers of the soft palate in the region of the pterygoid hamulus in infants have been referred to as Bednar's aphthae. A traumatic ulcer of the lips in children with erupting teeth has been termed Riga-Fede disease. Deep traumatic ulcers of the tongue associated with a granulomatous tumefaction and a pronounced eosinophilic myositis have been termed soft tissue eosinophilic granulomas, not to be confused with eosinophilic granuloma of bone, a specific form of histiocytosis X.

Microscopic Features: The epithelium is lacking, exposing bare connective tissue with an eosinophilic surface coagulum. The superficial layer is infiltrated with neutrophils, while the deeper and marginal connective tissues evince a round cell infiltrate. Soft tissue eosinophilic granuloma of the tongue is characterized by an avid eosinophil infiltrate interposed between muscle fibers.

Differential Diagnosis: Traumatic ulcers may be extensive and associated with tumefaction. In these cases carcinoma and specific granulomatous inflammation must be ruled out by biopsy.

Treatment: If a history of trauma is present or irritational factors are identified, they should be removed and 10 days should be allowed for healing. Failure to resolve necessitates a biopsy.

References

1. Abramson, M. and Dowrie, J. O.: Sublingual granuloma in infancy (Riga-Fede's disease). J. Pediatr. *24*:195, 1944.
2. Obermayer, M. E.: Cheek biting (Morsicatio buccarum). Arch. Dermatol. *90*:185, 1964.
3. Elzay, R.P.: Traumatic ulcerative granuloma with stromal eosinophilia (Riga-Fede's disease and traumatic eosinophilic granuloma). Oral Surg. *55*:497, 1983.

Necrotizing Sialometaplasia

Age: Adults
Sex: No predilection

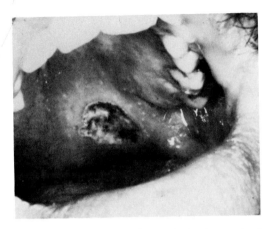

FIG. 4–12. Necrotizing sialometaplasia, characterized by a relatively deep-seated necrotic ulcer or bilateral ulcers of the palatal mucosa.

Clinical Features: The hard and soft palates show focal deep-seated ulceration, often bilateral. Occasionally other mucosal sites bearing minor salivary glands are affected. The ulcers are large, lack induration, and fail to show rolled margins; the necrotic center possesses a pebbly-surfaced gray membrane. Despite their extensiveness, they are generally painless. After biopsy the lesions generally heal spontaneously within two months. The etiology is unkown, but vascular occlusion of the arterioles supplying the palate and associated minor salivary glands has been suggested.

Microscopic Features: The ulcer bed is composed of necrotic debris and eosinophilic fibrinous material. The underlying salivary tissue is necrotic, with maintenance of cellular outlines reminiscent of ischemic necrosis. The salivary epithelium adjacent to the necrotic zone displays marked squamous metaplasia with loss of normal acinar morphology. The metaplastic islands are oval or linear with rounded margins. Lesions should not be confused with mucoepidermoid or epidermoid carcinoma.

Differential Diagnosis: Clinically, necrotizing sialometaplasia may be confused with carcinoma, adenocarcinoma, granulomatous ulcer, or traumatic ulcer. Lack of induration and rolled margins should divert suspicion of malignancy. Biopsy is required to obtain a definitive diagnosis.

Treatment: Once a definitive diagnosis is secured, no treatment is required. The lesions will spontaneously regress in 6 to 8 weeks. Palliation is not necessary since pain is generally not a problem.

References

1. Abrams, A. M., Melrose, R. J., and Howell, F. V.: Necrotizing sialometaplasia. Cancer 32:130, 1973.
2. Dunlap, C. L. and Barker, B. F.: Necrotizing sialometaplasia; report of five additional cases. Oral Surg. 37:722, 1974.
3. Samit, A. M., Mashberg, A., and Greene, G. W.: Necrotizing sialometaplasia. J. Oral Surg. 37:353, 1979.
4. Dunley, R. E. and Jacoway, J. R.: Necrotizing sialometaplasia. Oral Surg. 47:169, 1979.
5. Lynch, D. P., Crago, C. A., and Martinez, M.G.: Necrotizing sialometaplasia. Oral Surg. 47:63, 1979.

Specific Granulomatous Ulcer

Age: Adults
Sex: No predilection

Clinical Features: Specific granulomatous responses elicited by microorganisms are all primary pulmonary infections that involve oral mucous membranes secondarily by extrapulmonary dissemination; mycobacterium tuberculosum and the deep fungi are specifically implicated. Of the fungal infections, histoplasmosis, blastomycosis, cryptococcosis, and coccidiodomycosis are most common. The ulcers are always associated with a granulomatous, firm swelling that characteristically evinces a papillary or cobblestone surface pattern with patchy erythema. While any site may be affected, the tongue and buccal mucosa are favored. Often more than one lesion will be present. Since pulmonary infection is the dominant feature, chronic cough will be noted. Transmission of infection by physical contact with the lesions is remote but possible.

Microscopic Features: Subjacent to the ulcer-

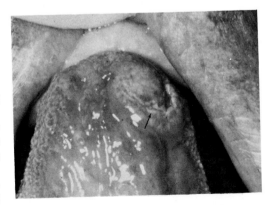

FIG. 4–13. Granulomatous ulcer represented by this case of oral histoplasmosis. It appears as a tumefaction with a central zone of ulceration.

ated zones are focal condensations of chronically inflamed granulation tissue with epithelioid cells and multinucleated giant cells showing a horse-shoe or wreath-like nuclear arrangement. Caseous necrosis is often, yet not always, seen in tuberculous granulomas. The deep fungal granulomas are noncaseating. Acid-fast stains disclose the presence of mycobacteria. Periodic acid-Schiff or methenamine silver will stain fungal cell walls.

Differential Diagnosis: Specific granulomatous ulcers may simulate carcinoma or traumatic ulcers. When predominantly papillary in appearance, they may be difficult to differentiate from papillary hyperplasia or verrucous carcinoma. Biopsy will show the characteristic features of granulomatous infection. Skin tests may also be indicated to demonstrate delayed hypersensitivity to a specific microorganism.

Treatment: Since oral granulomatous lesions are secondary to pulmonary disease, referral to an internist is indicated. Tuberculosis is treated with long-term isoniazid therapy. Deep fungi are managed with amphotericin B.

References

1. Levy, B. M.: Oral manifestations of histoplasmosis. J. Am. Dent. Assoc. *32*:215, 1945.
2. Yungco, J. C.: Tuberculosis of the tongue in patients with pulmonary tuberculosis. Dis. Chest *44*:638, 1963.
3. Mincer, H. H. and Oglesby, R.: Intraoral North American blastomycosis. Oral Surg. *22*:36, 1966.
4. Birkholz, H. and Riegler, H. C.: Tuberculosis of the tongue. J. Am. Dent. Assoc. *98*:60, 1979.
5. Fujibayashi, T., et al.: Tuberculosis of the tongue. A case report with immunologic study. Oral Surg. *47*:427, 1979.

Chancre (Primary Syphilis)

Age: Young adults
Sex: No predilection

Clinical Features: Primary syphilitic chancre of the oral mucosa arises subsequent to venereal contact as a consequence of orogenital sexual relationships. The lesion is most frequently seen on the lips or tongue and is typically a painless fungating tumefaction with central ulceration, firm to palpation. The examiner should wear gloves as the primary lesion is teeming with Treponema pallidum, the causative spirochetal microorganism. Chancres appear 5 to 6 weeks following sexual contact. The VDRL, fluorescent treponemal antibody test, or treponemal immobilization assay will usually be negative or only slightly reactive during the early stages of the disease and should therefore

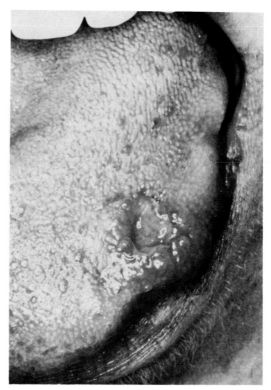

FIG. 4–14. Chancre of primary syphilis. A central zone of ulceration is surrounded by indurated, rolled, or swollen margins.

be assayed 1 to 2 weeks after appearance of the primary lesion.

Microscopic Features: The epithelium is lacking over the clinically ulcerated surface. Granulation tissue, which evinces an intense plasma cell infiltrate with a tendency for perivascular orientation, comprises the bulk of the tumefaction. A Warthin-Starry spirochete stain is required to visualize the microorganism. A smear with dark-field illumination discloses the presence of mobile spirochetes.

Differential Diagnosis: The granulomatous ulcer may resemble carcinoma, specific granulomatous ulcer of tuberculosis or the deep mycoses, and traumatic ulcer. A history of venereal transmission with rapid onset and growth should arouse suspicion of primary syphilis. VDRL, fluorescent treponemal antibody, or treponemal immobilization test will be positive 1 to 2 weeks after appearance of the chancre.

Treatment: Four million units of penicillin intramuscularly followed by oral penicillin 250 mg

4 times daily for 2 weeks is curative. Most states require that venereal disease cases be reported to the state board of health.

References

1. Meyer, I. and Shklar, G.: The oral manifestations of acquired syphilis. Oral Surg. 23:45, 1967.
2. Alexander, W. N.: Venereal disease and the dentist. J. Acad. Gen. Dent. 23:14, 1975.

Squamous Cell Carcinoma

Age: Elderly adults
Sex: Male predilection

Clinical Features: The most common presenting sign of oral cancer is the focal ulceration with indurated margins. Any oral ulcer without a readily apparent cause should be considered carcinoma until proven otherwise, particularly if the lesion has persisted longer than two weeks. Carcinomatous ulcers may arise in preexisting leukoplakia or erythroplasia, but there may be no history of a precedent precancerous lesion. The patients usually give a history of smoking or chewing tobacco and show a proclivity for overimbibing alcoholic beverages. The lateral border of the tongue, floor of the mouth, alveolar ridge, and lower lip are the sites of predilection; however, oral cancer can develop in any location. The ulcer is often, yet not always, painless. The growth rate is variable but usually progresses relatively rapidly. The larger the tumefactive ulceration, the more likely is the chance for nodal metastasis. Oral cancer spreads first to the submandibular and cervical lymph nodes. Regional metastatic disease in the neck, like the primary lesion, is indurated and fixed to adjacent tissues.

Microscopic Features: Subjacent and lateral to the zone of ulceration are invasive islands, cords, and nests of malignant epithelial cells that demonstrate varying degrees of pleomorphism, hyperchromatism, and increased mitoses, many of which are bizarre. Keratin and parakeratin pearls are often present.

Differential Diagnosis: Carcinoma appearing as an oral ulcer may be clinically indistinguishable from traumatic ulcer, chancre, or one of the specific granulomatous infections. Biopsy will provide a definitive diagnosis. Certainly, any ulcer without a cause, or one that fails to heal when a suspected cause is removed, requires microscopic examination.

Treatment: Cancer should be managed by an oncologist. Surgery, radiotherapy, or a combination of the two are the treatment modalities of choice.

References

1. Shafer, W. G., Hine, M. K., and Levy, B. M.: A Textbook of Oral Pathology, 4th Ed. Philadelphia, W. B. Saunders Co., 1983, pp. 112–127.
2. Tiecke, R. W. and Bernier, J. L.: Statistical and morphological analysis of four hundred and one cases of intraoral squamous cell carcinoma. J. Am. Dent. Assoc. 49:684, 1954.
3. Kremen, A.J. and Arhelger, S. W.: Early cancer of the oral cavity with special reference to cancer of the tongue. Postgrad. Med. 27:422, 1960.
4. Rossi, E. P. and Hirsch, S. A.: A survey of 4,793 oral lesions with emphasis on neoplasia and premalignancy. J. Am. Dent. Assoc. 94:883, 1977.
5. Nakissa, N., Hornback, N. B., Shidnia, H., and Sayoc, E. S.: Carcinoma of the floor of the mouth. Cancer 42:2914, 1978.

PERIORAL AND COMMISSURAL ULCERATIONS AND FISTULAE

Commissural Pits

Age: From infancy
Sex: No predilection

Clinical Features: Blind fistulae or pits located at the commissure of the lips are 1 to 2 mm in diameter and reach a depth of similar dimension.

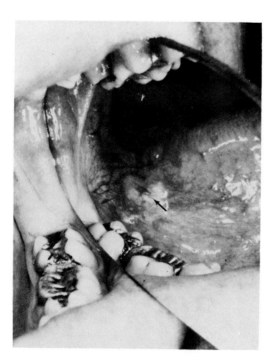

FIG. 4–15. Squamous cell carcinoma beginning as a focal ulceration with rolled borders, as seen here on the posterior lateral border of the tongue.

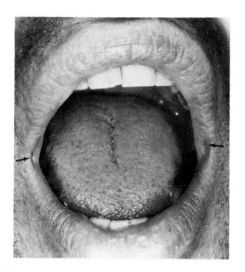

FIG. 4–16. Commissural pits: bilateral blind fistulae devoid of tumefactive margins.

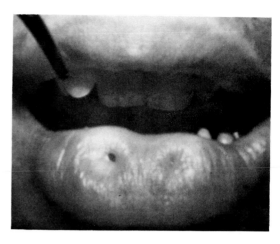

FIG. 4–17. Congenital lip pits. These may be bilateral blind ducts or they may communicate with salivary conduits. (Courtesy of Dr. Caesar Lopez.)

They may be unilateral or bilateral, show a familial tendency, and are more frequent among Negroes than whites. Their incidence has been reported to vary from 1 to 20 percent of the population.

Microscopic Features: Not applicable.

Differential Diagnosis: Commissural pits are clean, uninflamed depressions that can be easily differentiated from inflammatory or neoplastic lesions involving the angles of the mouth.

Treatment: No treatment is necessary.

References

1. Baker, W. R.: Pits of the lip commissures in caucasoid males. Oral Surg. *21*:56, 1966.
2. Everett, F. G. and Wescott, W. B.: Commissural lip pits. Oral Surg. *14*:202, 1961.

Congenital Lip Pits

Age: From infancy
Sex: Slight female predilection

Clinical Features: Developmental pits of the lower lip are blind fistulae located bilaterally on either side of the midline on the vermilion border. The fistulae may extend as deep as 2 cm and communicate with minor salivary ducts. The surrounding submucosa may be somewhat hyperplastic, producing a soft elevation of tissue around the broad sinuses. While lip pits may be an isolated finding, they are more often associated with cleft palate–cleft lip. This syndrome is inherited as an autosomal dominant trait.

Microscopic Features: Not applicable.

Differential Diagnosis: Lip pits lack ulceration and inflammation, allowing for easy recognition as a developmental anomaly, particularly in light

of their bilaterality and association with other developmental anomalies.

Treatment: Surgical removal may be undertaken for cosmetic purposes.

References

1. Watanbe, Y., et al.: Congenital fistulas of the lower lip. Oral Surg. *4*:709, 1951.
2. Van Der Woude, A.: Fistula labii inferious congenita and its association with cleft lip and palate. Am. J. Hum. Genet. *6*:244, 1954.
3. Bowden D. W.: Bilateral congenital fistulae of the lower lip. Br. J. Orthod. *4*:101, 1977.

Angular Cheilitis

Age: Adults
Sex: No predilection

Clinical Features: Located bilaterally at the commissures of the lips, angular cheilitis is characterized by weeping focal ulcerations showing cracking, keratosis, and mild erythema. In most instances, the disease is caused by or secondarily infected with Candida albicans. Predisposing factors are commonly encountered: decreased vertical intermaxillary dimension, pronounced an-

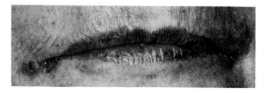

FIG. 4–18. Angular cheilitis characterized by commissural fissuring with keratotic, weeping lesions. (Courtesy of Dr. Alan Leider.)

gular skin folds, vitamin B complex deficiency, and pernicious anemia.

Microscopic Features: The surface epithelium shows zones of ulceration alternating with focal hyperkeratosis. Candida hyphae are aggregated in the superficial layers. The subjacent fibrous connective tissue displays a subacute or chronic inflammatory cell infiltrate.

Differential Diagnosis: The bilateral, weeping inflamed lesions devoid of tumefaction are characteristic. Underlying predisposing factors must be sought. A complete blood count and gastric analysis should be performed when pernicious anemia is suspected. Patients with pernicious anemia usually manifest atrophic glossitis in addition to angular cheilitis.

Treatment: The predisposing factors, be they local or systemic, must be eliminated or controlled. Topical application of nystatin cream or ointment 3 times daily will eliminate complicating candidal infection.

References
1. Finnerud, C.: Perleche: A study of 100 cases. Arch. Dermatol. Syph. 20:454, 1929.
2. Cawson, R. A.: Denture sore mouth and angular cheilitis. Br. Dent. J. 115:441, 1963.
3. Ritchie, G. M. and Fletcher, A. M.: Angular inflammation. Oral Surg. 36:358, 1973.
4. Lorentzer, S. H.: Angular cheilitis. Northwest Dent. 60:10, 1981.

Carcinoma

Age: Middle-aged and elderly adults
Sex: Male predilection

Clinical Features: Cancer of the lips may begin as a focal ulceration. Basal cell carcinomas are more often found on the upper lip than the lower,

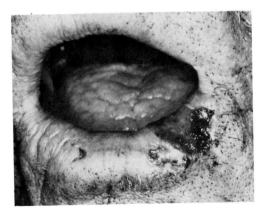

FIG. 4–19. Squamous cell carcinoma of the angle of the mouth appearing as an ulcer.

whereas squamous cell carcinoma is more frequent on the lower lip. Variant forms of squamous cell carcinoma, including the pseudoglandular type or adenoacanthoma of skin and spindle cell carcinoma, also favor the lower lip. These latter carcinomas are capable of metastasis whereas the basal cell carcinoma is only locally aggressive. Both cancers can appear ulcerative and may show rolled borders. Individuals of fair complexion and those with outdoor occupations, exposed to sunlight, are often affected.

Microscopic Features: Basal cell carcinomas show nests of tumor cells with monomorphic basiloid nuclei. Keratin pearl formation is also encountered. The microscopic features of squamous cell carcinoma have been enumerated elsewhere. The pseudoglandular variant shows islands of neoplastic squamous cells with cleft-like formations evincing acantholysis. The spindle cell variant is sarcomatoid with spindle-shaped cells seen to stream off from the basal cell layer.

Differential Diagnosis: Early carcinoma with focal ulceration may be confused clinically with traumatic and granulomatous ulcers. Biopsy is required to obtain a definitive diagnosis.

Treatment: Superficial squamous and basal cell carcinomas of the lips and commissure can be successfully managed by wide surgical wedge resection.

References
1. Bernier, J. L. and Clark, M. L.: Squamous carcinomas of the lip. Milit. Surg. 109:379, 1951
2. Greene, G. W., Jr., and Bernier, J. L.: Spindle-cell squamous carcinoma of the lip. Oral Surg. 12:1008, 1959.
3. Tomich, C. E. and Hutton, C. E.: Adenoid squamous cell carcinoma of the lip. Report of cases. J. Oral Surg. 30:592, 1972.
4. Ellis, G. L. and Corio, R. L.: Spindle cell carcinoma of the oral cavity. A clinicopathologic asessment of fifty-nine cases. Oral Surg. 50:523, 1980.
5. Nuutinen, J., et al.: Local and distant metastases in patients with surgically treated squamous cell carcinoma of the lip. Clin. Otolaryngol. 6:415, 1981.

ORAL FISTULAE

Periapical Abscess and Osteomyelitis

Age: No predilection
Sex: No predilection

Clinical Features: Drainage tracts resulting from infection of odontogenic and periodontal origin are the most frequent forms of oral fistulae. They are most often encountered on the gingiva in close proximity to the tooth, acting as the source

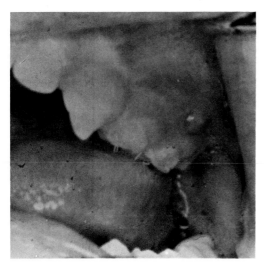

FIG. 4–20. Oral fistula associated with a periapical abscess.

of infection or adjacent to a focus of destructive or sclerosing osteomyelitis as evidenced radiographically. When a carious or traumatized noncarious tooth is present it will test nonvital with a vitalometer. The fistula contains a draining center from which a purulent exudate can often be expressed. Patients usually complain of a foul or metallic taste. Occasionally the fistula will be associated with a parulis.

Microscopic Features: The drainage tract is lined by subacutely inflamed granulation tissue and occasionally may evince a squamous epithelial lining. In either case, communication with inflamed granulation tissue in bone is observed.

Differential Diagnosis: A draining fistula may be clinically confused with traumatic ulcer, aphthous ulcer, or, rarely, carcinoma. Searching for an infectious source and probing the lesion with a periodontal probe or gutta-percha point will aid in obtaining a diagnosis.

When radiographic evidence of osteomyelitis exists, culture and sensitivity of the exudate, particularly for actinomycetes, should be pursued. When teeth are missing, search for a retained root tip is advisable.

Treatment: Infected teeth must be treated endodontically or, if nonrestorable, extracted. When osteomyelitis is present, antibiotic treatment with 250 mg of penicillin 4 times daily should be instituted and either maintaned or altered depending upon results of culture and sensitivity testing. When the patient is febrile with malaise and cel-

lulitis is present, hospitalization and intravenous antibiotic treatment may be indicated.

References

1. Shapiro, H. H., et al.: Spread of infection of dental origin. Oral Surg. 3:1407, 1950.
2. Smulson, M. H., Maggio, J. D., and Hagen, J. C.: Diseases of the pulp and periapex. In *Endodontic Therapy*, 3rd Ed., edited by F.S. Weine. St. Louis, C. V. Mosby Co., 1982, p. 142.

Periodontal Abscess

Age: Adults
Sex: No predilection

Clinical Features: An acute reaction to dental plaque irritants and bacteria may develop in periodontal pockets and in furcation areas. Whereas many periodontal abscesses drain via the sulcular pocket, others may spread through gingival tissues and perforate to form a fistula. The periodontally involved tooth may or may not be sensitive to percussion, and pain may be dull or severe. Constitutional signs of infection, including fever, malaise, and lymphadenopathy, may exist. Placing a probe into the periodontal pocket with mild manipulation will often elicit drainage of exudate

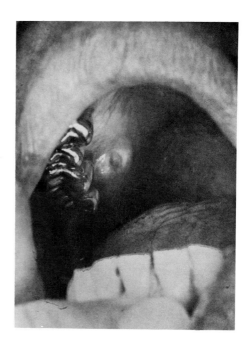

FIG. 4–21. Oral fistula associated with a periodontal abscess.

through the fistulous tract. When the pocket is deep and the abscess lies adjacent to lateral accessory root canals, retrograde pulpitis may ensue. Recurrent or multiple periodontal abscesses may be encountered in uncontrolled diabetics.

Microscopic Features: The zone of abscess formation shows infiltration by neutrophils and macrophages. Capillaries course through the abscess, and both necrotic debris and microbial colonies may be present. The fistula contains an acute inflammatory cell infiltrate and is usually lined by granulation tissue; however, epithelialization may develop.

Differential Diagnosis: Fistulae of periapical origin must be ruled out on a radiographic and clinical basis utilizing methods to ascertain pulp viability. Occasionally, a periodontal abscess may coexist with or indeed cause pulp necrosis. Specific infection by actinomycetes may be present and can be diagnosed by microbial anaerobic culture or biopsy.

Treatment: Periodontal curettage or flap surgery with elimination of the abscess is required. Root planing and periodontal therapy in general should be undertaken. If periodontal abscess exists in conjunction with pulp necrosis, either endodontic treatment or extraction is indicated.

References

1. Ray, H. G. and Orban, F.: Gingival structures in diabetes mellitus. J. Periodontol. 21:85, 1950.
2. Trott, J. R.: The acute periodontal abscess. J. Can. Dent. Assoc. 25:601, 1969.
3. Hall, B. W.: In *Oral Pathology*, edited by J. D. Spouge. St. Louis, C. V. Mosby Co., 1973, pp. 117–121.
4. O'Brien, J. J.: Diagnosis and treatment of periodontal and gingival abscesses. J. Ontario Dent. Assoc. 47:16, 1970.
5. Glickman, I.: *Clinical Periodontology*, 4th Ed. Philadelphia, W. B. Saunders Co., 1972, chap. 18.

Actinomycosis

Age: Young adults
Sex: Male predilection

Clinical Features: Either oral or extraoral fistulae may develop in an area of infection by Actinomyces israelii. The disease is most frequently encountered in the head and neck area and is acquired subsequent to tooth extraction or trauma. It usually manifests as an osteomyelitis with formation of granulation tissue and abscess in the submandibular region, producing so-called lumpy jaw. The infection may localize in periapical periodontal foci of inflammation. The organisms may be expressed though the fistulae and appear as

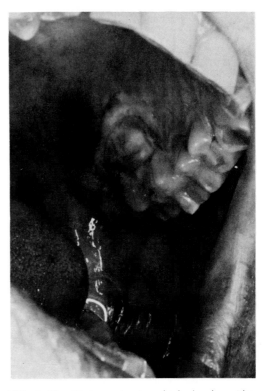

FIG. 4–22.   Drainage tracts, which develop either extraorally or intraorally in actinomycotic infection.

small yellow flecks termed sulfur granules. Anaerobic methods are required to culture the organism.

Microscopic Features: The granulation tissue in bone or underlying the fistulae shows foci of epithelioid histiocytes or localized abscesses. The microbial colonies are clove shaped, display a peripheral fringe, and are PAS-positive. They lie in the center of a sea of neutrophilic granulocytes.

Differential Diagnosis: Actinomycosis manifesting oral fistulae cannot be differentiated from nonspecific infection of pulpal or periodontal origin. Culture and biopsy will disclose the presence of actinomycotic microorganisms.

Treatment: The granulation tissue bed in bone should be curetted and the patient placed on antibiotics. Penicillin, one million units IM followed by 500 mg for 10 days, is the preferred treatment. In patients allergic to penicillin, erythromycin may be employed. If the disease fails to respond, massive intravenous doses of antibiotic may be required to achieve cure.

References

1. Porter, I.A.: Actinomycosis in the North-East of Scotland. Br. Med. J. 1:1360, 1951.

2. Kapsimalis, P., et al.: Actinomycosis of the periapical tissues. Oral Surg. 26:374, 1968.
3. Freeman, L. R., Zimmermann, E. E., and Ferrillo, P. J.: Conservative treatment of periapical actinomycosis. Oral Surg. 51:205, 1981.
4. Weir, J. C. and Buck, W. H.: Periapical actinomycosis; Report of a case and review of the literature. Oral Surg. 54:336, 1982.

Oroantral Fistula

Age: Adults
Sex: No predilection

Clinical Features: A fistula that traverses the maxillary alveolus, causing an oral-antral communication, may arise subsequent to tooth extraction in which a perforation of the antral floor developed. The fistula usually opens on the crest of the maxillary alveolar ridge, yet may exit in the mucobuccal fold area. The opening may be narrow or large and is usually devoid of erythema and purulent drainage. If residual inflammation exists in the maxilla or antral cavity, an exudate may be present. Occasionally, antral polyps will herniate through the fistula as a fluctuant bulbous tumefaction.

Microscopic Features: The fistula is lined by stratified squamous and often respiratory epithelium. The surrounding fibrous connective tissue evinces an inflammatory cell infiltrate of variable intensity.

Differential Diagnosis: Oroantral fistulae must be differentiated from fistulae developing from underlying osteomyelitis or actinomycosis. The location on the maxillary alveolus, history of extraction, and ability to probe through the defect into the antrum usually provide sufficient evidence to make the diagnosis. The presence of associated swelling or necrotic tissue could be indicative of a more serious disorder such as maxillary sinus carcinoma or mucormycosis. In this case a biopsy should be performed.

Treatment: The fistula should be curetted to disrupt the epithelialized communication, and a palatal flap can be rotated over the defect for primary closure. Gold or platinum foil may be employed during surgery to occlude the opening and facilitate tissue closure.

References
1. Clark, H. B., Jr.: *Practical Oral Surgery,* 3rd Ed. Philadelphia, Lea & Febiger, 1965, p. 168.
2. Anderson, M. F.: Surgical closure of oroantral fistula: report of a series. J. Oral Surg. 27:862, 1969.
3. Killey, H. C. and Kay, L. W.: An analysis of 250 cases of oro-antral fistula treated by buccal flap operation. Oral Surg. 24:726, 1967.
4. Goldman, E. H., Stratigos, G. T., and Arthur, A. L.: Treatment of oroantral fistula by gold foil closure: report of a case. J. Oral Surg. 27:875, 1969.
5. Wowren, N. V.: Oroantral communications and displacements of roots into the maxillary sinus: a follow-up of 231 cases. J. Oral Surg. 29:622, 1971.

Soft Tissue Abscess

Age: No predilection
Sex: No predilection

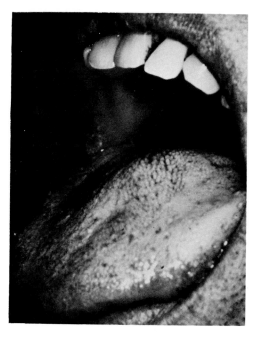

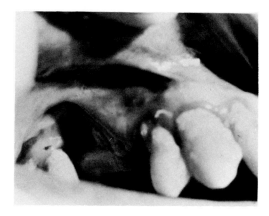

FIG. 4–23. Oroantral fistula representing a through-and-through communication between the oral cavity and antrum.

FIG. 4–24. Abscess formation in the soft tissues showing swelling with a focus of drainage.

Clinical Features: An abscess may develop in the submucosal connective tissues subsequent to a penetrating wound or introduction of a foreign body. Rarely, actinomyces may cause a soft tissue abscess. Any tissue site may be involved; however, the tongue and buccal mucosa are the most frequently affected locations. A tumefaction is usually palpable or visible subjacent to the site of drainage. Pain is often present, and compression of the area elicits exudation through the fistula.

Microscopic Features: Granulation tissue with foci of neutrophilic infiltration is observed. When a foreign body is present it is usually identifiable under ordinary or polarized light. Giant cells surround the foreign material. The fistulous tract is lined by granulation tissue.

Differential Diagnosis: A draining fistula in the soft tissues, since it is often associated with tumefaction, must be differentiated from specific granulomatous diseases and neoplasms that have become inflamed.

Treatment: Incision with curettage and drainage should be performed and the tissue submitted for microscopic examination to confirm the clinical impression.

If fever is present and the abscess is large, the patient should receive antibiotic therapy while culture and sensitivity are obtained.

Reference

1. Archer, W. H.: *Oral and Maxillofacial Surgery,* 5th Ed. Philadelphia, W. B. Saunders Co., 1975, pp. 490, 492.

Developmental Oral Sinuses

Age: From infancy
Sex: No predilection

Clinical Features: A variety of developmental fistulae and sinuses occur within the oral cavity. Some of these pits and fistulae fail to communicate with underlying structures or embryonic remnants whereas others do. Included in this group of developmental defects are: (1) fistula of the nasopalatine duct, (2) tonsilar faucial fistulae, (3) pits of the pterygomandibular fold, and (4) lingual thyroglossal sinus of the foramen cecum area. Most of these sinuses are blind and are devoid of inflammatory changes. Occasionally, oral pits and sinuses are associated with preauricular pits and deafness.

Microscopic Features: Not applicable.

Differential Diagnosis: The bilateral nature, location, and healthy tissue appearance allow for easy identification

Treatment: No treatment is necessary.

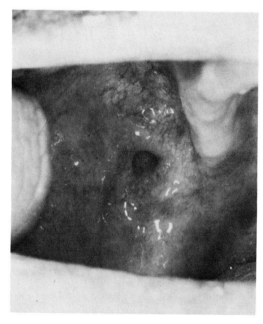

FIG. 4–25. Developmental sinus lateral to the pterygomandibular raphe.

References

1. Gorlin, R. J.: In *Thoma's Oral Pathology,* 6th Ed., edited by R. J. Gorlin and H. M. Goldman. St. Louis, C. V. Mosby Co., 1970, Vol. 1, pp. 46–47.
2. Claiborne, J. H., Jr.: Hiatus in the anterior pillar of the fauces of the right side with congenital absence of the tonsil on either side. Am. J. Med. Sci. *89*:490, 1885.
3. Campbell, E. H.: Perforation of the faucial pillars. Arch. Otolaryngol. *1*:503, 1925.
4. Hill, W. C. and Darlow, H. M.: Bilateral perforate nasopalatine communication in the human adult. J. Laryngol. Otolaryngol. *60*:160, 1945.
5. Leider, A. S., Lucas, J. W., and Eversole, L. R.: Sebaceous choristoma of the thyroglossal duct. Oral Surg. *44*:261, 1977.

Cutaneous Fistulae

Age: Developmental in the young, otherwise no predilection
Sex: No predilection

Clinical Features: Cutaneous fistulae of the face and neck represent a variety of pathologic processes; some are developmental, some are drainage tracts from infected teeth or underlying soft tissues, and others evolve secondary to trauma. Cutaneous draining fistulae of odontogenic origin are most common. The fistula is usually encountered over the chin or mandible and is associated with a periapically involved necrotic mandibular tooth. The

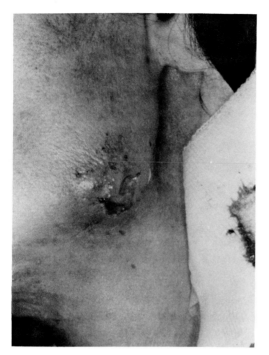

FIG. 4–26. Cutaneous fistula associated with odontogenic infection.

fistula will drain, then appear to heal, only to flare up again. Actinomycete infections will classically fester within the facial soft tissues and drain through fistulae on the skin. Actinomycosis is discussed in more detail in the chapter on extraoral swellings. Trauma or surgery to the parotid may inadvertently lead to duct severage with formation of a sialocele, which frequently drains onto the facial skin or into the ear or oral cavity. Lastly, a variety of developmental pits and sinuses are located on the face and neck including congenital aural sinuses, preauricular pits, second branchial sinuses or lateral cervical sinuses and thyroglossal sinuses. The sinuses are located, respectively, anterior to the ear, the upper lateral neck, and the anterior neck.

Microscopic Features: Sinuses of infectious or traumatic origin exhibit a linear tract filled with neutrophils and are lined by granulation tissue. Occasionally an epithelial lining develops. The developmental pits and sinuses are lined by epithelium, usually stratified squamous; however, the more interior recesses may evince a columnar or cuboidal appearance.

Differential Diagnosis: Sinuses of infectious origin usually present with a purulent discharge. All facial cutaneous sinuses should be evaluated for a dental source of infection. A parotid sinus is suspected when the tract exudes a clear fluid and overlies the gland. Sialography may aid in the diagnosis and, of course, a history of trauma or surgery to the gland is germane. Developmental sinuses, with the exception of the thyroglossal fistulae, usually fail to drain and are recognized by a lack of underlying soft tissue swelling along with a consideration of their location.

Treatment: Cutaneous sinuses of dental infectious origin require extraction or endodontic therapy of the incriminatory tooth. A plastic surgery procedure may then be required to correct the facial deformity. Parotid fistulae are treated surgically by duct anastomosis, ductoplasty, ligations, or tympanic neurectomy if repair procedures prove unsuccessful. Developmental pits and sinuses can be surgically excised and cosmetically corrected.

References

1. Pollock, W. F. and Stevenson, E. O.: Cysts and sinuses of the thyroglossal duct. Am. J. Surg. *112*:225, 1966.
2. Cowley, D. J. and Calman, J. S.: Pre-auricular fistulae in four generations: a study in heredity. Br. J. Plast. Surg. *24*:388, 1971.
3. Fradis, M., et al.: Actinomycosis of the face and neck. Arch. Otolaryngol. *102*:87, 1976.
4. Lewin-Epstein, J., Taicher, S., and Azaz, B.: Cutaneous sinus tracts of dental origin. Arch. Dermatol. *114*:1158, 1978.
5. Chadwick, S. J., Davis, W. E., and Templer, J. W.: Parotid fistula: current management. South. Med. J. *72*:922, 1979.
6. Avery, B. S.: A sialocele and unusual parotid fistulae—a case report. Brit. J. Oral Surg. *18*:40, 1980.

NECROTIC AND OSSEOUS DESTRUCTIVE LESIONS

Factitial Injury and Trauma

Age: No predilection
Sex: No predilection

Clinical Features: Self-inflicted wounds, chronic irritation and postsurgical defects may result in osseous or soft tissue perforations of the palate. Occasionally the palate will break down, leaving a defect after cleft palate repair. A large rhinolith may irritate the palatal roof, causing palatal perforation. The defects are usually clean with very little evidence of erythema, granulation tissue, or necrosis. Altered speech and difficulty in eating are found.

Microscopic Features: Not applicable.

Differential Diagnosis: Palatal perforations re-

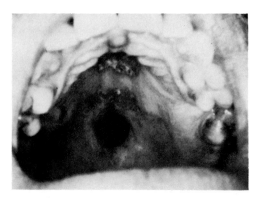

FIG. 4–27. Open communication between the oral cavity and nasal cavity that developed as a result of irritation from a large rhinolith.

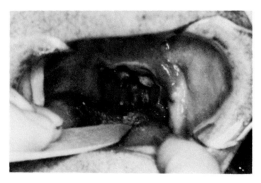

FIG. 4–28. Midline lethal granuloma showing destruction of the soft palate. (Courtesy of Dr. T. Daniels.)

sulting from factitial injury as a result of trauma or as sequelae to surgical intervention may simulate other osseous destructive lesions included in this section. The clean noninflamed character and a thorough history will usually provide information sufficient to secure the diagnosis. A biopsy will rule out other entities of a more serious nature.

Treatment: The defect may be occluded with a dental prosthesis or may be closed surgically with the aid of a palatal flap.

References

1. Grabb, W. C.: In *Cleft Lip and Palate,* edited by W. C. Grabb, S. W. Rosenstein, and K. R. Bzoch. Boston, Little, Brown & Co., 1971, p. 385.
2. Archer, W. H.: *Oral and Maxillofacial Surgery,* 5th Ed. Philadelphia, W. B. Saunders Co., 1975, pp. 1616, 1621.

Midline Lethal Granuloma and Wegener's Granulomatosis

Age: Adults
Sex: Female predilection

Clinical Features: Midline lethal granuloma is an immunopathologic collagen disease in which granulation tissue replaces normal osseous and soft tissues of the midline structure of the face, including the nasal septum, nose, palate, and nasopharynx. The palate may be perforated with an osseous destructive lesion bordered by inflamed granulation tissue. With time the entire midface may be destroyed with involvement of the orbits. Wegener's granulomatosis is a sytemic collagen disease that can manifest the same destructive and ulcerative lesions of the face and oral cavity. In addition, erythematous granular tumefactions may be encountered on the gingiva and other mucosal sites. Widespread manifestations are present with granulomatous and destructive lesions of the kidneys and lungs.

Microscopic Features: The granulomatous tissue surrounding the defects is infiltrated with mononuclear cells and a foreign-body type of multinucleated giant cell. Scattered eosinophils are occasionally observed. The sine qua non of the histomorphology is the presence of necrotizing vasculitis. Special stains fail to disclose the presence of specific bacterial or fungal microorganisms.

Differential Diagnosis: The palatal perforation and midfacial destructive lesions of these two granulomatous inflammations must be differentiated microscopically from malignant reticulosis, gummatous necrosis, mucormycosis, and antral carcinoma.

Treatment: These diseases are serious disorders, and Wegener's granulomatosis is lethal. They are treated with immunosuppressive drugs such as high-dose steroids or Imuran and should be managed by a physician.

References

1. Brown, H. A. and Woolner, L. G.: Findings referable to the upper part of the respiratory tract in Wegener's granulomatosis. Ann. Otol. 69:810, 1960.
2. Kassel, S. H., et al.: Midline malignant reticulosis (so-called lethal midline granuloma). Cancer 23:920, 1969.
3. Eichel, G. S. and Maybery, T. T.: The enigma of the lethal midline granuloma. Laryngoscope 78:1367, 1968.
4. Edwards, M. B. and Buckerfield, J. P.: Wegener's granulomatosis: A case with primary mucocutaneous lesions. Oral Surg. 46:53, 1978.
5. Flye, M. W., Mundinger, G. H., and Fauci, A. S.: Diagnostic and therapeutic aspects of the surgical approach to Wegener's granulomatosis. J. Thorac. Cardiovasc. Surg. 77:331, 1979.

Tertiary Syphilis

Age: Elderly adults

Sex: Male predilection

Clinical Features: Gummatous necrosis of the oral tissues frequently involves the palate. The gumma is rubbery with necrotic rolled margins and often sloughs, leaving a relatively clean vacant perforation of the palate. Following a course of antibiotic therapy, large masses of necrotic tissue may be lost (Herxheimer's reaction). Other signs of tertiary syphilis will be encountered: psychotic behavior with illusions of grandeur, luetic glossitis, other foci of gummatous necrosis, aortic aneurysm, peripheral neuropathy, and tabes dorsalis. The VDRL is positive at this late stage; however, the lesions are essentially noninfective.

Microscopic Features: The tissue adjacent to the zone of palatal perforation shows foci of eosinophilic necrotic aggregates, and the surrounding granulation tissue evinces a mononuclear inflammatory cell infiltrate. Treponemal organisms are usually not demonstrable.

Differential Diagnosis: Palatal perforation by syphilitic gumma may be confused clinically with Wegener's granulomatosis, midline lethal granuloma, malignant reticulosis, mucormycosis, and antral carcinoma. Other clinical signs and symptoms that aid in arriving at a diagnosis of syphilis are usually present. A VDRL serologic evaluation should be obtained.

Treatment: Tertiary syphilis should be managed by a physician because many of its ramifications involve various organ systems.

References

1. Huebsch, R. F.: Gumma of the hard palate with perforation. Oral Surg. 8:690, 1955.
2. Meyer, I. and Shklar, G.: The oral manifestations of acquired syphilis. Oral Surg. 23:45, 1967.
3. Penneau, M., et al.: Syphilitic necrosis of the incisive bone. Rev. Stomatol. Chir. Maxillofac. 81:392, 1980.
4. Ramstad, T. and Traaholt, L.: Destruction of the soft palate and nose by tertiary "benign" syphilis. A case report. J. Oral Rehabil. 7:111, 1980.

Osteoradionecrosis

Age: Elderly adults

Sex: Male predilection

Clinical Features: Patients who have received cancericidal radiation to the jaws experience a vascular derangement in the osseous tissues that severely compromises the inflammatory defense of the tissue to the onslaught of infection. Odontogenic or periodontal infection may become rampant and spread quickly through the bone. The mandible is much more susceptible than the maxilla. Oral fistulae develop in the involved area, with sequestration of large fragments of necrotic bone. Indeed, the entire alveolar ridge may show ulceration and drainage with exposure of nearly half the mandible. Lesions are usually exudative with a foul odor. Pain is invariably present. Radiographically, moth-eaten radiolucencies with opaque sequestra are observed. The risk of developing osteoradionecrosis is less with newer supravoltage radiation sources such as the linear accelerator, betatron, and cobalt 60 machines.

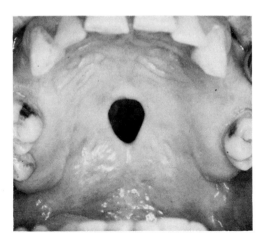

FIG. 4–29. Gumma formation in tertiary syphilis resulting in destruction of the midpalatal region. (Courtesy of Dr. V. Chalian.)

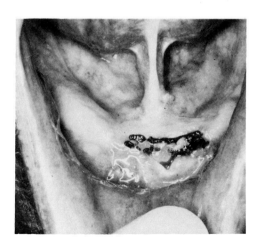

FIG. 4–30. Osseous sequestrum in a patient who received radiation for a mandibular alveolar ridge squamous cell carcinoma.

Microscopic Features: The soft tissues display necrosis with an acute or subacute inflammatory cell infiltrate. The osseous tissue lacks lacunar osteocytes; the marrow spaces contain necrotic debris, microbial colonies, and a neutrophilic infiltrate not unlike nonspecific acute osteomyelitis.

Differential Diagnosis: Since osteoradionecrosis is located chiefly in the mandible, it is not likely to be confused with the other osseous destructive draining lesions included in this section. At any rate, a history of radiation therapy in excess of 6000 rads will confirm a diagnosis of osteoradionecrosis. Recurrent tumor in the area must be ruled out by biopsy when tumefaction surrounds or infiltrates the involved osseous tissue.

Treatment: Sequestra should be carefully removed and the area debrided. When extensive areas of necrosis are present, surgical intervention should be delayed. The patient requires hospitalization with supportive care and intravenous antibiotic therapy. Hyperbaric oxygen therapy has been shown to be effective in facilitating healing in some cases. Prevention is the key to management. All pulpally or periodontally infected teeth should be extracted or treated prior to radiation; post-therapeutically, patients should be placed on a strict oral hygiene program with inclusion of daily topical application of fluoride gels to the remaining dentition.

References

1. Motila, E. and Westerholm, N.: Osteoradionecrosis of the jaw. Odontol. Tidskr. *73*:239, 1965.
2. Cook, H. P.: Tooth extraction and radiation therapy of the mouth. Br. Dent. J. *120*:372, 1966.
3. Pappas, G. C.: Bone changes in osteoradionecrosis. Oral Surg. *27*:622, 1969.
4. Hart, G. B. and Mainous, E. G.: The treatment of radiation necrosis with hyperbaric oxygen (OHP). Cancer *37*:2580, 1976.
5. Silverman, S., Jr.: Radiation effects. *In* Oral Cancer. New York, The American Cancer Society, 1981, p. 66.

Mucormycosis

Age: No predilection
Sex: No predilection

Clinical Features: Mucormycosis is an infection caused by one of the phycomycetes and is not pathogenic unless the patient is suffering from debilitating illness. Patients with diabetes or widespread lymphoma and those receiving antitumor chemotherapeutic agents are the most frequent sufferers. The antrum is usually the site of origin of the infection. As the antrum becomes progressively eroded by necrotic and granulation tissues,

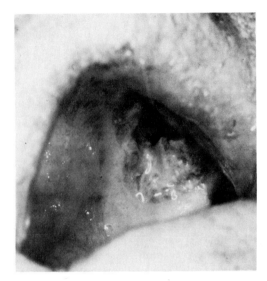

FIG. 4–31.   Necrotic osseous destruction of the palate in antral mucormycosis.

perforation ensues with osseous destruction and oroantral fistula formation. Anesthesia or paresthesia of the second division of the trigeminal nerve frequently occurs. The infected antrum is opacified on panoramic or Water's sinus radiographs, and evidence of bony erosion of the antral walls can be visualized, especially on tomograms. Aspergillosis may manifest features identical to those of mucormycosis when the antrum is involved.

Microscopic Features: The granulation and necrotic tissues contain colonies of large hyalinized basophilic hyphae that are devoid of septae. Inflammatory cells, chiefly neutrophils and eosinophils, prevail in the granulation tissue that is located peripheral to widespread zones of necrosis. Vascular invasion by the microorganism is common and results in ischemic necrosis with infarction.

Differential Diagnosis: Palatal osseous destructive lesions of mucormycosis may simulate nonspecific oroantral fistula, midline lethal granuloma, Wegener's granulomatosis, and malignant disease. A history of diabetes should arouse suspicion of mucormycosis. Biopsy will disclose the presence of the infectious agent.

Treatment: Since mucormycosis is a secondary invader, the underlying medical illness must be treated concurrently with the infection. Intravenous amphotericin B is the antibiotic of choice.

References

1. Savetsky, .L. and Waltner, J.: Aspergillosis of the maxillary antrum. Arch. Otolaryngol. 74:695, 1961.
2. Taylor, C. G., et al.: Mucormycosis (polycomycosis) involving the maxilla. Oral Surg. 27:806, 1969.
3. Blitzer, A., et al.: Patient survival factors in paranasal sinus mucormycosis. Laryngoscope 90:635, 1980.
4. Breiman, A., Sadowsky, D., and Friedman, J.: Mucormycosis. Discussion and report of a case involving the maxillary sinus. Oral Surg. 52:375, 1981.
5. Rosenberg, S. W, and Lepley, J. B.: Mucormycosis in leukemia. Oral Surg. 54:26, 1982.

Antral Carcinoma

Age: Elderly adults
Sex: Male predilection

Clinical Features: Cancer of the maxillary sinus develops insidiously and is extensive when per-

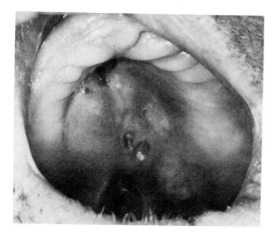

FIG. 4–32. Multiple sites of ulceration and palatal destruction in antral carcinoma.

foration of bone occurs. The carcinoma may extend and perforate through any of the antral walls. The palate is a frequent site, with formation of osseous destructive zones rimmed by necrotic tissue. Tumefaction may herniate through the perforation; however, the oroantral communication is more often a simple ulcerated perforation. The malar skin often shows erythema with facial swelling. Displacement of the nasal septum and globe is also frequently encountered. Second-division anesthesia or paresthesia is a frequent symptom. Water's sinus, panographic, and antral tomograms show opacification and osseous destruction of the sinus walls.

Microscopic Features: Tissue removed from around the site of perforation shows infiltrating islands, cords, and nests of tumor cells. Their morphology varies from squamous to adenomatous differentiation. Metastatic tumors and sarcomas may also arise in the antrum and invade the palate.

Differential Diagnosis: When antral carcinoma extends into the oral cavity with palatal perforation, other osseous destructive lesions including midline lethal granuloma, syphilitic gumma, and mucormycosis must be considered in the differential diagnosis.

Treatment: Antral carcinoma carries an extremely poor prognosis. It is treated surgically, radiotherapeutically, or with a combination of the two and should be managed by an oncologist.

References

1. Chaudhry, A. P., et al.: Carcinoma of the antrum. Oral Surg. 13:269, 1960.
2. Frazell, E. L. and Lewis, J. S.: Cancer of the nasal cavity and accessory sinuses; a report of the management of 416 patients. Cancer 16:1293, 1963.
3. Ahmad, K., Cordoba, R. B., and Fayos, J. V.: Squamous cell carcinoma of the maxillary sinus. Arch. Otolaryngol. 107:48, 1981.
4. Merrick, R. E., Rhone, D. P., and Chilis, T. J.: Malignant fibrous histiocytoma of the maxillary sinus. Arch. Otolaryngol. 106:365, 1980.

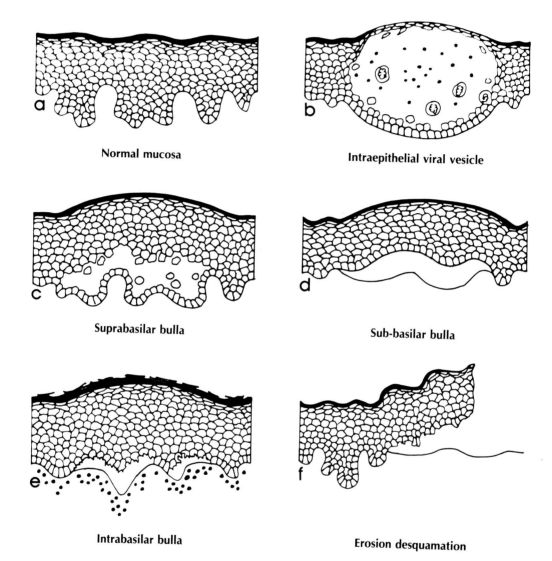

Normal mucosa

Intraepithelial viral vesicle

Suprabasilar bulla

Sub-basilar bulla

Intrabasilar bulla

Erosion desquamation

Vesiculobullous Lesions

5
Vesiculobullous and Desquamative Lesions

FEBRILE-ASSOCIATED VESICULAR ERUPTIONS

    Herpetic Gingivostomatitis
    Herpangina
    Hand-foot-and-mouth Disease
    Primary Varicella-zoster
    Secondary Varicella-zoster

NONFEBRILE-ASSOCIATED VESICULAR ERUPTIONS

    Recurrent Herpes Stomatitis
    Recurrent Herpes Labialis
    Contact Vesicular Stomatitis
    Impetigo

BULLOUS DISEASES

    Pemphigus Vulgaris
    Bullous Pemphigoid
    Benign Mucous Membrane Pemphigoid
    Bullous Lichen Planus
    Erythema Multiforme
    Stevens-Johnson Syndrome
    Epidermolysis Bullosa
    Dermatitis Herpetiformis

DESQUAMATIVE LESIONS

    Gingivosis
    Erosive Lichen Planus
    Toothpaste Idiosyncrasy Lesions

Vesicles are fluid-filled blisters measuring less than 5 mm; *bullae* are blisters in excess of 5 mm. On skin, vesicles and bullae are bleb-like and tense. In the oral cavity, both vesicles and bullae are more flattened with a smooth gelatinous surface. Because of chronic masticatory forces and a less rigid epithelial surface, oral vesicles and bullae are prone to rupture, leaving ulcerative and desquamative lesions later in the course of disease. When ulcers, erosions, and desquamations are observed in the mouth, a search should be made to detect intact fluid-filled surface lesions; the history should be investigated for indications that the early lesions were blister-like from onset.

When attempting to differentiate between a disease that is primarily vesicular and one that is bullous, the size of the individual lesions is the key to diagnosis. One must, however, be cognizant of the fact that vesicles often cluster together and may appear bullous. For this reason, close observation to detect a clustering phenomenon is necessary.

The vesicular diseases are primarily infectious and, specifically, most are the result of assault by viral organisms that propagate in epithelial cells and/or underlying nerve fibers. Of utmost importance in arriving at a definitive diagnosis is evaluation of the patient's temperature. For this reason, vesicular eruptions of the mouth have been divided into those associated with elevated temperature and those in which the patient is afebrile. The latter group may occasionally manifest mild elevation in temperature; if detected, it is invariably less than 100°F. When viral infections are suspected, a cytologic smear of intact vesicular contents often reveals the presence of viral-specific nuclear ballooning degeneration or inclusion bodies. The specific diagnosis of viral vesicular eruptions is obtained by observing the pattern of distribution of the lesions. These features are enumerated for each entity.

The bullous dermatoses are skin diseases characterized by bulla formation. All of the diseases included here manifest precedent or coexistent oral bullae. One disease, benign mucous membrane pemphigoid, is limited to the mucous membranes. The bullous lesions themselves may appear identical from one disease to the next. Biopsy is mandatory to arrive at a definitive diagnosis in most cases. Some of the entities in this group show specific site distributions or are accompanied by skin manifestations that evince a diagnostic pattern or configuration. These features are detailed in the text.

A final group of disorders in this chapter are those in which large areas of epithelial detachment occur. Bullae do not form; rather, diffuse zones of sloughing or desquamation ensue and are often accompanied by intense erythema.

The most common vesicular diseases are primary herpetic gingivostomatitis and secondary herpes labialis. Frequent recurrences of shingles may accompany underlying malignant lymphoma.

Most of the bullous dermatoses are rare. Erythema multiforme is the most common disease in this group. Pemphigus vulgaris and certain forms of epidermolysis bullosa are potentially lethal.

All three diseases included with the desquamative group are relatively common, erosive lichen planus being most prevalent. None is lethal.

FEBRILE-ASSOCIATED VESICULAR ERUPTIONS

Herpetic Gingivostomatitis

Age: Children and young adults
Sex: No predilection

Clinical Features: Primary infection with herpesvirus hominis type 1 of the oral cavity is characterized by multiple vesicular eruptions located on the attached gingiva and movable mucosa, chiefly the lips and buccal mucosa. Type 2 herpesvirus can also cause primary herpetic gingivostomatitis, being transmitted by either oral-oral or genito-oral routes. The vesicles rapidly rupture, leaving a raw or white pseudomembranous erosion. Erythema surrounds the vesicular and ulcerative zones. The oropharynx is involved only occasionally. The lesions are painful, and eating is a significant problem. The temperature is elevated

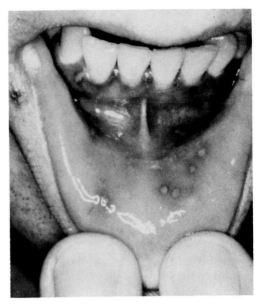

FIG. 5–1. Marginal gingivitis with ulceration accompanied by small vesicles with erythematous halos that rapidly desquamate to yield small ulcers in primary herpetic gingivostomatitis.

and may approach 103 to 104°F. Constitutional symptoms of inflammatory disease, including malaise and cervical lymphadenopathy, are present. The disease is contagious; however, most individuals exposed to it are either already immune or suffer only subclinical manifestations such as transient fever. During the course of infection antiherpes antibody titer is elevated. The disease runs its course in 10 to 14 days, and healing develops without scar formation. Rarely, complications develop, particularly in debilitated children and infants. The Pospischill-Feyrter syndrome and Kaposi's varicelliform eruption are disseminated herpes infections that are potentially lethal. Herpesvirus infections may also occur on the facial skin and conjunctiva. Contact with infected patients by dentists and oral health auxiliary personnel who have never been exposed to the disease may result in herpetic whitlow, a viral dermatitis of the finger.

Microscopic Features: Intraepithelial vesicle formation is seen with necrotic exudate and a neutrophilic infiltrate. Eosinophilic inclusion bodies (Lipshutz bodies) in the vesicular space are accompanied by epithelial cells showing nuclear ballooning degeneration. These viral-specific changes are not obvious in ulcerated vesicles.

Differential Diagnosis: The vesiculoulcerative

lesions of herpes are often confused with recurrent aphthae. Aphthae are not associated with a highly elevated temperature, and there is a history of recurrent episodes. Herpetic gingivostomatitis does not recur intraorally, with the exception of recurrent herpetic stomatitis, which manifests microvesicles localized unilaterally on the palatal gingiva. Primary herpes can be differentiated from Coxsackie virus infections on the basis of lesional distribution, the latter being localized to the oropharynx. Shingles, which is seen in older individuals and with unilateral lesions, can be ruled out on the basis of age and distribution. The gingival lesions of primary herpes can be confused with acute necrotizing ulcerative gingivitis; however, the latter fails to show vesicles on nongingival mucosa.

Treatment: Supportive care consists of prescribing a soft diet: milkshakes, baby foods, and liquids. Aspirin will reduce fever and pain. A soothing mouth rinse composed of equal parts of an antihistamine elixir with Kaopectate is useful in adults. One percent viscous lidocaine is recommended for children. Severe orofacial herpes infections may develop in immunocompromised patients; in such instances treatment with acyclovir is recommended. Whereas this antiviral medication is beneficial, cases have been reported in which a mutant organism evolves and escapes treatment with acyclovir.

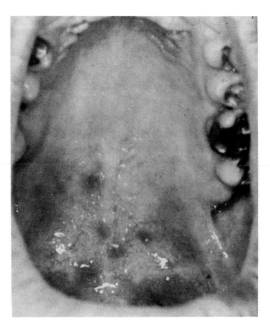

FIG. 5–2. Multiple erythematous vesicles limited to the soft palate and oropharynx in herpangina, a Coxsackie virus infection.

References

1. Lennette, E. H. and Magoffin, R. L.: Virologic and immunologic aspects of major oral ulcerations. J. Am. Dent. Assoc. 87:1055, 1973.
2. Silverman, S., Jr., and Beumer, J., III: Primary herpetic gingivostomatitis of adult onset. Oral Surg. 36:496, 1973.
3. Saral, R., et al.: Acyclovir prophylaxis of herpes-simplex-virus infections: a randomized, double-blind controlled trial in bone-marrow-transplant recipients. N. Engl. J. Med. 305:63, 1981.

Herpangina

Age: Children

Sex: No predilection

Clinical Features: Infection with Coxsackie viruses of both A and B groups may produce herpangina. The disease is limited to the oropharynx with vesicles located primarily on the soft palate and faucial pillars. Extension anteriorly is rare. The lesions are painful and are accompanied by generalized oropharyngitis evidenced by erythema of the throat. The vesicles tend to cluster and become ulcerated 3 to 4 days after onset. Fever, malaise, lymphadenitis, headache, and sore throat develop. The disease shows an incubation period of 1 week or less and runs its course in the same amount of time. Meningitis is a complication but is usually self-limited. The disease is contagious, and outbreaks among school-age children are common.

Microscopic Features: Intraepithelial vesicles contain an eosinophilic exudate, and nuclear ballooning degeneration of epithelial cells is a feature.

Differential Diagnosis: Herpangina must be differentiated from infection by herpesvirus and varicella-zoster virus and, when ulceration predominates, from aphthae. The limitation of lesions to the soft palate/faucial region is essentially diagnostic. Virus may be retrieved from stool specimens by tissue culture techniques.

Treatment: A palliative oral rinse such as an antihistamine elixir mixed 50:50 with Kaopectate is advised. Soft diet and antipyretics are recommended as well.

References

1. Cherry, J. D. and Hahn, C. L.: Herpangina: the etiologic spectrum. Pediatrics 36:632, 1965.
2. Lennette, E. H. and Magoffin, R. L.: Virologic and immunologic aspects of major oral ulcerations. J. Am. Dent. Assoc. 87:1055, 1973.
3. Chawareewong, S., et al.: Neonatal herpangina

caused by Coxsackie A-5 virus. J. Pediatr. 93:492, 1978.

Hand-foot-and-mouth Disease

Age: Children and young adults
Sex: No predilection

Clinical Features: Group A Coxsackie viruses of the enterovirus group are responsible for the vesicular eruption of hand-foot-and-mouth disease. The disease is more often seen in spring and summer in preschool and school children and is mildly contagious. The distribution of lesions is pathognomonic in that, after a short incubation period, vesicles with an erythematous halo appear in the oral cavity, on the hands, and on the feet. The oral lesions are located primarily on the lips and buccal mucosa, sparing the oropharynx. Within 24 to 48 hours the oral vesicles rupture, leaving erosions or ulcerations with a white or grey pseudomembrane. The extremity lesions are limited to the skin below the knees and elbows, are vesicular with circumferential erythema, and are located on both dorsal and ventral surfaces of the hands and feet. All lesions are painful, and constitutional signs of infection include elevated temperature, malaise, and lymphadenopathy.

Microscopic Features: Intraepithelial vesicles are seen in the early stages with intracytoplasmic eosinophilic inclusion bodies. Later stages are characterized by shallow ulcerations and erosions with regeneration of the marginal epithelium. A superficial inflammatory cell infiltrate is present in the submucosa.

Differential Diagnosis: The oral vesiculoulcerative lesions are similar to those encountered in herpetic gingivostomatitis, herpangina, varicella, and aphthous stomatitis. The distribution of lesions in hand-foot-and-mouth disease is diagnostic and eliminates these other entities from consideration. Coxsackie virus can be cultured from stool specimens.

Treatment: Antipyretic-analgesics, soft or liquid diet, fluids, and a soothing oral rinse such as an antihistamine elixir mixed 50:50 with Kaopectate are recommended. Viscous lidocaine may be employed in small children.

References

1. Cherry, J. D. and Jahn, C. L.: Hand, foot and mouth syndrome. Pediatrics 37:637, 1966.
2. Southam, J. C. and Colley, I. T.: Hand, foot, and mouth disease. Br. Dent. J. 125:298, 1968.
3. Cawson, R. A. and McSwiggan, D. A.: An outbreak of hand, foot and mouth disease in a dental hospital. Oral Surg. 27:451, 1969.
4. Buchner, A.: Hand, foot, and mouth disease. Oral Surg. 41:333, 1976.

Primary Varicella-zoster (Chickenpox)

Age: Children
Sex: No predilection

Clinical Features: Chickenpox is a dermal vesicular exanthem caused by the varicella-zoster virus. The incubation period lasts 2 to 3 weeks. The

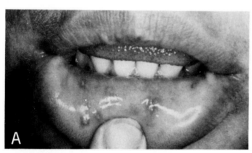

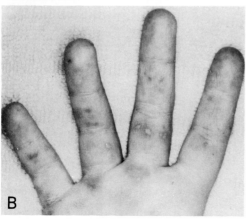

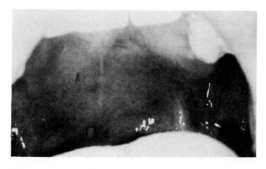

FIG. 5–3. Hand-foot-and-mouth disease, caused by a Coxsackie virus and showing vesiculoulcerative lesions of the oral mucous membranes *(A)* accompanied by a vesicular eruption of the hands *(B)* and feet.

FIG. 5–4. Focal vesicles seen in the mouth, usually the soft palate area in children with the typical dermal vesicular exanthem of chickenpox.

lesions are located primarily on the trunk and face, are vesicular with an erythematous boundary, and are extremely pruritic. Fever, malaise, and mild generalized lymphadenopathy are present. Oral manifestations are common, with early onset of vesicles that rapidly rupture and leave erosions with a surface pseudomembrane. These are limited in extent. The palatal mucosa is the predominant oral location. The lesions resolve within 5 to 8 days.

Microscopic Features: Superficial intraepithelial vesicle formation is present. The vesicular contents contain eosinophilic exudate, inflammatory cells, and epithelial cells. Nuclear ballooning degeneration is a feature. A superficial submucosal inflammatory cell infiltrate is discernible.

Differential Diagnosis: Oral vesiculoulcerative lesions of chickenpox resemble those of herpes, the Coxsackie viruses, and aphthae. The skin lesions predominate and must be differentiated from smallpox and Kaposi's varicelliform eruption, the latter caused by dermatotrophic herpesvirus. Antibody titers to varicella-zoster are elevated.

Treatment: Whereas complications are rare, it is nevertheless recommended that children with chickenpox be managed by a pediatrician. Oral lesions may be treated palliatively with viscous lidocaine.

References
1. Blank, H. and Rake, G.: *Viral and Rickettsial Diseases of the Skin, Eye, and Mucous Membranes of Man.* Boston, Little, Brown and Co., 1955.
2. Lennette, E. H. and Magoffin, R. L.: Virologic and immunologic aspects of major oral ulcerations. J. Am. Dent. Assoc. 87:1055, 1973.
3. Myers, M. G.: Varicella and herpes zoster: Comparisons in the old and young. Geriatrics 32:77, 1977.
4. Badger, G. R.: Oral signs of chickenpox (Varicella): Report of two cases. ASDC J. Dent. Child. 47:349, 1980.

Secondary Varicella-zoster (Shingles)

Age: Adults and elderly

Sex: Slight male predilection

Clinical Features: Shingles is caused by reactivation of varicella-zoster virus and may be conceptualized as a recurrent form of chickenpox. In the secondary or recurrent form, it is neurodermatropic. The virus propagates within ganglia, and the vesicular eruption follows the distribution of sensory nerves, being segmental and unilateral. Prodromal neuralgia is followed by clustered vesicular eruptions. Whereas the thoracic and abdominal nerves are most frequently involved, the

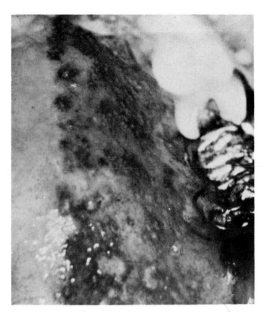

FIG. 5–5. Reactivation by the varicella-zoster virus, which causes shingles. The lesions begin as small vesicles that are unilateral, with a tendency to follow the sensory nerve pathways. (Courtesy of Dr. H. M. Cherrick.)

mucosa supplied by the second or third division of the trigeminal nerve may be the site of infection if the virus is harbored and propagated within the Gasserian ganglion. The vesicles are unilaterally distributed, stop at the midline, and are extremely painful. Patients experiencing multiple recurrent episodes of shingles have been shown to be at risk for lymphoma, leukemia, and carcinomatosis; a single episode does not connote any increased risk for malignancy. After healing of shingles post-herpetic neuralgia may develop. The disease has a 1- to 3-week incubation period, and the vesicular stage may persist for 1 to 5 weeks. Constitutional signs of infectious disease, including elevated temperature, malaise, and lymphadenitis, are apparent.

Microscopic Features: The epithelium manifests intraepithelial vesicles with epithelial nuclear ballooning degeneration. The subjacent submucosa contains a mononuclear inflammatory cell infiltrate.

Differential Diagnosis: Oral vesiculoulcerative eruptions of shingles mimic those observed in herpesvirus, Coxsackie virus, and aphthous stomatitis. Unilateral segmental distribution, prevalence in adults, and severe pain are features that allow for clinical differentiation. Antibody titers to varicella-zoster virus are elevated. Systemic malignancy should be ruled out.

Treatment: Varicella-zoster virus infections in the form of shingles restricted to the oral mucosa can be treated by prescribing soft or liquid diet, analgesic-antipyretic medication, and a palliative oral rinse such as an antihistamine elixir mixed with equal parts of Kaopectate. Should multiple recurrent episodes occur, referral to a physician or dermatologist is recommended; search for underlying lymphoma, leukemia, or widespread cancer must be undertaken.

References
1. Chaconas, C. P.: Herpes zoster, a primary manifestation of chronic lymphocytic leukemia. Oral Surg. *14*:942, 1961.
2. Nally, F. F. and Ross, I. H.: Herpes zoster of the oral and facial structures. Report of five cases and discussion. Oral Surg. *32*:221, 1971.
3. Eisenberg, E.: Intraoral isolated herpes zoster. Oral Surg. *45*:214, 1978.
4. Ragozzino, M. W., et al.: Risk of cancer after herpes zoster. A population-based study. N. Engl. J. Med. *307*:393, 1982.

NONFEBRILE-ASSOCIATED VESICULAR ERUPTIONS

Recurrent Herpes Stomatitis

Age: Young adults
Sex: No predilection

Clinical Features: Recurrent infection of the oral mucosa by herpesvirus hominis type 1 is uncommon. When it occurs, it is restricted to the palatal gingiva unilaterally and is characterized by the formation of microvesicles that rapidly rupture to leave small punctate ulcerations with a tendency to cluster. Even less common is the appearance of vesicles of the buccal mandibular gingiva in the vicinity of the mental foramen. The lesions are slightly painful and persist for only 5 to 7 days. Fever and malaise are usually not present.

Microscopic Features: The epithelium contains small vesicles with epithelial nuclear ballooning degeneration. The submucosa displays a mild mononuclear inflammatory cell infiltrate.

Differential Diagnosis: Recurrent oral herpetic vesicular eruptions are distributed unilaterally and must be differentiated from the lesions of shingles. Since pain is not severe and resolution is rapid, the distinction can usually be made. Antiherpes antibody titers are elevated during the course of infection. Differentiation from recurrent aphthae is not difficult; intraoral recurrent herpes lesions are microvesicles or tiny clustering punctate ul-

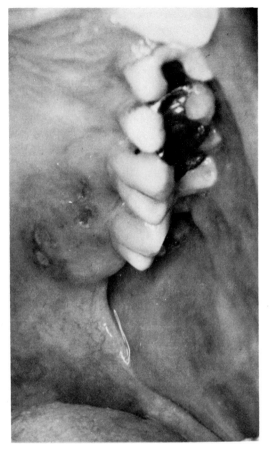

FIG. 5–6. Clustered painful microvesicles, which quickly rupture, classically confined to the palatal gingiva in recurrent intraoral herpes stomatitis.

cerations of attached mucosa, whereas aphthae do not tend to involve mucosa fixed to bone.

Treatment: No treatment is necessary. Elective palliative mouth rinses may be employed.

References
1. Griffin, J. W.: Recurrent intraoral herpes simplex virus infections. Oral Surg. *19*:209, 1965.
2. Southam, J. C.: Recurrent intraoral herpes simplex infections. Br. Dent. J. *127*:276, 1969.
3. Muller, S. A.: Recurrent herpes simplex of the hard palate. Arch. Derm. *98*:273, 1968.
4. Weathers, D. R. and Griffin, J. W.: Intraoral ulcerations of recurrent herpes simplex and recurrent aphthae: two distinct clinical entities. J. Am. Dent. Assoc. *81*:81, 1970.
5. Sheridan, P. J. and Herrmann, E. C.: Intraoral lesions of adults associated with herpes simplex virus. Oral Surg. *32*:390, 1971.

Recurrent Herpes Labialis

Age: Adults
Sex: No predilection

Clinical Features: Recurrent infection of the lips by herpesvirus hominis type I is herpes labialis. Vesicles occur in clusters on the vermilion border and adjacent perioral skin of the lips. Edema, which may be quite severe, and erythema underlie the vesicles. The patient is usually afebrile. The vesicles are associated with pain. Because of their location, they are unsightly. The oral cavity is free of disease. Various factors trigger the infection, including trauma and sunlight (ultraviolet light) exposure, even though the patients possess antiherpes antibody. Evidence implicates a latent property to the virus, which may remain sequestered from the immune system by residing in ganglia. During latent periods, no symptoms or lesions are encountered.

Microscopic Features: Cytologic smears of nonruptured vesicles disclose the presence of nuclear ballooning degeneration. Microscopic sections are represented by the presence of intraepithelial vesicles with the same cytologic changes already specified for primary herpes. The submucosa or dermis evinces an inflammatory cell infiltrate.

Differential Diagnosis: Recurrent herpes labialis shows vesicles that may be confused with impetigo or contact dermatitis. Focal clustering of lesions, history of trauma or sun exposure, tendency to occur in young adults, lack of linear streaking, and inability to correlate onset with contact by a potential allergen aid in eliminating these latter diseases from consideration. A cytologic smear of vesicular contents will disclose the presence of viral-specific cytologic alterations.

Treatment: Photoactivated dye treatments are contraindicated in light of studies implicating carcinogenic transformation. Topical application of 5-idoxyuridine to early lesions usually allows for early resolution; other topical antiviral agents have not been proven to be efficacious. Acyclovir has been effective topically in herpes genitalis, and both adenosine and L-lysine administered parenterally may inhibit formation of recurrent lesions in some patients. Subsequent to rupture of the vesicles, a topical steroid cream (one-quarter to one-half percent hydrocortisone) with antibiotic can be applied. Steroid-antibiotic preparations can be combined with 1 percent anesthetics to achieve pain control. Caution should be taken not to prescribe steroid creams during the early infective stage of the disease (i.e., the first 3 to 4 days).

References

1. Ship, I. I.: Virus and viral-like diseases of the mouth. Postgrad. Med. *38*:499, 1965.
2. Jaffe, E. C. and Lehner, T.: Treatment of herpetic stomatitis with idoxuridine. Brit. Dent. J. *125*:392, 1968.
3. Shklar, G.: Oral reflections of infectious diseases. 1. Postgrad. Med. *49*:87, 1971.
4. Sklar, S. H.: Adenosine in the treatment of recurrent herpes labialis. Oral Surg. *48*:416, 1979.
5. Corey, L. et al.: A trial of topical acyclovir in genital herpes simplex virus infections. N. Engl. J. Med. *306*:1313, 1982.

Contact Vesicular Stomatitis

Age: No predilection
Sex: No predilection

Clinical Features: Immediate or humoral-mediated immune reactions to allergens contacting the oral mucous membranes may manifest vesicle formation. The vesicles do not tend to cluster and are superimposed on a broad matted erythematous base. Pain or burning, rather than pruritus, is present. Vesicles arise in areas of allergenic contact and will therefore be seen on perioral skin if cosmetics are the offending substances. Intraorally, various substances may elicit hypersensitivity responses in patients who are allergic. Specifically, mouthwashes, dentifrices, acrylic, topical antibiotics, and foods can be incriminated. Perhaps more frequently, oral allergic eruptions of the immediate type arise subsequent to a systemically introduced allergen such as shellfish, berries, or drugs. Allergic stomatitis is much less common then atopic dermatitis. The lesions regress

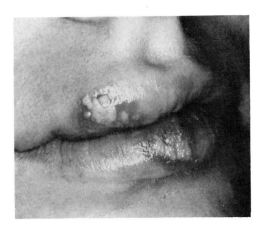

FIG. 5–7.   Vesicular eruptions of the lips with erythema and edema typically encountered in recurrent herpes labialis (cold sores).

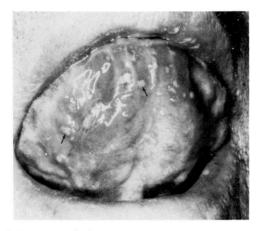

FIG. 5–8.   Multiple vesicles and small ulcers appearing as a manifestation of allergy to various mouth rinses, dentifrices, dental materials, foods, and drugs.

within 3 to 5 days providing repeated contact with allergen is avoided.

Microscopic Features: Intraepithelial vesicles are present. The vesicular contents are composed of an eosinophilic exudate and an acute inflammatory cell infiltrate composed of both neutrophils and eosinophils. The submucosa is traversed by dilated capillaries and is infiltrated with leukocytes.

Differential Diagnosis: The vesicular eruption of allergic mucositis may resemble primary herpes, hand-foot-and-mouth disease, and erythema multiforme. Since the patient is afebrile, this feature tends to eliminate the aforementioned diseases from the differential diagnosis. Questioning of the patient with regard to the use of newly contacted materials or chemicals will usually provide the necessary clue to the nature of the allergen. Those substances suspected of being allergenic may be applied to the buccal mucosa for epimucous patch testing. This is accomplished by mixing suspected allergens with Orabase and applying to the buccal mucosa. A positive reaction may be seen in 24 to 48 hours.

Treatment: Suspected contact allergens should be discontinued. Antihistamines, 50 mg of Benadryl or 12.5 mg of Phenergan twice daily will effect an early resolution of vesicles and associated discomfort.

References
1. Zakon, S. J., et al.: Lipstick cheilitis. Arch. Dermatol. Syph. *56:*499, 1947.
2. Laubach, J. L., et al.: Cheilitis caused by cinnamon oil in toothpaste. J. Am. Med. Assoc. *152:*404, 1953.

3. Goldman, L. and Farrington, J.: Stomatitis with glossitis following oral therapy with penicillin tablets. Arch. Dermatol. *57:*399, 1958.
4. Rickles, N. H.: Allergy in surface lesions of the oral mucosa. Oral Surg. *33:*744, 1972.
5. Eversole, L. R.: Allergic stomatitis. J. Oral Med. *34(4),* October-December, 1979.

Impetigo

Age: Children
Sex: No predilection

Clinical Features: Impetigo is a vesicular eruption seen on the perioral skin and vermilion border. Oral mucosa is not affected. The lesions are caused by staphylococci or a mixed staphylococcal-streptococcal infection. They are painful and pruritic and, since the patient scratches the lesions, they are excoriated and eroded. Scratching causes implantation of organisms, so that a linear or serpentine configuration of vesicles occurs. The disease is contagious.

Microscopic Features: Intraepithelial vesicles are engorged with neutrophils. The submucosa evinces a subacute inflammatory cell infiltrate.

Differential Diagnosis: Perioral vesicles of impetigo must be differentiated from those seen in recurrent herpes labialis and contact dermatitis. Involvement is usually more widespread with impetigo than with herpes, and the presence of linear tracks of vesicles is highly suggestive of impetigo. A cytologic smear of an intact vesicle will rule out viral-specific cytologic changes.

Treatment: Topical application of bacitracin, neomycin, and polymyxin is recommended.

References
1. Markowitz, M., et al.: The bacteriologic findings, streptococcal immune response, and renal compli-

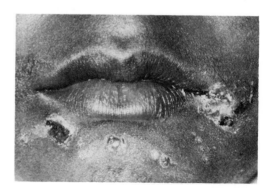

FIG. 5–9.   Excoriated clustering vesicles occurring in crops and linear streaks on the perioral skin in impetigo. (Courtesy of Drs. S. Rovin and W. Sabes.)

cations in children with impetigo. Pediatrics 35:393, 1965.

2. Hughes, W. T.: Impetigo contagiosa in children. GP 36:78, 1969.

3. Peter, G., et al.: Group A streptococcal infections of the skin and pharynx. N. Engl. J. Med. 297:311, 1977.

4. Fleisher, G.: Pediatric skin, soft tissue, and bone infections. Del. Med. J. 52:587, 1980.

BULLOUS DISEASES

Pemphigus Vulgaris

Age: Middle-aged and elderly adults

Sex: No predilection

Clinical Features: Pemphigus vulgaris is an immunopathologic dermatologic disease characterized by bulla formation. Oral lesions are invariably present at some time in the course of the disease and may actually precede the development of skin lesions in as many as 50 percent of the affected population. The oral bullae begin as bleb-like blisters or diffuse gelatinous plaques. Rupture of the bullae occurs within a few days, leaving broad areas of desquamation with associated erythema. The lesions are usually painful. Generalized desquamative lesions of the attached gingiva are commonly encountered. Rubbing uninvolved skin or mucosa may elicit the formation of a bullous lesion (Nikolsky's sign). Instances of pemphigus-like lesions have been reported to evolve subsequent to administration of certain drugs, particularly penicillamine. If left untreated, the disease may be fatal. Patients die from dehydration and septicemia through exposed denuded bullae of the skin.

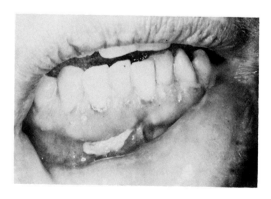

FIG. 5–10. Bullous lesion accompanied by a desquamative gingivitis with pemphigus vulgaris. (From Eversole, L. R., Kenney, E. B., and Sabes, W. R.: Oral lesions as the initial sign in pemphigus vulgaris. Oral Surg. 33:354, 1972.)

Microscopic Features: Biopsy should be performed on intact bullae when possible. The epithelium displays a suprabasilar cleft with round, smooth epithelial cells (acantholytic, Tzanck cells), found suspended in the bullous cavity. In vivo bound immunoglobulins can be detected in the intercellular cement regions, and patients with active disease have circulating antibodies directed to intercellular cementing substance.

Differential Diagnosis: When only oral bullae are present, pemphigus may be indistinguishable from the other bullous dermatoses listed in this section. A biopsy is required to confirm the diagnosis. Occasionally, pemphigus lesions are confined to the gingiva. If this is the case, gingivosis should be considered in the differential diagnosis.

Treatment: Pemphigus vulgaris should be treated by a general physician or dermatologist as high-dose, long-term systemic steroid therapy is required for control of the disease. With severe dermal involvement, fluid/electrolyte balance must be controlled and septicemia must be prevented. Levamisole in conjunction with prednisone allows for lower steroid dosage.

References

1. Beutner, E. H., et al.: Autoantibodies in pemphigus vulgaris: response to intercellular substance of epidermis. J. Am. Med. Assoc. 192:682, 1965.

2. Shklar, G.: The oral lesions of pemphigus vulgaris. Oral Surg. 23:629, 1967.

3. Eisenberg, E., et al.: Pemphigus-like mucosal lesions: A side effect of penicillamine therapy. Oral Surg. 51:409, 1981.

4. Laskaris, G.: Oral pemphigus vulgaris: An immunofluorescent study of fifty-eight cases. Oral Surg. 51:626, 1981.

5. Lozada, F., Silverman, S., and Cram, D.: Pemphigus vulgaris. A study of six cases treated wtih levamisole and prednisone. Oral Surg. 54:161, 1982.

Bullous Pemphigoid

Age: Adults

Sex: No predilection

Clinical Features: Bullous pemphigoid is an immunopathologic bullous dermatosis characterized by bulla formation of skin. Lesions are located primarily in the axillary and inguinal and abdominal regions. They begin as erythematous and eczematous plaques that ultimately progress to bullae. Occasionally, but not invariably, the oral mucosa is affected. The bullae are tense blebs or broad gelatinous plaques. As in the other oral bullous disorders, rupture with desquamation takes place shortly after the lesions appear. The disease

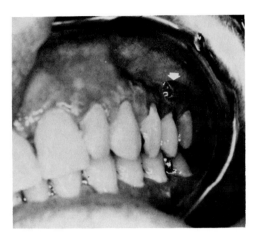

FIG. 5–11. Bullous pemphigoid, a bullous dermatosis of skin occasionally accompanied by oral bulla. (Courtesy of Dr. H. M. Cherrick.)

is annoying yet not usually fatal; nevertheless, septicemia may be a complication. There is some evidence that patients with bullous pemphigoid accompanied by oral lesions are more likely to develop malignancies elsewhere in the body.

Microscopic Features: The bullae are subepithelial. The bullous roof in an early lesion possesses well-aligned and polarized basal cells while the connective tissue floor is devoid of or shows only mild infiltration by mononuclear cells. Patients with active disease show high antibody titers of immunoglobulins that specifically bind to basement membrane.

Differential Diagnosis: Bullous pemphigoid must be differentiated from the other bullous dermatoses listed in this section. The restriction of lesions to the axillary and inguinal intertriginous zones is typical for pemphigoid. Biopsy is required to arrive at a definitive diagnosis. Immunofluorescent antibody testing to detect antibasement membrane antibodies may be useful in the diagnosis.

Treatment: Bullous pemphigoid is treated by systemic steroids. Dapsone has also been shown to be effective in the management of the disease; however, red cell suppression may be a complication. The disease, being a primary cutaneous disorder, should be managed by a dermatologist.

References

1. Beutner, E. H., et al.: The immunopathology of pemphigus and bullous pemphigoid. J. Invest. Dermatol. 51:63, 1968.
2. Shklar, G., et al.: Oral lesions in bullous pemphigoid. Arch. Dermatol. 99:663, 1969.
3. Person, J. R. and Rogers, R. S., III: Bullous pemphigoid responding to sulfapyridine and the sulfones. Arch. Dermatol. 113:610, 1977.
4. Hodge, L., et al.: Bullous pemphigoid: The frequency of mucosal involvement and concurrent malignancy related to indirect immunofluorescent findings. Br. J. Dermatol. 105:65, 1982.

Benign Mucous Membrane Pemphigoid

Age: Middle-aged and elderly adults
Sex: Female predilection

Clinical Features: Benign mucous membrane pemphigoid (BMMP) is a bullous disorder that resembles bullous pemphigoid, yet the bullae have a predilection for mucous membranes. The oral cavity and conjunctivas are favored sites, although

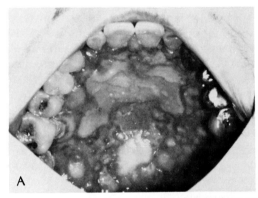

A

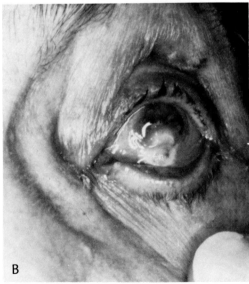

B

FIG. 5–12. *A:* Benign mucous membrane pemphigoid, a bullous disorder showing extensive oral bullae on an erythematous base. *B:* Accompanying bullae with a tendency for scarring of the bulbar and palpebral conjunctivas. (Courtesy of Dr. A. Leider.)

pharyngeal, anal, and vaginal lesions are present in half the patients. Bullae of the facial, neck, and genital skin are also occasionally present. The oral bullae develop slowly and vary in size. They are tense or gelatinous plaques. Desquamation of the gingiva is also a frequent finding. The eye lesions are found on both palpebral and bulbar conjunctivas and tend to heal with scarring. Fibrous bands extend from the lid to the sclera and are termed symblepharon. This finding, in conjunction with oral bullae, is essentially diagnostic for BMMP. The disease is not lethal and follows a protracted course. The major complication is entropion with blindness.

Microscopic Features: The bullous lesions are subepithelial with an intact basal cell layer on the roof. The submucosa in early lesions shows minimal inflammation. These features are identical to those encountered in bullous pemphigoid. Antibasement membrane antibodies in serum can be detected yet are present in very low titers.

Differential Diagnosis: The oral lesions of BMMP are similar in appearance to those of the other bullous dermatoses, but they develop more slowly and tend to be smaller and less extensive. The eye lesions are characteristic, and when oral biopsy discloses subepithelial bullae a clinicopathologic diagnosis can be obtained.

Treatment: Low-dose systemic steroid therapy consisting of 20 mg of prednisone in divided doses daily can be employed until control of lesions is achieved, after which medication is withdrawn until new lesions develop. Dapsone has also been found to be effective. Topical triamcinolone in Orabase or 0.05 percent Lidex mixed with equal parts of Orabase can be applied 4 to 6 times daily to oral bullous and desquamative lesions.

References

1. Harris, M.: Pemphigoid (benign mucous membrane pemphigus). Br. J. Oral. Surg. 5:42, 1967.
2. Shklar, G. and McMarthy, P. L.: Oral lesions of mucous membrane pemphigoid: a study of 85 cases. Arch. Otolaryngol. 93:354, 1971.
3. Dabelsteen, E., et al.: Demonstration of basement membrane autoantibodies in patients with benign mucous membrane pemphigoid. Acta Derm. Venereol. 54:189, 1974.
4. Person, J. R. and Rogers, R. S., III.: Bullous and cicatricial pemphigoid: Clinical, histopathologic, and immunopathologic correlations. Mayo Clin. Proc. 52:54, 1977.
5. Lozada, F.: Prednisone and azathioprine in the treatment of oral inflammatory mucocutaneous disease. Oral Surg. 52:257, 1981.
6. Rogers, R. S., III, Seehafer, J. R., and Perry, H. O.: Treatment of cicatricial (benign mucous membrane) pemphigoid with dapsone. J. Am. Acad. Dermatol. 6:215, 1982.

Bullous Lichen Planus

Age: Middle-aged adults
Sex: Slight female predilection

Clinical Features: Whereas lichen planus is typically a white lesion, erosive and bullous variants occur. The latter are quite uncommon. The oral bullae are most often encountered on the buccal mucosa and appear as flattened gelatinous bullous plaques surrounded by zones of erythema. Often, but not invariably, white lesions or striae can be found adjacent to bullae or in other intraoral locations. Burning discomfort or mild pain may be a complaint. Skin lesions are present in some instances. The disease is benign and chronic.

Microscopic Features: The diagnostic features of bullous lichen planus are most obvious on the margin of the lesion. A subepithelial separation is present. The roof of the bulla is composed of disoriented fragmented basal cells lacking polarization. The floor shows fragmented basal cells overlying fibrous tissue with a zonal superficial infiltrate of lymphocytes. The margin of the bulla blends with mucosa showing the microscopic features typical of the conventional type of lichen planus.

Differential Diagnosis: When white striae are present in conjunction with bullae, providing the microscopic features are typical, the diagnosis is easily determined. When only bullae are present,

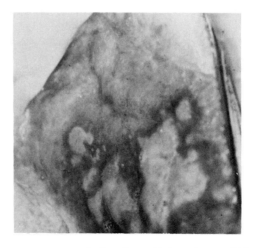

FIG. 5–13.   Rare bullous form of lichen planus, which may or may not show white striae in conjunction with the bullous lesions.

bullous lichen planus may be clinically indistinguishable from other bullous dermatoses. Biopsy is then required for a definitive diagnosis.

Treatment: Topical application of 1 percent triamcinolone in Orabase or 0.05 percent Lidex 50:50 with Orabase is useful in controlling the bullous and erythematous component of the disease but will not eliminate the white lesions that may be present.

References

1. Haselden, F. G.: Bullous lichen planus. Oral Surg. *24:*4, 1967.
2. Andreason, J. O.: Oral lichen planus. 1. A clinical evaluation of 115 cases. Oral Surg. *25:*31, 1968.
3. Goldstein, B. H.: Immunofluorescent findings in oral bullous lichen planus. J. Oral Med. *34(1):*8, 1979.

Erythema Multiforme

Age: Young adults

Sex: Male predilection

Clinical Features: Erythema multiforme is a dermatologic disorder that is often but not invariably precipitated by allergens such as sulfa drugs. Precedent herpes infection is a common finding in many instances in which no allergen can be

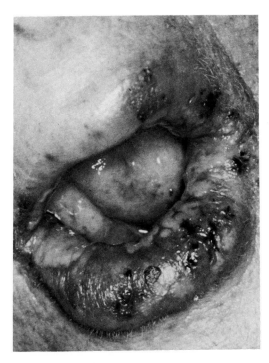

FIG. 5–14.   Vesiculobullous lesions with a tendency to hemorrhage seen throughout the oral mucosa, with predilection for the lips and vermilion border.

identified. The disease manifests a variety of lesions of skin and mucosa including bullae, macules, erosions, and, on skin, an erythematous circular wheal with a circumferential halo, the so-called target or iris lesion. The oral cavity is usually involved. Bullae develop and rapidly burst, leaving raw erosions with desquamation and underlying erythema. Whereas any oral tissue can be involved, the lips are almost constantly affected with painful exudative erythematous erosions. Occasionally oral lesions are seen without dermatologic manifestations. A slightly elevated temperature is commonly detected. The disease runs its course in 2 to 5 weeks.

Microscopic Features: The bullae or desquamating regions generally manifest a junctional separation; however, this feature is not consistent throughout, as zones of irregular intraepithelial separation are usually encountered. The upper spinous and parakeratin layers often contain vesicular pools of eosinophilic coagulum (mucopolysaccharide-keratin dystrophy). The subjacent fibrous connective tissue evinces a subacute inflammatory cell infiltrate.

Differential Diagnosis: The bullous lesions of erythema multiforme are clinically similar to those of the other bullous dermatoses. Severe involvement of the lips, target lesions of skin, and slight elevation of temperature are signs indicative of erythema multiforme. Biopsy should be performed to rule out the other bullous dermatoses. Localization of lesions on the oral, conjunctival, and genital mucous membranes are typical for Stevens-Johnson syndrome, a variant of erythema multiforme.

Treatment: Systemically administered antihistamines, antipyretics, and a palliative oral rinse such as antihistamine oral expectorant mixed 50:50 with Kaopectate are recommended. In more severe cases, 20 mg of prednisone in divided doses may be required. Fluid intake should be maintained and the patient should be placed on a soft diet.

References

1. Shelley, W. B.: Herpes simplex virus as a cause of erythema multiforme. J. Am. Med. Assoc. *201:*153, 1967.
2. Wooten, J. W., et al.: Development of oral lesions in erythema multiforme exudativum. Oral Surg. *24:*808, 1967.
3. Al-Ubaidy, S. S. and Nally, F. F.: Erythema multiforme: Review of twenty-six cases. Oral Surg. *41:*601, 1976.
4. Lozada, F. and Silverman, S., Jr.: Erythema multi-

forme: Clinical characteristics and natural history of fifty patients. Oral Surg. *46*:628, 1978.

5. Buchner, A., Lozada, F., and Silverman, S., Jr.: Histopathologic spectrum of oral erythema multiforme. Oral Surg. *49*:221, 1980.

Stevens-Johnson Syndrome

Age: Young adults
Sex: Male predilection

Clinical Features: Stevens-Johnson syndrome is a form of erythema multiforme in which bullous and erosive erythematous lesions are found in the oral cavity, on the bulbar and palpebral conjunctivae, and on the external genitalia (glans penis, vulva). Typical iris or target skin erythematous wheals are often present as well. The oral manifestations of Stevens-Johnson syndrome may be confused with other bullous dermatoses. The oral lesions invariably involve the lips as a diffuse hemorrhagic exudative bullous eruption. Sulfa drugs are often found to precipitate this syndrome, which may be fatal if no treatment is rendered.

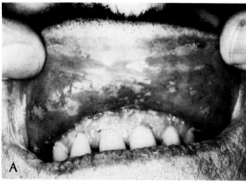

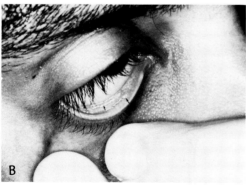

FIG. 5–15. The Stevens-Johnson syndrome, representing a specific form of erythema multiforme in which the oral mucosa *(A)*, conjunctiva *(B)*, and genital mucosa manifest a vesiculobullous eruption.

Microscopic Features: See erythema multiforme.

Differential Diagnosis: The bullous and erosive lesions of Stevens-Johnson syndrome may be confused with other bullous dermatoses. The triad of oral, eye, and genital involvement is classic for Stevens-Johnson syndrome. This distribution should not present a problem when differentiating this disease from the muco-oculocutaneous lesions of Behcet's syndrome and Reiter's disease since these latter two disorders manifest aphthous-like ulcerations rather than desquamating bullae of the oral cavity.

Treatment: Any allergenic drug or food should be withdrawn. The disease is then managed as outlined for erythema multiforme. Systemic steroids should be employed in severe cases, as fatalities in Stevens-Johnson syndrome associated with sulfa drugs have been recorded.

References

1. Robinson, H. M., Jr., and McCrumb, F. R., Jr.: Comparative analysis of the mucocutaneous-ocular syndromes. Arch. Dermatol. Syph. *61*:539, 1950.
2. Coursin, D. B.: Stevens-Johnson syndrome: Nonspecific parasensitivity reaction? J. Am. Med. Assoc. *198*:113, 1966.
3. Chanda, J. J., et al.: Erythema multiforme and the Stevens-Johnson syndrome. South. Med. J. *71*:566, 1978.
4. Yetiv, J. Z., et al.: Etiologic factors of the Stevens-Johnson syndrome. South. Med. J. *73*:599, 1980.

Epidermolysis Bullosa

Age: Children and young adults
Sex: No predilection

Clinical Features: An autosomally inherited disorder, epidermolysis bullosa simplex shows bulla formation of the skin over joints, primarily

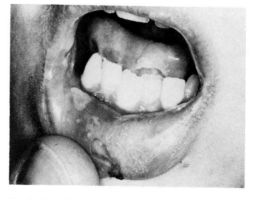

FIG. 5–16. Oral lesions accompanying bullous, scarring lesions located on skin over joints, a manifestation of epidermolysis bullosa. (Courtesy of Dr. J. Mink.)

the fingers, toes, knees, and elbows; bullae of the oral mucosa are encountered only rarely. The dystrophic type is subdivided into a mild and a severe form. The former is dominant, while the latter is inherited as a recessive trait. Lesions occur in the same regions as the simplex form, yet tend to burst and heal with scarring resulting in a cicatricial taut skin over joints. Oral lesions are more often present with the dystrophic forms. The fourth variant of epidermolysis bullosa, also transmitted recessively, is the lethalis form. This type develops during infancy, and death is imminent in a few months. (Indeed, all forms of epidermolysis bullosa have their onset at birth or during infancy.)

Microscopic Features: All forms show subepithelial bulla formation with an intact basal cell layer on the roof of the bulla. Nontraumatized bullae show only a minimal inflammatory cell infiltrate in the submucosa.

Differential Diagnosis: Oral bullae may appear similar to those of other bullous dermatoses; only epidermolysis bullosa, however, shows a predilection for children. Lesions located over joints and familial involvement are important clinical features differentiating this group of diseases from other dermatoses.

Treatment: No effective treatment can be offered. The parents of affected children should receive genetic counselling.

References

1. Winstock, D.: Oral aspects of epidermolysis bullosa. Br. J. Dermatol. 74:431, 1962.
2. Lowe, L. G., Jr.: Hereditary epidermolysis bullosa. Arch. Dermatol. 95:587, 1967.
3. Pearson, R. W., Potter, B., and Strauss, F.: Epidermolysis bullosa hereditaria lethalis. Arch. Dermatol. 109:349,1974.
4. Album, M. M., et al.: Epidermolysis bullosa dystrophica polydysplastica. Oral Surg. 43:859, 1977.

Dermatitis Herpetiformis

Age: Middle-aged adults
Sex: Male predilection

Clinical Features: Dermatitis herpetiformis is an immunopathologic vesiculobullous disease of skin rarely showing oral manifestations. The skin lesions are pruritic and are located primarily on the extremities and buttocks. They are vesicular with a tendency to rupture and desquamate. No specific intraoral tissue site predilection has been noted; the lesions may be bullous or erythematous. The disease is chronic, lasting for many years, yet is not life threatening.

Microscopic Features: The epithelium displays

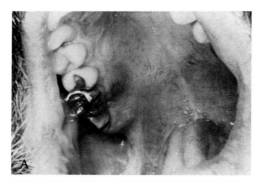

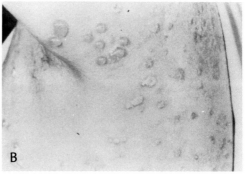

FIG. 5–17. *A:* Palatal gingiva bulla with erythematous halo in dermatitis herpetiformis. *B:* Bullous skin lesions. (Courtesy of Dr. H. Schneidman.)

a subbasilar separation with a subacute inflammatory infiltrate located in the dermal or submucosal papilla zones. The predominant cell type is the eosinophil. Lumps of immunoglobulin A can be demonstrated in the dermal papilla area with immunofluorescent staining.

Differential Diagnosis: The oral lesions of dermatitis herpetiformis are similar in appearance to those of the other bullous dermatoses. The clustered vesicles with pigmented base on the skin are highly suggestive, but not pathognomonic for the disease. Biopsy will disclose characteristic features.

Treatment: Since the disease is primarily a dermatologic disorder, referral to a dermatologist is recommended. Dermatitis herpetiformis responds to sulfapyridine therapy; steroids are not particularly useful.

References

1. Russotto, S. G. and Ship, I.I.: Oral manifestations of dermatitis herpetiformis. Oral Surg. 31:42, 1971.
2. Fraser, N. G., Kerr, N. W., and Donald, D.: Oral lesions in dermatitis herpetiformis. Br. J. Dermatol. 89:439, 1973.

3. Katz, S. I., et al.: Dermatitis herpetiformis: the skin and the gut. Ann. Intern. Med. 93:857, 1980.

4. Hall, R. P., et al.: Dermatitis herpetiformis. Springer Semin. Immunopathol. 4:33,1981.

DESQUAMATIVE LESIONS

Gingivosis (Desquamative Gingivitis)

Age: Middle-aged adults

Sex: Exclusive female predilection

Clinical Features: Gingivosis is a specific desquamative disease occurring after menopause and is confined to the attached gingiva. Since the clinical and microscopic features of the disease are very similar to those encountered in benign mucous membrane pemphigoid (BMMP), some investigators and clinicians have suggested that gingivosis is a form of BMMP that is merely confined to gingiva. True bullae do not develop; rather, the epithelium shows desquamation with a shaggy grey membrane. Bullae may be induced with an occlusally directed air jet or the tissue may be rubbed off with gauze. The underlying gingiva is edematous and erythematous. Contact with acidic or spicy foods may cause a severe burning sensation. The condition is not alleviated by dental prophylaxis. It persists for 1 to 5 years and eventually spontaneously resolves. Etiology is unknown.

Microscopic Features: A junctional separation occurs, with maintenance of an intact basal cell layer adherent to the desquamated tissue. The underlying submucosa manifests an intense chronic inflammatory cell infiltrate with numerous dilated capillaries.

Differential Diagnosis: The desquamation of the gingiva as seen in gingivosis may also occur in many of the bullous dermatoses including pemphigus vulgaris. Erosive lichen planus and toothpaste idiosyncrasy reactions may show features similar to gingivosis; however, the former usually shows extragingival lesions and the latter lacks an erythematous component.

Treatment: The patient should avoid spicy or acidic foods. A palliative mouth rinse may be used and topically applied triamcinolone in Orabase or 0.05 percent Lidex 50:50 with Orabase is sometimes, but not always, beneficial in minimizing the inflammatory component.

References

1. Ziskin, D. E. and Zegarelli, E. V.: Chronic desquamative gingivitis. Am. J. Orthod. Oral Surg. 31:1, 1945.

2. Scopp, I. W.: Desquamative gingivitis. J. Periodontol. 35:149, 1964.

3. Glickman, I. and Smulow, J. B.: Chronic desquamative gingivitis: Its nature and treatment. J. Periodontol. 35:297, 1964.

4. Nisengard, R. J., Alpert, A. M., and Krestow, V.: Desquamative gingivitis: Immunologic findings. J. Periodontol. 49:27, 1978.

Erosive Lichen Planus

Age: Middle-aged adults

Sex: Female predilection

Clinical Features: The erosive form of lichen planus is as frequently encountered as the nonerosive type. The lesions are most frequently located on the gingiva, mucobuccal fold, and buccal mucosa. The erosions and zones of desquamation are accompanied by erythema. Pe-

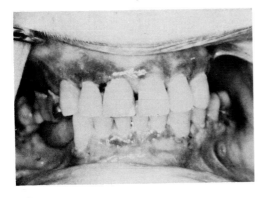

FIG. 5–18. Gingivosis characterized by an erythematous gingivitis accompanied by desquamation. The lesions are confined to the gingiva and fail to resolve following removal of dental plaque.

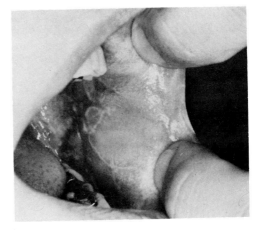

FIG. 5–19. The erosive form of lichen planus showing white striae accompanied by intense redness with superficial sloughing of the mucosa.

ripheral to the erosive lesions are white plaques or typical reticulated striae. Mild to moderate pain or burning is a common complaint. This form of lichen planus is also often associated with diabetes mellitus and hypertension, a triad known as the Grinspan syndrome. Instances of carcinomatous transformation in erosive lichen planus have been infrequently reported; the incidence is higher than that seen in nonaffected population. The disease runs a protracted course and may or may not be associated with skin manifestations. The oral lesions partially resolve in one region only to reappear at some new site. Many patients are prone to anxiety. Oral and cutaneous lesions identical to lichen planus are occasionally encountered in patients receiving gold therapy and other drugs such as antimalarials and penicillamine. Bone marrow graft recipients may also develop lichenoid mucocutaneous lesions.

Microscopic Features: At the margin of the erosions, the histomorphologic features typical of lichen planus are encountered. Transition is seen, whereby the epithelium becomes detached from the underlying chronically inflamed submucosa. Damage with disorientation of the basal cell layer is an important diagnostic feature.

Differential Diagnosis: When confined to gingiva, erosive lichen planus may simulate gingivosis. Erosive lichen planus is usually, however, multifocal and not localized to gingiva. Careful examination will usually disclose the presence of white striae. Since the microscopic features are pathognomonic, a biopsy should be performed.

Treatment: Topical application of 1 percent triamcinolone in Orabase or 0.05 percent Lidex mixed in equal parts with Orabase should be applied to lesional tissue 4 to 6 times each day. Maximal effects are observed if contact can be maintained overnight. The white component is not controlled with topical steroids.

References

1. Haselden, F. G.: Bullous lichen planus. Oral Surg. 24:472, 1967.
2. Silverman, S., Jr., and Griffith, M.: Studies on oral lichen planus. Oral Surg. 37:705, 1974.
3. Lozada, F. and Silverman, S., Jr.: Topically applied fluocinonide in an adhesive base in the treatment of oral vesiculoerosive diseases. Arch. Dermatol. 116:898, 1980.
4. Shulman, H. M., et al.: Chronic graft-versus-host syndrome in man. Am. J. Med. 69:204, 1980.
5. Seehafer, J. R., et al.: Lichen planus–like lesions caused by Penicillamine in primary biliary cirrhosis. Arch. Dermatol. 117:140, 1981.

Toothpaste Idiosyncrasy Lesions

Age: No predilection
Sex: No predilection

Clinical Features: Certain dentifrices, usually those containing fluoride salts, cause a superficial desquamation or slough of the cornified layer in susceptible patients. The reaction does not appear to represent a true form of allergy, but is more consistent with a mild irritant reaction; it is rather uncommon. The buccal mucosa and mucosal surfaces of the lips show a very thin white membrane that is easily dislodged by rubbing with gauze. Pain and erythema are lacking. The disease resolves when the causative agent is withdrawn.

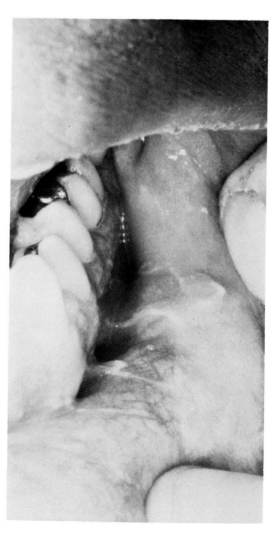

FIG. 5–20. Superficial sloughing of the mucosal cornified layer in response to specific dentifrices.

Microscopic Features: Biopsy at the margin of the zonal slough reveals a separation beneath the corneum without vesicle formation, and transmigration of leukocytes into epithelium and submucosa is not a feature.

Differential Diagnosis: Erosive lichen planus and gingivosis must be considered in the differential diagnosis. Absence of white striae, erythema, and pain or burning should limit the diagnosis to toothpaste idiosyncrasy reaction. The clinical diagnosis can be confirmed if the desquamation resolves after withdrawal of the suspected causative dentifrice.

Treatment: The patient should abstain from the use of toothpaste for one week, after which a bland nonfluoride dentifrice should be prescribed.

Reference

1. Kowitz, G., Lucatorto, F., and Bennett, W.: Effects of dentifrices on soft tissues of the oral cavity. J. Oral Med. *28*:105, 1973.

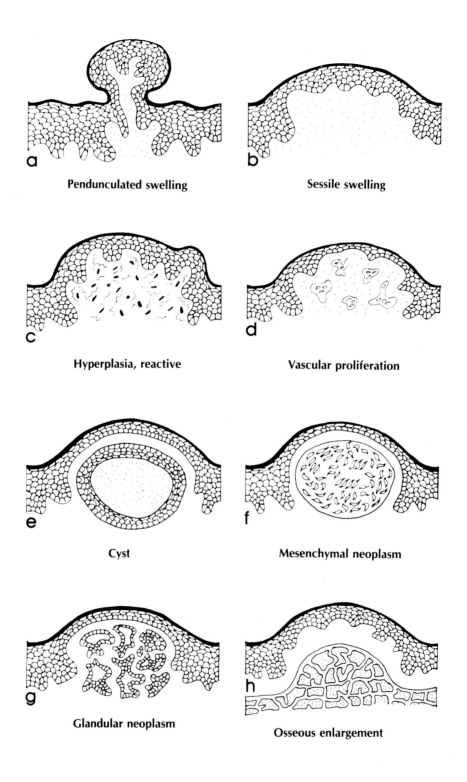

a Pendunculated swelling

b Sessile swelling

c Hyperplasia, reactive

d Vascular proliferation

e Cyst

f Mesenchymal neoplasm

g Glandular neoplasm

h Osseous enlargement

Soft Tissue Swellings

6
Intraoral Soft Tissue Swellings

LOCALIZED GINGIVAL TUMEFACTIONS

Parulis
Pyogenic Granuloma
Peripheral Giant Cell Granuloma
Peripheral Fibroma
Giant Cell Fibroma
Peripheral Ossifying Fibroma
Retrocuspid Papillae
Torus Mandibularis and Exostoses
Gingival Cyst
Eruption Cyst
Epulis Fissurata
Congenital Epulis
Peripheral Odontogenic Tumors
Squamous Cell Carcinoma
Mucoepidermoid Carcinoma

GENERALIZED GINGIVAL SWELLINGS

Fibromatosis Gingivae
Dilantin Hyperplasia
Hyperplastic Gingivitis
Wegener's Granulomatosis
Leukemia

SWELLINGS OF THE ORAL FLOOR

Ranula
Dermoid Cyst
Lymphoepithelial Cyst
Sialolithiasis with Sialadenitis
Salivary Gland Tumors
Mesenchymal Neoplasms
Ludwig's Angina
Squamous Cell Carcinoma

SWELLINGS OF THE LIPS AND BUCCAL MUCOSA

Mucous Retention Phenomenon
Minor Gland Sialolithiasis
Nasoalveolar Cyst
Cheilitis Granulomatosa

Cheilitis Glandularis
Angioneurotic Edema
Inflammatory Hyperplasia
Foreign Body Granuloma
Traumatic Neuroma
Mesenchymal Neoplasms
Herniated Buccal Fat Pad
Reactive Lymphoid Hyperplasia
Hemangioma and Varix
Keratoacanthoma
Squamous Cell Carcinoma
Monomorphic Adenoma
Other Salivary Neoplasms

TONGUE SWELLINGS

Median Rhomboid Glossitis
Ectopic Lingual Thyroid
Thyroglossal Duct Cyst
Lingual Cyst
Hemangioma and Lymphangioma
Neural Sheath Tumors
Granular Sheath Cell Lesions
Leiomyoma
Osteocartilaginous Choristoma
Sarcomas
Amyloid Nodules
Specific Granuloma
Squamous Cell Carcinoma

PALATAL SWELLINGS

Torus Palatinus
Cyst of the Incisive Papilla
Palatal Abscess
Adenomatous Hyperplasia
Pleomorphic Adenoma
Adenoid Cystic Carcinoma
Mucoepidermoid Carcinoma
Adenocarcinoma, NOS
Atypical Lymphoproliferative Disease
Carcinoma of the Antrum

Both epithelial and mesenchymal lesions can produce tumefaction in soft tissues. The swellings may be of developmental, inflammatory, or neoplastic origin, or they may reflect an oral representation of a generalized systemic disorder. When the physician develops a differential diagnosis for a given lump in the oral cavity, three parameters are of paramount importance in the limitation of the differential: location, consistency, and the presence or absence of pain. In this section, diseases that appear as tumefactions are categorized according to location. It should be emphasized that, while a disease is listed for a given topographic locale, that lesion is not limited exclusively to that region. To eliminate redundancies, the grouping of lesions according to location is based upon prevalence or a tendency for that lesion to occur in a given site.

When developing a differential diagnosis the physician must be aware both of the tendencies of a lesion to arise in a given locale and of the tissues normally present in a given region. For example, a swelling in the palate should suggest a diagnosis of salivary tumor, since the palate is replete with minor salivary glands. Nevertheless, salivary tissue is, with few exceptions, ubiquitous in oral mucous membranes. For this reason a swelling in any of the oral tissues could represent a salivary neoplasm. When a disease entity is restricted exclusively to a given location, this condition will be specified in the text.

The consistency of a swelling is of utmost importance when one considers diagnostic probabilities, determines procedures for securing a definitive diagnosis, and provides treatment. Tumefactions that are movable and firm yet not indurated are most consistent with benign neoplasms; tumefactions that are fixed, indurated, and ulcerated are more likely to be malignant neoplasms. Swellings that are tender or painful and may manifest fistulation are in all probability inflammatory conditions.

The most common tumefactions of the gingiva or alveolar ridge are the parulis of pulpal or periodontal origin, the pyogenic and peripheral giant cell granuloma, the peripheral fibroma, and the ossifying fibroma. It should be recalled that a central jaw lesion may perforate bone and manifest as a gingival growth or epulis.

The common swellings of the oral floor are the ranula, the dermoid cyst, and the lymphoepithelial cyst. The common swellings of the lips are mucoceles (lower lip) and benign salivary tumors (upper lip).

Commonly encountered swellings of the tongue include mesenchymal tumors, chiefly benign hemangiomas or lymphangiomas, neural sheath tumors, and granular cell myoblastomas. Lethal lesions include carcinoma and sarcoma. Systemic diseases that may cause death and produce tongue swellings include amyloidosis and specific granulomatous diseases such as tuberculosis and histoplasmosis.

The more common palatal swellings are tori, palatal abscesses, and benign or malignant salivary tumors, the latter of which are potentially lethal.

Common swellings in the cheek include benign mesenchymal tumors, fibrous hyperplasia, and salivary tumors. Malignant salivary tumors may cause death. Retromolar swellings include primarily dentigerous cysts from underlying impacted third molars, pericoronitis, and, importantly, mucoepidermoid carcinoma.

LOCALIZED GINGIVAL TUMEFACTIONS

Parulis

Age: No predilection
Sex: No predilection.

Clinical Features: Inflammation of pulpal or periodontal origin may drain peripherally, producing a fistula with submucosal abscess formation in the gingival tissues. The swelling is fluctuant and may be sore or painless. A parulis of odontogenic origin will be associated with a necrotic pulp, and periapical pathosis will be radiographically demonstrable. A parulis of periodontal origin is found adjacent to a deep periodontal pocket.

Microscopic Features: Abscess formation, which is composed of loose connective tissue, eosinophilic exudate, and neutrophils, may be ac-

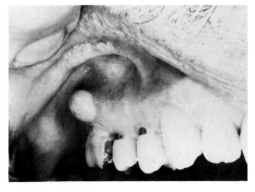

FIG. 6–1.   Gingival abscess or parulis overlies a necrotic molar with radiographic evidence of periapical inflammation.

companied by necrotic debris and scattered chronic inflammatory cells, chiefly macrophages.

Differential Diagnosis: Parulis can be differentiated from other gingival epulides by locating the source of infection. Periapical roentgenograms, pulp tests, and pocket probing are useful in this respect. A gutta-percha point may be inserted through the fistula feeding the parulis and radiographed to disclose the incriminating tooth when other clinical findings are equivocal.

Treatment: Elimination of the source of inflammation is curative; if pulpal, endodontics or extraction is required. If the source is periodontal, curettage or surgery with debridement of calculus and granulation tissue is indicated.

References

1. Darling, A. I.: In *Thoma's Oral Pathology*, 6th Ed., edited by R. J. Gorlin and H. M. Goldman. St. Louis, C. V. Mosby Co., 1970, Vol. 1, pp. 344–345.
2. Mitchell, D. F., Standish, S. M., and Fast, T. B.: *Oral Diagnosis/Oral Medicine*, 3rd Ed. Philadelphia, Lea & Febiger, 1978, p. 394.
3. Shafer, W. G., Hine, M. K., and Levy, B. M.: *A Textbook of Oral Pathology*, 4th Ed. Philadelphia, W. B. Saunders Co., 1983, p. 794.

Pyogenic Granuloma

Age: Teenagers and young adults
Sex: Female predilection

Clinical Features: The pyogenic granuloma is a reactive, exuberant overgrowth of granulation tissue resulting from irritation. It may occur anywhere on the mucocutaneous surfaces but is most common on the gingiva. The lesion is smooth or bosselated, usually ulcerated, hemorrhagic, and compressible. Pyogenic granulomas often reach large proportions yet generally emanate from a stalk originating at a gingival papilla. This lesion is commonly encountered among gravid females, hence the term *pregnancy tumor*. It has been suggested that the hormonal imbalance coincident with pregnancy heightens the organism's response to irritation.

Microscopic Features: The surface is usually ulcerated, and the tumor mass is composed of erythrocyte-engorged dilated vascular spaces. The intervening fibrous stroma is infiltrated with inflammatory cells.

Differential Diagnosis: Unlike parulis, the pyogenic granuloma does not contain a purulent exudate nor is there an inflammatory source of infection from dental origin. The lesion must be differentiated from other reactive gingival swellings and hemangioma.

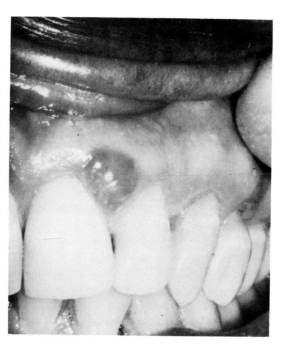

FIG. 6–2. Pyogenic granuloma of maxillary gingiva, usually erythematous and not related to pulp disease.

Treatment: Pyogenic granuloma is managed by excision and thorough scaling and curettage of the adjacent teeth and root surfaces. In the gravid patient, recurrence is likely and treatment, to be successful, should await parturition.

References

1. Bhaskar, S. N. and Jacoway, J. R.: Pyogenic granuloma—clinical features, incidence, histology, and result of treatment; report of 242 cases. J. Oral Surg. 24:391, 1966.
2. Lee, D. W.: The fibrous epulis and related lesions. Periodontics 6:277, 1968.
3. Angelopoulos, A. P.: Pyogenic granuloma of the oral cavity: statistical analysis of its clinical features. J. Oral Surg. 29:840, 1971.

Peripheral Giant Cell Granuloma

Age: No predilection
Sex: Female predilection

Clinical Features: Peripheral giant cell granuloma may arise on both dentulous and edentulous alveolar ridges and is restricted in location only to these regions of the mouth. The lesion may reach large size and may have a sessile base. The surface is either smooth or granular, often with a blue or purple tinge. It is somewhat firm to palpation. Giant cell granuloma is aggressive and has the potential to erode into underlying alveolar bone. Like other reactive gingival growths, it is

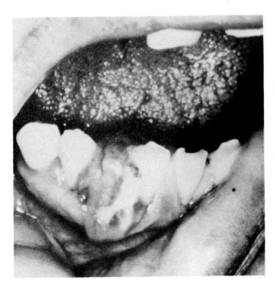

FIG. 6–3. Focal gingival enlargement with surface ulceration representing a peripheral giant cell granuloma.

commonly found in pregnant women and has a tendency to recur following excision.

Microscopic Features: A hypercellular fibrovascular stroma prevails; numerous giant cells are present, many of which line vascular spaces. The multinucleated cells show a random distribution of nuclei within the cytoplasm. The lesion is often lobulated with heavy deposits of of hemosiderin granules located about the periphery. Osteoid is also a common feature, elaborated within the granulomatous stroma.

Differential Diagnosis: Peripheral giant cell granuloma can clinically resemble any of the other gingival tumefactions, including reactive and neoplastic conditions. An infectious source is lacking.

Treatment: Giant cell granulomas originate from gingival tissues (i.e., periosteum) and require excision extending to bone. Recurrence can be anticipated if the lesion is not excised in its entirety. The adjacent teeth should be scaled in order to remove any irritants associated with plaque.

References
1. Giansanti, J. S. and Waldron, C. A.: Peripheral giant cell granuloma: Review of 720 cases. J. Oral Surg. 27:787, 1969.
2. Eversole, L. R., Sabes, W. R., and Rovin, S.: Reactive lesions of the gingiva. J. Oral Path. 1:30, 1972.
3. Shklar, G. and Cataldo, E.: The gingival giant cell granuloma. Histochemical observations. Periodontics 5:303, 1967.
4. Bhaskar, S. N. and Cutright, D. E.: Giant cell reparative granuloma (peripheral): report of 50 cases. J. Oral Surg. 29:110, 1971.
5. Sapp, J. P.: Ultrastructure and histogenesis of peripheral giant cell reparative granuloma of the jaws. Cancer 30:119, 1972.

Peripheral Fibroma

Age: Young adults
Sex: Female predilection

Clinical Features: Peripheral fibroma is merely a focal fibrous hyperplasia of the marginal gingiva and is analogous to the fibroma or inflammatory hyperplasia occurring elsewhere in the mouth. Peripheral fibroma may evolve as such or may represent a late sclerosing stage of a pyogenic granuloma. It is usually smooth, nonulcerated and firm, lacking discoloration. While peripheral fibromas may become quite large, they usually emanate from a slender stalk originating on a single gingival papilla.

Microscopic Features: Surface epithelium is distended by a mass of dense fibrous connective tissue that may contain mild diffuse inflammatory cell infiltrates or may be devoid of inflammation. Occasionally, multinucleated fibroblasts are encountered, the so-called *giant cell fibroma.*

Differential Diagnosis: The normal mucosal color and firm consistency help to differentiate the peripheral fibroma from pyogenic or peripheral giant cell granuloma. The clinical appearance may be identical to that of ossifying fibroma, gingival cysts, or peripheral odontogenic tumors.

Treatment: Excision with root scaling of adjacent teeth is recommended.

References
1. Lee, K. W.: The fibrous epulis and related lesions. Periodontics 6:277, 1968.
2. Bhaskar, S. N. and Jacoway, J. R.: Peripheral fibroma and peripheral fibroma with calcification. J. Am. Dent. Assoc. 73:1312, 1966.

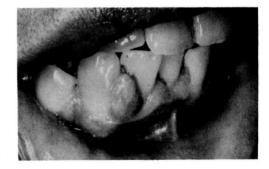

FIG. 6–4. Peripheral fibroma manifesting as a firm, normal-colored tumefaction of the dental papilla.

3. Eversole, L. R. and Rovin, S.: Reactive lesions of the gingiva. J. Oral Pathol. *1*:30, 1972.

Giant Cell Fibroma

Age: Teenagers and young adults
Sex: No predilection

Clinical Features: The giant cell fibroma is basically a fibrous proliferation with distinctive microscopic features and may represent a reactive or benign neoplastic process. It is smooth or papillary and usually pedunculated. Most lesions are small and normal in color. Half of these lesions are located on the gingiva, with mandibular lesions occurring more frequently than maxillary growths. They also arise on the tongue, palate, buccal mucosa, and lips. Similar lesions can be found on the skin and genitalia.

Microscopic Features: The mass may be papillary or smooth and is covered by a thin layer of stratified squamous epithelium. The bulk of the specimen is represented by irregular swirls of collagen fibers with interspersed plump stellate and spindle-shaped fibroblasts. Many of these cells exhibit a "manta ray" appearance and possess 2 to 5 oval nuclei.

Differential Diagnosis: Papillary-appearing lesions will be clinically indistinguishable from papilloma, condyloma, and other focal papillary lesions described in the next chapter. Dome-shaped lesions may be confused with the other localized gingival swellings listed here. Most giant cell fibromas arise on attached gingiva away from the interdental papilla and are normal in color, thereby eliminating most of the reactive proliferations from consideration. A biopsy is required to obtain a diagnosis.

Treatment: Most giant cell fibromas are pedunculated, and simple surgical excision is the treatment of choice. Recurrence is rare.

References

1. Weathers, D. R., and Callihan, M. D.: Giant-cell fibroma. Oral Surg. *37*:374, 1974.
2. Graham, J. H., Sanders, J. B., Johnson, W. C., and Helwig, E. B.: Fibrous papule of the nose: a clinicopathological study. J. Invest. Dermatol. *45*:194, 1965.
3. Ackerman, A. B. and Kornberg, R.: Pearly penile papules. Arch. Dermatol. *108*:673, 1973.
4. Regezi, J. A., Courtney, R. M., and Kerr, D. A.: Fibrous lesions of the skin and mucous membrane which contain stellate and multinucleated cells. Oral Surg. *39*:605, 1975.
5. Houston, G. D.: The giant cell fibroma. A review of 464 cases. Oral Surg. *53*:582, 1982.

Peripheral Ossifying Fibroma

Age: Young adults
Sex: Female predilection

Clinical Features: Peripheral ossifying fibroma is located exclusively on the gingiva and is rarely seen on edentulous ridges. Like other reactive proliferations of the gingivae, female predilection and association with pregnancy are encountered. The lesion is firm, usually not discolored. The surface is smooth, yet may occasionally be ulcerated. It emanates from one gingival papilla. Recurrence following excision is not uncommon.

Microscopic Features: Surface epithelium may be ulcerated, and the bulk of the tissue mass is composed of collagenous fibers with hypercellular plump fibroblasts. Osteoid or oval cementum-like deposits are randomly oriented within the fibrous element.

Differential Diagnosis: Peripheral ossifying fibroma resembles the other focal swellings included here; however, unlike pyogenic granu-

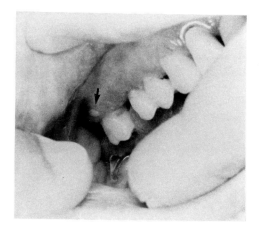

FIG. 6–5. Small gingival nodule representing a giant cell fibroma.

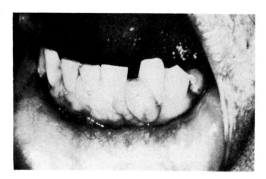

FIG. 6–6. Peripheral ossifying fibroma, which is a firm, usually normal-colored growth of the marginal gingiva.

loma and peripheral giant cell granuloma, it usually has a normal coloration. Microscopic examination is required for a definitive diagnosis.

Treatment: Since the lesion probably arises in the periodontal ligament, the excision should be deep, including periosteum and ligament, and thorough root scaling of adjacent teeth should be performed.

References

1. Bhaskar, S. N. and Jacoway, J. R.: Peripheral fibroma and peripheral fibroma with calcification. J. Am. Dent. Assoc. 73:1312, 1966.
2. Eversole, L. R., Sabes, W. R., and Rovin, S.: Reactive lesions of the gingiva. J. Oral Path. 1:30, 1972.
3. Cundiff, E. J.: Peripheral ossifying fibroma. A review of 365 cases. M.S.D. Thesis, Indiana University, 1972.
4. Gardner, D. G.: The peripheral odontogenic fibroma: An attempt at clarification. Oral Surg. 54:40, 1982.

Retrocuspid Papillae

Age: Young adults
Sex: No predilection

Clinical Features: Retrocuspid papillae are 2 to 4 mm papules located bilaterally on the lingually attached gingiva immediately posterior to the mandibular cuspids. They are soft, of normal color, and not associated with any causative factor. They probably represent developmental anomalies and may merely represent a variant of giant cell fibroma.

Microscopic Features: An epithelial-covered papule is composed of fibrous connective tissue. Fibroblasts may contain 2 or 3 nuclei, being stellate or spindle in shape.

Differential Diagnosis: The small papules may resemble a parulis or fistula; however, lack of an infectious source and bilateral location generally allow for a clinical diagnosis.

Treatment: No treatment is necessary.

References

1. Hirschfeld, I.: The retrocuspid papillae. Am. J. Orthod. (Oral Surg. Sec.) 33:447, 1947.
2. Everett, F. G., Hall, W. B., and Bennett, J. S.: Retrocuspid papillae. Periodontics 3:81, 1965.
3. Easley, J. R. and Weis, R. W.: Incidence of the retrocuspid papilla. J. Dent. Child. 37:523, 1970.
4. Berman, F. R. and Fay, J.: The retrocuspid papilla. Oral Surg. 42:80, 1976.

Torus Mandibularis and Exostoses

Age: Adults
Sex: Slightly more common among females

Clinical Features: Whereas tori and exostoses are hard tissue lesions, they are included with the soft tissue swellings because of their clinical resemblance to other gingival swellings. Mandibular tori are located bilaterally on the lingual mandibular gingiva in the cuspid-premolar region. Being bosselated and extremely hard, they represent bony excrescences. Unilateral instances occur less frequently. They are rather common among all races and are encountered in one third of the Eskimo population. Tori are inherited as an autosomal dominant trait. Progressive slow growth occurs throughout adulthood. Exostoses are multiple similar lesions located on the buccal aspect of the maxillary and mandibular alveolus. Both

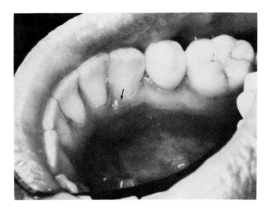

FIG. 6–7. The retrocuspid papilla, a developmental papule located on the lingual gingiva adjacent to mandibular cuspids.

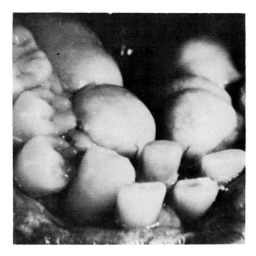

FIG. 6–8. Lingual tori. These are usually small, yet may reach the large proportions seen here.

may show oval-shaped radiopacities on dental roentgenograms.

Microscopic Features: Mature osseous trabeculae emanate from an outer cortex and are admixed with fibrous or adipose marrow.

Differential Diagnosis: The bony, hard consistency and bilaterality of tori are features sufficiently unique to allow for a clinical diagnosis.

Treatment: No treatment is required. Tori can be removed by chisel or burr should they interfere with fabrication of a dental prosthesis.

References

1. Kolas, S. and Halprin, V.: The occurrence of torus palatinus and torus mandibularis in 2,478 dental patients. Oral Surg. 6:1134, 1953.
2. Suzuki, M. and Sakai, T.: A familial study of torus palatinus and torus mandibularis. Am. J. Phys. Anthropol. *18*:263, 1960.
3. Summers, C. J.: Prevalance of tori. J. Oral Surg. 26:718, 1968.
4. Blakemore, J. R., Eller, D. J., and Tomaro, A. J.: Maxillary exostoses. Oral Surg. *40*:200, 1975.

Gingival Cyst

Age: Middle-aged adults
Sex: No predilection

Clinical Features: Submucosal cysts of the gingiva appear as firm or compressible smooth-surfaced nodules with a blanched appearance. The mandibular gingiva adjacent to the premolars is the most common location. The pathogenesis is variable as they may arise from rests of Serres or epithelial implantation, or they may be the peripheral counterpart of the central lateral periodontal cyst. Others may not be clinically obvious, but are discernible as microcysts in routine gingival surgical specimens. Regardless of their origin, all gingival cysts are relatively self-limited in terms of their growth potential. They are located in attached gingiva removed from the free gingival margin.

Microscopic Features: The cystic lining resembles that of nonkeratinizing lateral periodontal cyst. The microscopic features are unique. The lining epithelium is cuboidal and pursues a tortuous course with a multicystic pattern. Focal acanthotic excrescences are seen and are composed of clear cells. The multiple cystic cavities probably interconnect at various levels and are separated by dense fibrous tissue devoid of inflammation. Some gingival cysts show ameloblastic differentiation with ghost cells, keratinization, and calcification. Lesions of this nature represent peripheral calcifying and keratinizing (Gorlin) cysts.

Differential Diagnosis: Reactive proliferations generally arise in the gingival papillae area, whereas cysts are oriented away from the gingival margin. Parulis and peripheral odontogenic tumors may show identical clinical features; the former can usually be eliminated from consideration by ruling out a source of inflammation.

Treatment: Gingival cysts can be excised or enucleated.

References

1. Reeve, C. M. and Levy, B. P.: Gingival cysts: A review of the literature and a report of four cases. Periodontics 6:115, 1968.
2. Moskow, B. S., et al.: Gingival and lateral periodontal cysts. J. Periodontol. *41*:9, 1970.
3. Buchner, A. and Hansen, L. S.: The histomorphologic spectrum of the gingival cyst in the adult. Oral Surg. *48*:532, 1979.
4. Wysocki, G., et al.: Histogenesis of the lateral periodontal cyst and the gingival cyst of the adult. Oral Surg. *50*:327, 1980.
5. Freedman, P. D., Lumerman, H., and Gee, J. K.: Calcifying odontogenic cyst. A review and analysis of seventy cases. Oral Surg, *40*:93, 1975.

Eruption Cyst

Age: Children
Sex: No predilection

Clinical Features: The eruption cyst is a soft tissue dentigerous cyst arising from the reduced enamel epithelium and follicle of an erupting deciduous or permanent tooth. Therefore, it is seen directly overlying the alveolus at the site of eruption. It may be dark red when it is blood filled.

Microscopic Features: Lining stratified squamous or columnar epithelium is present, and the

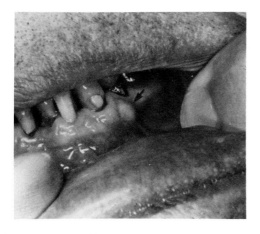

FIG. 6–9. Gingival cysts arising from the dental lamina or rests of Serres are either firm or fluctuant.

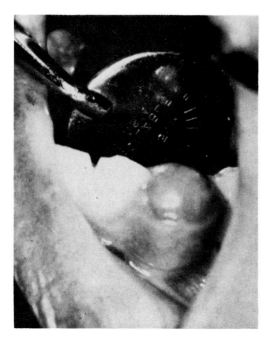

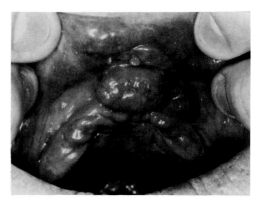

FIG. 6–11.   Redundant tissue folds underlying a denture flange, representing fibrous hyperplasia secondary to irritation.

FIG. 6–10.   An eruption cyst appearing as an inflamed mass of the gingiva overlying an erupting tooth. (Courtesy of Dr. S. Rovin.)

follicular wall evinces an avid inflammatory cell infiltrate.

Differential Diagnosis: The clinical features are diagnostic. Neoplasia has not been reported to arise from the lining of eruption cysts.

Treatment: The soft tissue cap can be excised to uncover the erupting tooth.

References

1. Anderson, B. B.: Hemorrhagic cysts associated with erupting teeth. Ann. Dent. *1*:114, 1942.
2. Clark, C. A.: A survey of eruption cysts in the newborn. Oral Surg. *14*:917, 1962.
3. Seward, M. H.: Eruption cyst: an analysis of its clinical features. J. Oral Surg. *31*:31, 1973.

Epulis Fissurata

Age: Adults
Sex: No predilection

Clinical Features: Flabby, redundant soft tissue masses, which are often fissured or bosselated, emanate from the base of the alveolar ridge and extend into the mucobuccal fold, as hyperplastic responses to ill-fitting dental prostheses. The hyperplastic tissue is located at the contact area of the denture flange and generally has a broad base of attachment. Epulis fissurata is usually of normal

color, yet may show foci of inflammation with ulceration. It is soft to palpation.

Microscopic Features: Surface epithelium overlies masses of dense fibrous connective tissue that contains variable amounts of inflammatory cells. Focal myxomatous zones and cartilaginous rests may be seen when the lesion is located on the interior maxillary alveolus and mucobuccal fold.

Differential Diagnosis: Redundant hyperplastic tissue must be differentiated from the other gingival tumefactions, including carcinoma. Its soft movability and broad base are usually sufficient to make this lesion clinically recognizable.

Treatment: The tissue should be excised and examined microscopically. A new set of dentures or a relining is required to prevent reestablishment of the hyperplastic response.

References

1. Shafer, W. G., Hine, M. K., and Levy, B. M.: *A Textbook of Oral Pathology,* 4th Ed. Philadelphia, W. B. Saunders Co., 1983, p. 552.
2. Cutright, D. E.: The histopathologic findings in 583 cases of epulis fissuratum. Oral Surg. *37*:401, 1974.

Congenital Epulis

Age: Present at birth
Sex: Female predilection

Clinical Features: The congenital epulis is a neoplasm of unknown origin found exclusively on the alveolar ridge. A large polypoid soft swelling, which may reach a diameter of several centimeters, emanates from a constricted stalk that attaches the tumor to the edentulous alveolus of newborns. Congenital epulis is more common on

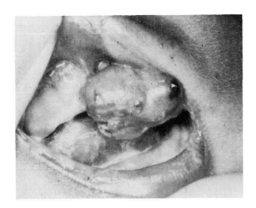

FIG. 6–12. Firm or rubbery gingival mass emanating from a constricted stalk in congenital epulis of the newborn. (Courtesy of Dr. S. Rovin.)

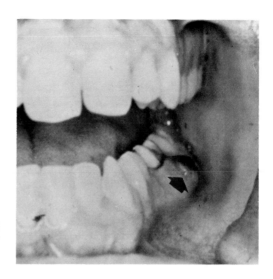

FIG. 6–13. Peripheral ameloblastoma of the mandibular buccal gingiva.

the maxillary anterior alveolar ridge. The tumor is somewhat firm yet may be compressible.

Microscopic Features: The overlying epithelium is intact and unremarkable. The tumor is composed of large swollen granular or foamy cells with a round pyknotic nucleus. The fibrous stroma is scant, only small vascular channels being seen. The cellular architecture is extremely monomorphic with no cytologic atypia, and organoid configuration is not featured. Recent evidence based on electron microscopy supports a pericyte origin for this lesion.

Differential Diagnosis: Congenital epulis is infrequently found. A pedunculated mass in the newborn on the gingiva may occur in congenital sarcoma or teratoma, both of which are extremely rare.

Treatment: Excision with inclusion of the stalk or base may be accomplished without danger of recurrence.

References

1. Custer, R. P. and Fust, J. A.: Congenital epulis. Am. J. Clin. Pathol. 22:1044, 1952.
2. Fuhr, A. H. and Krough, P. H.: Congenital epulis of the newborn: Centennial review of the literature and a report of case. J. Oral Surg. 30:30, 1972.
3. Blair, A. E. and Edwards, D. M.: Congenital epulis of the newborn. Oral Surg. 43:687, 1977.
4. Rohrer, M. D. and Young, S. K.: Congenital epulis (gingival cell tumor): ultrastructural evidence of origin from pericytes. Oral Surg. 53:56, 1982.

Peripheral Odontogenic Tumors

Age: Young adults
Sex: Depends on tumor type
Clinical Features: Tumors that arise from the odontogenic apparatus or remnants of the tooth germ are, as a rule, intraosseous. Occasionally, they arise in the extraosseous tissues of the alveolus. Clinically, they are nodular smooth-surfaced tumefactions of the gingiva that are firm to palpation. Soft tissue ossification may be detectable in radiographs in some of these tumors. The odontogenic tumors that can originate in the gingiva are the Gorlin cyst, Pindborg tumor, odontogenic adenomatoid tumor, ameloblastoma, peripheral odontogenic hamartoma, peripheral odontogenic fibroma, and ameloblastic fibrodentinoma.

Microscopic Features: The tumor cells may or may not be encapsulated and will vary, depending upon the type of tumor seen (see chapters dealing with radiolucencies and radiopacities). Two odontogenic tumors are characteristically extraosseous. The peripheral odontogenic hamartoma is composed of oval and linear islands of cuboidal epithelium resembling the rests of Malassez lying within a fibrovascular stroma. The other gingival tumor, ameloblastic fibrodentinoma, occurs in children and is represented by dental lamina-like epithelial cell rests, some of which show stellate reticulum. These cell rests are dispersed throughout a mesenchymal stroma that is poorly endowed with collagen. An eosinophilic dentin-like amorphous product is found in juxtaposition to the epithelial cell component.

Differential Diagnosis: Extraosseous odontogenic tumors show clinical features in common with the reactive proliferations and gingival cysts.

Treatment: Simple excision is the treatment of choice. Peripheral forms of odontogenic tumors, considered aggressive when located centrally, behave nonaggressively, with little tendency for recurrence.

References

1. Baden, E., Moskow, B. S., and Moskow, R.; Odontogenic gingival epithelial hamartoma. J. Oral Surg. 26:702, 1968.
2. Abrams, A. M., Melrose, R. J., and Howell, F. V.: Adenoameloblastoma: A clinical pathologic study of ten new cases. Cancer 22:175, 1968.
3. Gardner, D. G.: Peripheral ameloblastoma: a study of 21 cases, including 5 reported as basal cell carcinoma of the gingiva. Cancer 39:1625, 1977.
4. McKelvy, B. D. and Cherrick, H. M.: Peripheral ameloblastic fibrodentinoma. J. Oral Surg. 34:826, 1976.
5. Gardner, D. G.: The peripheral odontogenic fibroma: An attempt at clarification. Oral Surg. 54:40, 1982.

Squamous Cell Carcinoma

Age: Elderly
Sex: Male predilection

Clinical Features: Squamous cancer of the gingiva and alveolar ridge represents about 15 percent of all oral squamous cell carcinomas. The swelling is either red or keratotic and may appear granular or ulcerated. The lesion frequently extends into the mucobuccal fold or oral floor and is most prevalent on the mandibular arch. In addition, the marginal tissue is frequently leukoplakic or erythroplakic. The swelling is usually indurated. Palpation of the submandibular and cervical regions is essential in order to detect any clinical evidence of regional metastasis; a thorough medical workup should be pursued along

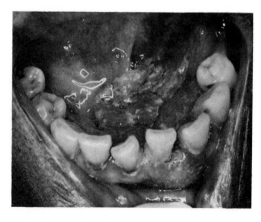

FIG. 6–14. Squamous cell carcinoma of the gingiva with extension into the floor of the mouth.

with a chest radiograph in order to evaluate for distant metastases. All squamous cell carcinomas in this location should be assessed for bone invasion of the alveolus by procuring panoramic and periapical radiographs.

Microscopic Features: Invasive nests and islands of squamous epithelium are encountered, and most tumors evince parakeratin pearls or squamous eddies. The individual cells show varying degrees of pleomorphism, hyperchromatism and mitoses. The fibrous stroma is frequently infiltrated by mononuclear cells.

Differential Diagnosis: Swellings of the gingiva or edentulous ridge representing carcinoma may be confused with reactive proliferations included in this section on gingival tumefactions. Usually the patient's age, when considered along with lesional induration, ulceration, and/or keratosis, supports a clinical impression of cancer. An incisional biopsy is essential to a definitive diagnosis.

Treatment: Squamous cell carcinoma must be treated aggressively in order to achieve a cure. Combined radiotherapy and surgery are generally employed along with regional node dissection in the presence of palpable nodes. Prophylactic neck dissecton or radiation therapy is usually indicated in the absence of palpable nodes. The prognosis is based on tumor size (T), the presence or absence of nodal metastasis (N), and the presence or absence of distant metastasis (M). The 5-year survival for patients with lesions under 3 centimeters is about 80 percent.

References

1. Martin, H. E.: Cancer of the gums (gingivae). Am. J. Surg. 54:765, 1941.
2. Tiecke, R.W. and Bernier, J. L.: Statistical and morphological analysis of four hundred and one cases of intraoral squamous cell carcinoma. J. Am. Dent. Assoc. 49:684, 1954.
3. Nathanson, A., Jakobsson, A., and Wersall, J.: Prognosis of squamous cell carcinoma of the gums. Acta Otolaryngol. 75:301, 1973.
4. Willen, R., et al.: Squamous cell carcinoma of the gingiva. Histological classification and grading of malignancy. Acta Otolaryngol. 79:146, 1975.

Mucoepidermoid Carcinoma

Age: Teenagers and adults
Sex: No predilection

Clinical Features: Mucoepidermoid carcinoma is included with gingival tumefactions because of the propensity of this tumor to arise at the posterior confines of the mandibular alveolus, the retromolar pad. It arises from salivary glands normally

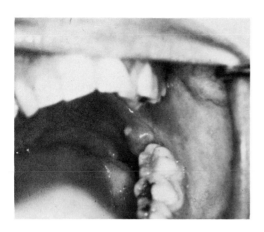

FIG. 6–15. Mucoepidermoid carcinoma, often observed as a swelling in the retromolar pad area.

present in this location and may be indurated or fluctuant and cystic, not unlike a mucocele. The surface mucosa is generally intact. Occasionally, cystic, mucin-filled spaces occur superficially, giving the tumor a vesicular or bleb-like appearance.

Microscopic Features: Neoplastic ductal, cuboidal, and squamous epithelia are present, as are mucous cells. The neoplastic islands may be solid or cystic with large dilated mucin-filled spaces.

Differential Diagnosis: The other tumefactions of the gingiva included in this section tend to occur anteriorly. Retromolar swellings, which appear clinically similar, include mucocele, eruption cyst from an impacted third molar, and mesenchymal neoplasms.

Treatment: Low-grade tumors are treated by wide local excision. High-grade malignancy requires wide excision and block resection of the underlying mandibular bone. Careful evaluation of the neck is necessary since nodal involvement will require in-continuity neck dissection or, at least, supraomohyoid dissection when submandibular nodes are palpable.

References
1. Eversole, L. R.: Mucoepidermoid carcinoma; review of 815 reported cases. J. Oral Surg. 28:490, 1970.
2. Bhaskar, S. N. and Bernier, J. L.: Mucoepidermoid tumors of major and minor salivary glands. Cancer 15:801, 1962.
3. Melrose, R. J., Abrams, A. M., and Howell, F. V.: Mucoepidermoid tumors of the intraoral minor salivary glands: a clinicopathologic study of 54 cases. J. Oral Pathol. 2:314, 1973.

GENERALIZED GINGIVAL SWELLINGS

Fibromatosis Gingivae

Age: Childhood onset
Sex: No predilection

Clinical Features: Transmitted as an autosomal dominant trait, hereditary fibromatosis gingivae becomes obvious soon after eruption of the primary teeth. The gingiva shows multinodular enlargement, most prominent in the interdental papillar regions. The tissue is firm and of normal color, and the hyperplasia may be so extensive that the entire coronal portion of the teeth is obliterated. Elimination of dental plaque does not significantly lessen the severity. Gingival fibromatosis may be accompanied by other disorders including splenomegaly, enlarged nasal and external ear soft tissues, shortened terminal phalanges, hyperflexia of joints, and hypoplasia of the nails, the so-called Laband syndrome.

Microscopic Features: Gingival epithelium is distended by massive accumulations of mature, dense collagenous tissue. Inflammation is minimal.

Differential Diagnosis: Dilantin hyperplasia, hyperplastic gingivitis, and leukemic infiltration of the gingiva may show signs clinically indistinguishable from fibromatosis gingivae. A history of familial involvement is of paramount importance in making the diagnosis.

Treatment: Periodic gingivectomy with placement of a gingival acrylic splint or prosthesis can be done for both cosmetic and functional reasons. Recurrence to some degree should be anticipated.

References
1. Savara, B. S., et al.: Hereditary gingival fibromatosis; study of a family. J. Periodontol. 25:12, 1954.
2. Emerson, T. G.: Hereditary gingival hyperplasia; a

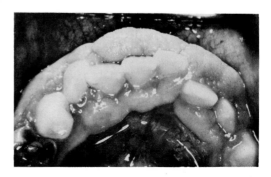

FIG. 6–16. Generalized fibrotic enlargement of the gingival tissues, a feature of hereditary fibromatosis gingivae.

family pedigree of four generations. Oral Surg. *19*:1, 1965.

3. Yurosko, J. J., et al.: Clinicopathological conference. Case 20, part 2. Idiopathic gingival fibromatosis. J. Oral Surg. *35*:820, 907, 1977.

4. Laband, P. F., Habib, G., and Humphreys, G. S.: Hereditary gingival fibromatosis. Report of an affected family with associated splenomegaly and skeletal and soft-tissue abnormalities. Oral Surg. *17*:339, 1964.

5. Oikawa, K., Cavaglia, A. M. V., and Lu, D.: Laband syndrome: report of case. J. Oral Surg. *37*:120, 1979.

Dilantin Hyperplasia

Age: Children and adults

Sex: No predilection

Clinical Features: Gingival enlargement occurring in seizure patients placed on sodium diphenylhydantoin is generalized. The gingiva shows bulbous fibrotic firm nodules emanating from the papillar regions and may be severe enough to obscure the crowns of the teeth. The condition is worsened when oral hygiene is poor and dental plaque accumulates. Hyperplastic tissue on edentulous ridge areas is extremely rare, yet has been reported to occur in edentulous patients.

Microscopic Features: Surface epithelium is distended by dense collagenous fibrous tissue. Long, slender so-called test-tube rete ridges extend deeply into the subjacent fibrous tissue.

Differential Diagnosis: A history of epilepsy controlled by diphenylhydantoin is necessary for the diagnosis. This drug-related gingival enlargement may be indistinguishable from fibromatosis gingivae and may resemble that seen in leukemia and nonspecific hyperplastic gingivitis.

Treatment: Cosmesis and function may be restored by gingivectomy followed by thorough pro-phylaxis and institution of a conscientious oral hygiene home care program.

References

1. Panuska, H. J., et al.: Effect of anticonvulsant drugs upon the gingiva: a series of analyses of 1048 patients. J. Periodontol. *31*:336, 1960; *32*:15, 1961.

2. Aas, E.: Hyperplasia gingivae diphenylhydantoinea; a clinical, histological and biochemical study. Acta Odontol. Scand. *21* (Suppl. 34):1, 1963.

3. Angelopoulos, A. P. and Goaz, P. W.: Incidence of diphenylhydantoin gingival hyperplasia. Oral Surg. *34*:898, 1972.

4. Dreyer, W. P. and Thomas, C. J.: Diphenylhydantoinate-induced hyperplasia of the masticatory mucosa in an edentulous epileptic patient. Oral Surg. *45*:701, 1978.

Hyperplastic Gingivitis

Age: Adults

Sex: No predilection

Clinical Features: Whereas most forms of non-specific gingivitis result in mild edema with erythema, an occasional response is one of marked swelling due to edema, fibroplasia, and inflammatory cell infiltration. This hyperplastic form of gingivitis is characterized by generalized enlargement, particularly interdentally; the tissues are boggy, and ulceration is not frequent. Erythema is generally present. Dental plaque is accumulated and periodontal disease with pocket formation is often present as well. The hyperplastic form may be uncomplicated by systemic disease; however, underlying medical problems such as uncontrolled diabetes mellitus or cyclic neutropenia must be ruled out. This form of gingivitis is frequently seen in gravid women.

Microscopic Features: Surface epithelium may

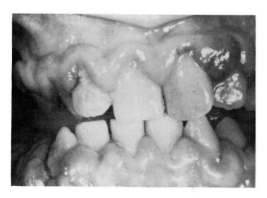

FIG. 6–17.   Generalized enlargement of the gingiva as a consequence of diphenylhydantoin therapy.

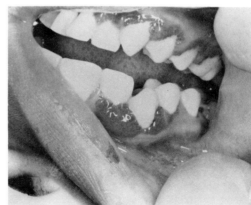

FIG. 6–18.   Nonspecific inflammatory enlargement of the gingival papillae in a pregnant female.

be unremarkable whereas the crevicular epithelium evinces anastomosing elongated rete ridges. The underlying tissues are fibrovascular with nonspecific inflammatory cell infiltrates. Fragments of calculus and microbial colonies are often found adherent to crevicular epithelium.

Differential Diagnosis: Leukemic infiltrates may show indistinguishable features. Fibromatosis gingivae and Dilantin hyperplasia can mimic hyperplastic gingivitis, yet the former two lesions are usually not boggy or erythematous. A blood count, fasting blood sugar, or, preferably, a glucose tolerance test can be obtained to rule out leukemia, cyclic neutropenia, and diabetes.

On rare occasions granulomatous inflammations such as Wegener's granulomatosis or tuberculosis can manifest generalized gingival enlargement. In these instances, the surface is pebbly or granular and ulceration is present. A biopsy will differentiate nonspecific hyperplastic gingivitis from these lesions and from leukemia.

Treatment: Dental prophylaxis with scaling and periodontal curettage will cause the hyperplastic tissue to subside. If the problem is complicated by systemic disease, systemic factors as well as local ones must be controlled.

References

1. Orban, B.: Classification and nomenclature of periodontal diseases (based on pathology, etiology, and clinical picture). J. Periodontol. *13*:88, 1942.
2. Silness, J. and Low, H.: Periodontal disease in pregnancy. I. Prevalence and severity. Acta Odontol. Scand. *21*:532, 1963.
3. Benvetiste, R., Bixler, D., and Conneally, P. M.: Periodontal disease in diabetics. J. Periodontol. *38*:271, 1967.
4. Bartolucci, E. G. and Parkes, R. B.: Accelerated periodontal breakdown in uncontrolled diabetes. Pathogenesis and treatment. Oral Surg. *52*:387, 1981.

Wegener's Granulomatosis

Age: Adults

Sex: No predilection

Clinical Features: Wegener's granulomatosis is a rare disorder with pathogenic features akin to many of the collagen diseases. The pathologic manifestations include destructive granulomas of both upper and lower respiratory tract, necrotizing angiitis, and glomerulonephritis signaled by sinusitis and rhinitis, cough with hemoptysis, and uremia. Other tissues that may be involved include the middle ear, urethra, skin, and salivary glands. Whereas osseous destructive lesions are sometimes observed in the nose, sinuses, and pal-

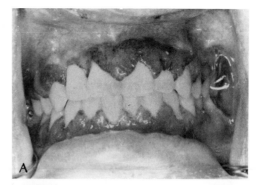

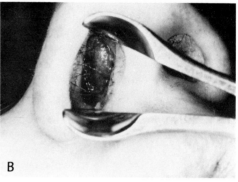

FIG. 6–19. A: Diffuse granular gingival enlargement in Wegener's granulomatosis. B: Nasal septum swelling.

ate, the gingival changes are unique and may, in fact, be pathognomonic of the disease. A generalized hyperplastic gingivitis is seen with a characteristic granular or pebbly telangiectatic appearance.

Microscopic Features: A gingival biopsy will disclose granulomatous inflammation with a mononuclear infiltrate. Multinucleated giant cells are present and some cases will be infiltrated by numerous eosinophils. The sine qua non on a microscopic basis is the presence of necrotizing vasculitis.

Differential Diagnosis: While the other entities included here as diffuse gingival enlargements may be considered, the granular telangiectatic appearance is classic for Wegener's granulomatosis. Other symptoms of the disease may be present, and altered laboratory findings include a markedly elevated sedimentation rate and elevated creatinine. Chest x-rays will disclose pulmonary involvement.

Treatment: Chemotherapy is the treatment of choice. Combined cyclophosphamide and prednisone will achieve resolution of lesions with remission in a few months. Some patients will enjoy fairly long-term remission even after cessation of treatment.

References

1. Wolff, S. M., et al.: Wegener's granulomatosis. Ann. Intern Med. *81*:513, 1974.
2. Flye, M. W., Mundinger, G. H., and Fauci, A. S.: Diagnostic and therapeutic aspects of the surgical approach to Wegener's granulomatosis. J. Thorac. Cardio. Surg. *77*:331, 1979.
3. Brooke, R. I.: Wegener's granulomatosis involving the gingivae. Br. Dent. J. *127*:34, 1969.
4. Scott, J. and Finch, L. D.: Wegener's granulomatosis presenting as gingivitis. Review of the clinical and pathologic features and report of a case. Oral Surg. *34*:920, 1972.
5. Israelson, H., Binnie, W. H., and Hurt, W. C.: The hyperplastic gingivitis of Wegener's granulomatosis. J. Periodontol. *52*:81, 1981.

Leukemia

Age: Children and young adults
Sex: No predilection

Clinical Features: Infiltration of leukemic cells into the gingiva occurs in approximately half of patients suffering from acute leukemia, particularly acute monocytic leukemia. The interdental papillae are greatly enlarged, red or bluish in color, and usually boggy, although they may occasionally feel firm to palpation. Ulceration with pseudomembrane is often seen. Other signs may accompany gingival enlargement: pallor of the skin and remaining mucosa, gingival hemorrhage, formation of petechiae and ecchymoses, joint swelling due to hemarthrosis, and general malaise.

Microscopic Features: The fibrous tissue underlying surface and sulcular epithelium displays a monomorphic, monotonous infiltrate of leukemic cells. In monocytic leukemia the cells are oval or round with vesicular nucleoplasm and prominent nucleoli.

Differential Diagnosis: Nonspecific hyperplastic gingivitis may show identical features. Fibromatosis gingivae and Dilantin hyperplasia, while usually not inflamed, should nevertheless be considered in the differential diagnosis. Other generalized signs and symptoms will arouse suspicion of leukemia. A biopsy and complete blood count should be obtained.

Treatment: Leukemia should be managed by a hematologist. Oral signs will diminish or resolve with successful treatment of the disease, usually with chemotherapeutic drugs.

References

1. Duffy, J. H. and Driscoll, E. J.: Oral manifestations in leukemia. Oral Surg. *11*:484, 1958.
2. Lynch, M. A. and Ship, I. I.: Oral manifestations of leukemia; a postdiagnostic study. J. Am. Dent. Assoc. *75*:1139, 1967.
3. Michand, M., et al.: Oral manifestations of acute leukemia in children. J. Am. Dent. Assoc. *95*:1145, 1977.

SWELLINGS OF THE ORAL FLOOR

Ranula

Age: More common in children
Sex: No predilection

Clinical Features: A ranula represents a mucin-filled cystic or pseudocystic cavity in the floor of the mouth. Since the mucin accumulation is superficial, the swelling appears fluid filled and has a bluish cast; the thin membranous surface is traversed by obvious capillary markings. It is compressible and usually located unilaterally in the vicinity of one of the submandibular ducts. Salivary flow on the affected side cannot be elicited

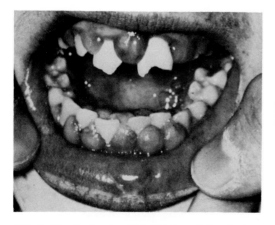

FIG. 6–20. Leukemic cell infiltration of the gingiva, producing a generalized enlargement.

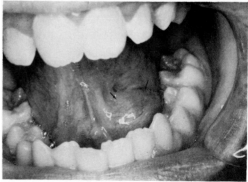

FIG. 6–21. Ranula, a mucocele of the oral floor, soft and fluctuant.

by milking the gland when a major duct is involved. When minor glands in the floor of the mouth are affected, salivary flow may be normal.

Microscopic Features: Most ranulas are fluid-(mucin-) filled spaces lined by a granulation tissue wall representing a large mucocele. Less frequently, they may be lined by cuboidal ductal epithelium with areas of oncocytic metaplasia.

Differential Diagnosis: The ranula may be differentiated clinically from other oral floor swellings by virtue of its compressible cystic nature, location lateral to the midline, and bluish fluid-filled character. It is conceivable that a low-grade cystic mucoepidermoid carcinoma in the floor of the mouth could resemble ranula in clinical appearance.

Treatment: Ranula is conventionally managed by marsupialization.

References

1. Olech, E.: Ranula. Oral Surg. 16:1169, 1963.
2. Catone, G. A., et al.: Sublingual gland mucous-escape phenomenon—treatment by excision of sublingual gland. J. Oral Surg. 27:774, 1969.
3. Mandel, L. and Baurmash, H.: Bilateral ranulas: report of a case. J. Oral Surg. 28:621, 1970.
4. Gormley, M. G., Jarrett, W., and Seldin, R.: Ranulas: a series of eighteen cases of extravasation cysts. J. Acad. Gen. Dent. 21:29, 1973.
5. Rees, R. T.: Congenital ranula. Br. Dent. J. 146:345, 1979.

Dermoid Cyst

Age: Adults
Sex: No predilection

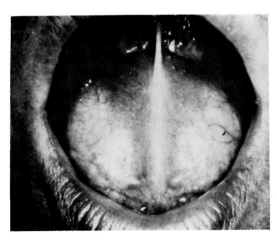

FIG. 6–22. Dermoid cysts arising from the oral floor in the midline—firm, rubbery tumefactions that elevate the tongue. (Courtesy of Dr. S. Rovin.)

Clinical Features: The dermoid cyst has been suggested to be derived from entrapped epithelium remaining from fusion of the embryonic processes forming the oral floor. It is located in the midline of the anterior floor of the mouth as a dome-shaped mass. It protrudes orally when localized above the mylohyoid muscle, submentally when arising below this muscle. Since dermoid cysts are filled with semisolid keratin and sebum, they are doughy on palpation.

Microscopic Features: The cyst lining is keratinizing stratified squamous epithelium. The luminal contents are eosinophilic, amorphous, and caseous. Respiratory epithelium is occasionally present. Within the fibrous wall are skin adnexal structures such as sebaceous glands, sweat glands, and hair follicles. Minor salivary tissue may be present as well. When other connective tissues and neural elements are encountered, the term *teratoid cyst* is preferable.

Differential Diagnosis: Most of the other lesions listed in this section as oral floor swellings arise lateral to the midline. The central location, doughy consistency, and tendency to elevate the tongue are classic signs of the dermoid cyst. As the cyst contents are semisolid, little or no fluid can be obtained on aspiration.

Treatment: The cyst can be delivered surgically by simple enucleation. When it is superior to the mylohyoid, an intraoral approach is preferred. Submylohyoid dermoids are removed by an extraoral approach.

References

1. Colp, R.: Dermoid cysts of the floor of the mouth. Surg. Gynecol. Obstet. 40:183, 1925.
2. New, E. B. and Erich, J. G.: Dermoid cysts of the head and neck. Surg. Gynecol. Obstet. 65:48, 1937.
3. Meyer, I.: Dermoid cyst of the floor of the mouth. Oral Surg. 8:1149, 1955.
4. Chakravorty, R. C. and Schatzki, P. F.: Lateral sublingual dermoid. Oral Surg. 39:862, 1975.
5. Lowry, R. E., Tempero, R. M., and Davis, L. F.: Epidermoid cyst of the floor of the mouth. J. Oral Surg. 37:271, 1979.

Lymphoepithelial Cyst

Age: Adults
Sex: No predilection

Clinical Features: The lymphoepithelial cyst arising in the oral floor is analogous to its extraoral counterpart, the branchial cleft cyst of the neck. The intraoral variety is generally small, located in the anterior oral floor, ventral tongue, or lingual frenum and is a doughy, well-circumscribed nod-

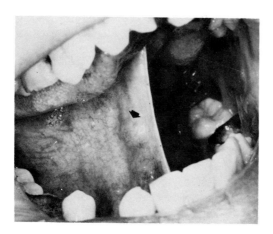

FIG. 6–23. Benign lymphoepithelial cysts, yellow nodules with a smooth surface usually located in the oral floor or ventral tongue.

ule. Because of the involved lymphoid tissue it may have a yellowish cast. The origin is obscure but may arise from confinement of salivary duct epithelium in a small lymph node. Alternatively, oral lymphoepithelial cysts have been suggested to represent tonsillar tissue with keratin-plugged cystic crypts.

Microscopic Features: Stratified squamous or, rarely, respiratory epithelium lines the cyst. When squamous epithelium is present, keratin fills the lumen. The wall of the cyst contains sheets of lymphocytes with germinal centers. Some examples show a microscopic communication with the oral epithelium.

Differential Diagnosis: The small nodule of lymphoepithelial cyst must be differentiated from salivary tumors, benign mesenchymal neoplasms, mucocele, and salivary stones.

Treatment: The nodule should be excised since a clinical diagnosis cannot unequivocably be made.

References

1. Knapp, M. J.: Oral tonsils: Location, distribution, and histology. Oral Surg. 29:155, 1970.
2. Knapp, M. J.: Pathology of oral tonsils. Oral Surg. 29:295, 1970.
3. Giunta, J. and Cataldo, E.: Lymphoepithelial cysts of the oral mucosa. Oral Surg. 35:77, 1973.
4. Buchner, A. and Hansen, L. S.: Lymphoepithelial cysts of the oral cavity: A clinicopathologic study of thirty-eight cases. Oral Surg. 50:441, 1980.
5. Toto, P. D., Wortel, J. P., and Joseph, G.: Lymphoepithelial cysts and associated immunoglobulins. Oral Surg. 54:59, 1982.

Sialolithiasis with Sialadenitis

Age: Adults
Sex: Male predilection

Clinical Features: Over 90 percent of all sialoliths occur within the submandibular duct. When they arise in the distal aspect, they do so as oral floor swellings. Duct occlusion will produce swelling and fibrosis of the affected gland. The duct is usually painless; however, pain on the affected side will be elicited when eating. Salivary flow from the sublingual orifice cannot be initiated upon milking of the gland. The dilated duct containing the stone is a rock-hard nodule. Occasionally, an occluded gland will become subject to secondary pathogenic bacteria with development of acute sialadenitis. The affected gland and duct will enlarge and be acutely tender to palpation. In addition, an exudate can often be milked from the Wharton's duct.

Microscopic Features: The decalcified specimen shows a stone with concentric laminations. The ductal lining shows metaplasia within the epithelium so that stratified squamous, mucous cell formation or oncocytic change may be discerned. Respiratory epithelium may be present.

Differential Diagnosis: The oral floor swelling may mimic neoplasm or cyst; however, the symptoms and indurated calcific nature of sialolithiasis are usually present, providing the information necessary to make a clinical diagnosis. An occlusal radiograph will disclose the presence of a radiopacity in the floor of the mouth.

Treatment: Small stones may be delivered through the duct orifice by manual manipulation. When they are large, surgical removal is indi-

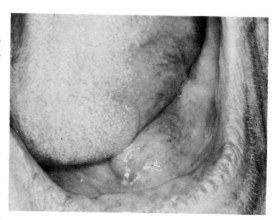

FIG. 6–24. Salivary stone causing swelling in the oral floor with distension of the submandibular salivary duct.

cated. Removal of the involved gland may be necessary, particularly if fibrosis and secondary infection exist.

References

1. Levy, B. M., ReMine, W. H., and Devine, K. D.: Salivary gland calculi: Pain, swelling associated with eating. J. Am. Med. Assoc. *181*:1115, 1962.
2. Seldin, H. M., et al.: Conservative surgery for removal of salivary calculi. Oral Surg. 6:579, 1963.
3. Narang, R. and Dixon, R. A.: Surgical management of submandibular sialadenitis and sialolithiasis. Oral Surg. 43:210, 1977.
4. El Deeb, M., Holte, N., and Gorlin, R. J.: Submandibular salivary gland sialoliths perforated through the oral floor. Oral Surg. *51*:134, 1981.

Salivary Gland Tumors

Age: Adults

Sex: Male predilection

Clinical Features: Salivary neoplasms, benign or malignant, may on rare occasions arise within the major or minor sublingual glands in the floor of the mouth. Salivary tumors of the oral floor are more commonly seen in the submandibular gland with evidence of a mass in the lateroposterior region. Submandibular tumors may not be visually noticeable intraorally but will become obvious on bimanual palpation. If the tumor is benign, it will be firm but encapsulated and movable. The most common tumor is the pleomorphic adenoma; however, both submandibular and sublingual gland neoplasms are more apt to represent malignancies than are parotid tumors. Adenocarcinomas may be of any type, yet adenoid cystic carcinoma or cylindroma and mucoepidermoid carcinoma are the more frequently encountered tumors. Malignant salivary tumors are nonencapsulated, indurated, and may or may not evince fixation.

Microscopic Features: The microscopic features vary, depending upon the type of tumor present. The major forms are discussed under palatal swellings.

Differential Diagnosis: Benign salivary tumors must be differentiated from mesenchymal neoplasms and sclerosing sialadenitis. Indurated swellings suspected of being salivary adenocarcinomas must be differentiated from submandibular lymph node metastasis from a primary oral carcinoma and from primary sarcomas.

Treatment: Benign tumors are treated by sialectomy. Malignant salivary neoplasms require resection with radical neck dissection when cervical or supraomohyoid nodes are palpable.

References

1. Eneroth, C. M. and Hjertman, L.: Benign tumors of the submandibular gland. Pract. Otorhinolaryngol. *29*:166, 1967.
2. Eneroth, C. M., et al.: Malignant tumors of the submandibular gland. Acta Otolaryngol. 64:514, 1967.
3. Hanna, D. C. and Clairmont, A. A.: Submandibular gland tumors. J. Plast. Reconstr. Surg. *61*:198, 1978.
4. Fu, K. K., et al.: Carcinoma of the major and minor salivary glands. Cancer 40:2882, 1977.
5. Shidnia, H., et al.: Carcinoma of major salivary glands. Cancer 45:693, 1980.

Mesenchymal Neoplasms

Age: More frequent in adults

Sex: Slight male predilection

Clinical Features: Benign or malignant connective tissue tumors may arise in any location. While mesenchymal neoplasms are more frequently seen in the tongue and buccal mucosa, they nevertheless will arise in the oral floor and appear as smooth-surfaced elevations. Reactive tumor-like proliferations, the fibromatoses, may also be located in the floor of the mouth. Benign mesenchymal tumors are encapsulated or well delineated, soft or firm, and movable. The more common entities include lipoma, fibroma, hemangioma, and neural sheath tumors. A special form of lymphangioma, the cystic hygroma, occurs in this location and usually bulges extraorally. The sarcomas are multinodular, indurated, and usually fixed. While all sarcomas are rare in this region, the entities most likely to be present include fibrosarcoma and lymphoma.

Microscopic Features: The histologic patterns found in mesenchymal neoplasms are extremely

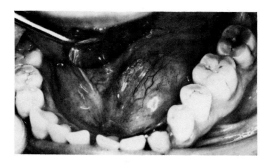

FIG. 6–25. Salivary neoplasms of the submandibular and sublingual glands often manifest unilateral oral floor swelling. (From Melrose, R. J. and Abrams, A. M.: *Oral Tumors: A Visual Instruction Course.* Los Angeles, Eureka Press, 1974, p. 51.)

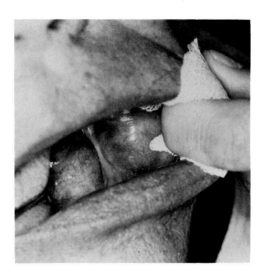

FIG. 6–26.   Neurofibroma in floor of mouth.

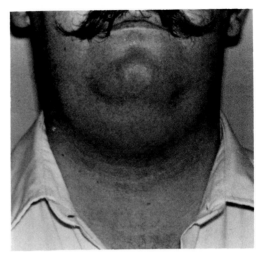

FIG. 6–27.   Ludwig's angina with diffuse swelling of the submandibular area, also showing elevation of the oral floor. (Courtesy of Dr. R. Middleton.)

varied depending upon the type of tumor and cell of origin. Some are described in the section on tongue swellings.

Differential Diagnosis: Oral floor swellings representing mesenchymal tumors are firm or indurated and must be differentiated from salivary tumors, sclerosing sialadenitis and metastatic lymphadenopathy. Those of vascular origin may be less encapsulated, particularly lymphangiomas, and therefore require wide excision. Sarcomas require radical excision. A diagnosis of lymphoma requires further workup to detect dissemination; the disease is managed by radiation and chemotherapeutic modalities.

Treatment: Well-localized nodules representing benign mesenchymal neoplasms are treated by simple surgical excision.

References

1. Watson, W. L. and McCarthy, W. D.: Blood and lymph vessel tumors; a report of 1,056 cases. Surg. Gynecol. Obstet. 71:569, 1940.
2. O'Day, R. A., et al.: Soft tissue sarcomas of the oral cavity. Mayo Clin. Proc. 39:169, 1964.
3. Vindenes, H.: Lipomas of the oral cavity. Int. J. Oral Surg. 7:162, 1978.
4. Brandjord, R. M., Reaume, C. E., and Wesley, R. K.: Leiomyosarcoma of the floor of the mouth: review of the literature and report of case. J. Oral Surg. 35:590, 1977.
5. Swart, J. G. N., et al.: Possible myxoma of the floor of the mouth: report of case. J. Oral Surg. 35:501, 1977.

Ludwig's Angina

Age: No predilection
Sex: No predilection

Clinical Features: Odontogenic infection with drainage into the fascial spaces of the oral floor will produce swelling. When bilateral involvement of the submandibular and sublingual spaces occurs in conjunction with cellulitis of the mylohyoid and tongue musculature, a diffuse board-hard swelling evolves and is obvious both extraorally and intraorally. The patient is febrile, with malaise. Pain is severe. Death may ensue from encroachment of edema and cellulitis on the airway or spread of infection into the paravertebral space and mediastinum.

Microscopic Features: The tissues are avidly and diffusely infiltrated with neutrophils and scattered histiocytes.

Differential Diagnosis: The only other disease that can extend into all regions of the oral floor as an indurated swelling resembling Ludwig's angina is infiltrating carcinoma or sarcoma. In these instances fever is not a dominant sign and conspicuous odontogenic infection with a carious or nonvital tooth is not featured unless it occurs as a coincidental finding. Whereas streptococci are usually cultured from the tissue, anaerobic organisms may be responsible either as concomitants or as primary agents.

Treatment: Antibiotic therapy with multiple incisions for drainage is required to prevent respiratory embarrassment. Intravenous antibiotic therapy with hospitalization and supportive care for infection are necessary.

References

1. Taffel, M. and Harvey, S. C.: Ludwig's angina. Surgery *11*:841, 1942.
2. Williams, A. C. and Guralnick, W. C.: Diagnosis and treatment of Ludwig's angina; report of 20 cases. N. Engl. J. Med. *228*:443, 1943.
3. Holland, C. S.: The management of Ludwig's angina. Br. J. Oral Surg. *13*:153, 1975.
4. Briggs, P. C.: Submandibular duct stenosis as a complication of Ludwig's angina. Oral Surg. *47*:14, 1979.

Squamous Cell Carcinoma

Age: Middle-aged and elderly adults

Sex: Male predilection

Clinical Features: Squamous cancer of the oral floor may appear red, white, mixed red and white, ulcerated, or tumefactive; the floor of the mouth represents the most common site for oral cancer. Invasive tumefactive lesions are indurated and usually ulcerated. They are most frequently located anteriorly overlying Wharton's duct. They may infiltrate laterally to involve the alveolar ridge or ventral tongue. About half the patients present with nodal involvement of the submandibular or cervical region.

Microscopic Features: Oral floor squamous cell carcinoma is characterized by invasive cords, nests, and islands comprised of squamous cells showing varying degrees of hyperchromatism, pleomorphism, and increased mitotic activity. Parakeratin pearl formation can usually be identified. Many oral floor tumors, particularly smaller lesions, will maintain carcinoma-in-situ changes

along the lateral margins. These changes frequently extend along salivary excretory ducts.

Differential Diagnosis: Most noncancerous oral floor swellings are soft and exhibit an intact mucosal surface. Any lesion that is indurated and ulcerated should be considered in all probability a carcinoma; immediate biopsy is indicated.

Treatment: Combined radiation therapy and surgery are preferable over a single modality. Lymph node dissection is advocated when palpable nodes are present and is usually advisable in the absence of palpable nodes. Survival is dependent upon extent of disease. Overall 5-year survival for this site is about 50 percent.

References

1. Martin, H. E. and Sugarbaker, E. L.: Cancer of the floor of the mouth. Surg. Gynecol. Obstet. *71*:347, 1940.
2. Feind, C. R. and Cole, R. M.: Cancer of the floor of the mouth and its lymphatic spread. Am. J. Surg. *116*:482, 1968.
3. Montana, G. S., et al.: Carcinoma of the tongue and floor of the mouth; results of radical radiotherapy. Cancer *23*:1284, 1969.
4. Ballard, B. R., et al.: Squamous cell carcinoma of the floor of the mouth. Oral Surg. *45*:568, 1978.

SWELLINGS OF THE LIPS AND BUCCAL MUCOSA

Mucous Retention Phenomenon (Mucocele)

Age: Young adults

Sex: Slight male predilection

Clinical Features: The mucocele is the most

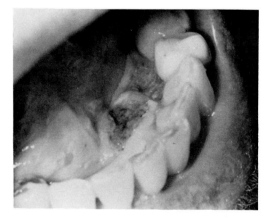

FIG. 6–28.   Squamous cell carcinoma of the oral floor showing an ulcerated tumefaction.

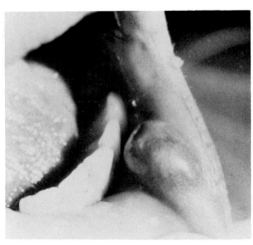

FIG. 6–29.   Mucocele, generally seen on the lower lip as fluctuant fluid-filled blebs. (Note that a papilloma also exists on the commissure.)

common swelling of the lower lip and arises secondary to traumatic severance of a minor salivary duct with pooling of extraductal mucin in the submucosa. It may be seen on the buccal mucosa as well. It is a dome-shaped elevation, which, if superficial, has a bluish fluid-filled appearance. If situated deep, it may be of normal color. A history of paroxysmal swelling and collapse is common.

Microscopic Features: The epithelium is distended by a pseudocystic space filled with mucin infiltrated with neutrophils and foamy histiocytes. The wall is composed of granulation tissue.

Differential Diagnosis: When mucoceles are superficial they may resemble bullae. The remaining oral tissues, conjunctivas, and skin must be examined to rule out bullous dermatoses. Mucoepidermoid carcinoma may clinically resemble mucocele yet is extremely rare in the lip. Deeply situated mucoceles may appear identical to fibrous hyperplasia or mesenchymal neoplasms. Occasionally blood enters the cystic cavity of a mucocele, giving the appearance of hemangioma or varix.

Treatment: Mucoceles cannot be unroofed and be expected to resolve. Excision with inclusion of the underlying salivary tissue will help minimize the chance for recurrence.

References

1. Standish, S. M. and Shafer, W. G.: The mucous retention phenomenon. J. Oral Surg. *17*:15, 1959.
2. Cohen, L.: Mucoceles of the oral cavity. Oral Surg. *19*:365, 1965.
3. Sela, J. and Ulmansky, M.: Mucous retention cysts of salivary glands. J. Oral Surg. *27*:619, 1969.
4. Cataldo, E. and Mosadomi, A.: Mucoceles of the oral mucous membrane. Arch. Otolaryngol. *91*:360, 1970.

Minor Gland Sialolithiasis

Age: Middle-aged adults
Sex: Slightly more common in males

Clinical Features: Salivary stones occasionally form within the ducts of minor glands, being most frequently detected in the buccal mucosa and upper lip. They are not always visible yet are easily detected by palpation. Larger stones may produce a nodular bulge; in all cases the lesion is hard and may give the impression of a foreign body such as a beebee or shot. They are usually asymptomatic.

Microscopic Features: Minor gland sialoliths are situated within a dilated duct that shows mucous, respiratory, or squamous metaplasia. The stone is composed of concentric acellular lami-

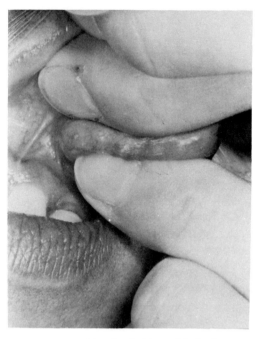

FIG. 6–30. Small hard palpable nodule in the upper lip representing a sialolith.

nations of basophilic amorphous material in decalcified specimens. Adjacent acini exhibit degenerative changes with fibrous and inflammatory changes.

Differential Diagnosis: These lesions are clinically typical in that a hard movable nodule can be palpated. They may, however, be confused with a foreign body.

Treatment: Surgical excision is the treatment of choice.

References

1. Eversole, L. R. and Sabes, W. R.: Minor salivary gland duct changes due to obstruction. Arch. Otolaryng. *94*:19, 1971.
2. Bahn, S. L. and Tabachnick, T. F.: Sialolithiasis of minor salivary glands. Oral Surg. *32*:371, 1971.
3. Pullon, P. A. and Miller, A. S.: Sialolithiasis of accessory salivary glands: review of 55 cases. J. Oral Surg. *30*:832, 1972.
4. Jensen, J. L.: Minor salivary gland calculi. A clinicopathologic study of forty-seven new cases. Oral Surg. *47*:44, 1979.

Nasoalveolar (Klestadt) Cyst

Age: Adults
Sex: Female predilection

Clinical Features: The nasoalveolar cyst is restricted in location to the submucosal tissues between and superior to the roots of the maxillary

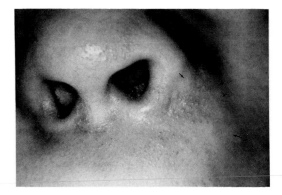

FIG. 6–31. Swelling with elevation of the ala of the nose in a nasolabial cyst. (Courtesy of Charles Tomich.)

lateral incisor and cuspid lying above the muco-buccal fold. It is soft and fluctuant or tense and often extends superiorly into the anterior nasal floor, producing a bulge below and anterior to the inferior turbinate. Bilateral cases have been reported. On aspiration a mucous fluid is obtained, and injection of radiopaque dye will clearly demonstrate its cystic nature on roentgenogram. The lesion is the soft tissue counterpart of the globu-lomaxillary cyst.

Microscopic Features: The cyst is lined by pseudostratified columnar epithelium. Cilia are demonstrable in most cases. Mucous metaplasia is frequently encountered. The fibrous wall usually lacks inflammatory cell infiltration.

Differential Diagnosis: A clinically cystic lesion in the location of the maxillary cuspid is almost invariably a nasoalveolar cyst. Nevertheless, it must be differentiated from a salivary or mesenchymal neoplasm and an abscess (parulis) due to drainage from odontogenic infection.

Treatment: Simple excision by enucleation generally is not followed by recurrence.

References

1. Klestadt, W. O.: Nasal cysts and the facial cleft theory. Ann. Otol. Rhinol. Laryngol. 62:84, 1953.
2. Roed-Peterson, B.: Nasolabial cysts; a presentation of five patients and review of the literature. Br. J. Oral Surg. 7:83, 1969.
3. Crawford, W. H. and Greskovich, F. J.: Nasolabial cysts: report of two cases. J. Oral Surg. 26:582, 1968.
4. Brandao, G. S., Ebling, H., and Souza, I. C.: Bilateral nasolabial cyst. Oral Surg. 37:480, 1974.

Cheilitis Granulomatosa

Age: Young adults
Sex: No predilection

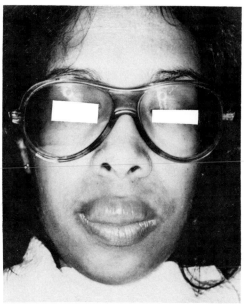

FIG. 6–32. Diffuse, firm enlargement of the upper lip seen in cheilitis granulomatosa.

Clinical Features: Either upper, lower, or both lips show a diffuse nodular enlargement that involves not just a portion but the entire lip from one commissure to the other. The lip is firm to palpation but devoid of any superficial inflammation or discoloration. Cheilitis granulomatosa accompanied by fissured tongue and facial paralysis constitutes the Melkersson-Rosenthal syndrome. The fissured tongue may also show nodular or papillary tumefactions. In actuality a spectrum of changes may be encountered in patients with cheilitis granulomatosa. Twenty percent exhibit facial paralysis, forty percent have fissured tongue; other oral sites, primarily the buccal mucosa and palate, are affected by multinodular lesions or erythematous or bluish edematous plaques. Cheilitis granulomatosa is of unknown origin but has been suggested to represent a regional form of sarcoidosis or an atypical granulomatous disease, possibly allergic in origin.

Microscopic Features: The swelling is accounted for by the presence of granulomatous inflammation with infiltration and replacement of the minor salivary glands. The granulomas are multinodular, being composed of swirled collagen fascicles with interspersed multinucleated giant cells.

Differential Diagnosis: The appearance is similar to that of angioneurotic edema or edema and cellulitis of odontogenic infectious origin. These two lesions are diffuse and soft to palpation, whereas cheilitis granulomatosa is firm and multinodular.

Treatment: Intralesional injection of triamcinolone or another steroid on 6 to 10 weekly occasions may result in significant diminution in the size of the lip. Intralesional steroids are not always effective, and surgical excision of lip granulomas may be followed by recurrence. Surprisingly, elimination of odontogenic and periodontal sources of infection often coincide with a diminution in signs and symptoms.

References
1. Rhodes, E. L. and Stirling, G. A.: Granulomatous cheilitis. Arch. Dermatol. 92:40, 1965.
2. Nally, F. M.: Melkersson-Rosenthal syndrome. Report of two cases. Oral Surg. 29:694, 1970.
3. Zecha, J. J., Van Dijk, L., and Hadders, H. N.: Cheilitis granulomatosa (Melkersson-Rosenthal syndrome). Oral Surg. 42:454, 1976.
4. Krutchkoff, D. and James, R.: Cheilitis granulomatosa. Successful treatment with combined triamcinolone injections and surgery. Arch. Dermatol. 114:1203, 1978.
5. Worsaae, N., et al.: Melkersson-Rosenthal syndrome and cheilitis granulomatosa. A clinicopathologic study of thirty-three patients with special reference to their oral lesions. Oral Surg. 54:404, 1982.

Cheilitis Glandularis

Age: Middle-aged and elderly adults
Sex: Male predilection

Clinical Features: Cheilitis glandularis is a disease of unknown etiology that represents both a superficial and deep (salivary) inflammatory disorder. Overexposure to sun with superimposed infection has been suggested to give rise to this uncommon condition. The vermilion border and mucosa may be of normal color, or diffuse keratosis with scaling may be featured. The lower lip is affected and a multinodular enlargement is seen. Multiple pits or fistulae representing dilated minor salivary ducts stipple the lip surface, and exudate may be expressed from these openings in some but not all instances. Carcinoma of the lip has been reported to complicate a number of cases.

Microscopic Features: The surface epithelium may be unremarkable; more often, hyperkeratosis and actinic changes are observed. The underlying salivary gland lobules show hypertrophy and sialadenitis, often of an acute nature.

Differential Diagnosis: Cheilitis glandularis may simulate the clinical features seen in cheilitis granulomatosa; however, the multiple dilated duct orifices along with multinodular enlargement are classic clinical findings. Biopsy should be performed, particularly in cases with foci of keratotic thickening or ulceration.

Treatment: Excision of the involved area can generally be accomplished without extending the surgical margin onto the vermilion, thereby avoiding cosmetic deformity.

References
1. Doku, H. C., Shklar, G., and McCarthy, P. L.: Cheilitis glandularis. Oral Surg. 20:563, 1965.
2. Weir, T. W. and Johnson, W. C.: Cheilitis glandularis. Arch. Dermatol. 103:433, 1971.
3. Oliver, I. D. and Pickett, A. B.: Cheilitis glandularis. Oral Surg. 49:526, 1980.
4. Stuller, C. B., et al.: Cheilitis glandularis. Oral Surg. 53:602, 1982.

Angioneurotic Edema

Age: No predilection
Sex   No predilection

Clinical Features: Angioneurotic edema represents a histamine-mediated immediate hypersensitivity reaction to some allergenic substance, usually a food or drug. An intraoral vesiculoerythematous reaction may accompany the edematous episode, which consists of diffuse, often massive swelling of the upper lip and face. The swelling, due to accumulation of edema fluid, is soft. Often the periorbital skin is involved and the swelling may be so marked that the eyelids cannot be opened. A hereditary form exists and is usually accompanied by generalized skin urticaria. The inherited variety shows a biochemical defect in the complement fixation pathway with a deficiency of C'1 esterase inhibitor.

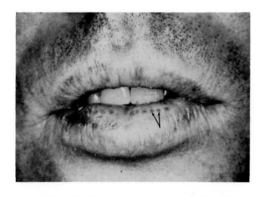

FIG. 6–33. Cheilitis glandularis characterized by enlargement of the lower lip accompanied by accentuation of the salivary excretory duct pores. (Courtesy of Dr. H. Cherrick.)

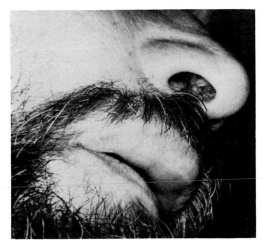

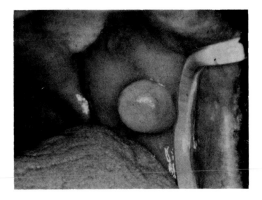

FIG. 6–35. Fibromas, usually seen on the cheek, are smooth-surfaced swellings and are well circumscribed.

FIG. 6–34. Angioneurotic edema, an allergic reaction, results in soft edematous enlargement of the upper lip and face.

Microscopic Features: Not applicable.

Differential Diagnosis: The rapid onset of swelling often preceded by pruritus is unique. The only other disease that may mimic angioneurotic edema is diffuse cellulitis with edema resulting from odontogenic infection in an anterior maxillary tooth. The hereditary form follows an autosomal dominant pattern with both skin and visceral manifestations.

Treatment: Any suspected allergens should be withdrawn. Systemically administered antihistamines will cause resolution within hours. Repeated exposure to the allergen can result in Quincke's edema and progress to anaphylactic shock. Patients with hereditary angioneurotic edema should be referred to an allergist. Three daily 200 mg doses of danazol on a maintenance schedule are employed in the hereditary form of the disease.

References

1. Reinberg, S. M. and Feinberg, A. R.: Allergy to penicillin. J. Am. Med. Assoc. *160*:778, 1956.
2. Donaldson, V. H. and Rosen, F. S.: Hereditary angioneurotic edema: A clinical survey. Pediatrics *37*:1017, 1966.
3. Sturdy, K. A., et al.: Hereditary angioedema controlled with danazol. Oral Surg. *48*:418, 1979.
4. Albright, B. W. and Taylor, C. G.: Hereditary angioneurotic edema: report of case. J. Oral Surg. *37*:888, 1979.

Inflammatory Hyperplasia (Traumatic Fibroma)

Age: No predilection
Sex: No predilection

Clinical Features: The traumatic fibroma may arise in any oral location. It represents the most common swelling of the buccal mucosa and is also extremely common on the mucosal surface of the lips. Traumatic fibroma represents reactive fibrous hyperplasia due to trauma and is not a true neoplasm. It is a sessile dome-shaped soft nodule, usually of normal color, and may be ulcerated from trauma as in cheek-biting.

Microscopic Features: The epithelium is distended by a mass of dense collagenous tissue with interspersed fibroblasts. Capillaries traverse the tissue, and there are few if any inflammatory cells. When stellate multinucleated cells are seen, the lesion represents a giant cell fibroma.

Differential Diagnosis: Traumatic fibroma may be clinically indistinguishable from true mesenchymal neoplasms, benign salivary tumor, a deeply situated mucocele, or an epidermoid cyst.

Treatment: Excisional biopsy is recommended to rule out the presence of a true neoplasm.

References

1. Shafer, W. G., Hine, M. K., and Levy, B. M.: A Textbook of Oral Pathology, 4th Ed. Philadelphia, W. B. Saunders Co., 1983, pp. 137–140.
2. Barker, D. S. and Lucas, F. B.: Localized fibrous overgrowths of the oral mucosa. Br. J. Oral Surg. *5*:86, 1967.

Foreign Body Granuloma

Age: No predilection
Sex: No predilection

Clinical Features: A variety of foreign bodies may be introduced into the oral submucosal tissues. Most foreign bodies are iatrogenic whereby a substance becomes implanted during an extraction or oral surgical procedure. Not all foreign agents and chemicals will elicit a granulomatous

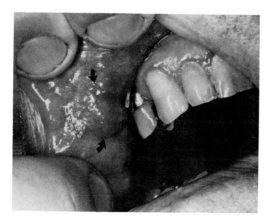

FIG. 6–36. Foreign body granuloma appearing as a mass in the buccal mucosa.

response. Common reactions of this nature occur with handpiece oil (oil granuloma), vegetable matter (pulse granuloma), dental cements. The true nature of the foreign agent often cannot be ascertained. The mucobuccal fold is probably the most common location; the lesions are soft or firm and either dome-shaped or multinodular.

Microscopic Features: The submucosa is fibrotic with chronically inflamed granulation tissue evincing a mild inflammatory cell infiltrate. Multinucleated giant cells are observed and usually phagocytosis of the foreign material can be seen. Oil granulomas appear as large vacant vacuoles. Pulse granulomas exhibit compartmentalized spaces with enveloping giant cells. When a foreign material is not readily identifiable, polarized lenses may be employed to detect refractile materials.

Differential Diagnosis: Foreign body granulomas are dome-shaped nodules that cannot usually be differentiated clinically from benign mesenchymal neoplasms, salivary neoplasms, or other granulomatous lesions. Whereas a history of trauma or previous surgery to the area would certainly arouse suspicion of a foreign body reaction, biopsy is required to obtain a definitive diagnosis.

Treatment: Local excisional biopsy is the treatment of choice.

References

1. Fine, L., et al.: Foreign body-type reaction following crown cementation. J. Periodontol. *48*:294, 1977.
2. Cataldo, E. and Santis, H.: Response of the oral tissue to exogenous foreign materials. J. Periodontol. *45*:93, 1974.
3. Wilson, D. F. and Garach, V.: Surgical glove starch granuloma. Oral Surg. *51*:342, 1981.

4. McMillan, M. D., et al.: Giant cell hyalin angiopathy or pulse granuloma. Oral Surg. *52*:178, 1981.

Traumatic (Amputation) Neuroma

Age: No predilection
Sex: No predilection

Clinical Features: An amputation neuroma evolves subsequent to severance of a nerve, whereby the distal segment undergoes Wallerian degeneration and the proximal segment attempts in vain to reunite with the distal nerve sheath. When the severed segments are displaced the proximal portion proliferates, pursuing a tortuous course resulting in tumefaction. The swelling is most frequently encountered in the mucobuccal fold adjacent to the mental foramen. The nodule is firm yet usually movable. Pain is often elicited when pressure is applied; however, cases have been reported in patients suffering from spontaneous facial pain. Most amputation neuromas measure less than 0.5 cm.

Microscopic Features: A tortuous array of axis cylinders accompanied by neurilemma sheath and enveloping perineurium is encountered, resembling an overabundance of normal nerve tissue.

Differential Diagnosis: The swelling observed with amputation neuroma is identical to that seen in mesenchymal neoplasms, salivary tumors, or foreign-body granulomas. A parulis may be considered in the differential diagnosis when the lesion lies directly below the attached gingiva. Firmness with pain on palpation should arouse clinical suspicion of neuroma. When multiple neuromas are identified, the neuropolyendocrine syndrome should be ruled out.

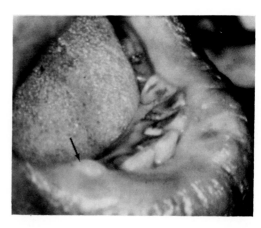

FIG. 6–37. Traumatic neuroma, a small nodule that arose on the lip after trauma.

Treatment: Simple surgical excision is rarely followed by recurrence.

References

1. Swanson, H. H.: Traumatic neuromas; a review of the literature. Oral Surg. *14*:317, 1961.
2. Robinson, M. and Slvakin, H. C.: Dental amputation neuromas. J. Am. Dent. Assoc. *70*:662, 1965.
3. Rasmussen, O. C.: Painful traumatic neuromas in the oral cavity. Oral Surg. *49*:191, 1980.
4. Sist, T. C., Jr., and Greene, G. W.: Traumatic neuroma of the oral cavity. Report of thirty-one new cases and review of the literature. Oral Surg. *51*:394, 1981.

Mesenchymal Neoplasms

Age: Young adults

Sex: No predilection

Clinical Features: Various neoplasms of mesenchymal origin may arise in the buccal mucosa and lips. Because of its prevalence, hemangioma is considered separately. The most common mesenchymal tumors in this location are neurofibroma, neurilemmoma, and lipoma. Less frequently encountered benign neoplasms or neoplastic-like swellings of connective tissue origin include leiomyoma, fibrous histiocytoma, and oral focal mucinosis. As a group, they vary considerably in size, may be soft or firm, movable, and well demarcated or encapsulated. Ulceration of the surface mucosa is unusual. In the cheek, a diffuse swelling composed of adipose tissue usually represents herniation of the buccal fat pad rather that a true lipoma. Rarely, sarcomas and lymphomas will be encountered; ulceration and induration will usually be present when the mass represents a mesenchymal malignancy.

Microscopic Features: The microscopic patterns vary with the tissue of orgin. Neural sheath tumors are described under tongue swellings.

Differential Diagnosis: Swellings of the cheek and lips due to mesenchymal tumors are identical to those of salivary neoplasm, traumatic fibroma, or deep mucocele. Indurated and ulcerated sarcomatous tumors may clinically resemble squamous cell carcinoma or malignant salivary neoplasms.

Treatment: Enucleation and excision are the treatments of choice for benign mesenchymal tumors. Sarcomas require radical wide excision.

References

1. Seldin, H. M., et al.: Lipomas of the oral cavity; report of 26 cases. J. Oral Surg. *25*:270, 1967.
2. Cherrick, H. M. and Eversole, L. R.: Benign neural sheath neoplasm of the oral cavity. Report on thirty-seven cases. Oral Surg. *32*:900, 1971.
3. Tomich, C. E.: Oral focal mucinosis: a clinicopathologic and histochemical study of eight cases. Oral Surg. *38*:714, 1974.
4. Vindenes, H.: Lipomas of the oral cavity. Int. J. Oral Surg. *7*:162, 1978.
5. DiLascio, J. P., Devlin, G. P., and Doyle, J. L.: Aggressive fibrous histiocytoma of perioral soft tissues: report of case. J. Oral Surg. *39*:134, 1981.

Herniated Buccal Fat Pad

Age: Middle-aged and elderly adults

Sex: No predilection

Clinical Features: The buccal fat pad lies external to the buccinator muscle. Trauma to this thin muscle from cheek biting or surgery may weaken or separate the muscle fibers allowing adipose tissue to herniate orally. Herniated fat pads are soft to palpation and may appear faintly yel-

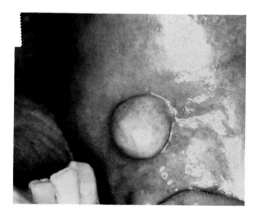

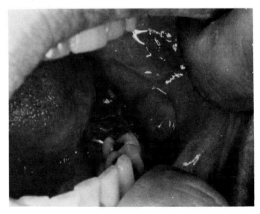

FIG. 6–38. Neurofibroma. Benign mesenchymal neoplasms such as lipoma, neurofibroma, and neurilemmoma are common tumefactions of the cheek.

FIG. 6–39. Soft mass in posterior aspect of buccal mucosa is composed of adipose tissue.

low. They are either dome-shaped tumefactions or exhibit surface lobulation.

Microscopic Features: The lesion is composed of normal-appearing adipose tissue traversed by capillary septae. They cannot usually be differentiated histologically from lipoma; however, scattered isolated muscle fibers are occasionally admixed with the adipose tissue, a feature not encountered in lipoma.

Differential Diagnosis: The buccal mucosal mass representing a herniated fat pad may clinically resemble the other mesenchymal and reactive lesions included in this section. The soft consistency and gross appearance do not allow for differentiation from lipoma. A history of trauma aids in arriving at a diagnosis in conjunction with biopsy.

Treatment: The excess fatty tissue should be excised; if the zone of buccinator perforation can be located, the fibers should be juxtaposed and sutured.

References

1. Clawson, R. J., Kline, K. K., and Armbrecht, E. C.: Trauma-induced avulsion of the buccal fat pad into the mouth. J. Oral Surg. 26:546, 1968.
2. Messenger, K. L. and Cloyd, W.: Traumatic herniation of the buccal fat pad: report of case. Oral Surg. 43:41, 1977.
3. Brooke, R. I.: Traumatic herniation of buccal pad of fat (traumatic pseudolipoma). Oral Surg. 45:689, 1978.

Reactive Lymphoid Hyperplasia

Age: No predilection
Sex: No predilection

Clinical Features: Facial nodes located adja-

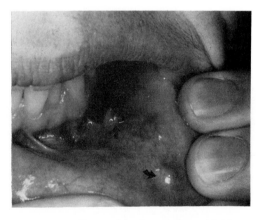

FIG. 6–40. Yellow nodules in mucobuccal fold area and lip represent hyperplastic lymphoid tissue.

cent to the facial vein and buccinator muscle are present in about 20 percent of the population. The nodes are usually not palpable unless stimulated to undergo reactive hyperplasia. Lymphoid hyperplasia of the buccal nodes may not be visible; yet the enlarged node will be firm, palpable, and movable, being located near Stenson's duct. The etiology is not always apparent yet may accompany generalized lymphadenopathy in viral infections or represent a local adenopathy secondary to oral or facial skin infections. Occasionally, an enlarged buccal node will represent a specific infection such as latent acquired toxoplasmosis. Handling of contaminated cat litter is usually the route of transmission; in gravid females, this could significantly endanger the developing fetus. Malignant lymphoma is extremely rare in this location.

Microscopic Features: The node is enlarged and encapsulated. Hyperplastic germinal centers are impacted with active large immunoblasts. The paracortical region may continue to possess a mature lymphocytic mantle; however, large blast cells may occupy this region. The medullary zone is often congested; in addition to mature lymphocytes, histiocytes showing phagocytosis and plasma cells may be present. Toxoplasma lymphadenitis is characterized by extrafollicular pale epithelioid histiocytes.

Differential Diagnosis: Reactive lymphoid hyperplasia is indistinguishable clinically from mesenchymal neoplasms, benign salivary tumors, and focal granulomas. For this reason, a biopsy is required to arrive at a definitive diagnosis.

Treatment: Provided no infectious source can be uncovered, further treatment, even for toxoplasma lymphadenitis, is not required. Generalized or systemic disease should be treated according to the nature of the process.

References

1. Doyle, J. L.: Benign lymphoid lesions of the oral mucosa. Oral Surg. 29:31, 1970.
2. Dorfman, R. F. and Warnke, R.: Lymphadenopathy simulating malignant lymphomas. Hum. Pathol. 5:519, 1974.
3. Weidman, B. and Warman, E.: Lymph nodes of the head and neck. J. Oral Med. 35:39, 1980.
4. Appel, B. N., Mendelow, H., and Pasqual, H. N.: Acquired Toxoplasma lymphadenitis. Oral Surg. 47:529, 1979.

Hemangioma and Varix

Age: Hemangiomas—children; Varix—adults
Sex: No predilection

Clinical Features: Vascular lesions are com-

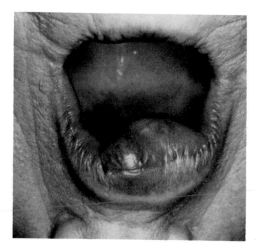

FIG. 6–41. Hemangioma of the lip. May be red, blue or of normal color when arising within deeper connective tissues.

monly located on the lips and buccal mucosa. In children, they represent hamartomatous proliferation of vascular channels (hemangiomas). Intramuscular hemangiomas may attain considerable dimensions; being situated in deeper tissues, they do not necessarily impart a red or bluish appearance to the distended overlying mucosa. In older patients, the clinical features are nearly identical but vascular growths generally represent aneurysmal-like dilations of venules known as varices. A localized varix may appear subsequent to trauma. Both hemangiomas and varices appear as smooth or slightly nodular soft swellings, red to purple in color, and will blanch on pressure. Hemangiomas of the oral mucosa may accompany facial skin angiomatoses or port-wine stain and can be a component of the Sturge-Weber syndrome. Angiomas or varices of long duration may contain radiographically demonstrable phleboliths. Aggressive or even malignant hemangioendotheliomas or hemangiopericytomas are rare, have a rapid growth rate, and are usually indurated.

Microscopic Features: Hemangiomas may be capillary in type, with numerous small-caliber vascular channels, or they may be cavernous with large dilated vessels. A varix may represent a single dilated tortuous venule, which, on microscopic section, will show numerous dilated channels similar to cavernous hemangiomas. Thrombi are frequently seen within the dilated vascular lumina.

Hemangioendotheliomas are very cellular with only slit-like vascular channels and sheets of plump endothelial cells. Likewise, hemangiopericytomas are hypercellular, yet reticulum stains disclose that the neoplastic cells proliferate beyond the confines of periendothelial reticulum. Additionally, the vascular spaces are irregular, evincing a "stag-horn" pattern.

Differential Diagnosis: Other swellings of the lips and cheek are not pigmented; however, deeply situated vascular lesions may not show a red color and therefore must be differentiated from mucocele, other mesenchymal neoplasms, salivary neoplasms, and inflammatory hyperplasia.

Treatment: Local excision is the treatment of choice for small lesions; excessive hemorrhage is generally not encountered. Large diffuse hemangiomas may be excised or sclerosed. If they do not interfere with function or are not a cosmetic problem, they may be left untreated. Hemangiomas in children may show spontaneous regression before or during pubescence. Wide excision with liberal margins is in order for hemangioendothelioma and hemangiopericytoma. When these turmors are encountered a thorough medical work-up is necessary, as they occasionally metastasize.

References

1. Watson, W. L. and McCarthy, W. D.: Blood and lymph vessel tumors; a report of 1,056 cases. Surg. Gynecol. Obstet. 71:569, 1940.
2. Shklar, G. and Meyer, I.: Vascular tumors of the mouth and jaws. Oral Surg. 19:335, 1965.
3. Weathers, D. R. and Fine, R. M. Thrombosed varix of the oral cavity. Arch. Dermatol. 104:427, 1971.
4. Walike, J. W. and Bailey, B. J.: Head and neck hemangiopericytoma. Arch. Otolaryngol. 93:345, 1971.
5. Kinni, M. E., Webb, R. I., and Christensen, R. W.: Intramuscular hemangioma of the orbicularis oris muscle: report of case. J. Oral Surg. 39:780, 1981.

Keratoacanthoma

Age: Adults
Sex: Male predilection

Clinical Features: The keratoacanthoma is a neoplasm-like swelling that occurs on skin and may involve the vermilion border. It has been reported to occur intraorally but rarely does so. On the lower lip, the lesion shows a smooth, raised, rolled border with a cental plug of hard heratin. Keratoacanthoma may clinically resemble carcinoma; however, the microscopic features are characteristic and, if left untreated, the lesion will spontaneously regress within 6 to 24 months.

Microscopic Features: The surface stratified

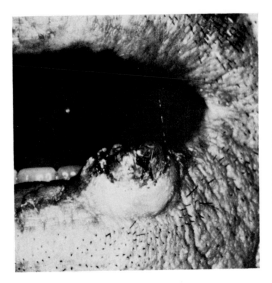

FIG. 6–42. Keratoacanthoma showing rolled margins with a central keratotic core. (From Kohn M. W. and Eversole, L. R.: Keratoacanthoma of the lower lip; report of cases. J. Oral. Surg. 30:522, 1972.)

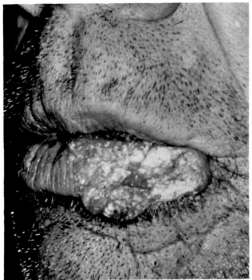

FIG. 6–43. Squamous cell carcinoma of the lower lip.

squamous epithelium is normal lateral to the tumor and at the margin evinces an abrupt transition whereby it invaginates with acanthosis and rete ridge formation. The central umbilicated zone overlying the acanthomatous spinous cell layer is characterized by a core of thickened parakeratin and orthokeratin. Cell atypia is minimal. The subjacent fibrous tissue shows a lymphocytic infiltrate.

Differential Diagnosis: Keratoacanthoma of the lower lip must be differentiated from keratinizing squamous cell carcinoma.

Treatment: Excisional biopsy is indicated to rule out malignancy. The scar remaining from excision is usually more cosmetic than that resulting from spontaneous regression.

References

1. Silberberg, I., Kopf, A. W., and Baer, R. L.: Recurrent keratoacanthoma of the lip. Arch. Dermatol. 86:44, 1962.
2. Reed, R. J.: Actinic keratoacanthoma. Arch. Dermatol. 106:858, 1972.
3. Bass, K. D.: Solitary keratoacanthoma of the lip. J. Oral Surg. 38:53, 1980.
4. Eversole, L. R., Leider, A. S., and Alexander, G.: Intraoral and labial keratoacanthoma. Oral Surg. 54:663, 1982.

Squamous Cell Carcinoma

Age: Elderly adults
Sex: Male predilection

Clinical Features: Early squamous cell carcinoma may appear as a focal ulcer on the lower lip and often shows actinic cheilosis. As tumefaction ensues, the surface may remain ulcerated or be encrusted with keratin. Usually, but not invariably, the mass is indurated and fixed to the adjacent soft tissues. Metastatic deposits may be detected in the submental, submandibular, or cervical nodes. Squamous cell carcinoma in the buccal mucosa will similarly be ulcerated and indurated. Not uncommonly, it may show a white keratinized surface.

Microscopic Features: The neoplastic epithelium is well differentiated when it involves the lip, showing minimal hyperchromatism or pleomorphism. Tumor islands display central parakeratin or keratin pearls. Two specific forms of squamous cancer occur on the lip and show unique histomorphologic features. Adenoid squamous cell carcinoma is characterized by acantholysis of cells, producing clefting within tumor islands. This change imparts an adenoid appearance. Spindle cell carcinoma is another variant of squamous cell cancer. Microscopically, the cells appear sarcomatoid with streams of invasive spindle cells that are usually in continuity with and emanate from the basal layer. Buccal mucosa carcinomas may not necessarily be well differentiated.

Differential Diagnosis: Small squamous cell carcinomas may be well localized and clinically appear identical to keratoacanthoma. Larger lesions are usually fungating and may resemble granulomatous lesions. Specific granulomatous infections of the lips and buccal mucosa are rare. Crusted or ulcerated lesions of the upper lip are more likely to represent basal cell carcinomas. Since they usually originate on the skin rather than on the vermilion border, basal cell carcinomas are dealt with in the section on soft tissue swellings of the neck and face. Ulcerated and indurated carcinoma of the buccal mucosa must be distinguished from malignant salivary or mesenchymal neoplasms.

Treatment: Biopsy must be performed to ensure a diagnosis of squamous cell carcinoma. Lip cancer is preferably treated with surgical excision and lip shave. Buccal mucosal carcinoma should be managed by a cancer specialist and may require both irradiation and surgery.

References

1. Cross, J. E., Guralnick, E., and Daland, E. M.: Carcinoma of the lip. Surg. Gynecol. Obstet. 87:153, 1948.
2. O'Brien, P. H. and Catlin, D.: Cancer of the cheek (mucosa). Cancer 18:1392, 1965.
3. Tomich, C. E. and Hutton, C. E.: Adenoid squamous cell carcinoma of the lip: report of cases. J. Oral Surg. 30:592, 1972.
4. Ellis, G. L. and Corio, R. L.: Spindle cell carcinoma of the oral cavity: A clinicopathologic assessment of fifty-nine cases. Oral Surg. 50:523, 1980.
5. Nuutinen, J. and Karja, J.: Local and distant metastases in patients with surgically treated squamous cell carcinoma of the lip. Clin. Otolaryngol. 6:415, 1981.

Monomorphic Adenoma

Age: Middle-aged and elderly adults
Sex: Female predilection

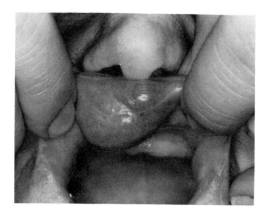

FIG. 6–44. Canalicular (monomorphic) adenoma of the upper lip.

Clinical Features: A variety of histologically distinct salivary neoplasms including canalicular adenoma, basal cell adenoma, and membranous adenoma are collectively grouped as monomorphic adenomas. These tumors arise most frequently in the minor glands of the upper lip, where they appear as movable nodules with either a fluctuant or soft consistency. Whereas most cases are solitary, some reported instances are multifocal. This finding would support a hamartomatous pathogenetic nature.

Microscopic Features: Three primary variations are encountered. The canalicular adenoma is characterized by anastomosing cords of basaloid cuboidal cells with an intervening delicate mucoid vascular stroma. Multicentric foci are frequently observed, and an intralobular origin can be documented in some cases. The basal cell adenoma is represented by cords and islands of basaloid cells showing duct formation. The stroma is fibrovascular without chondroid, adipose, or myxoid differentiation. The membranous adenoma is histologically similar to the basal cells type; however, the stroma is hyalinized. Interestingly, all three patterns may be identified within a single specimen.

Differential Diagnosis: Clinically, monomorphic adenoma will be indistinguishable from other salivary neoplasms or encapsulated mesenchymal tumors. A movable mass in the upper lip, however, will usually represent monomorphic adenoma.

Treatment: Excision of the tumor with an attempt to remove some of the adjacent marginal tissue is recommended.

References

1. Eversole, L. R.: Histogenic classification of salivary tumors. Arch. Pathol. 92:433, 1971.
2. Christ, T. F. and Crocker, D.: Basal cell adenoma of minor salivary gland origin. Cancer 30:214, 1972.
3. Nelson, J. F. and Jacoway, J. R.: Monomorphic adenoma (Canalicular type): Report of 29 cases. Cancer 31:1511, 1973.
4. Fantasia, J. E. and Neville, B. W.: Basal cell adenomas of the minor salivary glands: A clinicopathologic study of seventeen new cases and a review of the literature. Oral Surg. 50:433, 1980.
5. Mintz, G. A., Abrams, A. M., and Melrose, R. J.: Monomorphic adenomas of the major and minor salivary glands. Report of twenty-one cases and review of the literature. Oral Surg. 53:375, 1982.

Other Salivary Neoplasms

Age: Middle-aged adults
Sex: Female predilection

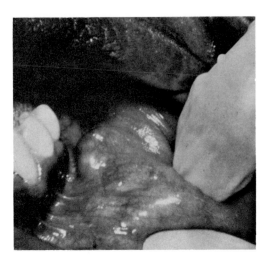

FIG. 6–45. Mucoepidermoid carcinoma. Benign or malignant salivary neoplasms are relatively common in the buccal mucosa as submucosal swellings.

Clinical Features: Salivary tumors are frequently seen in the cheek and upper lip; the lower lip is rarely the site of origin. The pleomorphic adenoma, which is most common, is a well-demarcated, encapsulated, soft-to-firm movable mass. Malignant salivary tumors infrequently arise in labial glands, but are often located in the buccal mucosa. They are firm or indurated and may or may not show ulceration. Specific tumors include adenocarcinoma, adenoid cystic carcinoma, and mucoepidermoid carcinoma. Acinic cell carcinoma is most often seen in the parotid; when it arises from oral minor glands, the buccal mucosa and lip are the more prevalent sites.

Microscopic Features: The histology varies depending upon the specific type of tumor. These features are separately enumerated in the section on palatal swellings.

Differential Diagnosis: Salivary neoplasms appearing as upper lip or buccal mucosal swellings resemble mucocele (which rarely occurs in the upper lip), mesenchymal neoplasm or inflammatory hyperplasia. Ulcerated and indurated adenocarcinomas must be differentiated from squamous cell carcinoma and sarcomas.

Treatment: Benign salivary tumors should be excised rather than merely enucleated, since the latter procedure often results in recurrence. Wide and often radical excision is necessary to eradicate malignant salivary tumors. Depending on the histologic designation, neck dissection may be indicated.

References

1. Spiro, R. H., et al.: Tumors of minor salivary origin; a clinicopathologic study of 492 cases. Cancer *31*: 117, 1973.
2. Krolls, S. O. and Hicks, J. L.: Mixed tumors of the lower lip. Oral Surg. *35*:212, 1973.
3. Main, J. H. P., et al.: Salivary gland tumors: review of 643 cases. J. Oral Pathol. *5*:88, 1976.
4. Gardner, D. G., et al.: Acinic cell tumors of minor salivary glands. Oral Surg. *50*:545, 1980.
5. Owens, O. T. and Calcaterra, T. C.: Salivary gland tumors of the lip. Arch. Otolaryngol. *108*:45, 1982.

TONGUE SWELLINGS

Median Rhomboid Glossitis

Age: Adults
Sex: Male predilection

Clinical Features: A smooth-surfaced, slightly nodular pink elevation that is devoid of papillae and is located immediately anterior to the foramen caecum and circumvallate papillae in the midline characterizes median rhomboid glossitis. This anomaly could represent a developmental defect: persistence of the tuberculum impar with failure to retrude during embryogenesis. This theory is equivocal in light of evidence that suggests the lesion is not congenital but arises later in life. Candida organisms are associated with this lesion and while some investigators feel they play a causative role, this has not been documented in all instances. It is innocuous, painless, and rarely warrants removal.

Microscopic Features: The surface epithelium

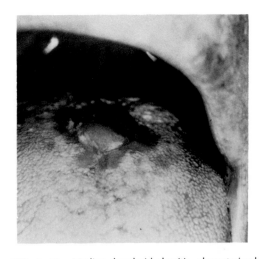

FIG. 6–46. Median rhomboid glossitis, characterized by a midline swelling located on the dorsum of the tongue.

is devoid of papillae and shows rete ridge extension into the submucosa. Candidal organisms are often present within the parakeratin layer. The subjacent fibrous tissue is mildly infiltrated with leukocytes.

Differential Diagnosis: Median rhomboid glossitis may clinically resemble mesenchymal neoplasms, lingual cyst, and glossal-oriented thyroglossal duct cyst. Generally, a clinical diagnosis is easily rendered by virtue of its configuration, lack of growth potential, and midline location.

Treatment: If the tumefaction is large, a biopsy is indicated to rule out neoplasia or cyst. When it is of limited size, periodic recall should be instituted to determine that no growth is taking place.

References

1. Martin, H. E. and Howe, M. E.: Glossitis rhombica mediana. Ann. Surg. *107*:39, 1938.
2. Baughman, R. A.: Median rhomboid glossitis: a developmental anomaly? Oral Surg. *31*:56, 1971.
3. Wright, B. A.: Median rhomboid glossitis: Not a misnomer. Review of the literature and histologic study of twenty-eight cases. Oral Surg. 46:806, 1978.
4. Wright, B. A. and Fenwick, B. A.: Candidiasis and atrophic tongue lesions. Oral Surg. *51*:55, 1981.

Ectopic Lingual Thyroid

Age: Early adulthood

Sex: Female predilection

Clinical Features: Ectopic thyroid tissue appears as a smooth, nodular, or occasionally cystic swelling posterior to the foramen caecum. Dysphagia may be a feature. In most patients, no thyroid tissue can be detected in the usual location. For this reason, excision could result in postsurgical hypothyroidism. An I[131] radioisotope scan is useful in the diagnosis of suspected lingual thyroid and will serve as an indication as to whether or not any thyroid tissue is present in the usual location. The ectopic location reflects the failure of normal developmental migration of the thyroglossal tract and gland primordium. Both adenoma and adenocarcinoma have been reported to arise in lingual thyroid nodules.

Microscopic Features: The oral epithelium is distended by mature thyroid follicles filled with colloid and lined by cuboidal epithelium.

Differential Diagnosis: The lingual thyroid nodule must be differentiated from thyroglossal duct cyst, a large superiorly displaced vallecular cyst, and mesenchymal neoplasm. An I[131] scan will outline the extent of the lesion and identify any normally located thyroid tissue.

Treatment: Incisional biopsy may be performed to aid in diagnosis; however, the entire mass should not be removed if normally located thyroid tissue cannot be demonstrated. Should the lesion show a history of recent growth, biopsy is indicated to rule out thyroid neoplasia.

References

1. Ashhurst, A. P. C. and White, C. Y.: Carcinoma in an aberrant thyroid at base of tongue. J. Am. Med. Assoc. *85*:1219, 1925.
2. Wible, L. E. and Freeman, G. R.: Lingual thyroid. Arch. Otolaryngol. *75*:168, 1962.
3. Baughman, R. A.: Lingual thyroid and lingual thyroglossal tract remnants. A clinical and histopathologic study with review of the literature. Oral Surg. *34*:781, 1972.
4. Reaume, C. E. and Sofie, V. L.: Lingual thyroid, review of the literature and report of a case. Oral Surg. 45:841, 1978.
5. Noyek, A. M. and Friedberg, J.: Thyroglossal duct and ectopic thyroid disorders. Otolaryngol. Clin. North Am. *14*:187, 1981.

Thyroglossal Duct Cyst

Age: Childhood onset

Sex: No predilection

Clinical Features: Thyroglossal cysts arise from remnants of the thyroid anlage and are generally seen above the thyroid in the vicinity of the hyoid bone in the midline of the neck. They may, however, arise in the substance of the tongue below the foramen caecum. They are compressible and yield a yellow fluid on aspiration. Dysphagia may develop. Carcinoma has been reported to arise from the cyst lining.

Microscopic Features: The cyst is lined by columnar, respiratory, or stratified squamous epithelium. Follicles of thyroid glandular epithelium are frequently located in juxtaposition to the cyst lining.

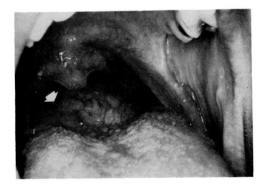

FIG. 6–47. Lingual thyroid nodule at base of tongue.

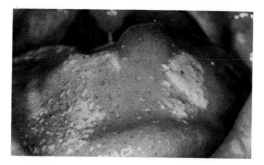

FIG. 6–48. Thyroglossal cyst in the tongue. (From Macdonald, D. M.: Thyroglossal cysts and fistulae. Int. J. Oral Surg. 3:342, 1974.)

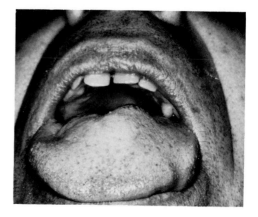

FIG. 6–49. Lingual developmental cyst.

Differential Diagnosis: Lingually localized thyroglossal duct cyst will show features similar to lingual thyroid nodule, mesenchymal neoplasms, and even a posteriorly located median rhomboid glossitis.

Treatment: The cyst should be surgically excised or enucleated.

References

1. Gross, R. E. and Connerly, M. L.: Thyroglossal cysts and sinuses; a study and report of 198 cases. N. Engl. J. Med. 223:616, 1940.
2. Nachlas, N. E.: Thyroglossal duct cysts. Ann. Otol. Rhinol. Laryngol. 59:381, 1950.
3. Snedecor, P. A. and Groshong, L. E.: Carcinoma of the thyroglossal duct. Surgery 58:969, 1965.
4. MacDonald, D. M.: Thyroglossal cysts and fistulae. Int. J. Oral Surg. 3:342, 1974.

Lingual Cyst

Age: Insufficient data to determine
Sex: Insufficient data to determine

Clinical Features: The lingual cyst is rare and is located in the anterior midline of the tongue. It is movable and compressible. Very few cases have been reported. It has been suggested to arise as a result of epithelial entrapment during fissural closure of the lateral lingual processes during development.

Microscopic Features: Most lingual cysts are lined by aberrant gastric epithelium and are referred to as gastric cysts or enterocystoma. Some cases are simply lined by columnar, respiratory, or stratified squamous epithelium.

Differential Diagnosis: The smooth nodular swelling protrudes dorsally so that confusion with dermoid cyst or ranula should be no problem. A lingual abscess or mesenchymal neoplasm may clinically resemble lingual cyst.

Treatment: Surgical excision is recommended.

References

1. Quinn, J. H.: Congenital epidermoid cyst of anterior half of tongue. Oral Surg. 13:1283, 1960.
2. Gorlin, R. J. and Jirasek, J. E.: Oral cysts containing gastric or intestinal mucosa; unusual embryologic accident or heterotopia. J. Oral Surg. 28:9, 1970.
3. Bury, H. P.: A cyst of the tongue containing gastric epithelium J. Pathol. Bact. 83:560, 1962.
4. Katz, A., Aimi, K., and Skolnik, E. M.: Enterocystoma of the head and neck. Laryngoscope 90:1441, 1980.

Hemangioma and Lymphangioma

Age: Children
Sex: No predilection

Clinical Features: Vascular tumors often arise within the tongue and manifest a swelling of the midline or lateral margins. When superficial, which is often the case, racemose nodules are present, and in hemangioma they will be red and will blanch on pressure. Lymphangiomas do not

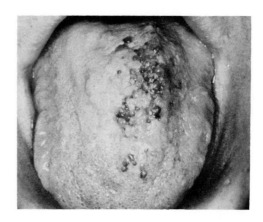

FIG. 6–50. Hemangioma of the tongue with racemose bluish nodules.

impart a color change to the mucosa. The entire tongue or only a portion of it may be occupied by neoplastic vessels. Calcified thrombi or phleboliths are often present in hemangiomas of long standing; the calcified nodules are demonstrable as soft tissue radiopacities on roentgenogram. The more aggressive vascular tumors, hemangioendothelioma and hemangiopericytoma, are more firm to palpation, have a rapid growth rate, and have metastatic potential.

Microscopic Features: Hemangioma and lymphangioma show similar microscopic characteristics. Dilated endothelial-lined channels course throughout the tongue stroma and are often intramuscular in location. When superficially oriented, exophytic extensions composed of vessels distend the surface epithelium. The vascular channels of hemangioma contain erythrocytes and occasionally thrombi. When the lesions are primarily cellular, they are designated as *cellular hemangioma* or *benign hemangioendothelioma*. These behave benignly, similarly to simple hemangiomas. Lymphangiomas contain lymph, an eosinophilic coagulum. The aggressive hemangioendothelioma is highly cellular, composed of monomorphic, plump elongated nuclei with very little pleomorphism. These cells line vacant clefts resembling stag horns. Hemangiopericytomas are composed of similar cells but are arranged in swirls around a small lumen.

Differential Diagnosis: Most vascular lesions are extensive so that confusion with focal midline tongue lesions such as median rhomboid glossitis, lingual thyroid, or cystic lesions is not probable. A racemose surface pattern is invariably a feature of vascular neoplasm. Deeply situated angiomas may be confused with other mesenchymal neoplasms.

Treatment: When the lesions are small, local excision is recommended. Lingual hemangiomas may bleed profusely. Extensive lesions, once diagnosed by biopsy, may be left untreated if asymptomatic. The aggressive angiomas (hemangioendothelioma, hemangiopericytoma) require wide local excision with periodic follow-up. Metastasis may develop late, but metastatic predictability is difficult, if not impossible, for aggressive angiomas based on microscopic evaluation.

References

1. Watson, W. L. and McCarthy, W. D.: Blood and lymph vessel tumors; a report of 1,056 cases. Surg. Gynecol. Obstet. *71*:569, 1940.
2. Shklar, G. and Meyer, L.: Vascular tumors of the mouth and jaws. Oral Surg. *19*:335, 1965.
3. Goldberg, M. H., Nemarich, A. N., and Danielson, P.: Lymphangioma of the tongue: medical and surgical therapy. J. Oral Surg. *35*:841, 1977.
4. Brockbank, J.: Hemangiopericytoma of the oral cavity: report of case and review of the literature. J. Oral Surg. *37*:659, 1979.
5. Khanna, J. N. and Khanapurkar, C. R.: Bilateral vascular lesion of the tongue, hemangioma, and lymphangioma. J. Ind. Dent. Assoc. *51*:139, 1979.

Neural Sheath Tumors

Age: Young adults
Sex: No predilection

Clinical Features: Benign neoplasms of cells that ensheath nerves include those derived from the neurilemma, neurilemmomas, and those derived by perineuronal fibroblasts, neurofibromas. Both types may arise anywhere in the mouth but are most frequently encountered in the tongue, where they appear as smooth-surfaced firm or rubbery painless nodules. Neurilemmomas are encapsulated yet may be multinodular. Neurofibromas are well defined, yet lack true encapsulation. When multiple oral neurofibromas are associated with similar lesions of skin and cafe-au-lait pigmentations, they represent a component of von Recklinghausen's neurofibromatosis. Oral neurofibromas are, however, most frequently solitary. Neural tumors occurring as multiple small nodules may be a component of the Sipple syndrome (see papillary and multiple polypoid swellings).

Microscopic Features: Neurilemmoma shows a fibrous capsule; the tumor cells are arranged in parallel rows, demonstrating palisading of nuclei, Antoni type A tissue. Palisaded nuclei are separated by a dense acellular fibrillar zone. Organoid swirls of Antoni A tissue constitute Verocay bodies. Antoni B tissue is composed of loosely ar-

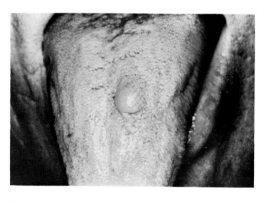

FIG. 6–51. Smooth nodule on dorsum of tongue representing a solitary neurofibroma.

ranged tissue with interfibrillar vacuolated foci. Neurofibromas are composed of elongated nuclei randomly dispersed in a fibrous background. The cellular pattern is winding, giving the appearance of intercoiled spaghetti noodles. Rare nerve sheath tumors include benign nerve sheath myxoma, palisaded encapsulated neuroma, and ancient neurilemmoma.

Differential Diagnosis: Neural sheath neoplasms tend to locate in the anterior one-third of the tongue, and the swelling must be differentiated from other mesenchymal neoplasms, lingual cysts, and salivary tumors, which occasionally arise from minor glands of the tongue.

Treatment: Simple excision is rarely complicated by recurrence.

References

1. O'Driscoll, P. M.: The oral manifestations of multiple neurofibromatosis. Br. J. Oral Surg. *3:22,* 1965.
2. Hatziotis, J. C. and Asprides, H.: Neurilemmoma (schwannoma) of the oral cavity. Oral Surg. *24:510,* 1967.
3. Cherrick, H. M. and Eversole, L. R.: Benign neural sheath neoplasm of the oral cavity; report of thirty-seven cases. Oral Surg. *32:900,* 1971.
4. Chen, S. and Miller, A. S.: Neurofibroma and schwannoma of the oral cavity. Oral Surg. *47:522,* 1979.
5. Sist, T. C., Jr., and Greene, G. W., Jr.: Benign nerve sheath myxoma: light and electron microscopic features of two cases. Oral Surg. *47:441,* 1979.

Granular Sheath Cell Lesions (Granular Cell Myoblastoma)

Age: No predilection
Sex: No predilection

Clinical Features: Granular cell tumors are derived from cells that ensheath other cells such as

neurilemma (Schwann) cells or sarcolemma. The term *granular cell myoblastoma* is usually used since most of these lesions are associated with muscle fibers. The lesions appear as small elevated nodules on the dorsum or lateral border of the tongue. They are painless and soft to palpation. The *rhabdomyoma,* a rare tumor of muscle origin, also arises in the tongue. These tumors are encapsulated and have limited growth potential.

Microscopic Features: Oval eosinophilic granular cells have pyknotic nuclei and are separated from one another by a scant stroma. When superficial, the epithelium may show extensive pseudoepitheliomatous hyperplasia. The granular cells may emanate from either muscle fibers or neural sheath. Rhabdomyomas are composed of large oval or elongated cells with eosinophilic granular cytoplasm showing evidence of cross-striations. The nuclei are eccentric.

Differential Diagnosis: Granular sheath cell lesions and rhabdomyoma may be clinically similar to median rhomboid glossitis or other mesenchymal neoplasms.

Treatment: Simple excision is recommended. Recurrence is almost nonexistent.

References

1. Day, R. C. B.: Granular cell myoblastoma. Br. J. Oral Surg. *2:65,* 1965.
2. Eversole, L. R., Sabes, W. R., Rovin, S.: Granular sheath cell lesions; report of cases. J. Oral Surg. *29:867,* 1971.
3. Regezi, J. A., Batsakis, J. G., and Courtney, R. M.: Granular cell tumors of the head and neck. J. Oral Surg. *37:402,* 1979.
4. Corio, R. L. and Lewis, D. M.: Intraoral rhabdomyomas. Oral Surg. *48:525,* 1979.

Leiomyoma

Age: Middle-aged adults
Sex: Male predilection

Clinical Features: Leiomyomas are smooth-surfaced tumefactions that may arise in any location. In the mouth, they are most frequently encountered in the tongue. The tumor is encapsulated, painless, firm, and may be multinodular.

Microscopic Features: The tumor cells possess elongated, blunt-ended nuclei with a vesicular nucleoplasm. The cells course in streams and fascicles, often evolving from vessels showing perivascular concentric laminations of spindle cells. The fibrillar background may be distinguished from collagen with a trichrome stain.

Differential Diagnosis: Leiomyoma may be clinically indistinguishable from other mesenchymal neoplasms.

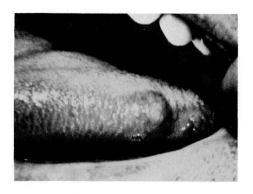

FIG. 6–52. Granular cell myoblastoma of the tongue, generally a smooth nodule with a sessile base.

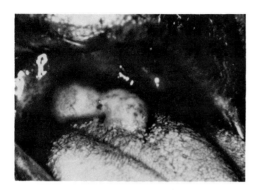

FIG. 6–53. Leiomyoma. These are rare in the mouth; when they occur, the tongue is the favored site. (Courtesy of Dr. H. Cherrick.)

Treatment: Simple surgical excision is recommeded. Recurrence is unlikely after complete excision.

References

1. MacDonald, D. G.: Smooth muscle tumors of the mouth. Br. J. Oral Surg. 6:207, 1969.
2. Cherrick, H. M. Dunlap, C. L., and Klug, O. H.: Leiomyomas of the oral cavity; review of the literature and clinicopathologic study of seven new cases. Oral Surg. 35:54, 1973.
3. Kelly, D. E. and Harrigan, W. F.: Leiomyoma of the tongue: report of a case. J. Oral Surg. 35:316, 1977.

Osteocartilaginous Choristoma

Age: Young adults
Sex: Female predilection

Clinical Features: Discrete nodules of osseous or osteocartilaginous tissue may form in the substance of the tongue. Whereas most are asymptomatic, some will cause dysphagia. They may be located in the anterior, mid, or posterior regions and are more often visualized or palpable on the dorsal aspect. They are firm or hard, sessile or pedunculated, and freely movable. Since there are no osteoprogenitor cells within the tongue their origin is obscure; hence, they represent choristomas. Their potential for growth is probably self-limited.

Microscopic Features: Some lesions are represented entirely by dense lamellar osseous tissue with a paucity of fibrous marrow or stroma. Others exhibit enclaved foci of chondroid tissue.

Differential Diagnosis: Clinically osseous or osteocartilaginous choristomas may resemble traumatic fibromas or other mesenchymal neoplasms. On palpation, however, a movable rock-hard nodule should arouse suspicion of osseous choristoma. An occlusal radiograph will show a radiopaque mass within the soft tissue of the tongue.

Treatment: Osseous and osteocartilaginous choristomas are easily enucleated from adjacent soft tissues. Pedunculated varieties can simply be excised at the base of the stalk.

References

1. Krolls, S. O., Jacoway, J. R., and Alexander, W. N.: Osseous choristomas (osteomas) of the intraoral soft tissues. Oral Surg. 32:588, 1971.
2. Zegarelli, D. J.: Chondroma of the tongue. Oral Surg. 43:738, 1977.
3. Wesley, R. K. and Zeilinski, R. J.: Osteocartilaginous choristoma of the tongue: clinical and histopathologic considerations. J. Oral Surg. 36:59, 1978.

Sarcomas

Age: Varies with tumor type
Sex: No predilection

Clinical Features: Sarcomas of the oral cavity are rare. They may arise in any locality, including the tongue. The more frequently encountered types include rhabdomyosarcoma and fibrosarcoma. All sarcomas show a rapid growth rate, are indurated and fixed and have a tendency toward ulceration. Hematogenous metastasis is the most frequent route of spread from sarcomas leading to pulmonary and widespread metastatic foci.

Microscopic Features: Histologic findings vary, depending upon differentiation of the tumor. Most sarcomas are composed of spindle, pleomorphic, and anaplastic cells with multiple and bizarre mitotic figures. Invasion of adjacent tissues is a constant feature. Microscopically, sarcomas must be differentiated from cellular fibromatoses and pseudosarcomas.

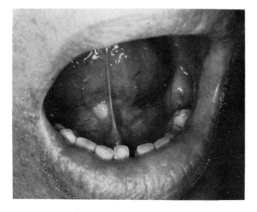

FIG. 6–54. Cartilaginous choristoma appearing as blanched nodule of ventral tongue.

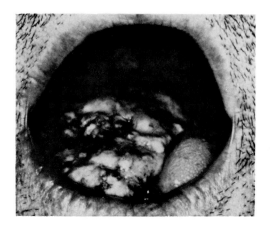

FIG. 6–55.   Rhabdomyosarcoma of the tongue.

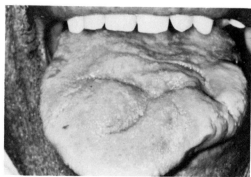

FIG. 6–56.   Amyloid nodules of the tongue. (Courtesy of Drs. S. Silverman and T. Daniels.)

Differential Diagnosis: Indurated fixed swellings in the tongue must be differentiated from carcinoma and salivary adenocarcinoma.

Treatment: Radical excision or glossectomy is required. Despite radical treatment, the prognosis is poor.

References

1. O'Day, R. A., Soule, E. H., and Gores, R. J.: Soft tissue sarcomas of the oral cavity. Proc. Mayo Clin. 39:169, 1964.
2. Masson, J. K. and Soule, E. H.: Embryonal rhabdomyosarcoma of the head and neck; report on eighty-eight cases. Am J. Surg. 110:585, 1965.
3. Eversole, L. R., Schwartz, D., and Sabes, W. R.: Central and peripheral fibrogenic and neurogenic sarcomas of the oral regions. Oral Surg. 36:49, 1973.
4. Ryan, M.D. and LaDow, C.: Primary fibrosarcoma of the tongue: report of case. J. Oral Surg. 30:135, 1972.

Amyloid Nodules

Age: Adults

Sex: No predilection

Clinical Features: Amyloidosis is a metabolic disorder characterized by deposition of a starch-like protein in the tissues. It may be primary, secondary to chronic infection such as tuberculosis or osteomyelitis, or associated with multiple myeloma. The tongue is the most common oral location for the accumulation of amyloid, and the areas of deposition appear as focal or multiple nodular elevations that are normal in color, nonulcerated, and painless.

Microscopic Features: Normal connective tissue is displaced by accumulations of amorphous eosinophilic deposits. The amyloid material stains with Congo red and exhibits dichroism with green birefringence under polarized light. Frequently the deposits are in perivascular distribution.

Differential Diagnosis: Solitary amyloid nodules may resemble inflammatory hyperplasia or mesenchymal neoplasm. Multiple nodules may be confused with those encountered in the Sipple syndrome or neurofibromatoses.

Treatment: Secondary amyloidosis and amyloidosis associated with myeloma must be managed by control of the primary disease process. All forms should be managed by a physician.

References

1. Barth, W. F.: Primary amyloidosis. Ann. Intern. Med. 69:787, 1968.
2. Stanback, J. S. and Peagler, F. D.: Primary amyloidosis. Review of the literature and report of a case. Oral Surg. 26:774, 1968.
3. Schwartz, H. C.: Amyloidosis: A rational approach to diagnosis by intraoral biopsy. Oral Surg. 39:837, 1975.
4. Kraut, R. A., et al.: Amyloidosis associated with multiple myeloma. Oral Surg. 43:63, 1977.
5. Meyer, I., et al.: Amyloidosis of the tongue secondary to multiple myeloma (CPC). J. Oral Surg. 36:372, 459, 1978.

Specific Granuloma

Age: Adults

Sex: No predilection

Clinical Features: Specific granulomatous infection is primary in the lungs and appears orally as a secondary manifestation of miliary spread. The infections most often encountered in the United States include tuberculosis, histoplasmosis and cryptococcosis. Less frequently, blastomycosis and coccidioidomycosis will have oral manifestations. The lesions may develop anywhere in the mouth and are frequently seen on the tongue.

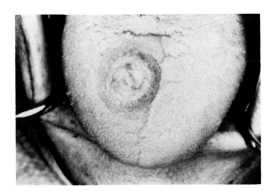

FIG. 6–57. Ulcerated nodule representing histoplasmosis, a granulomatous infection.

They are characterized by elevated nodular swellings with rolled margins and an ulcerated central region, or they are pebbly granular swellings. Pain is usually not a feature. Primary syphilitic chancre also occurs on the tongue, showing the same clinical features as the secondary granulomatous infections.

Microscopic Features: Granulation and fibrous tissues are admixed with macrophages and multinucleated giant cells. Fungi can usually be found free and within giant cells with routine stains. Acid-fast preparations are required for identification of tubercle bacilli and periodic acid-Schiff or methenamine silver will readily disclose the presence of mycotic microorganisms. A dense plasma cell infiltrate is suggestive of syphilis; however, a Warthin-Starry stain is required to demonstate spirochetes.

Differential Diagnosis: The ulcerated granulomas of tuberculosis or the deep mycoses may clinically resemble carcinoma or even sarcoma. Biopsy is required to establish a definitive diagnosis. When tuberculosis or deep mycotic infection is discovered, it should be recalled that the oral lesions represent secondary infection with primary pulmonary disease. Syphilitic chancre is not accompanied by positive serology; serologic testing should be performed 2 to 3 weeks following the appearance of the primary lesion. A darkfield smear will disclose the presence of spirochetes.

Treatment: Once a diagnosis of granulomatous infection is confirmed, a workup for pulmonary disease is in order and the patient should be placed under the care of a physician for management and therapy. Syphilis can be treated by penicillin therapy.

References

1. Weed, L. A. and Parkhill, E. M.: The diagnosis of histoplasmosis in ulcerative disease of the mouth and pharynx. Am. J. Clin. Pathol. *18*:130, 1948.
2. Franenfelder, D. and Schwartz, A. W.: Coccidioidomycosis involving head and neck. Plast. Reconstr. Surg. *39*:549,1967.
3. Agarwal, M. K., et al.: Tuberculosis of the tongue. Ann. Acad. Med. Singapore *8*:217, 1979.
4. Yusuf, H., Craig, G. T., and Allan, D.: Disseminated histoplasmosis presenting with oral lesions—report of a case. Br. J. Oral Surg. *16*:234, 1979.

Squamous Cell Carcinoma

Age: Elderly adults

Sex: Predominantly males

Clinical Features: The tongue is the second most common site for squamous cancer in the mouth, exceeded only by floor of the mouth. The posterior lateral border is the most common location; however, carcinoma may also affect the mobile and ventral regions. The dorsum is rarely involved; when it is, syphilitic glossitis is usually preexistent. The neoplasm may be red, white, mixed red and white, ulcerated, or tumefactive. Even tumefactive lesions are usually ulcerated and often have coexistent leukoplakia and/or erythroplakia on the margins. The mass is fixed and indurated and may have involved the oral floor or tonsilar pillar. These tumors are staged according to extent. Submandibular or cervical lymphadenopathy is frequently observed, particularly in association with larger tumors.

Microscopic Features: Invasive islands and cords of neoplastic cells extend into the underlying submucosa and muscle. Keratin pearl formation is usually present, and the individual cells exhibit pleomorphism, hyperchromatism, and increased mitotic activity. The stroma is infiltrated by plasma cells and lymphocytes.

Differential Diagnosis: Tongue swellings lo-

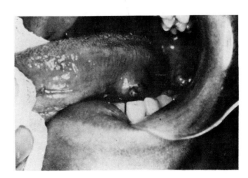

FIG. 6–58. Squamous cell carcinoma of the tongue.

cated on the lateral margin with ulceration and induration rarely represent benign lesions. Immediate biopsy is indicated.

Treatment: Combined radiation therapy and radical surgery, along with neck dissection and/ or radiation to the neck, are indicated for large tumors. Indeed, bilateral neck dissection should be undertaken as contralateral metastases are frequently found. Small stage I tumors are usually curable with either wide local excision or radiation therapy.

References

1. Martin, H. E., Munster, H., and Sugarbaker, E. D.: Cancer of the tongue. Arch. Surg. *41*:888, 1940.
2. Maddox, W. A., Sherlock, E. C., and Evans, W. B.: Cancer of the tongue: review of thirteen years experience. Am. Surg. *37*:642, 1971.
3. Spiro, R. H. and Strong, E. W.: Surgical treatment of cancer of the tongue. Surg. Clin. North Am. *54*:4, 1974.
4. Leipzig, B., et al.: Carcinoma of the anterior tongue. Ann. Otol. *91*:94, 1982.
5. Martis, C. S.: Carcinoma of the tongue: Evaluation of surgical treatment of 123 cases. J. Oral Surg. *40*:340, 1982.

PALATAL SWELLINGS

Torus Palatinus

Age: Young adults
Sex: Female predilection
Clinical Features: Palatal torus is a bone-hard

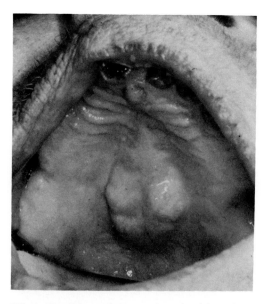

FIG. 6–59. Torus palatinus, a bone-hard bosselated swelling located in the palatal vault.

excrescence that develops after puberty in the midline of the palatal vault. It represents a developmental hereditary overgrowth of bone and is extremely hard to palpation. The surface mucosa is generally intact and often shows lobulation. Tori vary considerably in size and are common, occurring in 20 percent of the population. Orientals show a greater incidence than Caucasians and blacks. The palatal torus may be quite small, or it may grow to fill the entire palatal vault.

Microscopic Features: The excrescence is composed of an outer cortical plate with a central cancellous zone. The osseous tissues show normal histologic features.

Differential Diagnosis: The midline location, slow growth, and bone-hard nature of palatal tori allow for differentiation from palatal abscess or salivary tumors, which are softer and usually located somewhat lateral to the palatal raphe.

Treatment: Tori may be left untreated. When a torus interferes with fabrication of a maxillary dental prosthesis, it may be excised.

References

1. Kolas, S. and Halperin, V.: The occurrence of torus palatinus and torus mandibularis in 2,478 dental patients. Oral Surg. *6*:1134, 1953.
2. Gould, A. W.: An investigation of the inheritance of torus palatinus and torus mandibularis. J. Dent. Res. *43*:159, 1964.
3. Blakemore, J. R.: Maxillary exostoses: Surgical management of an unusual case. Oral Surg. *40*:200, 1975.
4. King, D. R. and Moore, G. E.: An analysis of torus palatinus in a transatlantic study. J. Oral Med. *31*:44, 1976.

Cyst of the Incisive Papilla

Age: Middle-aged adults
Sex: No predilection
Clinical Features: When epithelial remnants of the nasopalatine duct or incisive canal reside immediately subjacent to the incisive papilla and undergo proliferation with cystic change, they are termed *cysts of the incisive papilla*. They therefore represent the oral soft tissue counterpart of the incisive canal cyst. The cysts are usually small, soft, or fluctuant on palpation and may develop a draining fistula.

Microscopic Features: The cyst lining is stratified squamous epithelium, although on rare occasion respiratory epithelium is coexistent. The fibrous wall is rich in neurovascular elements, and an inflammatory cell infiltrate is not uncommon.

Differential Diagnosis: The location is characteristic; however, cysts of the incisive papilla

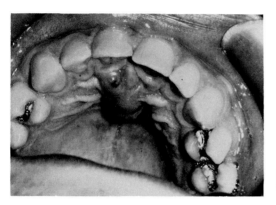

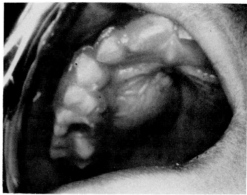

FIG. 6–60. Anterior palatal midline swelling representing a cyst of the incisive papilla. (Courtesy of Dr. A. Leider.)

FIG. 6–61. Firm palatal swelling adjacent to a carious molar, representing a subperiosteal abscess of odontogenic infectious origin.

References

1. Shafer, W. G., Hine, M. K., and Levy, B. M.: *A Textbook of Oral Pathology,* 4th Ed. Philadelphia, W. B. Saunders Co., 1983, chap. 8.
2. Shapiro, H. H., et al.: Spread of infection of dental origin. Oral Surg. *3:*1407, 1950.
3. Wood, N. K. and Goaz, P. W.: *Differential Diagnosis of Oral Lesions,* 2nd Ed. St. Louis, C. V. Mosby Co., 1980, pp. 138, 144.

must be differentiated from a central incisive canal cyst with draining fistula and palatal abscess arising from odontogenic infection.

Treatment: Simple excision is recommended.

References

1. Abrams, A. M., et al.: Nasopalatine cysts. Oral Surg. *16:*306, 1963.
2. Small, E. W.: Cysts. Dent. Clin. N. Amer. *15(2):*369, 1971.

Palatal Abscess

Age: No predilection
Sex: No predilection

Clinical Features: Palatal abscess is seen in the premolar-molar region lateral to the midline and is a tense yet compressible swelling. It represents palatally directed drainage of infection of odontogenic or periodontal origin. A palatal molar root is the most common source. Pain is a frequent finding. A purulent exudate may be aspirated from the swelling.

Microscopic Features: The palatal abscess is composed of necrotic debris, exudate and infiltration of neutrophils and histiocytes. The abscess is usually enveloped by a granulation tissue wall.

Differential Diagnosis: Palatal abscess can be clinically differentiated from salivary neoplasms by noting the presence of pain and identifying an odontogenic infectious source by vitalometer testing or a periapical lesion by radiographs.

Treatment: The source of infection must be identified and arrested by either extraction or pulpectomy. The abscess may be incised and drained to relieve pain.

Adenomatous Hyperplasia

Age: Adults
Sex: Male predilection

Clinical Features: Occasionally, a sessile mass on either the soft or hard palate, appearing to represent a neoplasm, is found to be comprised of normal-appearing mucous acini and accompanying ducts. These lesions are soft to palpation and usually do not exceed 2 centimeters. They are covered by normal-appearing mucosa and may represent a developmental anomaly or a focal glandular hyperplasia.

Microscopic Features: Lobules of normal-ap-

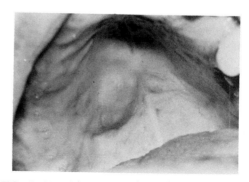

FIG. 6–62. Adenomatous hyperplasia at hard-soft palate junction.

pearing palatal minor mucous acini and associated ductal elements lie within the connective tissue under normal surface epithelium.

Differential Diagnosis: Benign salivary neoplasms and atypical lymphoproliferative disease should be considered in the differential diagnosis. A palatal abscess can be ruled out by virtue of location (adenomatous hyperplasia is usually not confluent with palatal gingiva) and absence of an odontogenic source of infection.

Treatment: Masses of this nature should be biopsied to rule out tumor. Once a diagnosis of adenomatous or glandular hyperplasia is made, no further treatment is required.

References

1. Giansanti, J. S., Baker, G. O., and Waldron, C. A.: Intraoral mucinous, minor salivary gland lesions, presenting clinically as tumors. Oral Surg. *32*:918, 1971.
2. Arafat, A., Brannon, R. B., and Ellis, G. L.: Adenomatoid hyperplasia of mucous salivary glands. Oral Surg. *52*:51, 1981.

Pleomorphic Adenoma

Age: Middle-aged adults
Sex: Female predilection

Clinical Features: Pleomorphic adenomas may arise in any of the major or minor salivary glands. When intraoral, the palate is the site of predilection. The tumor is located lateral to the midline in the hard or soft palate, is firm to palpation, and as a rule lacks surface ulceration.

Microscopic Features: Pleomorphic adenoma possesses a circumferential capsule. The tumor is composed of nests and sheets of cuboidal epithelium with ductal formations. Interspersed throughout are various mesenchymal tissues, which include fat, cartilage, and bone. Myxoid tissue is common and may be accompanied by proliferation of spindle-shaped myoepithelial cells.

Differential Diagnosis: Pleomorphic adenoma

can be differentiated from palatal abscess by failure to locate an infectious source; pain is not a feature. Clinically, it may simulate a malignant salivary tumor or a mesenchymal neoplasm; the latter is relatively uncommon in this location.

Treatment: Since tumor islands may actually perforate the capsule, simple enucleation may result in recurrence. Excision of the tumor and adjacent tissue is recommended. In the hard palate, the capsule may fuse with periosteum, necessitating subperiosteal dissection with excision.

References

1. Fine, G., et al.: Tumors of the minor salivary glands. Cancer *13*:653, 1960.
2. Chaudhry, A. P., et al.: Intraoral minor salivary gland tumors; analysis of 1,414 cases. Oral Surg. *14*:1194, 1961.
3. Naeim, F., et al.: Mixed tumors of the salivary glands. Arch. Pathol. Lab. Med. *100*:271, 1976.
4. Frable, W. J. and Elzay, R. P.: Tumors of minor salivary glands; a report of 73 cases. Cancer *25*:932, 1970.
5. Soskolne, A. et al.: Minor salivary gland tumors: a survey of 64 cases. J. Oral Surg. *31*:528, 1973.

Adenoid Cystic Carcinoma

Age: Middle-aged adults
Sex: No predilection

Clinical Features: Adenoid cystic carcinoma or cylindroma is the most common intraoral malignant salivary neoplasm and is most often seen in the hard palate. It appears as an indurated swelling lateral to the midline and frequently shows ulceration or surface telangiectasia. Pain is not uncommon. Despite this malignant behavior, it may show a lengthy growth progression. Metastasis is common late in the course of the disease and may not be detected for many years following initial

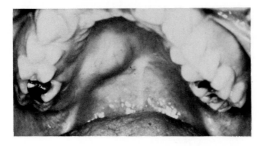

FIG. 6–63.   Pleomorphic adenoma located in the lateral hard palate.

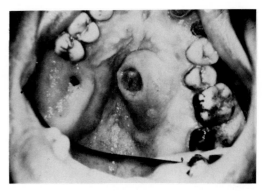

FIG. 6–64.   Adenoid cystic carcinoma with tumefaction showing surface ulceration.

therapy. It has an equal tendency for both regional and hematogenous spread.

Microscopic Features: The tumor lacks encapsulation and tends to invade adjacent hard and soft tissues. Tumor cells characteristically invade perineural lymphatics and may progress for extended distances along nerve sheaths. The classic pattern shows hyperchromatic, monomorphic cuboidal cells arranged in islands forming multicystic cribriform patterns resembling Swiss cheese. The cystic lumina often contain a basophilic hyaline substance, and the stroma may display eosinophilic hyalinization. When solid basaloid islands predominate, the tumor has a worse prognosis.

Differential Diagnosis: Cylindroma may be clinically identical to other benign or malignant salivary tumors, sarcomas, or antral carcinoma with palatal invasion.

Treatment: Wide excision with partial maxillectomy is necessary. Neck dissection is indicated when nodes are palpable. A clinically negative neck may not warrant node dissection as the tumor has great tendency to spread to distant sites. All patients with cylindroma should be evaluated with chest films. Adenoid cystic carcinoma pursues a slow rate of growth, and many years elapse before recurrence and distant metastases become detectable. The 5-year survival for palatal lesions is less than 35 percent; 10-year survival drops to about 15 percent.

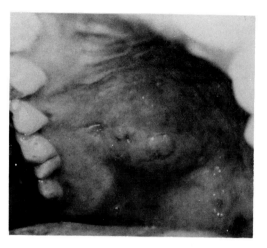

FIG. 6–65. Sessile palatal mass representing mucoepidermoid carcinoma.

References

1. Eneroth, C. M., et al.: Adenoid cystic carcinoma of palate. Acta Otolaryngol. 66:248, 1968.
2. Spiro, R. H., et al.: Tumors of minor salivary origin; a clinicopathologic study of 492 cases. Cancer 31:117, 1973.
3. Spiro, R. H., Huvos, A. Jr., and Strong, E. W.: Adenoid cystic carcinoma of salivary origin; a clinicopathologic study of 242 cases. Am. J. Surg. 128:512, 1974.
4. Conley, J. and Dingman, D. L.: Adenoid cystic carcinoma in the head and neck. Arch. Otolaryngol. 100:81, 1974.
5. Tarpley, T. M. and Giansanti, J. S.: Adenoid cystic carcinoma; analysis of fifty oral cases. Oral Surg. 41:484, 1976.

Mucoepidermoid Carcinoma

Age: Young and middle-aged adults
Sex: No predilection

Clinical Features: When minor glands give rise to mucoepidermoid carcinoma, the palate is the most frequent location. The tumor may be cystic or indurated to palpation and usually fails to show ulceration. Telangiectasia is not uncommon. The growth rate is often slow, and behavior is correlated with histologic grade of malignancy. Despite gradations, all mucoepidermoid carcinomas have metastatic potential. Recent studies appear to indicate that low-grade tumors in the oral cavity may not metastasize; however, this has not been completely documented. The higher-grade tumors spread by way of lymphatics; however, hematogenous metastasis often occurs in addition to or in lieu of nodal metastasis.

Microscopic Features: Tumor islands may be solid or may show large, dilated cystic formations. A capsule is lacking. The individual tumor cells show a biphasic differentiation with both an epidermoid and a mucous cell component. When the tumor is less cystic and epidermoid cells predominate, the prognosis is worse and the tumor is classified as high grade. Low-grade tumors are cystic with a preponderance of mucous and columnar cells.

Differential Diagnosis: Palatal abscess, other benign and malignant salivary tumors, antral cancer, and mesenchymal neoplasms are clinically similar in appearance to palatal mucoepidermoid carcinoma.

Treatment: Low-grade tumors can be treated successfully by wide local excision, making sure margins are free of tumor microscopically. High-grade lesions require more radical surgery. Maxillectomy is recommended for palatal tumors. Chest films should be ordered to rule out lung metastasis.

References

1. Eversole, L. R., Rovin, S., and Sabes, W. R.: Mucoepidermoid carcinoma of minor salivary glands: Report of 17 cases with follow-up. J. Oral Surg. 30:107, 1972.
2. Spiro, R. H., et al.: Tumors of minor salivary origin; a clinicopathologic study of 492 cases. Cancer 31:117, 1973.
3. Melrose, R. J., Abrams, A. M., and Howell, F. W.: Mucoepidermoid tumors of the intraoral minor salivary glands: a clinicopathologic study of 54 cases. J. Oral Pathol. 2:314, 1973.
4. Spiro, R. H., et al.: Mucoepidermoid carcinoma of salivary gland origin; a clinicopathologic study of 367 cases. Am. J. Surg. 136:461, 1978.

Adenocarcinoma, NOS

Age: Middle-aged adults

Sex: No predilection

Clinical Features: Adenocarcinomas, not otherwise specified (NOS), are malignant salivary gland tumors; they do not show microscopic features that allow specific classification into one of the recognized salivary tumor taxonomic categories. They appear as indurated, often ulcerated swellings lateral to the midline. Surface telangiectasia is common. These tumors behave aggressively and may metastasize regionally or distantly. Their behavior is similar to that of adenoid cystic carcinoma.

Microscopic Features: There is no capsule. Tumor cells show invasion and are arranged in sheets and cords showing ductal formations. Some are monomorphic while others evince anaplasia and pleomorphism. Rarely, a benign pleomorphic adenoma will undergo adenocarcinomatous trans-

formation; these lesions are referred to as malignant mixed tumors.

Differential Diagnosis: Adenocarcinomas clinically resemble other salivary neoplasms, mesenchymal tumors, antral carcinoma, or a palatal abscess.

Treatment: Wide surgical excision with resection of underlying bone is recommended. Radiographs of the chest should be obtained to rule out metastasis to lungs.

References

1. Spiro, R. H., et al.: Tumors of minor salivary origin; a clinicopathologic study of 492 cases. Cancer 31:117, 1973.
2. Koss, L. G., Spiro, R. H., and Hajdu, S.: Small cell (oat cell) carcinoma of minor salivary gland origin. Cancer 30:737, 1972.
3. Allen, M. S., Fitz-hugh, G. S., and Marsh, W. L.: Low-grade papillary adenocarcinoma of the palate. Cancer 33:153, 1974.
4. Livolsi, V. A. and Perzin, K.H.: Malignant mixed tumors arising in salivary glands. I. Carcinomas arising in benign mixed tumors. A clinicopathologic study. Cancer 39:2209, 1977.

Atypical Lymphoproliferative Disease

Age: Elderly adults

Sex: No predilection

Clinical Features: Lymphoid infiltration of salivary glands is generally a feature of benign lymphoepithelial lesion such as Sjögren's syndrome or Mikulicz's disease. This is true when the major salivary glands are involved; however, when the palatal salivary glands manifest diffuse lymphoid infiltration, the disease process in most instances represents non-Hodgkin's lymphoma. Atypical lymphoproliferative disease of the palate is a

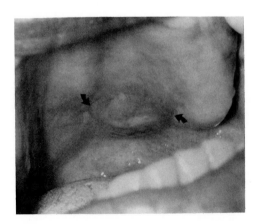

FIG. 6–66.   Adenocarcinoma, not otherwise specified, of the palate.

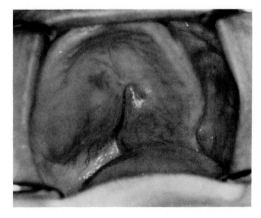

FIG. 6–67.   Diffuse soft swelling of hard palate representing lymphoproliferative disease.

unique entity because the microscopic features often suggest a benign lesion. The disease is characterized by diffuse soft tissue enlargement located unilaterally in the hard palate. Occasionally the lesion extends into the soft palate area and may cross the midline with bilateral swelling. The lesion is soft or spongy on palpation, and the mucosa either maintains normal coloration or manifests a bluish hue without evidence of ulceration or telangiectasia. Accompanying cervical lymphadenopathy is generally not noted at the time of diagnosis. Once the diagnosis has been secured, workup for malignant lymphoma is mandatory. Many patients will show evidence of lymphoma in other locations at the time that the palatal mass is detected; others may be free from disease in other sites yet will develop generalized lymphoma at a later date. In still other patients, the lesion remains static and progression to disseminated disease does not ensue, suggesting the palatal mass may represent pseudolymphoma. Insufficient long-term follow-up information exists in this latter group of patients to determine whether or not malignant lymphoma will eventually develop, given sufficient time.

Microscopic Features: The palatal salivary glands are infiltrated by lymphocytes that may be monomorphic and well differentiated or mildly pleomorphic and poorly differentiated. Interspersed thread-like basophilic strands with a tendency for compaction are common and probably represent degenerating lymphocytes. Reed-Sternberg cells are not encountered. The overall pattern of the infiltrate may be diffuse or nodular. The salivary tissue shows acinar replacement; however, ducts are often found intact, embedded in a sea of lymphocytes. These residual ducts often show pronounced periductal hyalinization. Epimyoepithelial islands encountered in benign lymphoepithelial lesions are not encountered in lymphoproliferative diseases of the palate.

Differential Diagnosis: A soft, spongy swelling of the hard palate that is diffuse and sessile should arouse suspicion of atypical lymphoproliferative disease, especially in elderly patients. Malignant salivary neoplasms are generally localized and indurated. Pleomorphic adenoma and palatal abscess will show clinical features in common with lymphoproliferative disease; palatal abscess can be eliminated from consideration when an infectious source is lacking.

Treatment: Once a diagnosis of atypical lymphoproliferative disease has been established, the patient should be referrred for complete evaluation in order to uncover evidence of malignant lymphoma in other reticuloendothelial tissues. Should the results prove negative, the patient should be subjected to periodic follow-up and reexamination semiannually in anticipation of probable dissemination of disease. The palatal lesion has been shown to respond favorably to radiation therapy; 800 to 1000 r is generally adequate to cause resolution. This treatment alone may not necessarily prevent the occurrence of lesions in other anatomic sites.

References

1. McNelis, F. L. and Pai, V. T.: Malignant lymphoma of the head and neck. Laryngoscope 79:1076, 1969.
2. Tomich, C. E. and Shafer, W. G.: Lymphoproliferative disease of the hard palate: A clinicopathologic entity. Oral Surg. 39:754, 1975.
3. Block, P., van Delden, L., and van der Waal, I.: Non-Hodgkin's lymphoma of the hard palate. J. Oral Surg. 47:445, 1979.
4. Harsany, D. L., Ross, J., and Fee, W. E., Jr.: Follicular lymphoid hyperplasia of the hard palate simulating lymphoma. Otolaryngol. Head Neck Surg. 88:349, 1980.

Carcinoma of the Antrum

Age: Elderly adults
Sex: Male predilection

Clinical Features: Cancer arising in the antrum generally becomes quite advanced before signs or symptoms occur. The tumor may erode any of the antral bony walls including the orbital floor, the lateral or medial wall, or often the palate. When the palate becomes eroded, a mass protrudes and is invariably ulcerated. A perforation or oroantral fistula is frequently encountered. Toothache, max-

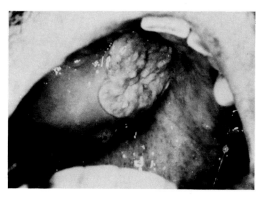

FIG. 6–68. Carcinoma of the antral mucosa invading the antral floor and producing a palatal swelling with ulceration.

illary division paresthesia, nasal obstruction, and loosening of teeth are common clinical symptoms. Radiographically, antral clouding and evidence of osseous erosion can be demonstrated employing Water's views or laminography.

Microscopic Features: Antral cancer is either typical epidermoid carcinoma or demonstrates glandular differentiation as an adenocarcinoma. Occasionally, one of the salivary tumors arises from antral submucosal glands.

Differential Diagnosis: Antral carcinoma will resemble the other malignant palatal swellings included here, necessitating biopsy with microscopic confirmation. Sinus radiographs are of diagnostic importance, and tomograms or CT scans will help determine the extent of the disease.

Treatment: Radiation therapy to the antrum and neck may be coupled with maxillectomy. When nodes contain tumor, any treatment should be considered palliative, as cures at this stage are almost nonexistent.

References

1. Chaudhry, A. P., et al.: Carcinoma of the antrum. Oral Surg. *13*:269, 1960.
2. Larsson, L. G. and Martensson, G.: Carcinoma of the paranasal sinuses and the nasal cavities. Acta Radiol. *42*:149, 1954.
3. Kadish, S. P., Goodman, M. L., and Wang, C. C.: Treatment of minor salivary gland malignancies of the upper food and air passage epithelium. A review of 87 cases. Cancer *29*:1021, 1972.
4. Ahmad, K., Cordoba, R. B., and Fayos, J. V.: Squamous cell carcinoma of the maxillary sinus. Arch. Otolaryngol. *107*:48, 1981.

7
Papillary, Papular, and Multiple Polypoid Lesions

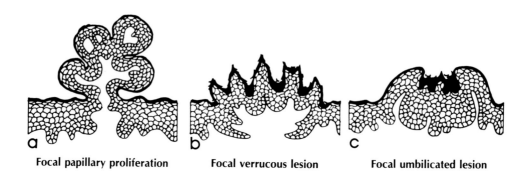

Focal papillary proliferation　　**Focal verrucous lesion**　　**Focal umbilicated lesion**

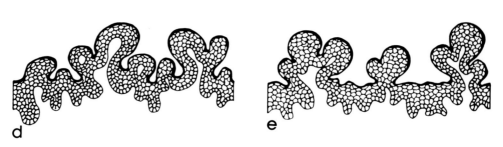
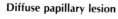
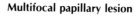

Diffuse papillary lesion　　　　　**Multifocal papillary lesion**

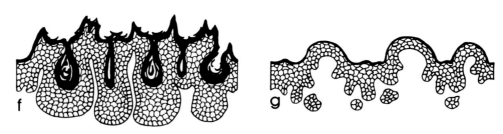

Diffuse verrucous lesion　　　　**Papular or multiple polypoid lesion**

Papillary, Papular, and Multiple Polypoid Lesions

7
Papillary, Papular, and Multiple Polypoid Lesions

FOCAL PAPILLARY LESIONS

Papilloma
Verruca Vulgaris
Condyloma Acuminatum*
Verruciform Xanthoma
Sialadenoma Papilliferum
Giant Cell Fibroma
Specific Granulomatous Infections

FOCAL AND UMBILICATED PAPULES

Keratoacanthoma
Warty Dyskeratoma
Molluscum Contagiosum

DIFFUSE AND MULTIFOCAL PAPILLARY LESIONS

Condyloma Acuminatum
Focal Dermal Hypoplasia

Nevus Unius Lateris
Oral Florid Papillomatosis
Verrucous Leukoplakia
Verrucous Carcinoma

DIFFUSE PAPULAR AND POLYPOID LESIONS

Papillary Hyperplasia
Stomatitis Nicotina
Acute Lymphonodular Pharyngitis
Keratosis Follicularis
Focal Epithelial Hyperplasia
Multiple Hamartoma Syndrome
Pyostomatitis Vegetans
Crohn's Disease
Amyloidosis
Hyalinosis Cutis et Mucosae
Hemangioma/Lymphangioma
Neuropolyendocrine Syndrome

*See Diffuse and Multifocal Papillary Lesions.

Papillary lesions represent swellings with finger-like projections imparting a cauliflower appearance; these microprojections are rounded and blunt like the fungiform papillae of the tongue. Verrucous lesions are similar, yet possess a more irregular surface. Indeed, differentiation between a papillary lesion and a verrucous one is based more on microscopic features rather than the clinical appearance. Umbilicated nodules are oval dome-shaped lesions with rolled margins and a central pit, which may be plugged with keratin. Papules are small, usually less than 0.5 cm, elevations that tend to occur in multiples or in crops. Polypoid lesions are similar in appearance to papules; however, they usually exceed 1.0 cm and, in the mouth, tend to be multifocal.

Most of the lesions in this chapter represent proliferations of the surface epithelium. Alternatively, some are the result of pathologic changes occurring in the lamina propria with secondary elevation of the epithelium. Whereas most papillary and focal umbilicated lesions are primary diseases of oral mucosa, some, particularly diffuse papular and polypoid lesions, represent oral markers of a systemic disorder. Biopsy is usually indicated to secure a definitive diagnosis; since some of these lesions herald the presence of an internal illness, the pathologist should be provided with data from the medical history.

Papilloma and giant cell fibroma are the most common focal papillary lesions. All lesions listed as focal umbilicated papules, extremely rare in the oral cavity, are more frequently encountered on skin.

Most of the diseases included as diffuse and multifocal papillary lesions are rare. Among these rarities is condyloma acuminatum, or venereal wart, which is fairly prevalent in homosexual males.

Papillary hyperplasia, also termed denture papillomatosis, is the most common entity observed as a diffuse papular lesion; stomatitis nicotina is also fairly common.

Most of the other diseases in this group are rare and are associated with either cutaneous or internal organ involvement.

FOCAL PAPILLARY LESIONS

Papilloma

Age: Young adults
Sex: No predilection

Clinical Features: Oral squamous papillomas are either pedunculated or sessile, show a cauliflower surface with finger-like projections, and may be white and keratotic or normal in color. These small epithelial neoplasms are most often encountered on the palate, uvula, tongue, and lip; they tend to reach a certain size, after which the growth essentially becomes arrested. A viral etiology, as seen in the common wart (verruca vulgaris), has not been confirmed in man.

Microscopic Features: The epithelium shows a thickened parakeratin layer and a papillary corrugated pattern. The epithelial projections are supported by fibrovascular cores, and inflammatory cells may be discernible.

Differential Diagnosis: A focal papilloma, by virtue of its papillary cauliflower surface, is readily recognized. Larger lesions must be differentiated

from verrucous carcinoma. On the lips papilloma may be indistinguishable from verruca vulgaris. Multiple confluent papillomas must be differentiated from condyloma acuminatum.

Treatment: Simple excision is recommended. Recurrence is extremely rare.

References

1. Kohn, E. M., et al.: Primary neoplasms of the hard and soft palates and the uvula. Proc. Staff Meet. Mayo Clin. 38:233, 1963.
2. Rose, H. P.: Papillomas of the oral cavity. Oral Surg. 20:542, 1965.
3. Greer, R. O. and Goldman, H. M.: Oral papillomas. Clinicopathologic evaluation and retrospective examination for dyskeratosis in 110 lesions. Oral Surg. 38:435, 1974.
4. Abby, L. M., Page D. G., and Sawyer, D. R.: The clinical and histopathologic features of a series of 464 oral squamous cell papillomas. Oral Surg. 49:419, 1980.

Verruca Vulgaris

Age: Children and young adults
Sex: No predilection

Clinical Features: Verruca vulgaris, the common wart, is a virus-induced neoplasm of the skin caused by a papovavirus. It may be seen on the vermilion border; lesions showing microscopic features indistinguishable from those of skin verrucae have been identified in the mouth. The le-

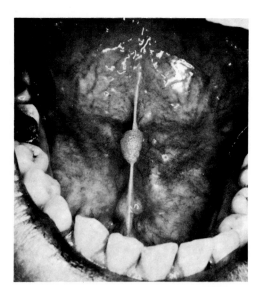

FIG. 7–1. Squamous papilloma showing a papillary cauliflower-like surface.

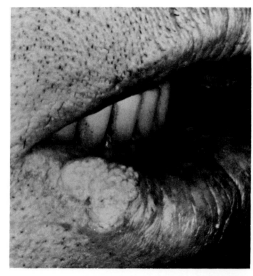

FIG. 7–2. Verruca vulgaris, rarely occurring on oral mucosa yet not particularly uncommon on the lip. The lesion is raised with a verrucous surface, which is white due to hyperkeratosis. (Courtesy of Dr. A. Leider.)

sion is white, with a keratotic surface and a well-delineated border. A stalk is not discernible. The papillary excrescences are composed of finger-like projections with a sharply angulated surface.

Microscopic Features: The epithelium possesses surface projections superficial to the normal tissue surface and showing no invagination. The projections are acute, pointed angles rather than bulbous or rounded, as with papillomas. Thickened keratin is a feature. Viral inclusion bodies are usually discernible in the upper spinous layer.

Differential Diagnosis: Verruca vulgaris is distinctive on vermilion border or skin, yet intraorally it may be clinically identical to papilloma.

Treatment: Simple local excision is recommended.

References

1. Orlean, S. and LaDoe, C., Jr.: Superficial keratoses, verruca vulgaris, and pachyderma oris. J. Dent. Med. *15*:108, 1960.
2. Clausen, F. P.: Rare oral viral disorders (molluscum contagiosum, localized keratoacanthoma, verrucae, condyloma acuminatum, and focal epithelial hyperplasia). Oral Surg. *34*:604, 1972.
3. Wysocki, G. P. and Hardie, J.: Ultrastructural studies of intraoral verruca vulgaris. Oral Surg. *47*:58, 1972.

Verruciform Xanthoma

Age: Adults
Sex: Female predilection

Clinical Features: Verruciform xanthoma is most often encountered on the alveolar ridge and buccal mucosa. It is keratotic yet may show a normal-colored pebbly surface. The lesion is well circumscribed, may be pedunculated, but more often is sessile and is under 1.5 cm in size. There is no known relationship between the occurrence

of this lesion and irritation, tobacco habits, or hyperlipidemia.

Microscopic Features: The surface epithelium is hypercornified and corrugated with small surface projections. The submucosal papillae extending between elongated rete ridges are diffusely infiltrated with foam cell histiocytes.

Differential Diagnosis: Clinically, verruciform xanthoma cannot be distinguished from verruciform hyperkeratosis. The lesion must also be differentiated from verrucous carcinoma; however, age differences are helpful in this case. A sessile papilloma may be grossly identical.

Treatment: Verruciform xanthoma can be locally excised. There is no known relationship between this type of xanthoma and the hyperlipoproteinemias.

References

1. Shafer, W. G.: Verruciform xanthoma. Oral Surg. *31*:784, 1971.
2. Miller, A. S. and Elzay, R. P.: Verruciform xanthoma of the gingiva: Report of six cases. J. Periodontol. *44*:103, 1973.
3. Neville, B. W. and Weathers, D. R.: Verruciform xanthoma. Oral Surg. *49*:429, 1980.
4. Nowparast, B., Howell, F. V., and Rick, G. M.: Verruciform xanthoma. A clinicopathologic review and report of fifty-four cases. Oral Surg. *51*:619, 1981.

Sialadenoma Papilliferum

Age: Elderly adults
Sex: Male predilection

Clinical Features: Sialadenoma papilliferum is a benign salivary tumor that presumably arises from the excretory duct system close to the surface mucosa when origin is from oral minor glands.

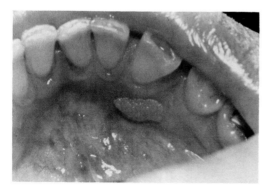

FIG. 7–3. Papillary gingival growth representing verruciform xanthoma. (Courtesy of Dr. A. Leider.)

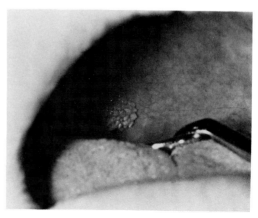

FIG. 7–4. Sialadenoma papilliferum.

Clinically, the lesion represents a well-localized sessile or pedunculated papillary growth, usually located on the hard palate. This tumor has also been observed to arise from the parotid gland and buccal mucosa minor glands. Since the proliferation extends down into the gland, the underlying base of the lesion is usually firm or indurated.

Microscopic Features: The papillary surface is usually represented by stratified squamous epithelium. These papillary folds extend into the deeper tissues undermining the surface. In this location, cystic channels are witnessed and the papillary projections protruding into the lumina are lined by ductal pseudostratified columnar epithelium. The individual cells are oncocytic with foci of mucous metaplasia. The base of the tumor lies directly over normal-appearing acinar tissue.

Differential Diagnosis: Sialadenoma papilliferum will clinically appear similar to most of the other focal papillary lesions included here. Localization to the palate along with palpation of a firm submucosal base are findings that would support the clinical diagnosis. Nevertheless, biopsy is required to secure the diagnosis.

Treatment: Since the lesion extends submucosally into salivary ducts, superficial excision will be inadequate. Once the diagnosis is provided histologically, a deeper wedge resection to include underlying glandular tissue is advisable.

References

1. Abrams, A. M. and Finck, F. M.: Sialadenoma papilliferum. A previously unreported salivary gland tumor. Cancer 24:1057, 1969.
2. Freedman, P. D. and Lumerman, H.: Sialadenoma papilliferum. Oral Surg. 45:88, 1978.
3. McCoy, J. M. and Eckert, E. F., Jr.: Sialadenoma papilliferum. J. Oral Surg. 38:691, 1980.
4. Nasu, M., Takagi, M., and Ishikawa, G.: Sialadenoma papilliferum: report of case. J. Oral Surg. 39:367, 1981.

Giant Cell Fibroma

Age: Teenagers and young adults
Sex: No predilection

Clinical Features: Whereas most oral traumatic fibromas are smooth-surfaced nodules, giant cell fibromas are usually multinodular or papillary. They may be pedunculated or sessile and are most frequently encountered on the gingiva, tongue, and palate.

Microscopic Features: The surface is multinodular and is covered by a thin layer of stratified squamous epithelium, which is distended by swirls of dense collagen fibers. The intervening fibroblasts are spindle or stellate in appearance,

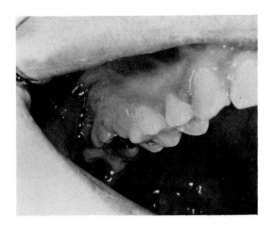

FIG. 7–5. Giant cell fibroma with papillary appearance.

and many have copious basophilic cytoplasm with 2 to 5 oval nuclei.

Differential Diagnosis: Papillary giant cell fibromas may be confused clinically with papillomas, verrucae, or condylomata. Biopsy is required to make the diagnosis.

Treatment: Complete surgical excision is the treatment of choice.

References

1. Weathers, D. R. and Callihan, M. D.: Giant-cell fibroma. Oral Surg. 37:374, 1974.
2. Regezi, J. A., Courtney, R. M., and Kerr, D. A.: Fibrous lesions of the skin and mucous membranes which contain stellate and multinucleated cells. Oral Surg. 39:605, 1975.
3. Houston, G. D.: The giant-cell fibroma: a review of 464 cases. Oral Surg. 53:582, 1982.

Specific Granulomatous Infections

Age: Adults
Sex: Equal distribution

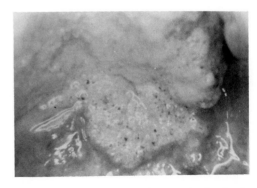

FIG. 7–6. Granular papillary lesion at hard-soft palate junction representing blastomycosis.

Clinical Features: Infectious and noninfectious granulomatous inflammatory lesions of the oral mucous membranes are usually localized and exhibit a granular or papillary surface. The lesions are usually raised and firm and may appear somewhat erythematous. Most of them are infectious in nature, representing hematogenous spread from a primary pulmonary focus. The deep fungal organisms such as histoplasmosis and blastomycosis are more apt to show pebbly granular lesions. The inherited disorder known as chronic granulomatous disease may manifest similar lesions. This disorder is characterized by ineffective phagocytolysis by leukocytes with recurrent and persistent infections accompanied by granulomatous inflammation. Oral lesions of sarcoidosis may also present in similar fashion clinically.

Microscopic Features: The epithelium may exhibit pseudoepitheliomatous hyperplasia; foci of granulomatous inflammation are located within the underlying connective tissue. Epithelioid histiocytes predominate, and multinucleated giant cells can be identified. Specific histochemical stains such as acid-fast, PAS, and methenamine silver demonstrate the presence of microorganisms in the infectious granulomas.

Differential Diagnosis: Most of the focal papillary lesions included here are small and fail to evince surface erythema. Granulomatous lesions are often large and are invariably sessile. A history of pulmonary disease or persistent cough and dyspnea should arouse suspicion of systemic granulomatous inflammatory disease.

Treatment: Depending on the organism identified, if any, the treatment is medical. Fungal infections are generally treated with amphotericin B or ketoconazole.

References

1. Tiecke, R. W., Baron, H. J., and Casey, D. E.: Localized oral histoplasmosis. Oral Surg. 16:441, 1963.
2. Kerr, M. W.: Sarcoidosis. Oral Surg. 20:166, 1965.
3. Wysocki, G. P. and Brooke, R. I.: Oral manifestations of chronic granulomatous disease. Oral Surg. 46:815, 1978.

FOCAL AND UMBILICATED PAPULES

Keratoacanthoma

Age: Adults
Sex: Male predilection

Clinical Features: The facial skin and lower lip, sun-exposed areas, are the common sites for keratoacanthoma, which rarely evolves from mucous membranes. Keratoacanthoma is a benign focal

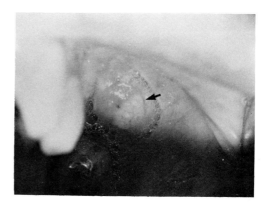

FIG. 7–7. Oral keratoacanthoma. (From Eversole, L. R., Leider, A. S., and Alexander, G.: Intraoral and labial keratoacanthoma. Oral Surg. 54:663, 1982.)

proliferation of surface epithelium that is classically dome shaped with a crateriform appearance. The lesion is round with rolled margins and possesses a central pit or core filled with a keratin plug that is frequently discolored, being yellowish brown. Oral examples usually possess a white core. Occasionally, the keratin plug exhibits a verrucous surface.

Microscopic Features: Keratoacanthoma is characterized by an abrupt marginal change with marked acanthosis and hyperparakeratosis or hyperorthokeratosis. The surface is verrucous. On low power, the lesion has a flask-shaped configuration with a superficial collarette and a bulbous expanded base. The individual cells are unremarkable, with one exception: the parabasilar cells may be hyperchromatic. Rarely, cytologic atypia may be a prominent feature, and differentiation from squamous cell carcinoma is problematical in these instances.

Differential Diagnosis: Squamous cancer may show similar clinical features; however, cancerous lesions usually fail to exhibit a smooth round regularity. Warty dyskeratoma and molluscum have gross features in common with keratoacanthoma; yet, they are usually small (less than 0.5 cm) while keratoacanthoma can attain dimensions of 1.0–2.0 cm.

Treatment: The lesion usually regresses spontaneously within a year or two. Despite this fact, it cannot be definitively diagnosed clinically, is unsightly, and if allowed to regress, often leaves a depressed scar. Surgical excision is the treatment of choice.

References

1. Kohn, M. W. and Eversole, L. R.: Keratoacanthoma of the lower lip. Report of cases. J. Oral Surg. 30:522, 1972.
2. Scofield, H. H., Werning, J. T., and Shukes, R. C.: Solitary intraoral keratoacanthoma. Oral Surg. 37:889, 1974.
3. Zegarelli, D. J.: Solitary intraoral keratoacanthoma. Oral Surg. 40:785, 1975.
4. Goodwin, R. E. and Fisher, G. H.: Keratoacanthoma of the head and neck. Ann. Otol. Rhinol. Laryngol. 89:72, 1980.
5. Eversole, L. R., Leider, A. S., and Alexander, G.: Intraoral and labial keratoacanthoma. Oral Surg. 54:663, 1982.

Warty Dyskeratoma

Age: Adults
Sex: No predilection

Clinical Features: Warty dyskeratoma, a localized lesion of skin, is occasionally encountered in the mouth. The oral lesion is usually found on the palate or alveolar ridge and appears as a small papule with a depressed central pit or as focal verrucous nodules. A variant, termed focal acantholytic dyskeratosis, manifests a similar appearance with two or three discrete lesions arising adjacent to one another.

Microscopic Features: Both warty dyskeratoma and focal acantholytic dyskeratosis display microscopic features that are nearly identical to those observed in keratosis follicularis. These two focal lesions have a keratinized surface with an invaginated central depression. The spinous layer is thickened and contains individually keratinized cells. The pathognomonic change is observed inferiorly where villous rete ridges pervade and exhibit acantholysis.

Differential Diagnosis: Other umbilicated or crateriform lesions listed here resemble or are clinically identical to warty dyskeratoma. When a pitted papule fails to show tumefaction, a traumatic lesion may be suspected clinically; therefore, the diagnosis requires a biopsy.

Treatment: Surgical excision of these small lesions is usually accomplished during biopsy.

References

1. Szymanski, F. J.: Warty dyskeratoma, a benign cutaneous tumor resembling Darier's disease microscopically. Arch. Derm. 75:567, 1957.
2. Tomich, C. E., and Burkes, E. J.: Warty dyskeratoma (isolated dyskeratosis follicularis) of the oral mucosa. Oral Surg. 31:798, 1971.
3. Harris, T. J., Murphy, G. F., and Mihm, M. C.: Oral warty dyskeratoma. Arch. Dermatol. 116:929, 1980.
4. Freedman, P. D., Lumerman, H., and Kerpel, S. M.: Oral focal acantholytic dyskeratosis. Oral Surg. 52:66, 1981.
5. Leider, A. S. and Eversole, L. R.: Focal acantholytic dyskeratosis of the oral mucosa. Oral Surg. In press 1984.

Molluscum Contagiosum

Age: Children and young adults
Sex: No predilection

Clinical Features: Molluscum contagiosum represents a unique type of viral wart, resulting from infection by a member of the poxvirus family. The disease is usually encountered on the skin of children or in the anogenital region in adults. It appears as a dome-shaped nodule that is usually, yet not invariably, characterized by a central pit or depressed core. The lesion is rare on the lips or in the mouth.

Microscopic Features: The histologic findings are unique and diagnostic. The epithelium exhibits an abrupt zone of acanthosis with a central para-

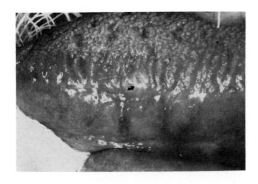

FIG. 7–8. Warty dyskeratoma appearing as crateriform lesion on the tongue. (Courtesy of Dr. J. Dittmer.)

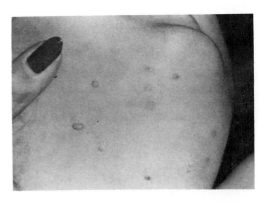

FIG. 7–9. Multiple lesions of cutaneous molluscum contagiosum. The rare oral instances show a similar appearance. (Courtesy of Dr. H. Schneidman.)

keratinized invagination. Large prominent eosinophilic globules, referred to as molluscum bodies, are located as conglomerates in the upper and middle spinous layers. Coalescing bulbous rete ridges are present, and the underlying connective tissue is often chronically inflamed.

Differential Diagnosis: Molluscum may clinically resemble a fistula or parulis, keratoacanthoma, or warty dyskeratoma when it occurs on lips or mucosa. Biopsy is required to make the diagnosis.

Treatment: Excisional biopsy is the treatment of choice.

References

1. Lynch, P. J. and Minkin, W.: Molluscum contagiosum of the adult. Arch. Dermatol. *98*:141, 1968.
2. Barsh, L. I.: Molluscum contagiosum of the oral mucosa. Oral Surg. *22*:42, 1966.
3. Nelson, J. F. and Tsaknis, P. J.: Molluscum contagiosum of the lower lip: Report of a case. J. Oral Med. *35*:62, 1980.

DIFFUSE AND MULTIFOCAL PAPILLARY LESIONS

Condyloma Acuminatum

Age: Adults
Sex: No predilection

Clinical Features: Condyloma acuminatum is a verrucous papillary lesion caused by a papovavirus. The lesions are generally confined to the anogenital intertriginous regions. They are autoinoculable and may also be transmitted as a venereal disease, accounting for the term *venereal warts.* Oral condylomata are similar in appearance to anogenital condylomata. The resemblance to the common oral papilloma is striking; however, condyloma tends to appear more racemose and also shows a tendency for multiplicity with clustering. A history of sexual contact as a source of transmission can usually be obtained.

Microscopic Features: Surface-stratified squamous epithelium displays a papillary pattern with rounded finger-like extension. A prominent parakeratin layer is present, and acanthosis is striking. Numerous mitotic figures can be encountered in the basal and parabasilar strata. Viral inclusion bodies are usually discernible in the upper spinous layer. The subjacent fibrous connective tissue is traversed by dilated vascular channels. Viral particles can be demonstrated with electron microscopy.

Differential Diagnosis: Condyloma acuminatum is most often confused with the common squamous papilloma. Differentiation can usually be made clinically by a history of sexual transmission. Multiplicity with clustering of lesions is also a feature in favor of a diagnosis of condyloma. In florid papillomatoses, the entire oral cavity is involved; in the Goltz syndrome, the dermal manifestations are characteristic.

Treatment: Biopsy is necessary to obtain a definitive diagnosis. Once the diagnosis has been secured, excision or cryotherapy with cotton applicators soaked in liquid nitrogen can be employed to remove the lesions. Recurrence is common, and the lesions are contagious.

References

1. Praetorius-Clausen, F.: Rare oral viral disorders (molluscum contagiosum, localized keratoacanthoma, verrucae, condyloma acuminatum, and focal epithelial hyperplasia). Oral Surg. *34*:604, 1972.
2. Doyle, J. L., Grodjesk, J. E., and Manhold, T. H., Jr.: Condyloma acuminatum occurring in the oral cavity. Oral Surg. *26*:434, 1968.
3. Seibert, J. S., Shannon, C. S., Jr., and Jacoway, J. R.: Treatment of recurrent condyloma acuminatum. Oral Surg. *27*:398, 1969.
4. McClatchey, K. D., Colquitt, W. N., and Robert, R. C., Jr.: Condyloma acuminatum of the lip: Report of case. J. Oral Surg. *37*:751, 1979.
5. Shaffer, E. L., Jr., Reimann, B. E. F., and Gysland, W. B.: Oral condyloma acuminatum. A case report with light microscopic and ultrastructural features. J. Oral Pathol. *9*:163, 1980.

Focal Dermal Hypoplasia (Goltz Syndrome)

Age: Children
Sex: No predilection

Clinical Features: Many defects accompany the skin lesions of the Goltz syndrome, including multiple papillomas of the lips and oral mucosa.

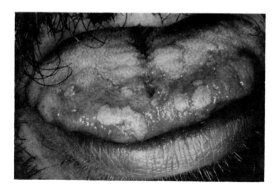

FIG. 7–10. Venereal warts, or condylomata, involving oral mucosa. They appear similar to papillomas with a tendency toward multiplicity and clustering.

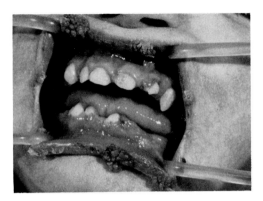

FIG. 7–11. Orolabial papillomas in focal dermal hypoplasia syndrome. (Courtesy of Dr. Robert Gorlin.)

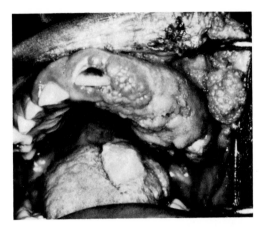

FIG. 7–12. Unilateral extensive papillary proliferations involving oral mucosa in nevus unius lateris. (From Kelly, J. E., Hibbard, E. D., and Giansanti, J. S.: Epidermal nevus syndrome; report of a case with unusual oral manifestations. Oral Surg. 34:774, 1972.)

The oral lesions consist of exophytic papillary outgrowths that are identical to the ordinary oral squamous papilloma, yet are prone to be multiple with tendency for confluency. The skin lesions located on the extremities are rubbery nodules with wrinkled pigmented surfaces and represent herniation of the subcutaneous tissues through a genetically deficient dermal layer. Other features of the syndrome include mental retardation, strabismus, syndactyly, and colobomas of the iris.

Microscopic Features: The oral papillomas of the Goltz syndrome show histomorphologic features indistinguishable from the ordinary squamous papilloma.

Differential Diagnosis: The various components of the syndrome allow differentiation from other diseases manifesting oral papillary or polypoid lesions.

Treatment: The papillomas should be excised, as they can be traumatized by mastication and thus hemorrhage.

References

1. Goltz, R. J., et al.: Focal dermal hypoplasia syndrome. Arch. Dermatol. 86:708, 1962.
2. Gorlin, R. J., et al.: Focal dermal hypoplasia syndrome. Acta. Dermatol. 43:421, 1963.

Nevus Unius Lateris

Age: Children
Sex: No predilection
Clinical Features: A developmental verrucous lesion of skin, nevus unius lateris (also termed the epidermal nevus syndrome) usually occurs on the arm as a keratotic washboard-rough lesion that conforms to a narrow linear configuration. When the face is involved, extension into the oral cavity may occur. The lesion continues its linear orien-

tation, yet its appearance assumes a pebbly papillary pattern identical to papilloma.

Microscopic Features: The skin lesion demonstrates acutely angulated verrucous epithelial hyperkeratotic projections not unlike those of verruca vulgaris. The oral lesion is microscopically indistinguishable from simple papilloma.

Differential Diagnosis: Nevus unius lateris must be differentiated from verrucous carcinoma, pyostomatitis vegetans, and florid papillomatosis. The linear configuration, extension onto facial skin, and development during childhood allow for differentiation from these entities.

Treatment: Following microscopic confirmation of the diagnosis, the lesion may be removed surgically or with electrocautery in stages. The facial lesions should be managed by a plastic surgeon.

References

1. Brown, H. M. and Gorlin, R. J.: Oral mucosal involvement in nevus unius lateris (ichthyosis hystrix). Arch. Dermatol. 81:509, 1960.
2. Kelly, J. E., Hibbard, E. D., and Giansanti, J. S.: Epidermal nevus syndrome; report of a case with unusual oral manifestations. Oral Surg. 34:774, 1972.
3. Ephraim, A. and Skeer, J.: Nevus unius lateris on the left cheek, scalp, and neck. Arch. Dermatol. Syph. 50:222, 1944.
4. Muller, J. T., Pickett, A. B., and Frederick, F. D.: Facial hemihypertrophy associated with nevus unius lateris syndrome. Oral Surg. 50:226, 1980.

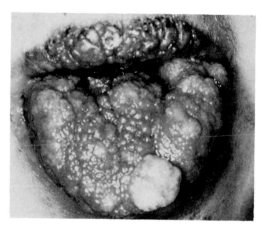

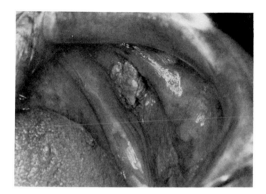

FIG. 7–14.   Verrucous leukoplakia in the mucobuccal fold.

FIG. 7–13.   Extensive involvement of oral mucosa and vermilion by papillomas in oral florid papillomatosis. (From Eversole, L. R. and Sorenson, H. W.: Oral florid papillomatosis in Down's syndrome. Oral Surg. 37:202, 1974.)

Oral Florid Papillomatosis

Age: Children

Sex: No predilection

Clinical Features: Rarely, squamous papillomas may be multiple and virtually involve the entire oral cavity. Extension into the larynx is also seen. It should be emphasized that earlier reports of this entity occurring in the elderly are for the most part now accepted as examples of verrucous carcinoma. Oral florid papillomatosis may manifest multiple isolated papillomas or, as previously mentioned, may be extremely extensive with profuse involvement of the mucous membranes. The papillomas are normal in color, failing to show significant keratinization.

Microscopic Features: The histomorphology is identical to that of simple squamous papilloma.

Differential Diagnosis: Oral florid papillomatosis may clinically appear identical to nevus unius lateris and similar to pyostomatitis vegetans. Age distinguishes this entity from verrucous carcinoma, as does lack of surface keratinization. Biopsy is required to confirm the clinical impression.

Treatment: Multistage excision is the treatment of choice. Electrosurgery may be employed.

Reference

1. Eversole, L. R. and Sorenson, H. W.: Oral florid papillomatosis in Down's syndrome. Oral Surg. 37:202, 1974.

Verrucous Leukoplakia

Age: Middle-aged and elderly adults

Sex: Slight female predilection

Clinical Features: Verrucous leukoplakia, also referred to as verrucous hyperplasia or verruciform leukoplakia, is a precancerous lesion that may be associated with or progress to verrucous carcinoma. Clinically, the lesion is a localized yet often diffuse verrucous or papillary lesion found most often on the gingiva, alveolar ridge, or mucobuccal fold. It may be white, pink, or speckled. Planar leukoplakia is frequently observed in association with the verrucous lesion, either in continuity or in separate locations.

Microscopic Features: Some examples exhibit sharp verrucous projections (acrokeratotic) or blunt rounded projections (polypoid and cryptic). The surface is frequently hyperortho- or hyperparakeratotic, and acanthosis is usually observed. There is a high incidence of dysplastic cytologic change, and many of these lesions lie adjacent to zones of verrucous carcinoma or invasive squamous cell carcinoma.

Differential Diagnosis: The clinical appearance of verrucous leukoplakia is similar if not identical to verrucous carcinoma, particularly when a white keratotic surface is present. Furthermore, occurrence in the elderly differentiates this lesion from other diffuse papillary lesions that occur in children.

Treatment: Once the diagnosis is made, other areas of a large lesion should be biopsied and examined for the presence of carcinoma. Wide local excision is recommended with periodic follow-up. If coexistent carcinoma is detected, the treatment must be more aggressive.

References

1. Bánóczy, J. and Sugar, L.: Longitudinal studies in oral leukoplakia. J. Oral Pathol. 1:265, 1972.
2. Adkins, K. F. and Monsour, F. N.: Verrucous leukoplakia. N. Z. Dent. J. 72:28, 1976.

3. Shear, M. and Pindburg, J. J.: Verrucous hyperplasia of the oral mucosa. Cancer 46:1855, 1980.
4. Eversole, L. R. and Shopper, T. P.: Oral leukoplakia: Prevalence of dysplastic and carcinomatous change in verruciform and planar patterns. Cal. Dent. Assoc. J. (Oct.):45, 1981.

Verrucous Carcinoma

Age: Elderly adults
Sex: Male predilection

Clinical Features: Verrucous carcinoma is a nonmetastasizing laterally spreading epithelial tumor, usually associated with tobacco chewing or snuff dipping. The lesion is typically fungating with a white verrucoid keratotic surface that has a shaggy appearance. It is most often encountered in the mucobuccal fold and buccal mucosa. In the later stages of disease, extensive lateral spread becomes manifest.

Microscopic Features: The histomorphology is distinctive. Massively enlarged bulbous acanthotic rete ridges invaginate into the connective tissue, yet extensions from the basal cell layer showing invasion do not exist. Apart from basilar and parabasilar hyperchromatism, cytologic atypia is not featured; rather, a normal maturation of epithelium exists. Deep crypts, filled with parakeratin, extend downward from the surface into the center of the bulbous rete ridge invaginations.

Differential Diagnosis: Verrucous carcinoma may clinically simulate papillary hyperplasia, pyostomatitis vegetans, and, importantly, epidermoid carcinoma that may be clinically verrucous in appearance. Only biopsy can differentiate between true verrucous carcinoma and a clinically verrucoid-appearing epidermoid carcinoma.

Treatment: Wide surgical excision is recommended; recurrence is common. Radiation therapy is contraindicated in verrucous carcinoma since anaplastic transformation has been reported to occur following such treatment.

References

1. Ackerman, L. V.: Verrucous carcinoma of the oral cavity. Surgery 23:670, 1948.
2. Perez, C. A., et al.: Anaplastic transformation in verrucous carcinoma of the oral cavity after radiation therapy. Radiology 86:108, 1966.
3. Shafer, W. G.: Verrucous carcinoma. Int. Dent. J. 22:451, 1972.
4. Jacobson, S. and Shear, M.: Verrucous carcinoma of the mouth. J. Oral Pathol. 1:66, 1972.
5. McCoy, J. M. and Waldron, C. A.: Verrucous carcinoma; analysis of fifty-six cases. Oral Surg. 52:623, 1981.

DIFFUSE PAPULAR AND POLYPOID LESIONS

Papillary Hyperplasia

Age: Adults
Sex: No predilection

Clinical Features: Confined to the palatal vault, papillary hyperplasia or papillomatosis is most often associated with a maxillary denture. Occasionally, it occurs in dentulous mouths in association with a partial denture. The lesion displays a cobblestone appearance and is either normal in color or erythematous. When the papillary lesions are reddened, secondary infection with Candida

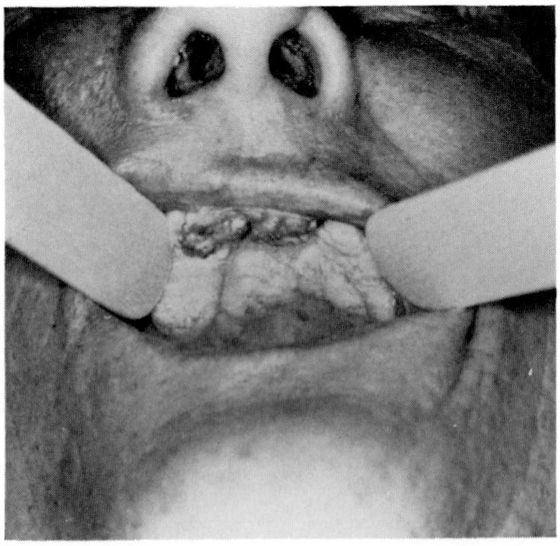

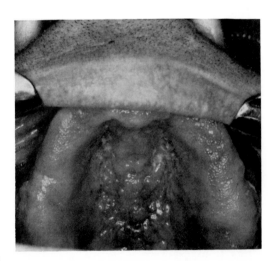

FIG. 7–15.   Verrucous carcinoma, a nonmetastasizing neoplasm of oral mucosa that shows a shaggy, verrucous keratotic surface.

FIG. 7–16.   Papillomatosis in the vault found under an ill-fitting maxillary denture. (Courtesy of Dr. A. Levere.)

is common. The cause is unknown but is probably related to trauma and may arise in response to negative pressure placed on the palatal tissues. The lesion is not premalignant.

Microscopic Features: The epithelium manifests multiple dome-shaped papules with elongated rete ridges and pseudoepitheliomatous hyperplasia. The submucosa contains a diffuse chronic inflammatory cell infiltrate.

Differential Diagnosis: The combination of dental prosthesis and palatal vault papillary outgrowth allows for a clinical diagnosis. If the lesion extends onto the alveolar ridge, it must be differentiated from verrucous carcinoma or a specific granulomatous infection.

Treatment: The hyperplastic tissue may resolve after removal of the old denture. If not, surgical removal is recommended prior to fabrication of a new prosthesis.

References

1. Schmitz, J. F.: A clinical study of inflammatory papillary hyperplasia. J. Prosthet. Dent. *14*:1034, 1964.
2. O'Driscoll, P. M.: Papillary hyperplasia of the palate. Br. Dent. J. *118*:77, 1965.
3. Uohara, G. I. and Federbush, M. D.: Removal of papillary hyperplasia. J. Oral Surg. 26:463, 1968.
4. Miller, E. L.: Clinical management of denture-induced inflammations. J. Prosthet. Dent. *38*:362, 1977.

Stomatitis Nicotina

Age: Middle-aged and elderly adults
Sex: Male predilection

Clinical Features: Pipe and cigar smokers will occasionally develop multiple white keratotic papules with red depressed centers that represent dilated, inflamed minor salivary ducts on the hard and soft palate. The papules do not coalesce and are separated from one another by intervening normal-appearing mucosa. It is not known whether these multifocal keratotic papules arise as a consequence of heat or tobacco tars. The lesion is rarely seen in cigarette smokers; evidence does not support a premalignant potential.

Microscopic Features: The surface epithelium is hyperkeratotic and usually acanthotic. The salivary excretory ducts are dilated and evince a periductal mononuclear inflammatory infiltrate.

Differential Diagnosis: White papules with a red center located on the palate of a pipe or cigar smoker are usually sufficient findings to permit establishment of the diagnosis on a clinical basis. Other papular lesions fail to show this combination of findings.

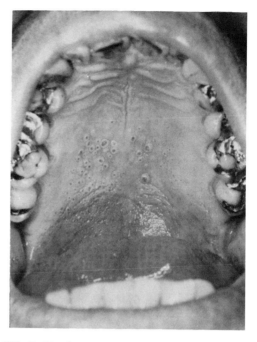

FIG. 7–17. Stomatitis nicotina, multiple crateriform papules.

Treatment: Abating the tobacco habit will allow for resolution. The oral cavity should be examined thoroughly in order to detect leukoplakic or erythroplakic foci, which may coexist.

References

1. Thoma, K. H.: Stomatitis nicotina and its effect on the palate. Am. J. Orthod. Oral Surg. 27:38, 1941.
2. Saunders, W. H.: Nicotine stomatitis of the palate. Ann. Otol. Rhinol. Laryngol. 67:618, 1958.
3. Schwartz, D. L.: Stomatitis nicotina of the palate. Oral Surg. *20*:306, 1965.

Acute Lymphonodular Pharyngitis

Age: Children and young adults
Sex: No predilection

Clinical Features: Coxsackie virus infections manifest a variety of clinical presentations. Lymphonodular pharyngitis is unique and is usually diagnosed clinically, based on lesion morphology and location. Multiple yellowish-pink papules are distributed over the soft palate, tonsilar fauces, and oropharynx. The patient fails to show a cutaneous exanthem. Fever, lymphadenopathy, and sore throat are the typical symptoms. Epidemics among school children are common.

Microscopic Features: Surface epithelium is distended by focal aggregates of lymphocytes, and

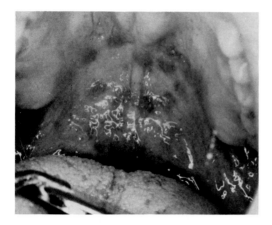

FIG. 7–18. Multiple red papules of the soft palate and oropharynx characteristic of lymphonodular pharyngitis, a Coxsackie virus infection.

attempts at germinal center formation can be observed in some of these lymphoid papules.

Differential Diagnosis: None of the other entities listed as papular or multiple polypoid lesions are restricted to the oropharynx, nor are they associated with constitutional symptoms of infectious disease. A clinical diagnosis can be made. If confirmation is required, a stool culture for Coxsackie virus can be ordered.

Treatment: The disease is self-limited and resolves in 7 to 10 days. Antipyretic medication may be used along with a palliative mouth rinse or gargle.

References

1. Steigman, A. J., Lipton, M. M., and Braspennickx, H.: Acute lymphonodular pharyngitis: A newly described condition due to coxsackie A virus. J. Pediatr. 61:331, 1963.
2. Lennette, E. H. and Magoffin, R. L.: Virologic and immunologic aspects of major oral ulcerations. J. Am. Dent. Assoc. 87:1055, 1973.

Keratosis Follicularis

Age: Adults
Sex: Male predilection

Clinical Features: A primary disease of skin, keratosis follicularis or Darier-White's disease frequently affects the oral mucous membranes. This autosomal dominantly inherited disorder affects epithelial maturation and keratinization. Orange-brown keratotic papules appear on the skin and often keratinize progressively, resulting in diffuse white verrucoid plaques. The oral lesions may be white or may exhibit normal coloration; they diffusely affect the buccal mucosa and palate, thus

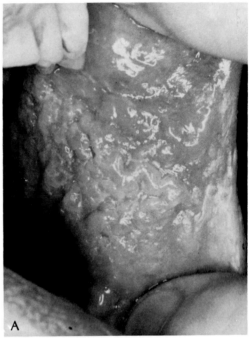

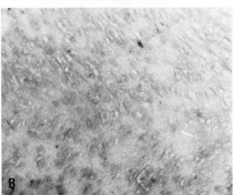

FIG. 7–19. Keratosis follicularis. A: Oral papular lesions. (From Weathers, D. R. and Driscoll, R. M.: Darier's disease of the oral mucosa. Oral Surg. 37:711, 1974.) B: Cutaneous scaley papules.

appearing as multiple confluent papules with a cobblestone pattern.

Microscopic Features: Hyperkeratosis occurs, and the spinous cell layer contains individually keratinized cells, many of which are enveloped by spinous layer cells (corps ronds). The rete ridges assume a villous pattern with suprabasilar acantholytic cleavage.

Differential Diagnosis: The cobblestone pattern resembles that seen in Cowden's disease, papillary hyperplasia, and pyostomatitis vegetans. The occurrence of papular and keratotic cutaneous lesions suggests keratosis follicularis clinically, and the microscopic features will confirm this impression.

Treatment: Retinoids have been employed with moderate success for the cutaneous lesions. No effective treatment exists for the oral lesions.

References

1. Spouge, J. D., et al.: Darier-White's disease: a cause of white lesions of the mucosa. Oral Surg. *21*:441, 1966.
2. Weathers, D. R. and Driscoll, R. M.: Darier's disease of the oral mucosa. Oral Surg. *37*:711, 1974.
3. Prindville, D. E. and Stern, D.: Oral manifestations of Darier's disease. J. Oral Surg. *34*:1001, 1976.

Focal Epithelial Hyperplasia (Heck's Disease)

Age: Children
Sex: No predilection

Clinical Features: Focal polypoid nodules appear primarily on the lips and buccal mucosa during the prepubescent period in Heck's disease. These peculiar lesions occur in clusters and in isolated crops, which eventually manifest spontaneous regression. They are pale to normal in color and show a flattened surface. American Indians and other ethnic groups of Athapaskan descent are often afflicted, but cases have also been reported in other ethnic groups, including Europeans. A viral etiology has been suggested.

Microscopic Features: The epithelium displays an exophytic nodular surface with thickened parakeratin. The major portion of the outgrowth is accounted for by epithelial hyperplasia with acanthosis and elongated anastomosing rete ridges. Inclusion bodies may be seen in cells occupying the spinous cell layer.

Differential Diagnosis: The appearance of multifocal polypoid lesions on the lips of Indian children is characteristic. Lack of total confluency aids in differentiating Heck's disease from the other lesions included in this section.

Treatment: No treatment is required; spontaneous regression occurs.

References

1. Archard, H. O., et al.: Focal epithelial hyperplasia: an unusual oral mucosa lesion found in Indian children. Oral Surg. *20*:201, 1965.
2. Witkop, C. J., Jr. and Niswander, J. D.: Focal epithelial hyperplasia in Central and South American Indians and Latinos. Oral Surg. *20*:213, 1965.
3. Borghelli, R. F., et al.: Focal epithelial hyperplasia. Oral Surg. *40*:107, 1975.
4. Buchner, A., Bubis, J. J., and Ramon, Y.: Ultrastructural study of focal epithelial hyperplasia. Oral Surg. *39*:622, 1975.
5. Acevedo, A., Gonzales, G. M., and Nelson, J. F.: Focal epithelial hyperplasia. Oral Surg. *51*:524, 1981.

Multiple Hamartoma Syndrome

Age: Adults
Sex: No predilection

Clinical Features: Also known as Cowden's disease, the multiple hamartoma syndrome appears to represent an autosomal dominant hereditary disease characterized by widespread hamartomas and neoplasms of skin, mucosa, and internal organs. The oral lesions are found on the attached gingiva. Multiple papular nodules yield a cobblestone pebbly surface. Cutaneous papu-

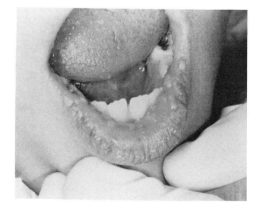

FIG. 7–20. Multiple sessile papules of the lips and buccal mucosa characteristic of focal epithelial hyperplasia.

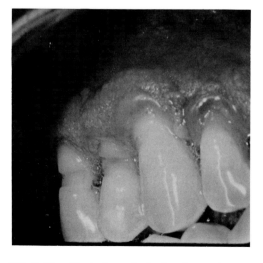

FIG. 7–21. Gingival papules in Cowden syndrome.

lonodular lesions are seen around the nares, lip commissures and palmar surface of the hands. Patients with Cowden's disease also develop goiter or thyroid adenomas and fibrocystic disease of the breast, which may progress to malignancy. Other organs may also be involved.

Microscopic Features: The oral papules exhibit microscopic features of fibroepithelial polyps. The epithelium is somewhat hyperplastic with acanthosis and elongated, anastomosing rete ridges. Supporting this epithelium is a mature fibrous connective tissue core.

Differential Diagnosis: The cobblestone lesions of multiple hamartoma syndrome may appear similar to the papular lesions observed in Sipple syndrome, pyostomatitis vegetans, keratosis follicularis, and focal epithelial hyperplasia. Localization to the gingiva, observed papules on the facial skin, and a history of thyroid or breast disease in conjunction with familial involvement lead to the diagnosis.

Treatment: No treatment is necessary for the oral lesions. A complete medical workup for organ-system involvement is recommended.

References

1. Weary, P. E., et al.: Multiple hamartoma syndrome (Cowden's disease). Arch. Dermatol. *105*:682, 1972.
2. Gentry, W. C., Jr., Eskritt, N. E., and Gorlin, R. J.: Multiple hamartoma syndrome (Cowden disease). Arch. Dermatol. *109*:521, 1974.
3. Gertzman, G. B. R., Clark, M., and Gaston, G.: Multiple hamartoma and neoplasia syndrome (Cowden's syndrome). Oral Surg. *49*:314, 1980.

Pyostomatitis Vegetans

Age: Middle-aged adults
Sex: Slight female predilection

Clinical Features: Pyostomatitis vegetans is a vegetating disease of oral mucosa characterized by multifocal polypoid lesions of the lips and buccal mucosa. While it may occur in the absence of systemic disease, it is more often associated with either ulcerative colitis or regional enteritis, thereby representing the oral mucosal counterpart to the skin disease pyodermatitis vegetans of Hallopeau. The individual polyps vary in size and are usually inflamed. Pain is not a prominent feature.

Microscopic Features: The surface epithelium is acanthotic with polypoid extensions of submucosal connective tissue. A subacute inflammatory cell infiltrate prevails, with foci of eosinophilic abscesses located in the papillae and at the epithelial connective tissue junction.

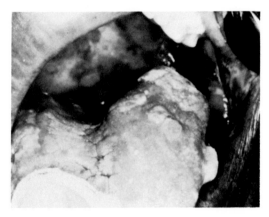

FIG. 7–22.   Multiple papules in pyostomatitis vegetans. (Courtesy of Drs. S. Silverman and P. Merrell.)

Differential Diagnosis: The lesion must be differentiated from verrucous carcinoma, oral florid papillomatosis, mycotic granuloma, and focal epithelial hyperplasia (Heck's disease). Biopsy with identification of eosinophilic abscesses and medical workup for ulcerative colitis are recommended to aid in arriving at a definitive diagnosis.

Treatment: Treatment is empirical. Systemic steroids (25 to 30 mg prednisone daily) with standard care for ulcerative colitis will usually result in diminution of the oral lesions. Ulcerative colitis is managed by a general physician or gastroenterologist.

References

1. McCarthy, F. P. and Shklar, G.: A syndrome of pyostomatitis vegetans and ulcerative colitis. Arch. Dermatol. *88*:913, 1963.
2. Forman, L.: Two cases of pyodermite vegetante (Hallopeau); an eosinophilic pustular and vegetating dermatitis with conjunctival, oral and colonic involvement. Proc. R. Soc. Med. *58*:244, 1965.
3. Cataldo, E., Covino, M. C., and Tesone, P. E.: Pyostomatitis vegetans. Oral Surg. *52*:172, 1981.
4. Hansen, L. A., Silverman, S., Jr., and Daniels, T. E.: The differential diagnosis of pyostomatitis vegetans and its relation to bowel disease. Oral Surg. *55*:363, 1983.

Crohn's Disease

Age: Middle-aged adults
Sex: No predilection

Clinical Features: Regional enteritis or Crohn's disease is a segmental granulomatous disease of the ileum and ascending colon. Oral lesions are occasionally present and consist of bosselated multiple polyps usually located in the buccal mucosa or mucobuccal fold. They are firm, usually normal in color, and painless. Gingival swellings

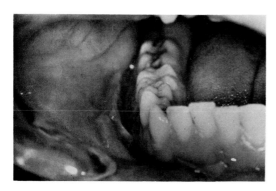

FIG. 7–23. Multiple polypoid tumefactions of the mucobuccal fold in Crohn's disease. (From Varley, E. W. B.: Crohn's disease of the mouth; report of three cases. Oral Surg. *33*:570, 1972.)

and erythematous pebbly lesions may also be encountered. Patients will complain of gastrointestinal irregularity, mild chronic diarrhea, and abdominal discomfort.

Microscopic Features: The epithelium is distended by an underlying mass of organized granulation tissue with lymphoid infiltration, epithelioid histiocytes, and giant cells yielding a noncaseating specific granulomatous reaction. Special stains fail to disclose the presence of microorganisms.

Differential Diagnosis: The polypoid masses in Crohn's disease are broader and, overall, larger than most of the other polypoid or papillary lesions included in this section. They must be differentiated from denture hyperplasia, pyostomatitis vegetans, and mycotic granuloma.

Treatment: The oral lesions may be excised. Crohn's disease is managed by a general physician or gastroenterologist.

References

1. Eisenbud, L., Katzka, I., and Platt, N.: Oral manifestations in Crohn's disease. Oral Surg. *34*:770, 1972.
2. Bottomley, W. K., Giorgini, G. L., and Julienne, C. H.: Oral extension of regional enteritis (Crohn's disease). Oral Surg. *34*:417, 1972.
3. Varley, E. W. B.: Crohn's disease of the mouth; report of three cases. Oral Surg. *33*:570, 1972.
4. Snyder, M. B. and Cawson, R. A.: Oral changes in Crohn's disease. J. Oral Surg. *34*:594, 1976.
5. Bernstein, M. L. and McDonald, J. S.: Oral lesions in Crohn's disease: report of two cases and update of the literature. Oral Surg. *46*:234, 1978.

Amyloidosis

Age: Middle-aged adults

Sex: Male predilection

Clinical Features: Amyloidosis is a systemic disease in which a peculiar glycoprotein accumulates within the connective tissues and around vascular walls. The disease may be primary or secondary. Secondary forms are more common and arise in conjunction with multiple myeloma or, occasionally, in association with a chronic granulomatous disease. The tongue is the most common intraoral site, yet deposits of amyloid protein may also be identified in the lips and buccal mucosa. The lesions are usually multifocal and appear as sessile, deep nodules that are indurated.

Microscopic Features: Globular aggregates of acellular eosinophilic proteinaceous material distend the surface epithelium and are deposited within the underlying connective tissues. Congo red staining with polarization microscopy will allow visualization of green birefringence, confirming the presence of amyloid.

Differential Diagnosis: Large nodular deposits causing macroglossia are usually observed, and these features do not closely parallel those seen in the other papular or multiple polypoid lesions listed here. Microscopically, amyloidosis resembles hyalinosis cutis et mucosae. A biopsy along with Congo red staining will provide a definitive diagnosis.

Treatment: Once amyloidosis is diagnosed, a thorough medical workup is indicated to uncover myeloma or granulomatous disease. In the former, cytologic chemotherapeutic drugs are employed. Large amyloid nodules interfering with speech or deglutition can be removed surgically.

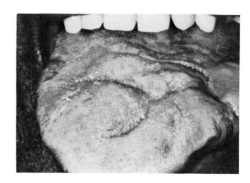

FIG. 7–24. Multiple tongue nodules in amyloidosis. (Courtesy of Dr. T. Daniels.)

References

1. Akin, R. K., Barton, K., and Walters, P. J.: Amyloidosis, macroglossia and carpal tunnel syndrome associated with myeloma. J. Oral Surg. 33:690, 1975.
2. Kraut, R. A., et al.: Amyloidosis associated with multiple myeloma. Oral Surg. 43:63, 1977.
3. Meyer, I., et al.: Amyloidosis of the tongue secondary to multiple myeloma (CPC). J. Oral Surg. 36:372, 1978.
4. Flick, W. G. and Lawrence, F. R.: Oral amyloidosis as initial symptom of multiple myeloma. A case report. Oral Surg. 49:18, 1980.

Hyalinosis Cutis et Mucosae

Age: Young adults

Sex: No predilection

Clinical Features: Also known as lipoid proteinosis or the Urbach-Wiethe syndrome, hyalinosis cutis et mucosae represents a rare autosomal recessive disorder involving many organ systems. Diffuse deposits of hyaline glycoprotein and acid as well as neutral glycosaminoglycans occur in the mucosal tissues, skin, and vessel walls. Deposits are also found in the brain with calcifications of the dorsum sellae. The oral tissues show infiltrated plaques, papules, and nodules that are yellowish-white and are distributed in multiple array over the lips, tongue, buccal mucosa, and pharynx with occasional gingival involvement. The larynx is frequently involved as well. Cutaneous lesions may commence as vesicles; upon healing, acneiform scars develop. Subsequently, pale yellow nodules may form. The face, neck, and eyelids are most often involved. Hypodontia involving the maxillary lateral incisors and premolars is also a feature of the syndrome.

Microscopic Features: A biopsy of one of the mucosal nodules shows diffuse connective tissue hyalinization with prominent hyalin perivascular cuffing. These deposits are PAS positive and show equivocal reactions for amyloid.

Differential Diagnosis: Neuropolyendocrine syndrome, focal epithelial hyperplasia, Cowden syndrome, and amyloidosis may show similar clinical features. A dermatologic examination should be performed. The clinical findings in conjunction with microscopic and histochemical findings will provide a definitive diagnosis.

Treatment: There is no known treatment for this syndrome. Most patients enjoy normal longevity of life. Gingivectomy is recommended when diffuse hyperplastic-appearing gingival infiltration is present.

References

1. Laymon, C. W. and Hill, E. M.: An appraisal of hyalinosis cutis et mucosae. Arch. Dermatol. 75:55, 1967.
2. Williams, R.: Lipoid proteinosis (report of a case). Oral Surg. 31:624, 1971.
3. Simpson, H. E.: Oral manifestations in lipoid proteinosis. Oral Surg. 33:528, 1972.
4. Finkelstein, M. W., Hammond, H. L., and Jones, R. B.: Hyalinosis cutis et mucosae. Oral Surg. 54:49, 1982.

Hemangioma/Lymphangioma

Age: Children and young adults

Sex: No predilection

Clinical Features: Both blood and lymph vessel hamartomas may appear as diffuse polypoid

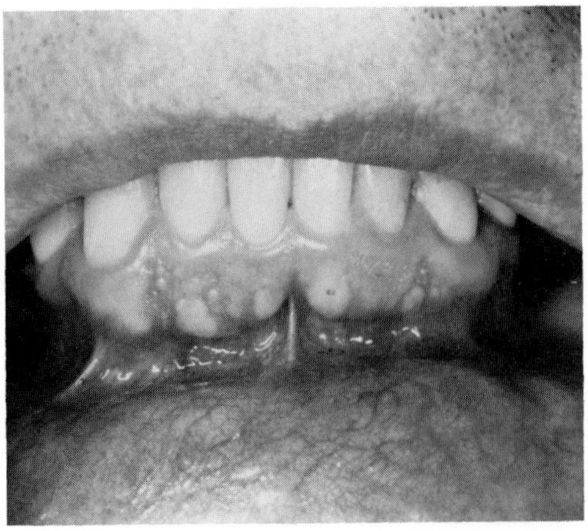

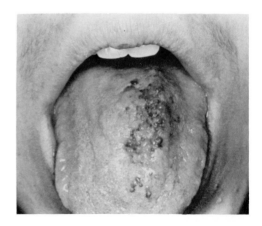

FIG. 7–25. Multiple gingival papules in hyalinosis cutis et mucosae.

FIG. 7–26.   Hemangioma showing grape-like clustered papules.

masses yielding a grape cluster configuration. These lesions are most often observed on the tongue and buccal mucosa. Hemangiomas are red, blue, or purple, while lymphangiomas will often mimic a mass of clustered vesicles. Most vascular hamartomas are present from early childhood; however, some lesions don't begin to proliferate until the patient is in the second decade of life.

Microscopic Features: Racemose exophytic papules are covered by a thin layer of stratified squamous epithelium, which is distended by dilated, endothelial-lined vascular channels. These channels usually extend into the deeper connective tissues and may course between skeletal muscle fibers. In hemangioma, the vascular channels are filled with erythrocytes, whereas lymphangiomas are represented by ectatic vessels filled with an eosinophilic coagulum.

Differential Diagnosis: Most of the vascular hamartomas are distinctive and are not often confused clinically with other diffuse papular and polypoid lesions. The clustered grape pattern and localization are typical features. Nevertheless, a biopsy should be procured to confirm the clinical impression.

Treatment: Hemangiomas and lymphangiomas may be treated by injection of sodium morrhuate as a sclerosing agent or excised by scalpel or electrocautery. The surgeon should bear in mind the tendency for these lesions to extend into underlying muscle.

References
1. Shklar, G. and Meyers, I.: Vascular tumors of the mouth and jaws. Oral Surg. *19*:335, 1965.
2. Dingman, R. O. and Grabb, W. C.: Lymphangioma of the tongue. Plast. Reconstr. Surg. *27*:214, 1961.
3. Goldberg, M. H., Nemarich, A. N., and Danielson, P.: Lymphangioma of the tongue: medical and surgical therapy. J. Oral Surg. *35*:841, 1977.

Neuropolyendocrine (Sipple) Syndrome

Age: Teenagers and young adults
Sex: No predilection

Clinical Features: Inherited as an autosomal dominant trait, the neuropolyendocrine syndrome represents one of the phacomatoses in that the lesions do not evolve until the second decade or late childhood. There are numerous forms of the syndrome; type III shows oral lesions. The oral manifestations are multiple isolated polyps or nodules on the lips and tongue that represent plexiform neuromatous hamartomas. These neural tu-

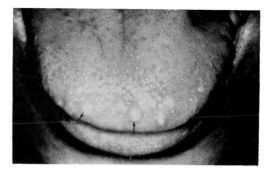

FIG. 7–27. Multiple papular neuromas of the tongue accompanied by medullary carcinoma of the thyroid and adrenal pheochromocytoma. (Courtesy of Dr. S. Rovin.)

mors are also seen on the eyelids. A Marfanoid facies is present. The importance of uncovering this syndrome lies with the more serious manifestations that coexist, including malignant tumors of various endocrine glands. Adrenal pheochromocytoma and medullary carcinoma of the thyroid are the most frequently encountered cancers.

Microscopic Features: The oral neuromas are characterized by an organoid, plexiform arrangement of nerve and nerve sheath elements similar to those of traumatic neuroma. The neural elements are enveloped by perineurium and are separated from one another by intervening fibrous stroma.

Differential Diagnosis: Multiple mucosal neuromas of the Sipple syndrome may clinically simulate focal epithelial hyperplasia and Crohn's disease. A biopsy will disclose their true nature.

Treatment: The oral lesions may be excised or left untreated once a diagnosis is obtained. Referral to an internist is recommended to detect or anticipate the occurrence of endocrine malignancies.

References
1. Williams, E. D. and Pollack, D. J.: Multiple mucosal neuromata with endocrine tumors; a syndrome allied to von Recklinghausen's disease. J. Pathol. Bacteriol. *91*:71, 1966.
2. Schemke, R. N., et al.: Syndrome of bilateral pheochromocytoma, medullary thyroid carcinoma and multiple neuromas. N. Engl. J. Med. *279*:1, 1968.
3. Bartlett, R. C., et al.: A neuropolyendocrine syndrome: mucosal neuromas, pheochromocytoma, and medullary thyroid carcinoma. Oral Surg. *31*:206, 1971.
4. Wright, B. A. and Wysocki, G. P.: Traumatic neuroma and multiple endocrine neoplasia type III. Oral Surg. *51*:527, 1981.

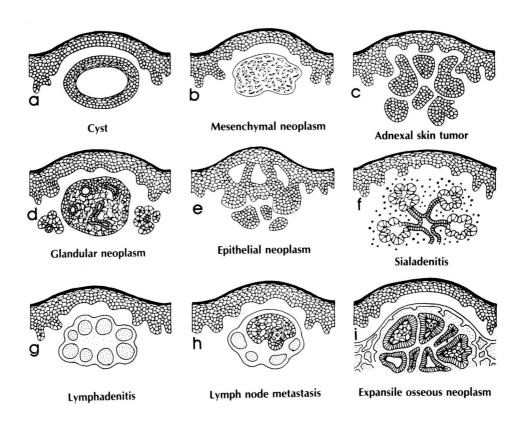

a — Cyst

b — Mesenchymal neoplasm

c — Adnexal skin tumor

d — Glandular neoplasm

e — Epithelial neoplasm

f — Sialadenitis

g — Lymphadenitis

h — Lymph node metastasis

i — Expansile osseous neoplasm

Extraoral Swellings

8
Soft Tissue Swellings of the Neck and Face

LATERAL NECK SWELLINGS

Branchial Cleft Cyst
Cervical Rib and Transverse Process
Nonspecific Lymphadenitis
Infectious Mononucleosis
Tuberculous Lymphadenitis
Cat-scratch Fever
Actinomycosis
Reactive Proliferations
Sinus Histiocytosis
Benign Mesenchymal Tumors
Cystic Hygroma
Carotid Body Tumor
Metastatic Carcinoma
Sarcomas
Malignant Lymphoma

UNILATERAL PAROTID AND SUBMANDIBULAR SWELLINGS

Acute Sialadenitis
Sialolithiasis and Obstructive Sialadenitis
Intraparotid Mesenchymal Tumors
Lymphoma
Pleomorphic Adenoma
Papillary Cystadenoma Lymphomatosum
Oncocytoma
Miscellaneous Adenomas
Adenoid Cystic Carcinoma
Mucoepidermoid Carcinoma
Acinic Cell Carcinoma
Adenocarcinoma NOS and Miscellaneous
  Malignancies

BILATERAL PAROTID AND SUBMANDIBULAR SWELLINGS

Endemic Parotitis
Sjögren's Syndrome
Mikulicz's Disease
Sarcoid Sialadenitis and Heerfordt's Syndrome
Tuberculosis
Metabolic Sialadenosis
Papillary Cystadenoma Lymphomatosum*

MIDLINE NECK SWELLINGS

Thyroglossal Tract Cyst
Goiter
Thyroid Neoplasia
Dermoid Cyst

GROWTHS AND SWELLINGS OF THE FACIAL SKIN

Nevi
Sebaceous Cyst
Seborrheic Keratosis
Adnexal Skin Tumors
Basal Cell Carcinoma
Keratoacanthoma
Mesenchymal Tumors

DIFFUSE FACIAL SWELLINGS

Cellulitis and Space Infections
Emphysema
Angioneurotic Edema
Cushing's Syndrome
Facial Hemihypertrophy
Fibrous Dysplasia and Other Bone Lesions
Masseteric Hypertrophy

*See Unilateral Parotid and Submandibular Swellings.

As with swellings located anywhere in the body and particularly in the subcutaneous tissues, neck and facial swellings may represent neoplasms, inflammatory disorders, hyperplastic reactions, or developmental defects. If the mass is painful or tender, soft and movable, and associated with fever, the process is probably inflammatory. If the mass is painless, well circumscribed, soft or firm yet not indurated, and can be grasped and moved freely, a benign neoplastic or reactive process should be foremost in the mind of the examiner. Indurated fixed swellings with a history of progressive enlargement are prime suspects for malignancy.

Anatomic localization of the tumefaction is perhaps the most germane consideration when attempting to diagnose masses in the

163

head and neck region. In this chapter the nosology of extraoral swellings is approached in this fashion. The rationale for grouping lesions according to site rests with regional anatomic considerations. For example, the lateral neck is riddled with lymph nodes; most swellings in the lateral neck, located along the course of the sternomastoid muscle, include developmental cysts, specific infectious diseases of lymphoid tissue, and various mesenchymal and lymphoid neoplasms. Midline neck swellings are more likely to represent thyroid disease. Swellings located at the mandibular angle or just anterior to the ear in the parotid region are usually salivary neoplasms or inflammatory diseases of the parotid gland. When a swelling of the parotid region is detected and the mass is clinically consistent with neoplasia, it should be emphasized that needle biopsy or incisional biopsy through the facial skin is contraindicated because it may result in seeding of the tumor. The preferred approach is to admit the patient for a partial lobectomy and obtain frozen sections at the time of surgery. Depending on the diagnosis, this procedure may be adequate or further surgery may be indicated.

Localized swellings on the facial skin often represent skin adnexal or dermal neoplasms. Diffuse facial swellings produce asymmetry and may be caused by soft tissue enlargement or expansion of the underlying osseous tissue of the maxilla or mandible.

When extraoral swellings are encountered a source of disease should be sought. Infections of the upper air passages or odontogenic infection are the most common causes of lymphadenopathy in the neck. The workup should consist of physical evaluation of the mass itself, noting its location, consistency, relationship to adjacent tissues, and whether or not it is tender. The patient's temperature should be obtained. A complete oral soft tissue examination should be performed; if it is negative, the larynx, nasopharynx, and nasal cavity should be inspected. The dentition should be evaluated for necrotic teeth and periodontal abscesses. Jaw roentgenograms

and, if all else proves negative or if symptoms warrant, sinus radiographs and tomograms may be ordered. If no source of disease can be found and the mass fails to resolve in 2 weeks, the patient should be referred to an appropriate specialist for biopsy.

The most frequently encountered lateral neck swellings are lymphadenitis of dental origin, infectious mononucleosis, lipoma, metastatic tumor, and lymphoma. The latter two, as well as sarcoma and tuberculosis, are potentially lethal.

The most common midline neck swellings are goiter and thyroglossal tract cyst. Thyroid carcinoma is potentially lethal. Common parotid region swellings include obstructive sialadenitis, pleomorphic adenoma, and adenocarcinoma, the latter being potentially life threatening. Localized facial swellings generally represent nevi, sebaceous cyst, seborrheic keratosis, or basal cell carcinoma. The latter may be lethal if left untreated. The most common diffuse facial swellings are cellulitis and underlying expansile bone lesions such as fibrous dysplasia or benign intraosseous neoplasms.

LATERAL NECK SWELLINGS

Branchial Cleft Cyst

Age: Onset in childhood or early adulthood
Sex: No predilection
Clinical Features: The lymphoepithelial or branchial cleft cyst is believed to be derived from

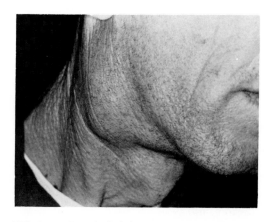

FIG. 8–1. Branchial cleft cyst, a compressible, movable mass overlying the sternomastoid.

epithelial remnants of the embryonic branchial clefts that become entrapped within cervical lymph nodes. An alternative theory implicates intranodal entrapment of salivary epithelial elements. The cyst may reach impressive proportions and can be located anywhere along the anterior surface of the sternomastoid muscle within the subcutaneous tissues. It is doughy or firm and movable on palpation. Rarely, cysts similar to the branchial cleft cyst yet derived from cervically migrating thymus or parathyroid anlagen localize in the lateral neck.

Microscopic Features: The cyst lining consists of either stratified squamous or respiratory epithelium or alternating zones of both. The cyst wall is composed of lymphoid tissue, which often contains germinal centers. Carcinomatous change (so-called branchiogenic carcinoma) has been reported to occur from the lining of such cysts; however, the probability that the carcinoma represents metastatic disease to nodal tissue from an upper respiratory or facial skin primary tumor must be considered.

Differential Diagnosis: The compressible, movable mass of branchial cleft cyst must be differentiated from benign mesenchymal neoplasms, specific infectious lymphadenitis, and carotid body tumors. Lymphomas may also, albeit rarely, show clinical features of a benign lesion. Biopsy will afford a definitive diagnosis.

Treatment: The lesion may be excised.

References

1. Bhaskar, S. N. and Bernier, J. L.: Histogenesis of branchial cysts; a report of 468 cases. Am. J. Pathol. 35:407, 1959.
2. Proctor, B.: Lateral vestigial cysts and fistulas of the neck. Laryngoscope 65:355, 1955.
3. Rickles, N. H. and Little, J. W.: The histogenesis of the branchial cyst. Am. J. Pathol. 50:533, 765, 1967.
4. Schewitsch, I., et al.: Cysts and sinuses of the lateral head and neck. J. Otolaryngol. 9:1, 1980.
5. Howie, A. J. and Proops, D. W.: The definition of branchial cysts, sinuses and fistulae. Clin. Otolaryngol. 7:51, 1982.

Cervical Rib and Transverse Process

Age: Childhood onset

Sex: No predilection

Clinical Features: Although rare, an extension of the transverse process of a cervical vertebra may appear as an anomalous rib. Clinically, a bone-hard swelling can be palpated directly behind the sternomastoid muscle or in the parotid region. To the unwary examiner, the lump has all the features

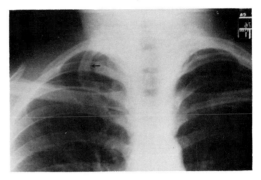

FIG. 8–2. Cervical rib emanating from lower cervical vertebra. Similar anomalies on the upper cervical vertebrae are palpable.

of malignant or metastatic disease. An anteroposterior radiograph through the neck will disclose the presence of the elongated transverse process. Occasionally, symptoms may accompany this anomaly as a result of neurovascular compression in the region of the branchial plexus and subclavian vessels. Neural compression may result in neuralgia, paresthesia, and paralysis of the skin in the areas supplied by the eighth cervical and first thoracic nerves. These latter symptoms are usually seen with a cervical rib from C7, which is not palpable.

Microscopic Features: Not applicable.

Differential Diagnosis: The rock-hard character of a cervical rib may allow for easy confusion with lymphoma, primary sarcoma, or metastatic carcinoma. A radiograph of the neck will quickly eliminate these from consideration.

Treatment: No treatment is necessary.

References

1. Gray, H. and Goss, C. M.: *Anatomy of the Human Body (Gray's Anatomy),* 29th Ed. Philadelphia, Lea & Febiger, 1973, pp. 119, 132.
2. Brannon, E. W.: Cervical rib syndrome. J. Bone Joint Surg. 45A:977, 1963.
3. Einstein, R. A. and Katz, A. D.: Parotid area swelling caused by a prominent transverse process of atlas. Arch. Otolaryngol. 101:558, 1975.
4. Match, R. M.: Neck mass caused by a cervical rib. J. Pediatr. 92:508, 1978.

Nonspecific Lymphadenitis

Age: No predilection

Sex: No predilection

Clinical Features: Tender soft-to-firm swellings of the lateral neck are usually indicative of regional lymphadenopathy subsequent to upper respiratory or odontogenic infection. The swellings are often bilateral when upper respiratory inflammation

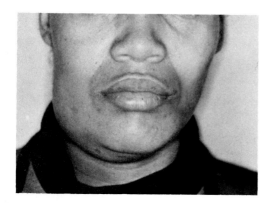

FIG. 8–3. Nonspecific lymphadenitis associated with a necrotic mandibular molar.

occurs and are generally unilateral in the face of acute odontogenic or periodontal inflammation. The upper cervical nodes located just inferior to the angle of the mandible are most frequently affected by this reactive hyperplastic swelling. The patient is usually slightly or moderately febrile. A search should be made for inflammatory change in the pharynx or oropharynx; tonsillar enlargement is often present. A variety of specific viral or bacterial infectious diseases may be responsible. In the absence of upper respiratory infection, the dentition should be evaluated clinically and radiographically to disclose the presence of pulpal or periodontal inflammatory disease.

Microscopic Features: The lymph node is grossly enlarged and shows enlargement of the germinal centers. The reticulum cells may show evidence of mitosis, and a prominent lymphoid mantle is obvious. The medullary sinusoids are impacted with small and large lymphocytes.

Differential Diagnosis: Soft tender swellings, typical of cervical lymphadenopathy, must be differentiated from specific inflammatory lymphadenitides such as infectious mononucleosis, cat-scratch fever, actinomycosis, and tuberculous lymphadenitis. The latter two diseases are often accompanied by fistulous tracts onto the skin surface. Failure of the neck swellings to subside after conventional treatment for cervical lymphadenopathy (i.e., control of upper respiratory infection or odontogenic infection) warrants further workup to rule out the aforementioned entities.

Treatment: Cervical lymphadenitis is a secondary reactive manifestation of infectious disease elsewhere. Throat infections should be managed by an otolaryngologist or general physician. Per-

iodontal infection should be managed by surgery and/or curettage, whereas pulpal infection can be treated by therapeutic pulp canal exposure with subsequent endodontics or extraction. If fever is present the patient should be given antibiotics, preferably penicillin 250 mg q.i.d. for 7 days, and local control of the infection should be instituted.

References

1. Darling, A. I., Ruben, M. P., Goldman, H. M., and Schulman, S. M.: In *Thoma's Oral Pathology*, 6th Ed., edited by R. J. Gorlin and H. M. Goldman. St. Louis, C. V. Mosby Co., 1970, Vol. I, pp. 340–341, 423–426.
2. Mitchell, D. F., Standish, S. M., and Fast, T. B.: *Oral Diagnosis/Oral Medicine*, 3rd Ed. Philadelphia, Lea & Febiger, 1978, pp. 337–338.
3. Shafer, W. G., Hine, M. K., and Levy, B. M.: *A Textbook of Oral Pathology*, 4th Ed. Philadelphia, W. B. Saunders Co., 1983, Chapters 6, 8.
4. Weidman, B. and Warman, E.: Lymph nodes of the head and neck. J. Oral Med. *35(2):*39, 1980.

Infectious Mononucleosis

Age: Teenagers and young adults
Sex: No predilection

Clinical Features: Caused by the Epstein-Barr virus, a form of herpesvirus, infectious mononucleosis is a relatively common infectious disease that is transmitted by oral droplet contamination and frequently develops after kissing. It is not as contagious as many of the childhood exanthems. The disease is characterized by extreme malaise, intense painful pharyngitis, and moderate to severe lymphadenopathy. The submandibular, upper cervical, and occipital lymph nodes may be markedly enlarged, are painful, and are usually soft or rubbery. Tonsillar enlargement and pharyngeal ulceration with formation of a pseudomembrane are evident. Petechial lesions of the soft

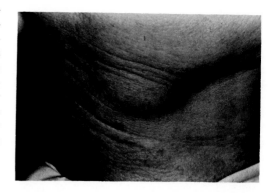

FIG. 8–4. Lymphadenitis in a patient with infectious mononucleosis.

palate are present in nearly half of the instances. The patients are febrile. The disease persists from 2 to 5 weeks.

Microscopic Features: Lymph nodes show marked hypertrophy with hyperplasia of the germinal centers. Both the germinal centers and medullary sinusoids contain epithelioid-appearing atypical lymphocytes.

Differential Diagnosis: The enlarged nodes in infectious mononucleosis are usually bilateral. The presence of lymphadenopathy in conjunction with intense pharyngitis and malaise must be differentiated from streptococcal sore throat, scarlet fever, diphtheria, and lymphoma. A swab culture may be obtained to rule out bacterial infection. The peripheral blood in infectious mononucleosis shows atypical "Downey" lymphocytes, and the Paul-Bunnell or heterophil antibody titer is positive by the second or third week of the disease.

Treatment: Bed rest and supportive care with fluids, soft diet, an anesthetic gargle, an analgesic-antipyretic, and systemic antibiotics to control secondary bacterial pharyngitis are recommended.

References

1. Fraser-Moodie, W.: Oral lesions in infectious mononucleosis. Oral Surg. *12*:685, 1959.
2. Dunnett, W. N.: Infectious mononucleosis. Br. Med. J. *1*:1187, 1963.
3. Ragab, A. H. and Vietti, T. J.: Infectious mononucleosis, lymphoblastic leukemia, and the E B virus. Cancer 24:261, 1969.

Tuberculous Lymphadenitis (Scrofula)

Age: Children and young adults

Sex: No predilection

Clinical Features: The lateral neck is the most common location for tuberculous inflammation of lymph nodes. As opposed to other mucocutaneous manifestations of tuberculosis that are secondary to pulmonary disease, cervical node tuberculosis or scrofula is often primary and may be associated with a portal of entry in the throat. It may be contracted by ingestion of contaminated milk. While Mycobacterium tuberculosis is usually responsible, atypical tuberculosis may be acquired by infection with less common strains of mycobacteria. The lesion is located in the submandibular or cervical nodes, is usually unilateral, and eventually manifests exudative drainage via a fistula. The swelling is initially painless and on palpation is firm, generally movable, and of normal temperature, hence the designation *cold abscess.* Mycobacteria can be cultured from the exudate.

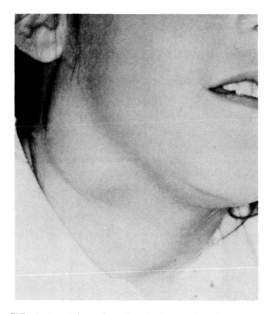

FIG. 8–5. Tuberculous lymphadenopathy of cervical nodes. (Courtesy of Dr. Willard Fee.)

Microscopic Features: The lymph node is replaced by focal granulomas evincing epithelioid cells and Langhans' giant cells. Caseation necrosis with neutrophil infiltration is seen in fistulating lesions. Acid-fast bacilli are detected with the appropriate special stains.

Differential Diagnosis: The isolated swelling with fistula must be differentiated from actinomycosis. When a fistula is not present scrofula may simulate other specific granulomatous lymphadenitides or benign neoplasms. The exudate can be smeared and stained for acid-fast organisms, and definitive identification can be obtained by culture. A complete workup to define the systemic extent of the disease is warranted.

Treatment: The caseating granuloma can be excised; however, this does not necessarily remove all infectious microorganisms. The patient requires conventional isoniazid therapy and should be managed by a physician.

References

1. Knewitz, F. W., Devine, K. D., and Waite, D. E.: Differential diagnosis of cervicofacial swellings. Oral Surg. 25:43, 1968.
2. Mulay, S. G. and Hiranandani, L. H.: A clinical study: Surgical management of 250 cases of tuberculous cervical lymphadenitis. J. Laryngol. Otol. 89:781,1970.
3. Ord, R. J. and Matz, G. J.: Tuberculous cervical lymphadenitis. Arch. Otolaryngol. 99:327, 1974.

4. Mair, I. W. and Elverland, H. H.: Cervical myco-bacterial infection. J. Laryngol. Otol. *89*:933, 1975.
5. Popowich, L. and Heydt, S.: Tuberculous cervical lymphadenitis. J. Oral Surg. *40*:522, 1982.

Cat-scratch Fever

Age: Children and young adults
Sex: No predilection

Clinical Features: As the term implies, the disease is contracted after scratch by a cat. Many patients do not report a scratch, yet have been in contact with cats. The causative agent is thought to be a pleomorphic, gram-negative bacillus. A papule develops in the zone of contact, and subsequently lymph node swelling in the region draining the scratch site develops; other nodes may enlarge as well. In the head and neck area, the submandibular, cervical, or occipital nodes are involved. The nodes are sore, somewhat firm, and movable. Occasionally a fistula is encountered. Fever, malaise, headache, and nausea become manifest early in the course of the disease.

Microscopic Features: The involved node or nodes are replaced by focal granulomas that are characterized by epithelióid histiocyte infiltration and multinucleated giant cells that surround central zones of granular eosinophilic necrotic material. The organism may be demonstrable with a Wharthin-Starry or Giemsa's stain.

Differential Diagnosis: The cervical swelling

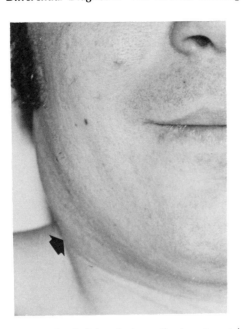

FIG. 8–6. Cervical lymphadenopathy in cat-scratch fever. (Courtesy of Dr. Willard Fee.)

of cat-scratch fever must be differentiated from actinomycosis, scrofula, and other rare granulomatous lymphadenitides such as tularemia, lymphogranuloma venereum, atypical tuberculosis, and neoplasms. A history of scratch or contact with a cat is, of course, helpful in making the diagnosis. A definitive diagnosis is obtained by noting a positive intracutaneous reaction with Mollaret's antigen or a positive complement-fixation test.

Treatment: The disease does not respond to antibiotics. Supportive care with fluids, good diet, bed rest, and administration of antipyretics is recommended. Extremely tender nodes may require incision with drainage.

References
1. Rickles, N. H. and Bernier, J. R.: Cat-scratch disease. Oral Surg. *13*:282, 1960.
2. Brooksaler, F. S., et al.: Cat-scratch disease. Postgrad. Med. *36*:366, 1964.
3. Margileth, A. M.: Cat scratch disease: nonbacterial regional lymphadenitis. Pediatrics *42*:803, 1968.
4. Gross, B. D. and Case, D.: Cat scratch disease. Report of a case. Oral Surg. *43*:698, 1977.
5. Wear, D. J., et al.: Cat scratch disease: a bacterial infection. Science *221*:1403, 1983.

Actinomycosis

Age: Young adults
Sex: Male predilection

Clinical Features: The submandibular and lateral neck regions are the most commonly involved areas in cervical-facial actinomycosis. Caused by infection with Actinomyces israelii, actinomycosis is characterized by a firm, often indurated multinodular tumefaction that has a tendency to develop drainage. The exudate contains clumped colonies of the microorganisms that appear crystalline and are yellow in color, hence the term *sulfur granules.* The mass usually develops after trauma or tooth extraction, which apparently provides a portal of entry for the fungus-like bacillus. The lesion develops within a few weeks to months with slow progressive enlargement. It is more frequently encountered among rural than urban inhabitants.

Microscopic Features: The focus of inflammation is characterized by surrounding fibroplasia with extensive vascular proliferation. Focal abscesses are distributed throughout and are characterized by sheets of neutrophils that surround amphophilic club-shaped colonies that manifest a peripheral fringe. These colonies are positively stained with the periodic acid-Schiff technique. In the early stages, microbial colonies may elicit a

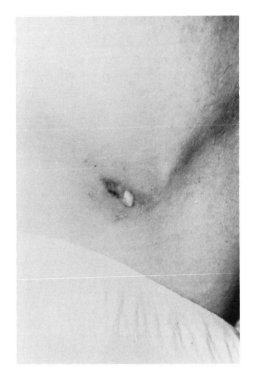

FIG. 8–7.   Swollen cervical fistula in actinomycosis.

granulomatous response with epithelioid histiocytes and multinucleated giant cells.

Differential Diagnosis: The indurated swelling of the neck seen in actinomycosis is often "woody" and must be differentiated from a neoplasm by biopsy. Once a fistula has developed, suspicion of actinomycosis is high. Nevertheless, other lateral neck swellings with drainage, such as scrofula or less common granulomatous infections, must be considered as possibilities. Identification of tiny yellow sulfur granules (usually measuring less than 2 mm) from the exudate or curettage of the lesion is of diagnostic aid. Anaerobic methods of culture will provide a definitive diagnosis.

Treatment: Actinomyces infection responds to penicillin therapy. High-dose therapy—10 to 20 million units IV for 5 to 6 weeks—is required in many instances. Erythromycin may be utilized in patients with allergy to penicillin.

References

1. Perlstein, W. H.: Cervico-facial actinomycosis. N. Engl. J. Med. 248:67, 1963.
2. Rud, J.: Cervicofacial actinomycosis. J. Oral Surg. 25:229, 1967.
3. Towns, T. M.: Actinomycosis: Case report. Oral Surg. 46:615, 1978.

4. Dusek, J. J., et al.: Cervicofacial actinomycosis (Case 37, Parts I & II). J. Oral Surg. 40:38, 113, 1982.

Reactive Proliferations

Age: Children and young adults
Sex: No predilection

Clinical Features: Various fibroproliferative lesions such as fibromatosis, pseudosarcomatous fasciitis, and dermatofibrosarcoma protuberans, collectively grouped as the fibrous histiocytomas, often arise within the subcutaneous tissues of the lateral neck. These swellings are multinodular and firm but are usually somewhat movable within the surrounding tissues. They often grow rapidly and may become large if not removed. Clinically, they appear to represent neoplasms, yet are more likely to evolve as a reaction to injury.

Microscopic Features: All of the fibroproliferative reactions are similar in their histomorphology. Spindle cells are grouped into fascicles or form pinwheel-like swirls (storiform pattern) with variable amounts of collagen. Epithelioid or foam cell histiocytes are often present but are usually sparse and randomly distributed among fibroblastic cells. Many of these tumors are cellular and, under these circumstances, may closely mimic sarcoma.

Differential Diagnosis: Reactive proliferations are clinically indistinguishable from a variety of mesenchymal neoplasms, actinomycosis, or specific granulomatous enlargements. They may be indurated and suggest lymphoma, sarcoma, or metastatic disease. Multinodularity is suggestive of a reactive proliferation. A biopsy is required for a definitive diagnosis.

Treatment: While encapsulation is common, a merging with adjacent fascia or connective tissue is also frequently encountered. For this reason,

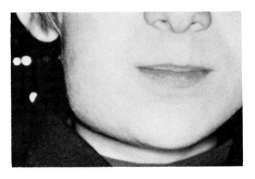

FIG. 8–8.   Fibrous histiocytoma of the lateral neck.

wide local excision is generally required to eradicate the disease and circumvent recurrence.

References

1. Price, E. G., Jr., et al.: Nodular fasciitis: a clinicopathologic analysis of 65 cases. Am. J. Clin. Pathol. 35:122, 1961.
2. Taylor, H. B. and Helwig, E. B.: Dermatofibrosarcoma protuberans; a study of 115 cases. Cancer 15:717, 1962.
3. Stout, A. P. and Lattes, R.: Tumors of the soft tissues. In Atlas of Tumor Pathology, Sec. II, Fasc. 1. Washington, Armed Forces Institute of Pathology, 1967.
4. Werning, J. T.: Nodular fasciitis of the orofacial region. Oral Surg. 48:441, 1979.
5. Dahl, I. and Jarlstedt, J.: Nodular fasciitis in the head and neck. A clinicopathological study of 18 cases. Acta Otolaryngol. 90:152, 1980.

Sinus Histiocytosis

Age: Children
Sex: No predilection

Clinical Features: Sinus histiocytosis with massive lymphadenopathy is a childhood disease that occurs more frequently among Negroes than among whites. The affected children show enlargement of the cervical and submandibular nodes, usually bilaterally, and these nodal swellings often reach massive proportions. The neck is distended by bosselated, nodular confluent masses that are firm, painless, and may become fixed to adjacent tissues. Other node groups (axillary, inguinal, hilar, and retroperitoneal lymph nodes) often show enlargement; however, the size is not comparable to that of the cervical adenop-

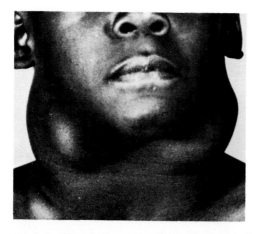

FIG. 8–9.   Sinus histiocytosis with massive lymphadenopathy of the cervical lymph nodes. (From Rosai, J. and Dorfman, R. F.: Sinus histiocytosis with massive lymphadenopathy: A pseudolymphomatous benign disorder. Analysis of 34 cases. Cancer 30:1174, 1972.)

athies. Cutaneous nodules and lytic lesions of long bones may also occur. Fever is a constant finding; however, other constitutional signs of infectious disease, such as anorexia and malaise, are not present. Neutrophilic leukocytosis, elevated erythrocyte sedimentation rate, normocytic anemia, and hypergammaglobulinemia are present.

The disease persists for months or even years, shows no tendency for malignant change, and eventually undergoes spontaneous resolution. Elevated antibodies to the Epstein-Barr virus have been demonstrated in this disease, yet a cause-and-effect relationship has not been proven.

Microscopic Features: Capsular fibrosis is a constant finding. The lymph node architecture is obliterated by dilated sinusoids lined by oval histiocytes with abundant granular or foamy cytoplasm; multinucleated forms are common. A hallmark of the disease is a marked tendency for phagocytosis of both lymphocytes and erythrocytes.

Differential Diagnosis: Bilateral multinodular lymphoid swelling seen in sinus histiocytosis must be differentiated from similar changes encountered in other infectious lymphadenitides such as tuberculosis or cat-scratch fever, malignant lymphoma, and metastatic carcinoma. The absence of positive skin tests for specific microorganisms, presence of fever without malaise, and laboratory data as designated earlier point to a diagnosis of sinus histiocytosis. Biopsy will disclose the characteristic features.

Treatment: Neither antibiotics nor steroids show any therapeutic value. Radiation therapy likewise is of no benefit in reducing the size of the tumefactions. Since the etiology is essentially unknown, no treatment can be rendered. The lesions eventually regress, even though the disease persists for many months or even years.

References

1. Azoury, F. J. and Reed, R. J.: Histiocytosis. N. Engl. J. Med. 274:928, 1966.
2. Rosai J. and Dorfman, R. F.: Sinus histiocytosis with massive lymphadenopathy: A pseudolymphomatous benign disorder. Analysis of 34 cases. Cancer 30:1174, 1972.
3. Lober, M., et al.: Sinus histiocytosis with massive lymphadenopathy; report of a case associated with elevated EBV antibody titers. Cancer 32:421, 1973.
4. Walker, P. D., Rosai, J., and Dorfman, R. F.: The osseous manifestations of sinus histiocytosis with massive lymphadenopathy. Am. J. Clin. Pathol. 75:131, 1981.
5. Penneys, N. S., et al.: Sinus histiocytosis with massive lymphadenopathy: a case with unusual skin

involvement and a therapeutic response to vinblastine-loaded platelets. Cancer 49:1994, 1982.

Benign Mesenchymal Tumors

Age: Adults
Sex: Depends upon specific histologic type

Clinical Features: A variety of connective tissue tumors arise in the lateral neck region. The more common forms are lipoma, neurilemmoma, neurofibroma, and lymphangioma (cystic hygroma). The mass is either soft or firm, yet not indurated, and is movable on palpation. The neoplasms are slow growing and are usually painless. If left untreated they may become quite large. Ulceration, surface telangiectasia, and fistulization of the overlying skin are extremely rare with benign mesenchymal neoplasms.

Microscopic Features: The histomorphologic features vary depending upon the tissue cell of origin. Nearly all are well differentiated and have well-defined margins or are encapsulated. Lipomas are tumor masses composed of normal adipose tissue, whereas the neural sheath neoplasms are composed of benign-appearing spindle cells associated with varying amounts of collagen.

Differential Diagnosis: The firm or soft movable nonulcerated mass representing a benign mesenchymal neoplasm must be differentiated

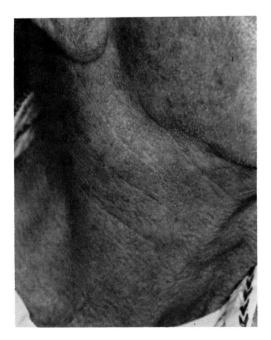

FIG. 8–10.   Neurofibroma appearing as a lateral neck mass.

from branchial cleft cyst, carotid body tumor, and nonfistulating granulomatous inflammations of lymph nodes. Biopsy is required to obtain a definitive diagnosis.

Treatment: Practically all benign mesenchymal neoplasms of the neck can be treated by conservative surgical excision. For most, recurrence rates after simple excision are low.

References

1. Oberman, H. A. and Sullenger, G.: Neurogenous tumors of the head and neck. Cancer 20: 1992, 1967.
2. Adair, F. E., Pack, G. T., and Farrior, J. H.: Lipomas. Am. J. Cancer 16:1104, 1932.
3. Batsakis, J. G., Regezi, J. A., and Rice, D. H.: The pathology of head and neck tumors: fibroadipose tissue and skeletal muscle. Part 8. Head Neck Surg. 3:45, 1980.
4. Garfinkle, T. J. and Handler, S. D.: Hemangiomas of the head and neck in children—a guide to management. J. Otolaryngol. 9:439, 1980.
5. Hawkins, D. B. and Luxford, W. M.: Schwannomas of the head and neck in children. Laryngoscope 90:1921, 1980.

Cystic Hygroma (Lymphangioma)

Age: Infancy and childhood
Sex: No predilection

Clinical Features: Cystic hygroma is considered separately from the other benign mesenchymal neoplasms because of its marked propensity to arise in the soft tissues of the neck in children. The tumor mass may be present at birth or develop during the early childhood years. It may reach large proportions, becoming pendulous. The mass is soft and pliable on palpation. The neoplastic lymphatic channels may infiltrate between muscle and the contiguous soft tissues, thus making it difficult to determine the extent of the condition.

Microscopic Features: Cystic hygroma is composed of dilated endothelial-lined lymphatic channels. The channels lie in juxtaposition to one another with very little intervening fibrous stroma. Infiltration of adjacent tissues is common; however, the endothelial cells show no signs of cellularity, pleomorphism, or hyperchromatism.

Differential Diagnosis: Cystic hygroma must be differentiated from branchial cleft cyst, sinus histiocytosis, and lipoma. When the mass is small, it may simulate one of the specific granulomatous inflammations such as tuberculosis. When a large, soft, pliable mass is detected in the lateral neck in a child, the foremost diagnostic consideration is cystic hygroma. Biopsy is required for a definitive diagnosis.

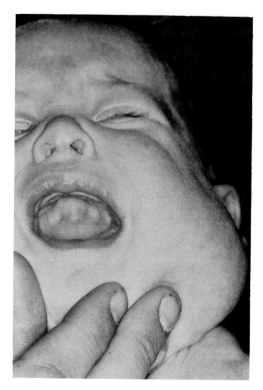

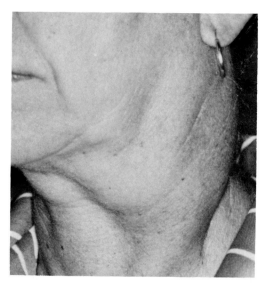

FIG. 8–12. Carotid body tumor causing large tumefaction overlying carotid bifurcation. (Courtesy of Dr. Willard Fee.)

FIG. 8–11. Lymphangioma (cystic hygroma) of the neck in an infant. (Courtesy of Dr. Willard Fee.)

Treatment: The mass requires surgical excision with careful dissection from surrounding tissues, which it may infiltrate.

References

1. Watson, W. L. and McCarthy, W. D.: Blood and lymph vessel tumors; a report of 1,056 cases. Surg. Gynecol. Obstet. 71:569, 1940.
2. Bill, A. H., Jr., and Summer, D. S.: A unified concept of lymphangioma and cystic hygroma. Surg. Gynecol. Obstet. 120:79, 1965.
3. Batsakis, J. G. and Rice, D. H.: The pathology of head and neck tumors: vasoformative tumors, Part 9A, B. Head Neck Surg. 3:231, 326, 1981.
4. Nussbaum, M. and Buchwald, R. P.: Adult cystic hygroma. Am. J. Otolaryngol. 2:159, 1981.
5. Pounds, L. A.: Neck masses of congenital origin. Pediatr. Clin. North Am. 28:841, 1981.

Carotid Body Tumor (Chemodectoma)

Age: Middle-aged adults
Sex   No predilection

Clinical Features: Neoplasms originating in the carotid body are rarely malignant. Tumors are located in the upper lateral neck adjacent to the angle of the mandible. They are firm and movable anteroposteriorly, yet cannot be manipulated in a superoinferior direction because of their attachment to the carotid bifurcation. The tumors are generally asymptomatic, yet a bruit may be detected, the overlying skin may be warm, and medial growth may constrict the airway. Rarely, paralysis of cranial nerves X or XII may be observed. Occasionally, chemodectomas arise more inferiorly from other chemoreceptors located along the carotid and aortic arteries. The mass may be somewhat tender, yet is usually asymptomatic.

Microscopic Features: Carotid body tumors typically mimic the morphology of the normal carotid body with organoid nests of polygonal cells. Two cell types are seen: the more prevalent vesicular with similarly vesicular oval nuclei, the other pyknotic and hyperchromatic. The organoid nests are separated from one another by a prominent vascular network. Fibrous stroma is extremely sparse.

Differential Diagnosis: Carotid body tumors, by virtue of their location, must be differentiated from lymphadenopathy, other mesenchymal tumors, and lymphoma. Their unique clinical features with regard to limited movement in a vertical plane with movability in the horizontal plane, while not pathognomonic, are certainly highly suggestive. Angiography will disclose a well-circumscribed vascular "blush" in the carotid bifurcation area.

Treatment: Surgical excision is recommended.

The tumor must be removed with great care to avoid carotid perforation and therefore should be managed by an experienced head and neck surgeon.

References

1. McGuirt, W. F. and Harker, L. A.: Carotid body tumors. Arch. Otolaryngol. *101*:58, 1975.
2. Wilson, H.: Carotid body tumors. Surgery 59:483, 1966.
3. Conley, J. J.: The carotid body tumors. Arch. Otolaryngol. *81*:187, 1965.
4. Ruby, R., Gullane, P. J., and Mintz, D.: Chemodectomas of the head and neck. J. Otolaryngol. *10*:126, 1981.
5. Parry, D. M., et al.: Carotid body tumors in humans: genetics and epidemiology. J. N. C. I. 68:573, 1982.

Metastatic Carcinoma

Age: Teenagers (nasopharyngeal) and elderly adults (squamous cell carcinoma)

Sex: Male predilection

Clinical Features: The first depot of metastatic carcinoma from primary lesions of the upper respiratory tract and face is the regional cervical and submandibular group of lymph nodes. While usually unilateral, malignant disease with more longevity may manifest bilateral metastases. The mass is usually yet not invariably fixed to the adjacent fascia or sternomastoid muscle and is almost always indurated. Nasopharyngeal carcinomas occur more frequently in teenagers than in adults. The neck metastases may be the first sign of disease, as they may be considerably larger than the primary tumor itself. When an indurated swelling is detected in the lateral neck, a diligent search for a primary tumor in the oral cavity, nose, throat, nasopharynx, and paranasal sinuses is mandatory. Carcinomas of the skin of the face and scalp may also metastasize to cervical lymph nodes. When nodal metastases are encountered, the prognosis is considerably worsened. It should be noted that primary adenocarcinomas of salivary origin and melanoma of the head and neck frequently manifest cervical metastasis.

Microscopic Features: The metastatic tumor is essentially identical microscopically to the primary lesion. Tumor cells tend to localize first in the subcapsular region and later replace the entire node. Infiltration into the adjacent tissues ensues.

Differential Diagnosis: The indurated fixed node containing metastatic cancer must be differentiated from malignant lymphoma, primary sarcoma, and certain inflammatory diseases such as actinomycosis and scrofula, which may also be hard and immovable. Detection of a primary tumor in the head and neck region will determine the diagnosis. Occasionally, no primary tumor can be found when intranodal carcinoma is discovered on biopsy. Most lesions of this nature arise in the nasopharynx, which must again be examined with scrutiny.

Treatment: The primary tumor may be treated surgically or with radiation therapy. Metastatic disease to nodes may be treated by cervical node dissection, often in continuity with the primary lesion, or may be radiated. These treatment modalities must be carefully selected for each case by the oncologist or head and neck team.

References

1. Frazell, E. L. and Lucas, J. C., Jr.: Cancer of the tongue. Cancer *15*:1085, 1962.
2. Mustard, R. A. and Rosen, I. B.: Cervical lymph node involvement in oral cancer. Am. J. Roentgenol. Radium Ther. Nucl. Med. 90:978, 1963.
3. Robertson, M. S. and Snape, L.: The malignant gland in the neck as a presenting sign in head and neck cancer. N. Z. Med. J. 92:303, 1980.
4. Sharpe, D. T.: The pattern of lymph node metastases in intra-oral squamous cell carcinoma. Br. J. Plast. Surg. *34*:97, 1981.
5. Roseman, J. M. and James, A. G.: Metastatic cancers to the neck from undetermined primary sites: long-term follow-up. J. Surg. Oncol. *19*:247, 1982.

Sarcomas

Age: Children and young adults

Sex: No predilection

Clinical Features: Primary sarcomas of the head and neck region are quite rare, yet when they occur the orbit and lateral neck are the most frequently affected sites. In the neck, the most frequently encountered tumors are fibrosarcoma, rhabdomyosarcoma, and synovial sarcoma. The

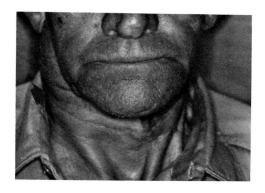

FIG. 8–13.   Metastatic cancer in a cervical node from a primary carcinoma of the tongue.

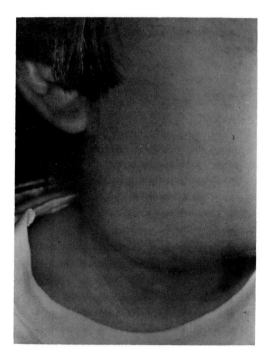

FIG. 8–14.   Fibrosarcoma appearing as an indurated neck mass.

swellings are firm or indurated and fixed to adjacent tissues. They may or may not be painful. When large, telangiectasia and erythema of the overlying skin may be seen. Growth is progressive and often rapid.

Microscopic Features: The histomorphology varies depending on the cell of origin. The mesenchymal malignancies are as a group spindle cell neoplasms with marked cellularity, pleomorphism, and nuclear hyperchromatism or vesiculation. Encapsulation is lacking, and invasion of muscle and fascia is an almost constant feature.

Differential Diagnosis: Primary sarcomas of the neck, being fixed and indurated, must be differentiated from lymphoma, metastatic carcinoma, some of the reactive proliferations, and specific granulomatous inflammations, which are occasionally hard to palpation. Biopsy is required to determine the diagnosis and ascertain the tissue of origin.

Treatment: Wide radical excision is required and should be undertaken by an oncologic surgeon. Even with radical surgery, recurrences may ensue and the prognosis is generally poor.

References

1. Conley, J., et al.: Clinicopathologic analysis of eighty-four patients with an original diagnosis of fibrosarcoma of the head and neck. Am. J. Surg. 114:564, 1967.
2. Masson, J. D. and Soule, E. H.: Embryonal rhabdomyosarcoma of the head and neck; report on eighty-eight cases. Am. J. Surg. 110:585, 1965.
3. Healy, G. B.: Malignant tumors of the head and neck in children: diagnosis and treatment. Otolaryngol. Clin. North Am. 13:483, 1980.
4. Farr, H. W.: Soft part sarcomas of the head and neck. Semin. Oncol. 8:185, 1981.
5. Otte, T. and Kleinsasser, O.: Liposarcoma of the head and neck. Arch. Otorhinolaryngol. 232:285, 1981.
6. Feldman, B. A.: Rhabdomyosarcoma of the head and neck. Laryngoscope 92:424, 1982.

Malignant Lymphoma

Age: Young and middle-aged adults
Sex: Male predilection

Clinical Features: Two basic types of lymphoid malignancy, Hodgkin's disease and non-Hodgkin's lymphoma, involve the cervical lymph nodes. Indeed, the cervical nodes are one of the most frequently involved node groups in the entire body. The swelling is occasionally unilateral, but is more often bilateral. The tumor masses may be multinodular and are, as a rule, fixed and indurated. Growth is progressive and may be rapid. The two forms of lymphoma manifest similar clinical features, yet differ in prognosis; Hodgkin's lymphomas as a group progress more slowly, and longevity is greatly increased over the non-Hodgkin's group. As the disease progresses, more extensive node involvement occurs with axillary and inguinal enlargement. Hilar node enlargement becomes apparent radiographically. Hepatospleno-

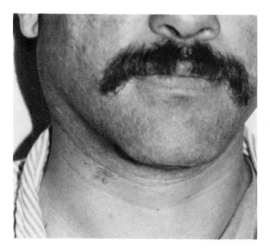

FIG. 8–15.   Cervical mass in malignant lymphoma. (Courtesy of Dr. Robert Middleton.)

megaly eventually occurs, and extranodal involvement with visceral, central nervous system, and osseous tumor is seen in the terminal stages. Low-grade fever, malaise, weight loss, frequent night sweats, and pruritus are common symptoms. Shingles is a frequent complication.

Microscopic Features: The microscopic changes in the lymph nodes are highly variable. The sine qua non for Hodgkin's disease is the presence of a binucleated large histiocyte with prominent central nucleoli known as the Reed-Sternberg cell. The non-Hodgkin's lymphomas show either well or poorly differentiated lymphocytes arranged in follicular patterns or in monotonous cell sheets. The various subtypes in both groups have different natural histories and prognoses.

Differential Diagnosis: Unilateral neck node enlargement in lymphoma must be differentiated from sarcoma, metastatic carcinoma and certain inflammatory enlargements such as scrofula and actinomycosis. Bilateral enlargements must be differentiated from sinus histiocytosis, metastatic carcinoma, and nonspecific lymphadenopathy. A complete physical examination, which includes hematologic studies, chest radiographs, and lymphangiography, is required to determine the extent of the disease.

Treatment: Lymphomas should be treated by a hematologist, oncologic chemotherapist, and/or radiotherapist. The disease is managed by radiotherapy in combination with multiphasic antitumor chemotherapy.

References

1. Butler, J. J.: Relationship of histological findings to survival in Hodgkin's disease. Cancer Res. *31*:1770, 1971.
2. Rappaport, H.: Tumors of the hematopoietic system. *Atlas of Tumor Pathology*, Fasc. 8. Sect. 3, Washington, Armed Forces Institute of Pathology, 1966.
3. Aisenberg, A. C.: Malignant lymphoma. N. Engl. J. Med. *288*:883, 1973.
4. Evans, C.: A review of non-Hodgkin's lymphomata of the head and neck. Clin. Oncol. *7*:23, 1981.
5. Plantenga, K. F., et al.: Non-Hodgkin's malignant lymphomas of upper digestive and respiratory tracts. Inst. J. Radiat. Oncol. Biol. Phys. *7*:1419, 1981.

UNILATERAL PAROTID AND SUBMANDIBULAR SWELLINGS

Acute Sialadenitis (Surgical Mumps)

Age: Elderly adults
Sex: Male predilection
Clinical Features: Acute inflammatory disease

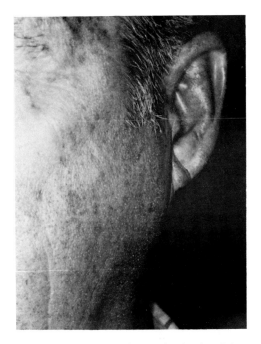

FIG. 8–16. Parotitis developing shortly after abdominal surgery.

of the major salivary glands most commonly affects the parotid. Unilateral involvement is more frequent than bilateral. Staphylococci and streptococci are the causative organisms. The disease is uncommon; when present it is seen primarily in debilitated patients and those who are recovering from major surgery. It has also been reported to occur in patients with xerostomia complicating the use of phenothiazine drugs. The patients are febrile, the swelling is painful, and a purulent exudate can be milked from the salivary ducts.

Microscopic Features: The acinar parenchyma shows degeneration and necrosis with diffuse infiltration by neutrophils. The ducts display ectasia and are impacted with necrotic debris and neutrophils.

Differential Diagnosis: Acute parotitis of bacterial origin must be differentiated from endemic parotitis and duct occlusion phenomenon (sialolithiasis). Pain and swelling are common to all three disorders. Purulent drainage from the duct orifice is more common in acute parotitis; bacteria can be cultured from this exudate and, in addition, a history of recent surgery or a predisposing debilitating condition can be obtained.

Treatment: Fluid and electrolyte balance should be maintained in postsurgical patients. Efforts to control any debilitating disease should be made in consultation with the patient's physician. The parotitis is treated with penicillin therapy in nonallergic patients while results from culture and sensitivity testing are awaited.

References
1. Carlson, R. G. and Glas, W. E.: Acute suppurative parotitis; twenty-eight cases at a county hospital. Arch. Surg. 86:659, 1963.
2. Banning, G. L.: Postoperative suppurative parotitis. Arch. Surg. 89:653, 1964.
3. Zollar, L. M. and Mufson, M. A.: Parotitis of non-mumps etiology. Hosp. Pract. 5:93, 1970.

Sialolithiasis and Obstructive Sialadenitis

Age: Middle-aged adults
Sex: Male predilection

Clinical Features: The formation of salivary calculi within the ducts of the major salivary glands is overwhelmingly more common in the submandibular ducts. The stone develops on some sort of nidus, perhaps a mucous plug, and calcium salts become deposited in a concentric fashion. When the stone reaches sufficient size, the duct becomes occluded, mucin is retained, and the gland develops sclerosing sialadenitis. Clinically, the gland becomes enlarged and firm but is still movable. Pain is often severe or stabbing during mealtime, when salivation is stimulated. The stone can often be palpated within the duct or demonstrated radiographically. The parotid duct is only occasionally involved. Rarely, the intraoral minor glands develop a calculus. Occasionally, developmental or post-traumatic strictures develop in the duct system. The clinical signs and symptoms simulate sialolithiasis, and sialography aids in identifying the stricture.

Microscopic Features: The stone, when decalcified, is composed of concentric laminations of amorphous basophilic matrix. The occluded gland shows acinar degeneration with replacement by fibrous tissue and mononuclear cells. Ducts are dilated, contain impacted mucin, and show oncocytic, mucous, and squamous metaplasia.

Differential Diagnosis: Sclerosing sialadenitis associated with sialolithiasis may show features that can be confused with endemic parotitis, salivary neoplasm, or mesenchymal neoplasm. Presence of pain that is increased at mealtime, failure to obtain flow when milking the gland, and presence of a palpable indurated mass in the complementary duct lead to a diagnosis of sialolithiasis. Submandibular duct stones are visualized with mandibular occlusal radiographs, while parotid

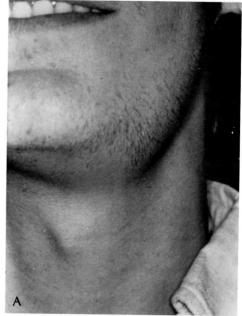

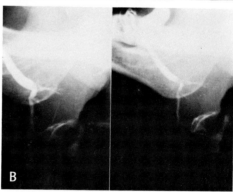

FIG. 8–17.   A: Submandibular swelling in sialadenitis secondary to duct blockage by a sialolith. B: Localized stricture at convergence of secondary ducts.

duct stones can be detected on panographic jaw radiographs.

Treatment: The stone can often be digitally manipulated out of the duct orifice. If this cannot be achieved, surgical removal is indicated. If pain, induration, and lack of function persist, particularly in cases of long-standing occlusion, sialectomy is indicated.

References
1. Harrison, G. R.: Calculi of the salivary glands and ducts. Surg. Gynecol. Obstet. 43:431, 1926.
2. Seldin, H. M., et al.: Conservative surgery for removal of salivary calculi. Oral Surg. 6:579, 1953.

3. Elmostehy, M. R.: Parotid salivary calculus: report of case. Oral Surg. *26*:18, 1968.
4. Brusati, R. and Fiamminghi, L.: Large calculus of the submandibular gland. Report of a case. J. Oral Surg. *31*:710, 1973.
5. Bullock, K. N.: Parotid and submandibular duct calculi in three successive generations of one family. Postgrad. Med. J. *58*:35, 1982.

Intraparotid Mesenchymal Tumors

Age: Infants and children

Sex: Female predilection

Clinical Features: Neoplasms arising from the supportive stroma of the salivary glands are much less common than parenchymal tumors. When they do occur, they are primarily seen in children. Vascular tumors are the most frequently encountered mesenchymal tumors. Juvenile nevoxanthoendotheliomas and neurilemmomas also arise from salivary stromal progenitor cells. Sarcomas in major glands are extremely rare. The benign tumor(s) may be present at birth or develop slowly during childhood. The gland substance is unilaterally affected and may evince a soft to firm diffuse swelling, or the neoplasm may be well localized and encapsulated. The masses are painless, and no erythema or skin surface changes are found. Spontaneous regression of vascular tumors by puberty is a frequent occurrence with skin; however, intraparotid lesions do not tend to involute.

Venous aneurysms, although not neoplastic, represent other mesenchymal lesions occurring within parotid tissue. They are nonpulsatile soft swellings that appear when the head is lowered below the level of the heart. The swelling resolves in 2 to 3 minutes after the patient elevates the head.

Microscopic Features: Intraparotid hemangiomas and lymphangiomas are characterized by infiltrative endothelial-lined channels of variable cellularity that tend to course between lobules and acini. Neurilemmomas are typically encapsulated and are composed of spindle-shaped nuclei and condensed collagen with foci of microcyst formation (Antoni B) and nuclear palisading (Antoni A) zones.

Differential Diagnosis: The slowly enlarging tumor mass seen with mesenchymal neoplasms must be differentiated from tuberculosis and unilateral mumps. The latter has an acute course with pain and fever. Primary parenchymal salivary tumors, particularly benign ones, show identical clinical features, but are rarely seen in children. Biopsy is required to provide a definitive diagnosis.

Treatment: Vascular tumors, being infiltrative, lack encapsulation and therefore require lobectomy or parotidectomy, depending upon the extent. Treatment should be deferred until after puberty, as regression may occur; however, parotid vascular tumors are less prone to involute spontaneously than are angiomas of skin. Neurilemmomas may be locally excised.

References

1. Campbell, J. S.: Congenital capillary hemangiomas of parotid gland; a lesion characteristic of infancy. N. Engl. J. Med. *254*:56, 1956.
2. Roos, D. B., et al.: Neurilemomas of facial nerve presenting as parotid gland tumors. Ann. Surg. *144*:258, 1956.
3. Bhaskar, S. N. and Lilly, G.E.: Salivary gland tumors of infancy; report of 27 cases. J. Oral Surg. *21*:305, 1963.
4. Krolls, S. O., Trodahl, J. N., and Boyers, R. C.: Salivary gland lesions in children. A survey of 430 cases. Cancer *30*:459, 1972.
5. Castro, E. B., et al.: Tumors of the major salivary glands in children. Cancer *29*:312, 1972.
6. Jensen, J. L. and Reingold, I. M.: Venous aneurysms of the parotid gland. Arch. Otolaryngol. *103*:493, 1977.

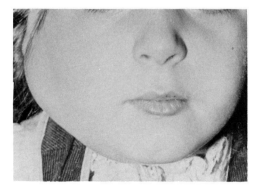

FIG. 8–18. Intraparotid lymphangioma. (Courtesy of Dr. Willard Fee.)

Lymphoma

Age: Middle-aged adults

Sex: Male predilection

Clinical Features: Whereas lymphomas generally make their initial appearance in the cervical nodes of the lateral neck, intraparotid nodes may also be the site of original tumefaction, producing enlargements anterior to the ears and over the mandibular angle. They are often bilateral and are indurated. Salivary flow is usually not affected and can be milked from the ducts. Pain is uncommon.

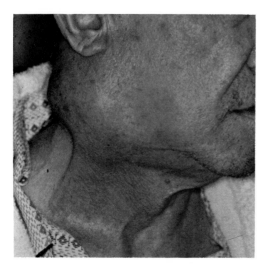

FIG. 8–19. Intraparotid malignant lymphoma.

When both parotids are enlarged in conjunction with lymphomatous swelling of the lacrimal glands, the disease is said to represent Mikulicz's syndrome (not to be confused with Mikulicz's disease, which is one of the benign lymphoepithelial lesions). Most instances of intraparotid lymphoma are of the non-Hodgkin's type. Cases of lymphomatous transformation in parotid glands with Sjögren's syndrome have been reported.

Microscopic Features: Both acini and ducts within salivary lobules are replaced by diffuse sheets of lymphocytes. Epimyoepithelial islands seen in benign lymphoepithelial lesions are not encountered in parotid lymphomas. The individual lymphocytes are either well or poorly differentiated, and follicular patterns are uncommon.

Differential Diagnosis: Bilateral parotid swellings seen in acute sialadenitis and endemic parotitis may be differentiated from lymphoma on the basis of high fever, pain, lack of induration, and rapid onset. Lymphoma may be confused clinically with Sjögren's syndrome, Mikulicz's disease, Heerfordt's syndrome, and tuberculosis. However, in these disorders the glandular swellings are soft or only moderately firm and lack fixation. Biopsy is required to obtain a definitive diagnosis. Once a diagnosis of malignant lymphoma is established, thorough physical examination, laboratory evaluation, and radiologic survey are required to determine the extent of disease.

Treatment: The patient should be managed by an oncologist, a hematologist, and a radiotherapist. Combination chemotherapy and radiotherapy are employed in treatment.

References

1. Gravanis, M. B. and Giansanti, J. S.: Malignant histopathologic counterpart of the benign lymphoepithelial lesion. Cancer 26:1332, 1970.
2. Freedman, S. I.: Malignant lymphomas of the major salivary glands. Arch. Otolaryngol. 93:123, 1971.
3. Hyman, G. A. and Wolfe, M.: Malignant lymphomas of the salivary glands. Review of the literature and report of 33 new cases, including four cases associated with the lymphoepithelial lesion. Am. J. Clin. Pathol. 65:421, 1976.
4. Colby, T. V. and Dorfman, R. F.: Malignant lymphomas involving the salivary glands. Pathol. Ann. 14:307, 1979.

Pleomorphic Adenoma

Age: Middle-aged adults
Sex: Female predilection

Clinical Features: The pleomorphic adenoma or mixed tumor is the most common neoplasm of the major salivary glands. Over 80 percent arise in the parotid, and most of the remainder in the submandibular gland and minor salivary glands. The tumor is generally located superficially overlying the angle of the mandible. It is firm or soft, movable, slow growing, and usually free from pain even on palpation. It has a great growth potential in that long-standing tumors may become so enormous that they hang to the shoulders. Malignant transformation is uncommon but does occur.

Microscopic Features: The term *pleomorphic* refers to the stromal element of the tumor and is the paramount pathologic feature. Monomorphic basophilic epithelial cells grow in diffuse sheets or are grouped into clusters showing duct formation. A spindle cell element is seen to proliferate in juxtaposition to the epithelial cell component and may actually be the predominant cell

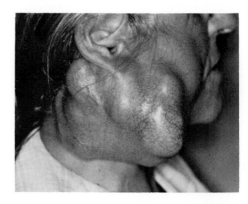

FIG. 8–20. Pleomorphic adenoma of the parotid gland.

type. These myoepithelial spindle cell proliferations merge with stromal components that differentiate into myxomatous, cartilaginous, osseous or adipose tissues. Some tumors contain hyaline cells with a plasmacytoid appearance, and occasionally tyrosine crystals are encountered. Encapsulation is a constant finding; however, multiple extracapsular satellite cell nests or a multinodular pattern are frequently noted.

Differential Diagnosis: Pleomorphic adenoma must be differentiated from papillary cystadenoma lymphomatosum, oncocytoma, mesenchymal neoplasms, and adenocarcinomas, all of which may appear well circumscribed. While the clinical features may appear to be typical for pleomorphic adenoma, biopsy is required to rule out these other entities.

Treatment: Simple excision is contraindicated, as recurrence is a common complication. Lobectomy or incontinuity gland extirpation is the treatment of choice. Facial nerve palsy and the auriculotemporal syndrome are common complications subsequent to parotid gland surgery.

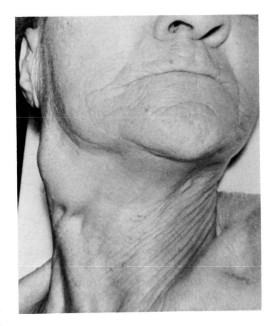

FIG. 8–21. Parotid nodule representing papillary cystadenoma lymphomatosum. (Courtesy of Dr. R. Bowles.)

References

1. Eneroth, C. M.: Histological and clinical aspects of parotid tumors. Acta Otolaryngol. *191* (Suppl.): 5, 1964.
2. Davies, J. N. P., et al.: Salivary gland tumors in Uganda. Cancer *17*:1310, 1964.
3. Krolls, S. O. and Boyers, R. C.: Mixed tumors of salivary glands: long-term follow-up. Cancer *30*:276, 1972.
4. Clairmont, A. A., Richardson, G. S., and Hanna, D. C.: The pseudocapsule of pleomorphic adenomas (benign mixed tumors). Am. J. Surg. *134*:242, 1977.
5. Conley, J. and Clairmont, A. A.: Facial nerve in recurrent benign pleomorphic adenoma. Arch. Otolaryngol. *105*:247, 1979.

Papillary Cystadenoma Lymphomatosum

Age: Middle-aged and elderly adults
Sex: Significant male predilection

Clinical Features: Papillary cystadenoma lymphomatosum or Warthin's tumor is a benign tumor of salivary origin that probably represents a hamartomatous enlargement rather than a true neoplasm. Credence is given to this concept on the basis of the clinical features of the lesion. It is very slow growing and is self-limited. Once it reaches 2 to 4 cm, growth ceases in most cases. Another feature supporting the concept of a hamartomatous lesion is its frequent bilateral occurrence. The tumor is restricted to the parotid gland(s) and is not found in other major or minor glands. It tends to be superficial, well circumscribed, movable, and classically feels doughy and compressible on palpation.

Microscopic Features: The lesion is well encapsulated and shows cystic spaces lined by papillary projections of columnar oncocytes with a double row of nuclei. The stroma is composed of lymphocytes with scattered germinal centers. A variant contains nests of squamous epithelial islands showing cyst formation and sebaceous acinar differentiation. The variant is termed *sebaceous lymphadenoma*.

Differential Diagnosis: Warthin's tumor must be differentiated from other benign salivary neoplasms of parenchymal and stromal origin and enlarged parotid lymph nodes. Occurrence in males, doughy compressible consistency, and indolent growth are typical features. Bilateral swellings with these characteristics are almost invariably Warthin's tumors; nevertheless, biopsy should be performed to confirm the clinical diagnosis.

Treatment: Simple local excision is recommended.

References

1. Chaudhry, A. P. and Gorlin, R. J.: Papillary cystadenoma lymphomatosum (adenolymphoma); a review of the literature. Am. J. Surg. *95*:923, 1958.
2. McGavran, M. H., et al.: Sebaceous lymphaden-

oma of the parotid salivary gland. Cancer 13:1185, 1960.

3. Dietert, S. E.: Papillary cystadenoma lymphomatosum (Warthin's tumor) in patients in a general hospital over a 24-year period. Am. J. Clin. Pathol. 63:866, 1975.
4. Blatnick, D. S., Kurtin, J. B., and Lehman, R. H.: Multicentricity of Warthin's tumors. Wis. Med. J. 75:61, 1976.
5. Shugar, J. M., Som, P. M., and Biller, H. F.: Warthin's tumor, a multifocal disease. Ann. Otol. Rhinol. Laryngol. 91:246, 1982.

Oncocytoma

Age: Elderly adults

Sex: Female predilection

Clinical Features: Oncocytoma or oxyphilic adenoma is a rare benign salivary tumor that rarely occurs before the age of 60. It arises most frequently in the parotid gland but may be located in the submandibular region as well. The mass is firm, well demarcated, and movable. It has a slow growth rate.

Microscopic Features: Solid sheets or trabecular cords of rectangular cells show voluminous amounts of granular eosinophilic cytoplasm with pyknotic or small nuclei containing a central nucleolus. Cystic spaces or duct formations may be encountered, yet rarely predominate. Oncocytic metaplasia in ductal cells is common in both major and minor salivary glands with ensuing age; however, this represents reactive rather than neoplastic change.

Differential Diagnosis: The well-localized movable swelling of oncocytoma must be differentiated from Warthin's tumor, pleomorphic adenoma, mesenchymal neoplasm, and enlarged parotid lymph node. Age is highly significant, and a swelling of this nature in an elderly patient is strongly suggestive of oncocytoma. Microscopic examination is required to make the diagnosis.

Treatment: Simple local excision is recommended.

References

1. Chaudhry, A. P. and Gorlin, R. J.: Oxyphilic granular cell adenoma (oncocytoma). Oral Surg. 11:897, 1958.
2. Hamperl, H.: Benign and malignant oncocytoma. Cancer 15:1019, 1962.
3. Eneroth, C. M.: Oncocytoma of major salivary glands. J. Laryngol. 79:1064, 1965.
4. Blanck, C., Eneroth, C. M., and Jacobsson, P. A.: Oncocytoma of the parotid gland: Neoplasm or nodular hyperplasia? Cancer 25:919, 1970.

Miscellaneous Adenomas

Age: Adults

Sex: Female predilection

Clinical Features: A variety of histologically distinct benign glandular tumors, other than the more common types included in this chapter, arise within the major salivary glands, usually the parotid. Most of them are rare. Included in this group are basal cell adenoma, membranous adenoma, sialadenoma papilliferum, myoepithelioma, sebaceous lymphadenoma, and papillary cystadenoma. Generally located within the superficial parotid, they appear as movable soft or somewhat firm nodules. Facial nerve compression resulting in paralysis is rare. Sialadenoma papilliferum may

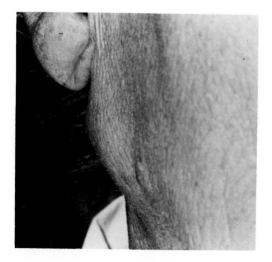

FIG. 8–22. Oncocytoma of the parotid in an elderly female. (Courtesy of Dr. Sheldon Rovin.)

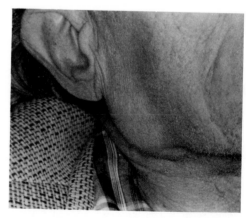

FIG. 8–23. Basal cell adenoma of the parotid gland.

extend through skin with an overlying cutaneous cauliflower-like papillomatous mass.

Microscopic Features: Each tumor exhibits characteristic histomorphologic patterns. Basal cell adenomas are composed of tumor islands, which are comprised of polygonal monomorphic cells with oval or round nuclei. Ductal elements are often encountered. Membranous adenomas appear similar to basal cell adenomas with zones of hyalinization encompassing individual nests or islands of monomorphic-appearing cells. Sialadenoma papilliferum shows cystic areas lined by papillary interconnecting projections lined by oncocytic columnar cells. When surface skin is involved, the ductal-appearing cells merge with papillary projections covered with stratified squamous epithelium. Myoepitheliomas are characterized by diffuse sheets of spindle cells resembling mesenchymal cells; thorough search of the specimen reveals streaming of spindle cells around small ducts. Sebaceous lymphadenomas, a variant of Warthin's tumor, show ducts, sebaceous acini, and lymphoid stroma. Papillary cystadenomas are cystic with papillary projections into the lumina.

Differential Diagnosis: These miscellaneous adenomas are soft or firm movable masses that are clinically indistinguishable from the other benign adenomas included here.

Treatment: The recurrence rate after excision is not known for most of these less commonly encountered tumors. It would probably be advisable to perform excision with in-continuity lobectomy.

References

1. Batsakis, J. G. and Brannon, R. B.: Dermal analogue of the major salivary glands. J. Laryngol. Otol. 95:155, 1981.
2. Headington, J. T., et al.: Membranous basal cell adenoma of parotid gland, dermal cylindromas, and trichoepitheliomas: comparative histochemistry and ultrastructure. Cancer 39:2460, 1977.
3. Abrams, A. M. and Finck, F. M.: Sialadenoma papilliferum: a previously unreported salivary gland tumor. Cancer 24:1057, 1969.

Adenoid Cystic Carcinoma

Age: Middle-aged adults

Sex: Slight female predilection

Clinical Features: Adenoid cystic carcinoma or cylindroma occurs more frequently in adults than in children. Unlike other malignant tumors of the salivary glands, it is just as likely to be encountered in the submandibular as in the parotid gland. The tumor mass is firm or indurated, often fixed, and does not necessarily grow rapidly. Unlike benign

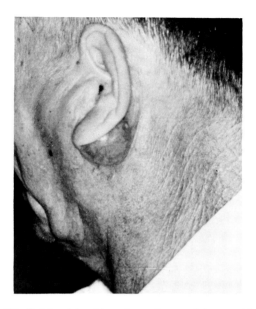

FIG. 8–24. Adenoid cystic carcinoma of the parotid gland appearing as an indurated erythematous mass below the ear lobe.

tumors, pain is often a symptom. In the parotid gland, facial nerve paralysis is encountered in nearly one-third of the patients. When the tumor lies in close proximity to the overlying skin, erythema, telangiectasia, and ulceration may be seen. The tumor metastasizes to regional cervical nodes and distantly by hematogenous spread with about equal frequency. A feature typical of adenoid cystic carcinoma is its slow rate of metastasis. Many tumors have been known to manifest metastatic foci 10 or 15 years after treatment.

Microscopic Features: The tumor cells are cuboidal, uniform, and hyperchromatic. Pleomorphism is uncommon. The cells are arranged in cords, solid sheets, or, typically, a multicystic honeycombed or cribriform pattern. The cystic areas contain a basophilic secretion product; the outer margin of the tumor islands, in the basal lamina region, evince a thickened hyaline rim. Tumor cells show a tendency for invasion of perineural lymphatic vessels. The leading margins lack encapsulation, and invasion of contiguous tissues is a constant finding. Histologic grading has been undertaken whereby the typical cribriform pattern is grade I, cribriform with admixed solid sheets is grade II, and basaloid or anaplastic predominance is grade III.

Differential Diagnosis: Because cylindromas are not always solidly fixed, they may simulate benign salivary neoplasms and mesenchymal tumors. When indurated and fixed they must be differentiated from other malignant salivary tumors such as mucoepidermoid carcinoma, acini cell carcinoma, and adenocarcinoma. Microscopic examination is required to make the diagnosis.

Treatment: Depending upon location, total parotidectomy or excision of the entire submandibular gland is mandatory. If the gland capsule is invaded, inclusion of adjacent tissues is necessary. In-continuity neck dissection should be performed when nodes are palpable; because hematogenous spread is frequent, chest radiographs must be obtained. Twenty percent of patients with major gland tumors exhibit nodal metastasis, while 50 percent present with or eventually develop distant metastases. The recurrence rate is high (over 50 percent) when wide excision (not gland extirpation) is performed. The determinate 5-year survival is about 30 percent; 10-year survival, 20 percent; and 15-year survival, 10 percent. Histologic grading is not highly correlated with prognosis.

References

1. Eneroth, C. M. and Hjertman, L.: Adenoid cystic carcinoma of the submandibular gland. Laryngoscope 76:1639, 1966.
2. Eby, L. S., Johnson, D. S., and Baker, H. W.: Adenoid cystic carcinoma of the head and neck. Cancer 29:1160, 1972.
3. Conley, J. and Dingman, D. L.: Adenoid cystic carcinoma in the head and neck (Cylindroma). Arch. Otolaryngol. 100:81, 1974.
4. Spiro, R. H., Huvos, A. G., and Strong, E. W.: Adenoid cystic carcinoma of salivary origin, a clinicopathologic study of 242 cases. Am. J. Surg. 128:512, 1974.
5. Grahne, B., Lauren, C., and Holsti, L. R.: Clinical and histological malignancy of adenoid cystic carcinoma. J. Laryngol. Otol. 91:743, 1977.

Mucoepidermoid Carcinoma

Age: Middle-aged adults

Sex: Slight female predilection

Clinical Features: Mucoepidermoid carcinoma is most common in adults; however, a significant number of cases can be found in children. The parotid gland is by far the most frequent site of origin. The tumors are divided microscopically into low- and high-grade varieties. Low-grade tumors are cystic and on palpation may be soft and compressible, whereas the more cellular high-grade lesions are often fixed and indurated. The skin overlying a superficially oriented tumor may be ulcerated, erythematous, and telangiectatic. Low-grade tumors have metastatic potential if left

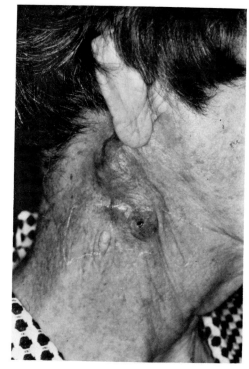

FIG. 8–25. Nodular inflamed mass of parotid representing a mucoepidermoid carcinoma.

untreated, yet as a group the prognosis is good when treatment is adequate. High-grade tumors show a more rapid growth rate and metastasize by both lymphatic and hematogenous routes. It should be noted that nearly 15 percent of patients have other salivary primaries or cancer of other organs.

Microscopic Features: Low-grade tumors show a tendency for demarcation but lack a capsule. The tumor nests show large cystic spaces lined by stratified squamous epithelium, columnar ductal cells, and mucus-secreting cells. Pleomorphism is not a feature. High-grade tumors contain a preponderance of epidermoid cells with a low population of mucous cells. Cyst formation is less frequent, with a tendency for tumor cells to grow in sheets. Clear cells are commonly seen admixed with the epidermoid component. In fact, some tumors are predominantly clear cell tumors and closely resemble renal cell carcinoma. Rarely, a pure epidermoid carcinoma arises from salivary epithelium.

Differential Diagnosis: Cystic or low-grade mucoepidermoid carcinomas are soft, compressible, and often demarcated and movable. In these instances, clinical differentiation from pleomorphic adenoma and other benign tumors is impossible. Indurated fixed carcinomas are clinically identical to other salivary adenocarcinomas. Biopsy is necessary to obtain a definitive diagnosis.

Treatment: Surgical removal of the entire gland with the tumor is required for both low- and high-grade tumors. Nearly one-third of both varieties recur after simple excision. Nodal metastases are observed at admission in 30 percent of patients with parotid tumors and over 50 percent when the tumor arises in the submandibular gland. According to histologic grade, less than 10 percent wih low-grade tumors present with positive nodes, whereas almost 60 percent of patients with high-grade tumors exhibit positive palpable nodes. If palpable nodes are present, a neck dissection should be performed. Radiation therapy is not as effective as surgery in obtaining a cure. Five-year survival for low-grade tumors is quite good, exceeding 90 percent. Five-year survival for high-grade tumors is less than 50 percent. Ten-year survival rates are lower, but the precipitous decrease seen in other salivary malignancies is not a feature of mucoepidermoid carcinoma.

References

1. Eversole, L. R.: Mucoepidermoid carcinoma; review of 815 reported cases. J. Oral Surg. 28:490, 1970.
2. Jakobsson, P. A., et al.: Mucoepidermoid carcinoma of the parotid gland. Cancer 22:111, 1968.
3. Thackray, A. C. and Lucas, R. B.: Tumors of the major salivary glands. In Atlas of Tumor Pathology, 2nd ser., Fasc. 10. Washington, Armed Forces Institute of Pathology, 1974.
4. Prior, P. and Waterhouse, A. H.: Second primary cancers in patients with tumors of the salivary glands. Br. J. Cancer 36:302, 1977.
5. Spiro, R. H., et al.: Mucoepidermoid carcinoma of salivary gland origin. A clinicopathologic study of 367 cases. Am. J. Surg. 136:461, 1978.

Acinic Cell Carcinoma

Age: Middle-aged adults

Sex: Female predilection

Clinical Features: Acinic cell carcinoma occurs primarily in the substance of the parotid gland, appearing as a firm nodule, which may be fixed or somewhat movable. Vague pain is often a symptom, as is some degree of facial muscle weakness on the affected side. The duration is often long, with a history of slow progressive enlargement. Despite its early indolent course, the tumor is prone to recur after simple excision and is capable of both nodal and distant metastases.

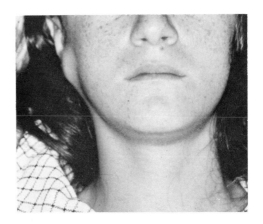

FIG. 8–26.   Acinic cell carcinoma of the parotid.

Microscopic Features: Neoplastic tumor cells are arranged in acinus-like clusters, and cystic spaces are often a prominent feature. When present, these cystic cavities are lined by cells that are not ductal cell types, but have a cobblestone pattern and resemble those cells arranged in the acinar organoid groupings. The individual cells contain copious amounts of clear or finely granular cytoplasm or may be filled with zymogen granules. Whereas the tumor margins are often well defined, neoplastic islands extend beyond the body of the tumor mass.

Differential Diagnosis: Because of its slow growth potential, acinic cell carcinoma may mimic the clinical features of benign salivary neoplasms, stromal tumors, and enlarged lymph nodes. When a firm, slowly enlarging mass in the parotid is accompanied by pain and facial weakness, acinic cell carcinoma should be the primary consideration. Biopsy must be performed to secure a definitive diagnosis.

Treatment: Local excision or even superficial parotidectomy results in recurrence in over 50 percent of the cases, whereas total parotidectomy will significantly lower the propensity for recurrence. Overall 5-year survival exceeds 75 percent.

References

1. Abrams, A. M., et al.: Acinic cell adenocarcinoma of the major salivary glands; a clinicopathologic study of 77 cases. Cancer 18:1145, 1965.
2. Chong, G. C., Beahrs, O. H., and Woolner, L. B.: Surgical management of acinic cell carcinoma of the parotid gland. Surg. Gynecol. Obstet. 138:65, 1974.
3. Spiro, R. H., Huvos, A. G., and Strong, E. W.: Acinic cell carcinoma of salivary origin, a clinicopathologic study of 67 cases. Cancer 41:924, 1978.

4. Perzin, K. H. and LiVolsi, V. A.: Acinic cell carcinomas arising in salivary glands: a clinicopathologic study. Cancer *44*:1434, 1979.

Adenocarcinoma NOS and Miscellaneous Malignancies

Age: Middle-aged adults
Sex: Female predilection

Clinical Features: Adenocarcinomas not otherwise specified (NOS) do not show microscopic

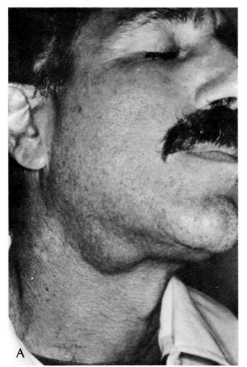

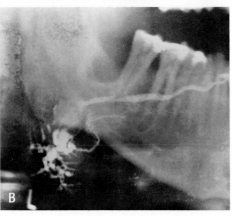

FIG. 8–27. Adenocarcinoma, not otherwise specified (NOS). *A:* Submandibular mass. *B:* Sialogram showing ductal compression and sialectasia.

features that allow classification with the other salivary tumors included here. Their frequency of occurrence is on a parity with adenoid cystic carcinoma with a predilection for the parotid gland. They are indurated and fixed to adjacent tissue, may be associated with erythema and telangiectasia of the overlying facial skin, and may compress the facial nerve, thus causing paralysis. Approximately 2 percent of pleomorphic adenomas either develop adenocarcinomatous transformation (carcinoma ex pleomorphic adenoma), are malignant from onset, or metastasize despite a benign histologic appearance. Among the adenocarcinomas not associated with mixed tumors are histologically distinct subcategories, which have been more clearly defined during the last decade. They include primary squamous cell carcinoma of salivary origin, small (oat) cell carcinoma, clear cell myoepithelioma of intercalated ducts, and papillary cystadenocarcinoma. Other malignant tumors arising in salivary glands are quite rare. Primary melanomas and sarcomas of stromal origin are included among these rarities. These uncommon salivary neoplasms all show rapid growth, fixation, and induration.

Microscopic Features: Adenocarcinoma not otherwise specified is infiltrative, lacking a capsule. The histomorphology is protean. Tumor cells may be arranged in trabecular cords, sheets, or ductal formations. The cytologic features are also variable, some tumors showing hyperchromatic monomorphic cells, others being pleomorphic or anaplastic. Malignant mixed tumors (carcinoma ex pleomorphic adenoma) show the classic features of benign pleomorphic adenoma with foci of malignant transformation displaying the aforementioned characteristics. Salivary squamous cell carcinomas exhibit similar features to those of surface mucosa origin. Small (oat) cell carcinomas are characterized by solid islands of small pleomorphic hyperchromatic nuclei without overt evidence of ductal differentiation. Clear cell myoepitheliomas fail to show pleomorphism; rather, they manifest small ducts lined by eosinophilic cuboidal cells enveloped by sheets of clear cells. Papillary cystadenocarcinomas are cystic with papillary proliferations of columnar cells displaying pleomorphism, hyperchromatism, and mitotic figures.

Differential Diagnosis: Adenocarcinoma and the other rare salivary malignancies (epidermoid carcinoma, melanoma, and sarcoma) are indurated and fixed. They must be differentiated from the other specific malignant salivary neoplasms and malignant lymphoma by microscopic evaluation.

Treatment: Wide surgical excision including the entire gland is required. Neck dissection should be performed in continuity when palpable nodes are detected clinically. Adenocarcinoma NOS is moderately radiosensitive, so combined radiation therapy and surgery may be considered in the treatment plan. Chest radiographs should be procured, as adenocarcinoma shows a tendency for both regional and distant metastasis. The survival figures for most adenocarcinomas NOS are similar to those for adenoid cystic carcinoma.

References

1. Greene, G. W., Jr., and Bernier, J. L.: Primary malignant melanomas of the parotid gland. Oral Surg. *14*:108, 1961.
2. Rosenfeld, L., et al.: Malignant tumors of salivary gland origin: 37 year review of 184 cases. Ann. Surg. *163*:726, 1966.
3. Spiro, R. H., Huvos, A. G., and Strong, E. W.: Malignant mixed tumor of salivary origin. A clinicopathologic study of 146 cases. Cancer *39*:388, 1977.
4. Batsakis, J. G.: Malignant mixed tumor. Ann. Otol. *91*:342, 1982.
5. Corio, R. L., et al.: Epithelial-myoepithelial carcinoma of intercalated duct origin. A clinicopathologic and ultrastructural assessment of sixteen cases. Oral Surg. *53*:280, 1982.

BILATERAL PAROTID AND SUBMANDIBULAR SWELLINGS

Endemic Parotitis (Mumps)

Age: Children

Sex: No predilection

Clinical Features: Mumps virus, a paramyxovirus, has an incubation period of 2 to 3 weeks. The initial parotid swelling is usually unilateral; enlargement of the opposite gland follows shortly thereafter. Frequently only one gland remains involved. The swelling is diffuse and soft and causes elevation of the ear lobe. Submandibular involvement is also common. The swelling is accompanied by moderate to severe pain. An exudate may be expressed from the parotid duct in some cases, but not always. Sour-tasting foods are intolerable, eliciting severe pain. Patients manifest other signs of infectious disease, including malaise, headache, and fever. The virus is not limited to salivary tissue; pancreatitis and meningitis are complications, while orchitis may lead to sterility in males. Orchitis develops within 3 to 5 days

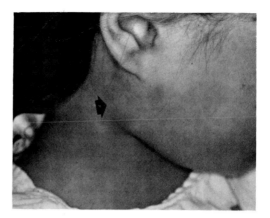

FIG. 8–28. Endemic parotitis showing diffuse parotid enlargement in a febrile child.

following parotid swelling if spread to the testes occurs.

Microscopic Features: The parotid ducts are dilated and contain secretion products with inflammatory cells. The acini manifest degenerative changes such as degranulation and vacuolization with a mononuclear inflammatory cell infiltrate.

Differential Diagnosis: Mumps must be differentiated from bacterial or occlusive salivary inflammatory disease, the benign lymphoepithelial lesions (Sjögren's syndrome, Mikulicz's disease), Heerfordt's syndrome, and parotid lymphoma. Most of these entities occur in adults, while mumps is more common in childhood. Serum amylase is elevated early in mumps, and leukopenia is a common finding.

Treatment: The patient is infectious and should be confined to bed. A bland diet with added liquids and prescription of antipyretics and analgesics are recommended. Because of the possibility of orchitis and meningitis, the patient's physician should be consulted.

References

1. Wolman, I. J., et al.: Amylase levels during mumps; the findings in blood and saliva. Am. J. Med. Sci. *213*:477, 1947.
2. Banks, P.: Nonneoplastic parotid swellings: a review. Oral Surg. *25*:732, 1968.
3. Marcy, S. M. and Kibrick, S.: Mumps. In *Infectious Diseases*, 2nd Ed., edited by P. D. Hoeprich. Hagerstown, Md., Harper & Row, 1977, p. 621.
4. Elvin-Lewis, M.: Paramyxoviridae. In *Oral Microbiology and Infectious Diseases*, 2nd Ed., edited by G. S. Schuster. Baltimore, Williams & Wilkins, 1983, ch. 42, p. 429.

Sjögren's Syndrome

Age: Middle-aged adults
Sex: Marked female predilection

Clinical Features: Sjögren's syndrome is a collagen disease of the rheumatoid group of immunopathologic disorders. The syndrome triad consists of xerostomia, xerophthalmia, and rheumatic joint disease. The parotid glands show slight to

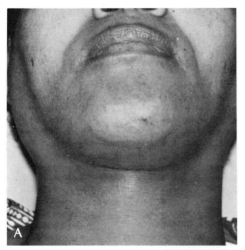

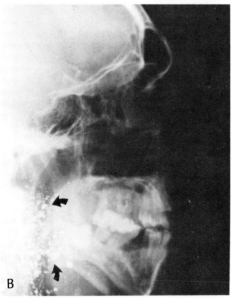

FIG. 8–29. A: Bilateral parotid enlargement associated with xerostomia, xerophthalmia and rheumatoid arthritis characterizing Sjögren's syndrome. (Courtesy of Dr. R. Provencher.) B: Sialogram in Sjögren's syndrome showing "bird-shot" appearance representing multifocal ectasia.

moderate enlargement bilaterally, and milking the glands fails to elicit flow from the ducts. Pain is occasionally a symptom. The mouth feels dry, the oral mucosa is often erythematous, and eventually cervical dental decay develops. The conjunctivae are also dry because of the lacrimal gland involvement with cessation of secretion, producing keratoconjunctivitis sicca. Classic signs of rheumatoid arthritis, including joint pain and swelling, are present in most patients. All three components of the syndrome are not necessarily coexistent in any one patient. Sjögren's syndrome may accompany other collagen-immune diseases such as lupus erythematosus, polyarteritis nodosa, and scleroderma. Malignant lymphoma is more common among patients with Sjögren's syndrome, and the lymphoid malignancies are usually found in extrasalivary locations.

Microscopic Features: The acini are replaced by diffuse infiltrative sheets of well-differentiated small and large lymphocytes. Ductal elements are not destroyed, but manifest cellular proliferation in the form of epimyoepithelial islands. Fluorescent antibody studies show immunofluorescence of ductal epithelium. Intraoral minor salivary glands show multifocal lymphoid aggregates dispersed throughout the gland lobules and in periductal arrangement.

Differential Diagnosis: Diffuse enlargement of the parotid glands in Sjögren's syndrome is clinically similar to that seen in Mikulicz's disease, Heerfordt's syndrome, parotid lymphoma, and metabolic sialadenosis. The occurrence in females and existence of other components of the syndrome are essentially classic features of Sjögren's syndrome. The disease may be confirmed by evaluation of parotid flow rates, use of the Shirmer lacrimation test, and evaluation of serum for the presence of rheumatoid (RA) factor. Sialograms reveal multifocal microsialectasia with a "birdshot" appearance of contrast medium retention. Labial gland biopsy is also useful in diagnosis.

Treatment: Patients with Sjögren's syndrome should be thoroughly evaluated for the presence of malignant lymphoma and other collagen diseases. The patient should be managed by a physician. The disease is treated with steroids or other immunosuppressive therapeutic agents.

References

1. Henderson, J. W.: Keratoconjunctivitis sicca; review with survey of 121 additional cases. Am. J. Ophthalmol. 33:197, 1950.
2. Bertram, U. and Halberg, P.: A specific antibody against the epithelium of the salivary ducts in sera

from patients with Sjögren's syndrome. Acta Allergol. *19*:458, 1964.

3. Pinkus, G. S. and Dekker, A.: Benign lymphoepithelial lesion of the parotid glands associated with reticulum cell sarcoma. Cancer *25*:121, 1970.

4. Dijkstra, P. F.: Classification and differential diagnosis of sialographic characteristics in Sjögren syndrome. Semin. Arthritis Rheum. *10*:10, 1980.

5. Scharf, J., Scharf, Y., and Nahir, M.: Sjögren's syndrome. Compr. Ther. *8*:40, 1982.

Mikulicz's Disease

Age: Middle-aged and elderly adults
Sex: Male predilection

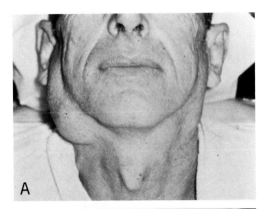

Clinical Features: Mikulicz's disease is a benign lymphoepithelial lesion of the parotid and lacrimal glands that occurs in males and is probably a localized form of Sjögren's syndrome. The disease in males is rarely associated with rheumatoid arthritis. The parotid swellings are soft, movable, and painless. Xerostomia is present, yet is rarely as severe as in women with Sjögren's syndrome. The term *Mikulicz's disease* is synonymous with localized benign lymphoepithelial lesion and should not be confused with *Mikulicz's syndrome*, which refers to parotid and lacrimal enlargement, which may represent malignant lymphoma.

Microscopic Features: The microscopic changes in Mikulicz's disease are identical to those encountered in Sjögren's syndrome.

Differential Diagnosis: Mikulicz's disease is differentiated from Sjögren's syndrome on the basis of sex and limitation of extent, rheumatoid disease being absent. In all probability, both diseases are merely variations of the same process. Other disorders that must be considered in the differential diagnosis are malignant lymphoma, Heerfordt's syndrome, disseminated tuberculosis, and metabolic sialadenosis. Parotid biopsy discloses the classic benign lymphoepithelial morphology. Sialographic changes are identical to those seen in Sjögren's syndrome.

Treatment: Moderate doses of steroids (e.g., 20 to 30 mg prednisone daily) may help control the immune process. The patient may require the use of a water bottle periodically to relieve xerostomia.

References

1. Morgan, W. S. and Castleman, B. C.: Clinicopathologic study of "Mikulicz's disease." Am. J. Pathol. *29*:471, 1953.

2. Bernier, J. L. and Bhaskar, S. N.: Lymphoepithelial lesions of salivary glands. Histogenesis and classi-

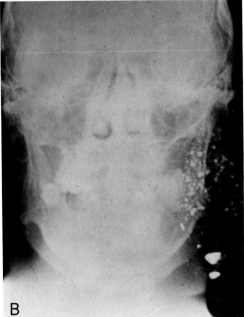

FIG. 8–30. *A*: Bilateral benign lymphoepithelial lesions of the parotid in Mikulicz's disease. *B*: Sialogram showing a lack of ductal arborization in Mikulicz's disease.

fication based on 186 cases. Cancer *11*:1156, 1958.

3. Romero, R. W., Nesbitt, L. T., Jr., and Ichinose, H.: Mikulicz disease and subsequent lupus erythematosus development. J. Am. Med. Assoc. *237*:2507, 1977.

4. Kahn, L. B.: Benign lymphoepithelial lesion (Mikulicz's disease) of the salivary gland: an ultrastructural study. Hum. Pathol. *10*:99, 1979.

5. Maynard, J.: Recurrent swellings of the parotid gland, sialectasis and Mikulicz's syndrome. J. R. Soc. Med. *72*:591, 1979.

Sarcoid Sialadenitis and Heerfordt's Syndrome

Age: Middle-aged adults
Sex: No predilection

Clinical Features: Sarcoidosis of the salivary glands occurs in less than 5 percent of patients suffering from the generalized form of the disease. When the sarcoid granulomas are present within the salivary tissue, parotid and lacrimal enlargement and induration are the primary signs. The enlarged glands are firm to palpation and free from pain, and the patients are often slightly febrile. The enlargement evolves slowly, requiring many months to manifest clinically obvious signs. It is usually bilateral but rarely symmetrical. Diminished flow of saliva from the involved glands is a common finding, and if the granulomatous infiltration is extensive, xerostomia with widespread cervical caries may be seen. Sialography discloses pathologic findings with deficient secondary and tertiary ducts and dye pooling, which yields a clouded pattern that represents terminal ectasia. Extensive lacrimal infiltration leads to xerophthalmia and conjunctivitis. Other manifestations of generalized sarcoidosis, such as hilar node enlargement on chest radiographic examination, are frequently identifiable. The cause for this tuberculoid granulomatous disease is unknown. It is most commonly encountered in middle European countries.

Microscopic Features: Sarcoid sialadenitis is characterized by multifocal granulomatous infiltration of the gland. The epithelioid histiocytes are admixed with multinucleated giant cells, and the former are arranged in fasciculated whorls. The granulomas are devoid of caseation necrosis.

Differential Diagnosis: The enlargement seen in Heerfordt's syndrome may clinically resemble that seen in Sjögren's syndrome, Mikulicz's disease, tuberculosis, or lymphoma. A search for other signs of generalized sarcoidosis should be pursued. Serum calcium is often elevated. Biopsy will show the features of noncaseating granulomas. The Kveim test uses specific antigen to detect delayed hypersensitivity and is positive in most cases.

Treatment: Since generalized sarcoidosis is often present, a thorough physical examination is required. The disease is treated with steroids or other immunosuppressive agents and should be managed by an internist or general physician.

References

1. Michelson, H. E.: Uveoparotitis. Arch. Dermatol. Syph. *39*:329, 1939.
2. Hamner, J. E., III, and Scofield, H. H. L.: Cervical lymphadenopathy and parotid swelling in sarcoidosis; a study of 31 cases. J. Am. Dent. Assoc. *74*:1224, 1967.
3. Chisholm, D. M., et al.: Salivary gland function in sarcoidosis. Oral Surg. *31*:766, 1971.
4. Mitchell, D. N. and Scadding, J. G.: Sarcoidosis. Am. Rev. Respir. Dis. *110*:774, 1974.
5. Nitzan, D. W. and Shteyer, A.: Sarcoidosis of the parotid salivary glands. J. Oral Maxillofacial Surg. *40*:443, 1982.

Tuberculosis

Age: Middle-aged and elderly adults
Sex: Male predilection

Clinical Features: Both the parotid and submandibular glands may show involvement with Mycobacterium tuberculosis. Diffuse enlargement occurs in conjunction with disseminated or miliary tuberculosis, along with extensive pulmonary disease. The enlargement may be unilateral or bilateral and is more common in the parotid gland. Pain and fistula formation are unusual findings. As in the case of cervical node scrofula, primary tuberculosis in the absence of pulmonary infection may develop in parotid lymph nodes. In this form of the disease, the enlargement is unilateral and manifests as a firm circumscribed tumefaction. A drainage tract may appear on the skin. The tonsil

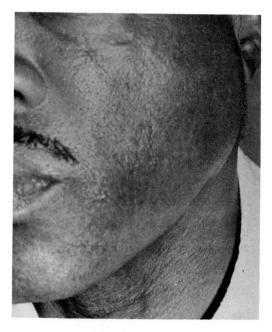

FIG. 8–31. Parotid swelling in sarcoidosis. (Courtesy of Dr. Willard Fee.)

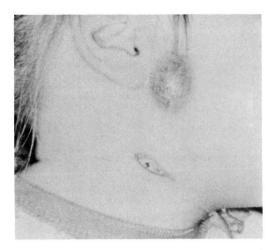

FIG. 8–32. Erythematous parotid enlargement and cervical fistula in atypical tuberculous sialadenitis. (Courtesy of Dr. R. Bowles.)

or pharynx is the probable portal of entry in this form.

Microscopic Features: Tuberculosis granulomas with epithelioid histiocytes and Langhans' giant cells are present. Zones of caseous necrosis are often but not invariably present. Focal abscess formation with neutrophilic infiltrates is often present, particularly in the localized primary form.

Differential Diagnosis: The firm parotid swelling of disseminated tuberculosis must be differentiated from Mikulicz's disease, Sjögren's syndrome, Heerfordt's syndrome, and malignant lymphoma. Sialography reveals lakes of pooled contrast medium and foci of ductal stenosis. Tuberculin skin tests and chest radiographs will be required to obtain a definitive diagnosis and determine the extent of disease. The localized form of intrasalivary tuberculosis must be differentiated from salivary tumor, mesenchymal neoplasms, or sclerosing sialadenitis. Biopsy will disclose specific granulomatous inflammation. Acid-fast stains will demonstrate the bacilli.

Treatment: Isoniazid therapy is the treatment of choice for typical tubercular lesions.

References

1. Patey, D. H. and Thackray, A. C.: Tuberculosis of the parotid gland. Arch. Middlesex Hosp. 4:256, 1954.
2. Allen-Mersh, M. G. and Forsyth, D. M.: Primary tuberculosis of the parotid gland. Tubercle 39:108, 1958.
3. Kant, R., et al.: Primary tuberculosis of the parotid gland. J. Indian Med. Assoc. 68:212, 1977.
4. Mankodi, R. C. and Shah, N. B.: Salivary gland granulomas—report of two cases. Indian J. Pathol. Microbiol. 20:275, 1977.

Metabolic Sialadenosis

Age: Middle-aged and elderly adults
Sex: Female predilection

Clinical Features: Metabolic sialadenosis is not a single specific disorder but, rather, an alteration both clinically and functionally of the salivary glands that accompanies a variety of generalized metabolic disorders. The most common of these diseases are hormonal imbalances (including changes evolving in conjunction with menopause, pregnancy, and menarche) and a salivary manifestation of diabetes mellitus. Similar changes may also be seen in hypothyroidism, cirrhosis, and ure-

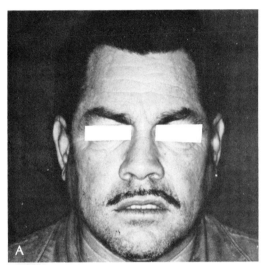

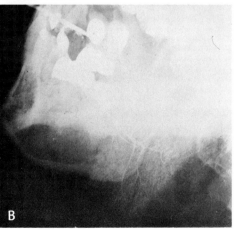

FIG. 8–33. *A:* Metabolic sialadenosis. *B:* Sialogram showing thin, filamentous ducts.

mia. In all of these disorders, the parotid is the salivary gland most often affected. Preauricular soft movable swellings are seen bilaterally in sex hormonal sialadenosis, whereas the swellings are more prominent below and behind the mandibular angle in diabetic sialadenosis. Salivary flow is diminished, there is no pain, and the patients are afebrile.

Microscopic Features: Both acinar and ductal cells appear edematous with cloudy swelling. Degranulation of zymogen secretory granules is a prominent feature, and extensive fatty infiltration of the stroma is observed.

Differential Diagnosis: The slow-growing soft enlargement seen in metabolic diseases with salivary involvement is unusual; however, the disease must be differentiated from other chronic sialadenopathies manifesting bilateral enlargement such as Sjögren's syndrome, Mikulicz's disease, Heerfordt's syndrome, tuberculosis, and lymphoma. Sialograms may appear normal; however, close scrutiny will usually disclose a filamentous, fine network of ducts. Analysis of parotid electrolytes is helpful, as potassium is elevated and sodium is decreased in the metabolic sialadenosis. A thorough history and physical evaluation are required to uncover the underlying, coexisting metabolic disorder.

Treatment: Treatment consists of correcting the underlying metabolic disturbance and should be managed by a physician.

References

1. Rauch, S. and Gorlin, R. J.: In *Thoma's Oral Pathology*, 6th Ed., edited by R. J. Gorlin and H. M. Goldman. St. Louis, C. V. Mosby Co., 1970, Vol. II, pp. 986–997.
2. Lyon, E.: Swelling of parotid gland and diabetes mellitus. Gastroenterologia 68:139, 1943.
3. Rothbell, E. N. and Duggan, J. J.: Enlargement of parotid gland in disease of the liver. Am. J. Med. 22:367, 1957.
4. Suzuki, S. and Kawashima, K.: Sialographic study of diseases of the major salivary glands. Acta Radiol. 8:456, 1969.
5. Chilla, R.: Sialadenosis of the salivary glands of the head. Studies on the physiology and pathophysiology of parotid secretion. Adv. Otorhinolaryngol. 26:1, 1981.

MIDLINE NECK SWELLINGS

Thyroglossal Tract Cyst

Age: Children and young adults
Sex: No predilection
Clinical Features: Derived from epithelium that

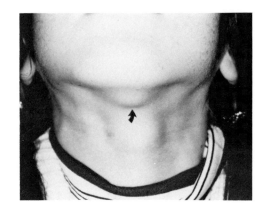

FIG. 8–34.   Thyroglossal tract cyst appearing as a small nodule in the flexure of the midline of the neck.

coursed through the neck during thyroid organogenesis, the thyroglossal tract cyst may be localized anywhere between the foramen caecum at the base of the tongue and the mature thyroid gland in the lower midline of the neck. The cyst is firm or soft and compressible, freely movable (unless entwined with the hyoid bone), and frequently develops a fistula. Most are located below the hyoid bone. If localized in the tongue or hyoid region, dysphagia may be a symptom. Rarely, thyroid carcinoma may arise from remnants of the tract.

Microscopic Features: The cyst is lined by stratified squamous or respiratory epithelium. The fibrous wall may evince a mild mononuclear inflammatory cell infiltrate, and both mucous glands and thyroid follicles can be observed.

Differential Diagnosis: Cysts located high in the midline of the neck must be differentiated from the dermoid cyst; if they are located low in the neck, goiter and thyroid neoplasms must be considered in the differential diagnosis.

Treatment: Simple excision is the treatment of choice. When the cyst is intimately associated with the hyoid bone, it may be necessary to remove a portion of the bone to ensure complete excision and avoid recurrence.

References

1. Gross, R. E. and Connerly M. L.: Thyroglossal cysts and sinuses; a study and report of 198 cases. N. Engl. J. Med. 223:616, 1940.
2. Bollock, W. F. and Stevenson, E. O.: Cysts and sinuses of the thyroglossal duct. Am. J. Surg. 112:225, 1966.
3. Butler, E. C., et al.: Carcinoma of the thyroglossal duct remnant. Laryngoscope 70:264, 1969.

4. Wampler, H. W., Krolls, S. O., and Johnson, R. P.: Thyroglossal-tract cyst. Oral Surg. 45:32, 1978.
5. Brereton, R. J. and Symonds, E.: Thyroglossal cysts in children. Br. J. Surg. 65:507, 1978.

Goiter

Age: Middle-aged adults

Sex: Female predilection

Clinical Features: Goiter refers to benign thyroid enlargement. Many forms exist, including iodine deficiency goiter, adenomatous goiter, and hyperthyroidism with exophthalmos (Graves' disease). When hypothyroidism accompanies goiter, the patients are dull, lethargic, and if the condition is severe, show diffuse myxedema of the soft tissues. The enlargement, located below the thyroid cartilage in the midline, is firm or compressible, movable, and in adenomatous goiter, multinodular. In Graves' disease, the metabolic rate is elevated, the patients are nervous and tense, and the goitrous swelling lacks nodularity, being diffuse.

Microscopic Features: The histology varies depending upon the type of goiter. In iodine deficiency and adenomatous goiter, the thyroid follicles are markedly enlarged and impacted with thyroglobulin. In Graves' disease, the follicular epithelium shows hyperplasia.

Differential Diagnosis: The goitrous conditions must be differentiated from one another on the basis of clinical signs and symptoms. Metabolic studies evaluating I^{131} uptake and radioactive thyroid scan are useful, as is evaluation of serum T_3 and T_4 levels. The diffuse nature of the swelling usually allows differentiation from tumor; however, when the swelling is small or located just lateral to the midline, neoplasia in the thyroid gland must be considered.

Treatment: Some goiters can be treated surgically, others medically. Referral to an internist or endocrinologist is recommended.

References

1. Bell, G. O. and Eisenbeis, C. H., Jr.: The nontoxic nodular hyperplastic goiter. N. Engl. J. Med. 253:812, 1955.
2. Taylor, S.: Genesis of the thyroid nodule. Br. Med. Bull. 16:102, 1960.
3. Miller, J. M., Horn, R. C., and Block, M. A.: The evolution of toxic nodular goiter. Arch. Intern. Med. 113:72, 1964.
4. Hennemann, G.: Non-toxic goitre. Clin. Endocrinol. Metab. 8:167, 1979.
5. Beckers, C.: Thyroid nodules. Clin. Endocrinol. Metab. 8:181, 1979.

Thyroid Neoplasia

Age: Middle-aged adults

Sex: Female predilection

Clinical Features: Thyroid neoplasms may be benign adenomas or malignant adenocarcinomas. They are classified according to their histomorphology. The benign adenomas arise in one pole of the gland so that they are located slightly lateral to the laryngeal cartilage. The tumors are generally small and may not be visually obvious; rather, they are often detected by palpation. They are soft or slightly firm and movable. Adenocarcinomas manifest a similar localization, but tend to be firm or indurated and fixed to adjacent tissues. They, too, may be small when first detected. Indeed, cervical node metastasis may be detected before a noticeable thyroid enlargement presents itself.

Microscopic Features: It is beyond the scope of this book to outline the microscopic features of thyroid tumors. The more common benign neoplasms are fetal and follicular adenomas. Papillary

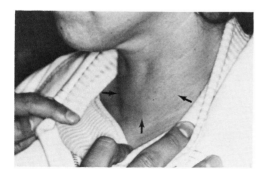

FIG. 8–35. Diffuse swelling in the thyroid area representing nontoxic goiter.

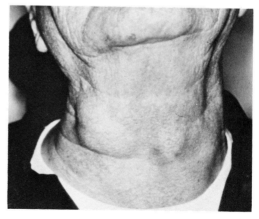

FIG. 8–36. Papillary carcinoma of the thyroid gland.

carcinoma is the most common form of thyroid cancer. Medullary carcinoma may arise in conjunction with oral neuromas and other endocrine neoplasms as a component of the neuropolyendocrine syndrome.

Differential Diagnosis: Neoplastic swellings in the thyroid region must be differentiated from one another by microscopic evaluation. Rarely, they must be differentiated from goiter.

Treatment: Most thyroid tumors are treated surgically. Those that take up iodine may be treated with I[131] radiotherapy. An oncologic surgeon or otolaryngologist should manage patients with thyroid neoplasms.

References

1. Willis, J.: Incidence and aetiology of thyroid carcinoma. Br. Med. J. 1:1646, 1961.
2. Liechty, R. D., Graham, M., and Freemeyer, P.: Benign solitary thyroid nodules. Surg. Gynecol. Obstet. *121*:571, 1965.
3. Meissner, W. A. and Warren, S.: Tumors of the thyroid gland. In *Atlas of Tumor Pathology,* Fasc. 4. Washington, Armed Forces Institute of Pathology, 1969.
4. Hawk, W. A. and Hazard, J. B.: The many appearances of papillary carcinoma of the thyroid. Cleve. Clin. Q. *43*:207, 1976.
5. Harwick, R. D.: Thyroid cancer—surgical decision making. Semin. Oncol. *7*:392, 1980.

Dermoid Cyst

Age: Adults

Sex: No predilection

Clinical Features: The dermoid cyst is usually encountered in the oral floor. When it arises inferior to the mylohyoid muscle it will protrude inferiorly, as an extraoral swelling in the upper midline of the neck in the submental flexure area. The mass is movable and has a doughy consistency on palpation.

Microscopic Features: The cyst is lined by keratinizing stratified squamous epithelium. Skin adnexal tissues such as sebaceous glands, sweat glands, and hair follicles are present within the fibrous wall.

Differential Diagnosis: A superiorly located thyroglossal tract cyst may simulate the dermoid cyst. Sebaceous cyst should also be considered in the differential diagnosis.

Treatment: Simple excision using an extraoral approach is recommended for dermoid cysts located below the mylohyoid muscle.

References

1. New, E. B. and Erich, J. B.: Dermoid cysts of the head and neck. Surg. Gynecol. Obstet. 65:48, 1937.
2. Seward, G. R.: Dermoid cysts of the floor of the mouth. Br. J. Oral Surg. 3:36, 1965.
3. Kinnman, J. and Suh, K. W.: Dermoid cysts of the floor of the mouth: report of three cases. J. Oral Surg. 26:190, 1968.
4. Sanders, B. and McKelvy, B.: Submental dermoid cyst of unusual size and duration. J. Oral Med. 32(2):38, 1977.
5. Lowry, R. E., Tempero, R. M., and Davis, L. F.: Epidermoid cyst of the floor of the mouth. J. Oral Surg. 37:271, 1979.

GROWTHS AND SWELLINGS OF THE FACIAL SKIN

Nevi

Age: Childhood onset

Sex: No predilection

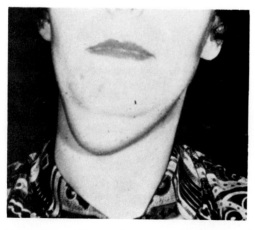

FIG. 8–37.   Midline swelling of neck and submandibular region representing a dermoid cyst. (Courtesy of Dr. I. Meyer.)

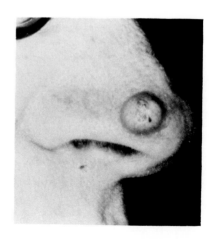

FIG. 8–38.   Nonpigmented nevus of nasal skin.

Clinical Features: Moles or nevi are the most common swellings of the facial skin. They are usually less than 1 cm in diameter, may be multiple, and are either brown, blue, or nonpigmented. Nonpigmented nevi are focal nodules that may contain hair; they lack ulceration and surface telangiectasia. Once they reach a certain size, they stop growing.

Microscopic Features: Nevi may be junctional, compound, or intradermal. The nevus cells contain variable amounts of melanin pigment if clinically pigmented. Nonpigmented nevi are composed of sheets and theques of polygonal epithelioid cells devoid of melanin granules.

Differential Diagnosis: Pigmented nevi are differentiated from melanoma on the basis of history and clinical appearance. A long duration with arrested growth and lack of ulceration are indicators of a benign lesion. Should a pigmented lesion continue to grow or ulcerate, a biopsy is indicated. Nonpigmented nevi must be differentiated from basal cell carcinoma, adnexal skin tumors, and sebaceous cysts. Basal cell carcinomas show progressive growth and often ulcerate. If they are not ulcerated, they will usually show surface telangiectasia.

Treatment: Skin nodules that are pigmented or nonpigmented and lack ulceration or telangiectasia, if they have persisted unchanged for many years, are probably nevi. No treatment is required. Excisional biopsy is recommended if recent growth has occurred, if the lesion is ulcerated, or if surface telangiectasia is encountered.

References

1. Beerman, H., Lane, R. A. G., and Shaffer, B.: Pigmented nevi and malignant melanoma of the skin. A survey of some of the recent literature. Am. J. Med. Sci. 229:444, 583, 1955.
2. Lund, H. Z. and Kraus, J. M.: Melanotic tumors of the skin. In *Atlas of Tumor Pathology*, Sec. 1, Fasc. 3. Washington, Armed Forces Institute of Pathology, 1962.
3. Castilla, E. E., da Graca Dutra, M., and Orioli-Parreiras, I. M.: Epidemiology of congenital pigmented naevi: I. Incidence rates and relative frequencies. Br. J. Dermatol. *104*:307, 1981.
4. Kamino, H. and Ackerman, A. B.: A histologic atlas of some common benign pigmented lesions of the skin. J. Dermatol. Surg. Oncol. *5*:718, 1979.
5. Jacobs, A. H.: Birthmarks: II. Melanocytic and epidermal nevi. Pediatrics *64*:47, 1979.

Sebaceous Cyst

Age: Young adults
Sex: No predilection

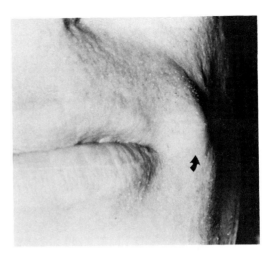

FIG. 8–39. Sebaceous cyst of the cheek.

Clinical Features: Sebaceous and epidermoid cysts are derived from the pilosebaceous apparatus. Similar cysts result from implantation of surface epithelium after a cut or laceration. The cysts are often quite superficial and small; however, they can exceed 2 to 3 cm in diameter. When superficial, they have a pearly, blanched quality. Larger cysts are fixed to the dermis yet can be moved about over the subcutaneous tissues and are compressible; they have a doughy consistency. Multiple sebaceous cysts are not uncommon; when they are encountered, workup for Gardner's syndrome should be undertaken.

Microscopic Features: The lumen is filled with an eosinophilic caseous material, and shredded keratin fibers are seen to desquamate from the keratinizing stratified squamous epithelium. The wall is often ruptured with keratin and epithelial cells embedded within the fibrous wall. A foreign-body reaction with multinucleated giant cells is seen under these circumstances. A specific type of cyst is derived from the hair follicle, which contains basophilic epithelial cells and luminally oriented ghost cells (eosinophilic epidermal cells with vacuolated spaces in place of nuclei). This specific type of pilar cyst is known as the calcifying epithelioma of Malherbe.

Differential Diagnosis: Sebaceous and epidermoid cysts, particularly when superficial, will resemble basal cell carcinoma, adnexal skin tumors, or benign mesenchymal tumors.

Treatment: Surgical enucleation of the cyst is the treatment of choice.

References

1. Erich, J. B.: Sebaceous, mucous, dermoid and epidermoid cysts. Am. J. Surg. *50:*672, 1940.
2. Love, W. R. and Montgomery, H.: Epithelial cysts. Arch. Dermatol. Syph. *47:*185, 1943.
3. McGavran, M. H. amd Binnington, B.: Keratinous cysts of the skin. Arch. Dermatol. *94:*499, 1966.
4. Leppard, B. J., Sanderson, K. V., and Wells, R. S.: Hereditary trichilemmal cysts. Hereditary pilar cysts. Clin. Exp. Dermatol. *2:*23, 1977.
5. Holmes, R. and Black, M. M.: Steatocystoma multiplex with unusually prominent cysts on the face. Br. J. Dermatol. *102:*711, 1980.

Seborrheic Keratosis

Age: Middle-aged and elderly adults
Sex: No predilection

Clinical Features: Seborrheic keratoses usually occur in multiples. They are focal papular or nodular lesions with a brown waxy character, so superficial that they appear to have been "stuck on" to the skin. They are not encountered in young individuals, but become more numerous with advancing age. Etiology is unknown.

Microscopic Features: The epithelium evinces acanthosis that is exophytic, with a smooth surface. Invagination of epidermal cells into the dermis is not a feature. The acanthotic epithelium may contain keratin pearls and cysts or may evince a retiform pattern with accompanying dermal connective tissue papillae.

Differential Diagnosis: Because of their pigmentation, seborrheic keratoses may be confused with nevi. Nevi are not as superficial, lack the waxy or oily character of seborrheic keratosis, and do not become prevalent with advancing age.

Treatment: No treatment is necessary. If cosmesis is a problem, the keratosis can be shaved superficially or cauterized.

References

1. Becker, S. W.: Seborrheic keratosis and verruca, with special reference to the melanotic variety. Arch. Dermatol. Syph. *63:*358, 1951.
2. Rowe, L.: Seborrheic keratosis. I. "Pseudoepitheliomatous hyperplasia" (Weidman). J. Invest. Dermatol. *29:*165, 1957.
3. Morales, A. and Hu, F.: Seborrheic verruca and intraepidermal basal cell epithelioma of Jadassohn. Arch. Dermatol. *91:*342, 1965.
4. Sanderson, K. F.: The structure of seborrheic keratosis. Br. J. Derm. *80:*588, 1968.
5. Molokhia, M. M. and Portnoy, B.: A study of dendritic cells in seborrheic warts. Br. J. Derm. *85:*254, 1971.

Adnexal Skin Tumors

Age: Middle-aged and elderly adults
Sex: Male predilection

Clinical Features: Tumors of skin that are derived from or differentiate along the lines of the skin appendages commonly arise on the face. Hair follicle tumors (trichoepithelioma), sebaceous cell adenomas, and sweat gland adenomas (eccrine acrospiroma, hidradenoma) are all benign neoplasms. Malignant counterparts occur but are rare. The adnexal skin tumors as a group may be either uninodular or multinodular. Most are firm, painless, and nonulcerated; however, malignant varieties are often ulcerated.

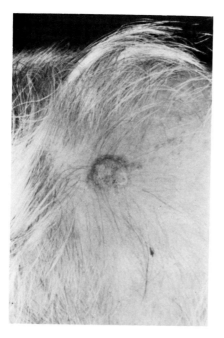

FIG. 8–40.   Scaly nodule of scalp in an elderly male representing seborrheic keratosis.

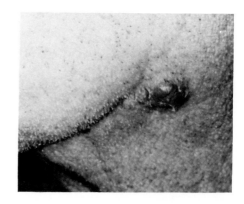

FIG. 8–41.   Trichoepithelioma of facial skin.

Microscopic Features: The adnexal skin tumors vary considerably in their histomorphology. They are composed of epithelial cells that differentiate along pilar, sebaceous, or adenomatoid lines.

Differential Diagnosis: The nodular swellings of adnexal skin tumors must be differentiated microscopically from one another. Clinically, they have features in common with basal cell carcinomas, mesenchymal dermal neoplasms, and sebaceous cysts.

Treatment: Surgical excision is the treatment of choice.

References

1. Lever, W. F.: Pathogenesis of benign tumors of cutaneous appendages and of basal cell epithelioma. Arch. Dermatol. Syph. *57*:679, 1948.
2. Kligman, A. M. and Pinkus, H.: The histogenesis of nevoid tumors of the skin. Arch. Dermatol. *81*:922, 1960.
3. Johnson, B. L. and Helwig, E. B.: Eccrine acrospiroma; a clinicopathologic study. Cancer *23*:641, 1969.
4. Mellette, J. R., et al.: Carcinoma of sebaceous glands on the head and neck. A report of four cases. J. Dermatol. Surg. Oncol. *7*:404, 1981.
5. King, A. I., Klima, M., and Johnson, P.: Sweat gland tumors of the head and neck. Arch. Otolaryngol. *108*:48, 1982.

Basal Cell Carcinoma

Age: Middle-aged and elderly adults

Sex: Male predilection

Clinical Features: The basal cell carcinoma is an aggressive yet nonmetastasizing neoplasm of the skin; rare instances of metastasis have been reported. Over 90 percent of all basal cell carcinomas are encountered on the skin of the upper face and forehead. The tumor may be solitary or multiple; it tends to occur in patients with fair complexions and in those who are constantly exposed to solar radiation. The early tumor may be a smooth-surfaced nodule with telangiectasia, a focal ulcer, or a nodule with central keratosis. Large lesions are ulcerative with rolled, indurated margins. Multiple basal cell tumors that show a slow growth rate or reach a given size and become static may be seen in children and young adults suffering from odontogenic keratocysts of the jaws and a bifid rib. This triad, in conjunction with other anomalies, constitutes the nevoid basal cell carcinoma syndrome.

Microscopic Features: Surface epithelium shows a transition, whereby neoplastic cords and islands of hyperchromatic monomorphic basaloid-appearing epithelial cells demonstrate invasion into the dermis. The center of the neoplastic cell nests may contain keratin pearls; however, acanthotic squamous cells mimicking the normal spinous cell layer are not typically present. Adenoid forms with tubular rete-ridge cords and ductal patterns are occasionally encountered. The morphea type shows extensive desmoplasia.

Differential Diagnosis: Early basal cell carcinomas lacking ulceration must be differentiated from nonpigmented nevi, adnexal skin tumors, mesenchymal dermal tumors, and sebaceous cysts. Surface telangiectasia is strongly indicative of basal cell carcinoma. Larger lesions with ulceration and rolled margins must be differentiated from squamous cell carcinoma, which is significantly less prevalent on the face. Specific granulomatous infection must also be considered in the differential diagnosis. Biopsy is required to obtain a definitive diagnosis.

Treatment: Basal cell carcinoma requires excision with a 1-cm margin from the clinically obvious tumor. This is necessary to avoid recurrence, since the neoplasm commonly displays microscopic invasion or multicentricity that is often not visually detectable clinically. Microscopic examination of the margins is required to ensure complete excision.

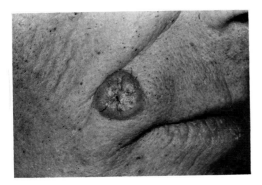

FIG. 8–42. Basal cell carcinoma of the face showing rolled margins with central ulceration.

References

1. Creschickter, C. F. and Koehler, H. P.: Ectodermal tumors of the skin. Am. J. Cancer *23*:804, 1935.
2. Gellin, G. A., Kopf, A. W., and Garfinkel, L.: Basal cell epithelioma. Arch. Dermatol. *91*:38, 1965.
3. Levine, H. L. and Bailin, P. L.: Basal cell carcinoma of the head and neck: identification of the high risk patient. Laryngoscope *90*:955, 1980.
4. Goepfert, H., Arredondo, R., and McNeese, M. D.: Cancers of the skin of the nose. Otolaryngol. Head Neck Surg. *90*:237, 1982.

Keratoacanthoma

Age: Middle-aged adults
Sex: Male predilection

Clinical Features: Keratoacanthoma is a benign tumor of epithelial origin. It may be solitary or multifocal. Multiple keratoacanthoma is a dominantly inherited disorder. The tumor is characterized by an elevation with rolled margins and a central keratotic core; the margins are sharply delineated. The lesion may occur anywhere, but is most frequently seen on the extremities and the face. The tumor proliferates rapidly, becomes static with regard to growth, and within 6 to 12 months spontaneously involutes, leaving a depressed scar.

Microscopic Features: The histologic features are similar to those of a well-differentiated squamous cell carcinoma. A central zone composed of voluminous strata of keratin and parakeratin is observed. The spinous cell layer is thickened and rete-ridge formation is present, yet invasion of the dermis is not observed. Pathognomonic features of this tumor are identifiable at the lateral margins. The acanthotic central core shows lipping at the margins, and at this point an abrupt transition into normal epithelium is observed.

Differential Diagnosis: The umbilicated nodule with a keratin plug, typical for keratoacanthoma, may also be encountered with basal and squamous cell carcinomas and with some adnexal tumors of skin.

Treatment: Excision is the treatment of choice. Waiting for spontaneous involution is not advisable for two reasons: (1) one cannot be assured clinically that the lesion does indeed represent keratoacanthoma rather than cancer, and (2) the scar remaining after surgery is often more cosmetic than that which develops after spontaneous regression.

References

1. Ghadially, F. N., Barton, B. W., and Kerridge, D. F.: The etiology of keratoacanthoma. Cancer *16*:603, 1963.
2. Garrett, W. S., et al.: Keratoacanthoma. Arch. Surg. *94*:853, 1967.
3. Reed, R. J.: Actinic keratoacanthoma. Arch. Dermatol. *106*:858, 1972.
4. Flannery, G. R. and Muller, H. K.: Immune response to human keratoacanthoma. Br. J. Dermatol. *101*:625, 1979.
5. Goodwin, R. E. and Fisher, G. H.: Keratoacanthoma of the head and neck. Ann. Otol. Rhinol. Laryngol. *89*:72, 1980.

Mesenchymal Tumors

Age: Young and middle-aged adults
Sex: No predilection

Clinical Features: Mesenchymal neoplasms arising in the dermal and subcutaneous connective tissues of the face are uncommon. The superficial dermatofibroma shows a smooth or slightly keratotic surface and a pale brown or pink color, which may blanch on pressure. Hemangiomas are also seen on the face, may be flat or tumefactive, are reddish-purple, and blanch on pressure. Lipomas and neural sheath neoplasms arise on the facial skin. The former are quite soft, compressible, and movable. The latter are uninodular or multinodular, firm, and movable. Multiple neurofibromatous nodules and brown café-au-lait macules are encountered in von Recklinghausen's disease of skin. Other mesenchymal tumors also arise here, but are rare.

Microscopic Features: The benign connective

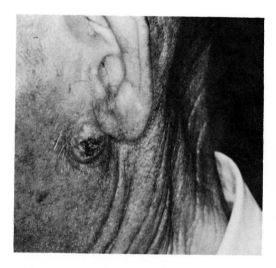

FIG. 8–43. Keratoacanthoma of facial skin showing rolled borders with a central keratotic plug.

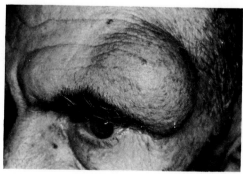

FIG. 8–44. Lipoma of the facial subcutaneous tissues.

tissue tumors are encapsulated or well localized and fail to show pleomorphism. Their differentiation is dependent upon the tissue cells of origin.

Differential Diagnosis: Benign mesenchymal tumors have a smooth surface and are soft or firm. These features may be seen with sebaceous cysts, nonpigmented nevi, and adnexal tumors of skin. Microscopic examination is required to determine the cell of origin.

Treatment: Local excision is the treatment of choice. Recurrence rate for most mesenchymal neoplasms of the skin is quite low.

References

1. Adair, F. E., Pack, G. T., and Farrior, J. H.: Lipomas. Am. J. Cancer 16:1104, 1932.
2. Watson, W. L.: Blood and lymph vessel tumors in children. J. Pediatr. 15:401, 1939.
3. Ross, D. E.: Skin manifestations of von Recklinghausen's disease and associated tumors (neurofibromatosis). Am. Surg. 31:729, 1965.
4. Meigel, W. N. and Ackerman, A. B.: Fibrous papule of the face. Am. J. Dermatopathol. 1:329, 1979.
5. Horn, K. L., Crumley, R. L., and Schindler, R. A.: Facial neurilemmomas. Laryngoscope 91:1326, 1981.

DIFFUSE FACIAL SWELLINGS

Cellulitis and Space Infections

Age: No predilection
Sex: No predilection

Clinical Features: Cellulitis of the facial tissues usually arises subsequent to spread of odontogenic infection. The swelling is diffuse, firm, or indurated and warm. The overlying skin may display erythema. Moderate to severe pain is present. The patient is febrile and complains of malaise, and cervical lymphadenopathy is a frequent finding. Examination of the teeth or dental radiographs will

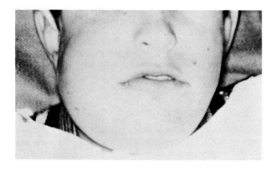

FIG. 8–45. Diffuse soft tissue swelling of face subsequent to spread of odontogenic infection represents cellulitis.

disclose a carious tooth and periapical radiolucency. Cellulitis will localize in the soft tissue adjacent to the infected tooth. When a question exists with regard to the incriminating tooth, vitalometer testing is in order. Anterior maxillary teeth may drain into the soft tissues of the upper face and orbit while posterior maxillary and mandibular teeth are associated with cellulitis in the masseter region. The soft tissue inflammation may ultimately point and drain, or may progress through fascial planes and spaces. If the mediastinum becomes involved, the process may be lethal.

Microscopic Features: Muscle and fascial connective tissue fibers are diffusely infiltrated with neutrophils and scattered histiocytes. Tissue edema is not prominent.

Differential Diagnosis: Because of its induration, cellulitis may simulate malignant neoplasm or underlying bone disease. Fever, constitutional signs of infectious disease, and localization of infectious sources, either in the dentition or periodontium, allow for a clinical diagnosis of cellulitis.

Treatment: The patient should be placed on analgesics and antipyretics. Penicillin is the drug of choice, provided that the patient is not allergic to it. The source of infection should be eliminated either by pulp exposure or extraction. Hot packs can be applied to the swelling in an attempt to localize the infection, after which incision and drainage can be performed. Failure of the processes to show resolution in 48 hours requires routine and anaerobic culture and sensitivity tests of an aspirate from the inflamed tissues.

References

1. Kent, H. A.: Cellulitis. Am. J. Orthod. Oral Surg. 25:172, 1939.
2. Shapiro, H. H., Sleeper, E. L., and Guralnick, W. C.: Spread of infection of dental origin. Oral Surg. 3:1407, 1950.
3. Shafer, W. G., Hine, M. K., and Levy, B. M.: A Textbook of Oral Pathology, 3rd Ed. Philadelphia, W. B. Saunders Co., 1974, p. 464.
4. Moose, S. M., and Marshall, K. J.: In Textbook of Oral and Maxillofacial Surgery, 5th Ed., edited by G. O. Kruger. St. Louis, C. V. Mosby Co., 1979, ch. 11.

Emphysema

Age: No predilection
Sex: No predilection

Clinical Features: Emphysema of the oral and facial soft tissues arises as the result of entrapment of air introduced into tissue or fascial spaces. This phenomenon is usually iatrogenic, following some

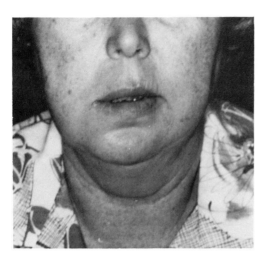

FIG. 8–46. Diffuse soft swelling of the cheek due to air entrapment in the facial tissues.

dental or surgical procedure rendered in conjunction with application of positive-pressure air introduction into a wound, periodontal pocket, surgical flap, or root canal. As the air becomes trapped within tissues it causes diffuse swelling, which yields a bubbly sensation with soft crepitus when palpated. Pain is often a complaint.

Microscopic Features: Not applicable.

Differential Diagnosis: Soft tissue emphysema is easily differentiated from other diffuse facial swellings on the basis of the bubbly consistency detected on palpation. Occasionally, emphysema may be confused with the soft swellings seen in edema, particularly angioneurotic edema. A complete history with consideration of potential etiologic factors will allow for differentiation on a clinical basis.

Treatment: Soft tissue emphysema may be complicated by venous air embolism, which is often fatal, or by soft tissue abscess; in the latter, antibiotic therapy is indicated. Emphysema generally resolves in 4 to 7 days with no treatment. If the swelling is significant, negative-pressure needle aspiration may aid in resolution.

References

1. Rhymes, R., Jr.: Postextraction subcutaneous emphysema. Oral Surg. 17:271, 1964.
2. Lantz, B.: Cervicofacial emphysema. A report of three cases with periodontal etiology. Odontol. Revy 15:279, 1964.
3. Longenecker, C. G.: Venous air embolism during operations on the head and neck; report of a case. Plast. Reconstr. Surg. 36:619, 1965.
4. Cardo, V. A., Jr., Mooney, J. W., and Stratigos, G. T.: Iatrogenic dental air emphysema: report of a case. J. Am. Dent. Assoc. 85:144, 1972.
5. Spaulding, C. R.: Soft tissue emphysema. J. Am. Dent. Assoc. 98:587, 1979.

Angioneurotic Edema

Age: No predilection
Sex: No predilection

Clinical Features: Patients allergic to certain foods or drugs exhibit urticaria in most instances; however, for unknown reasons, the allergic manifestations may be localized to the facial area. The facial swelling may also be accompanied by urticaria. The facial swelling of angioneurotic edema is the result of histamine-mediated profuse capillary permeability with a resultant diffuse often massive, edematous swelling of the upper lip, face, and periorbital area. The tissue is soft, pliable, and usually pruritic. The reaction is a manifestation of immediate immunoglobulin-mediated hypersensitivity that takes place within 1 or 2 hours after antigenic challenge, which is usually venom from a localized spider bite or bee sting to the face. Ingestion of food allergens may also result in angioneurotic edema. A hereditary form of angioneurotic edema occurs. Patients with this form are genetically deficient in an enzyme that inhibits an esterase responsible for a certain reaction in the complement-fixation process.

Microscopic Features: Not applicable.

Differential Diagnosis: The diffuse swelling of angioneurotic edema must be differentiated from emphysema and facial cellulitis associated with spread of odontogenic infection. Cellulitis may show an early edematous phase prior to cellular infiltration with induration. Infection of dental origin should be ruled out with appropriate radiologic and clinical evaluations. Diligent questioning is required to uncover the suspected allergen, and reexposure to the suspected agent may be necessary to confirm the etiology.

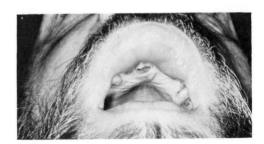

FIG. 8–47. Diffuse soft swelling of the lips in angioneurotic edema.

Treatment: The suspected allergen should be withdrawn and avoided in the future. The disease can be treated by prescribing 50 mg of diphenhydramine or 12.5 mg of promethazine q.i.d. for 3 days. Progression to anaphylactic shock may develop but is not a frequent complication.

References
1. Donaldson, V. H. and Rosen, F. S.: Hereditary angioneurotic edema: a clinical survey. Pediatrics 37:1017, 1966.
2. Sturdy, K. A., et al.: Hereditary angioedema controlled with Danazol. Oral Surg. 48:418, 1979.
3. Albright, W. B. and Taylor, C. G.: Hereditary angioneurotic edema: report of a case. J. Oral Surg. 37:888, 1979.

Cushing's Syndrome

Age: Adults
Sex: No predilection

Clinical Features: Cushing's syndrome is characterized by bilateral edematous swelling of the face, upper torso adiposity (buffalo hump), abdominal stria, hypertension, and hyperglycemia. These signs and symptoms are the result of adrenal hypercorticism. The disease may be due to an adrenal cortical adenoma or hyperplasia, pituitary adenoma, or steroid-secreting malignancies of other organs. The most common cause is prolonged steroid drug therapy, producing the so-called moon facies or cushingoid facies. The soft tissues of the cheeks are bilaterally puffy and edematous, yielding a round face.

Microscopic Features: Not applicable.

Differential Diagnosis: The soft bilateral swellings, being bilateral and of slow onset, are quite characteristic. A history of steroid therapy will confirm the impression. Cushing's syndrome occurring in patients who are not taking steroid medication requires a complete medical workup with laboratory studies in order to determine the cause of elevated steroid levels. Obtaining a high blood pressure reading (secondary to mineralocorticoids) and fasting sugar (elevated due to glucocorticoids) represents the initial phase of the workup.

Treatment: The cause of the disease must be determined initially; treatment rests with medical and/or surgical intervention.

References
1. Hunder, G. G.: Pathogenesis of Cushing's disease. Mayo Clin. Proc. 41:29, 1966.
2. Rovitt, R. L., and Duane, T. D.: Cushing's syndrome and pituitary tumors. Pathophysiology and ocular manifestations of ACTH-secreting pituitary adenomas. Am. J. Med. 46:416, 1969.
3. McArthur, R. G., et al.: Cushing's disease in children. Findings in 13 cases. Mayo Clin. Proc. 47:318, 1972.

Facial Hemihypertrophy

Age: Childhood onset
Sex: Male predilection

Clinical Features: Hypertrophy of the facial tissues is a developmental defect of unknown origin, which has been suggested to be related to an anomalous vascular supply. The disease is unilateral, with enlargement of both osseous and soft tissues. The opposite side of the face is normal, whereas the affected side shows enlargement of the facial bones and mandible. The eye is laterally displaced. Half of the tongue is enlarged, and the cheek tissues are thickened. The enlarged osseous tissues do not show an alteration of trabeculation on radiographs. Teeth on the affected side may be larger than those on the normal side. In nearly half the cases of this peculiar syndrome, the remainder of the body shows a similar unilateral involvement. Syndactyly and polydactyly are present in some instances, and one-fifth of the patients with hemihypertrophy are retarded. A familial or genetic trend is not encountered.

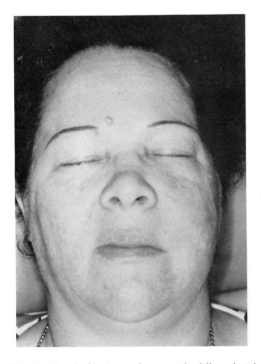

FIG. 8–48.   Cushing's syndrome with diffuse facial edema.

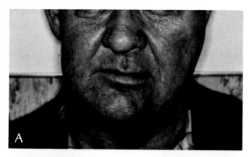

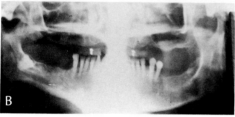

FIG. 8–49. Facial hemihypertrophy. *A:* Unilateral enlargement of the maxilla and mandible. *B:* Panorex shows osseous asymmetry.

Microscopic Features: The affected tissues do not show any histopathologic changes.

Differential Diagnosis: The history of long-standing facial asymmetry helps to limit the differential diagnosis. Facial hemihypertrophy must be differentiated from fibrous dysplasia and other osseous enlargements. This can be accomplished by obtaining radiographs, since no radiologic changes in osseous trabeculation occur in facial hemihypertrophy.

Treatment: The disease is self-limiting but is certainly a cosmetic dilemma. Cosmetic surgical osseous contouring may be performed, with plastic surgical correction for the soft tissue enlargement.

References

1. Ward, J. and Lerner, H. H.: A review of the subject of congenital hemihypertrophy and a complete case report. J. Pediatr. *31:*403, 1947.
2. Gorlin, R. J. and Meskin, L. H.: Congenital hemihypertrophy. J. Pediatr. *61:*870, 1962.
3. Ringrose, J. T., Jabbour, J. T., and Keels, D. K.: Hemihypertrophy. Pediatrics *36:*434, 1965.
4. Kirks, D. R. and Shackeford, G. D.: Idiopathic hemihypertrophy with associated ipsilateral benign nephromegaly. Radiology *115:*145, 1975.
5. Burchfield, D. and Escobar, V.: Familial facial asymmetry (autosomal dominant hemihypertrophy?). Oral Surg. *50:*321, 1980.

Fibrous Dysplasia and Other Bone Lesions

Age: Children and young adults
Sex: No predilection

Clinical Features: Diffuse facial swellings not related to soft tissue enlargement are included here for the sake of differential diagnosis because their clinical appearance may simulate the other entities included in this section. Any central lesion of the jaws that induces cortical expansion can distort the facial contour, producing enlargement and asymmetry. Fibrous dysplasia of bone is one of the more frequent diseases to appear in such a fashion. The maxilla is more often affected than the mandible. The swelling is usually obvious over the malar eminence, zygoma, or lateroinferior orbital rim. The other features of fibrous dysplasia are discussed in the chapter on radiopaque lesions of the jaws. Neoplasms of mesenchymal or odontogenic origin often cause bony expansion and facial enlargement. These specific neoplasms are also described in detail in subsequent chapters, which categorize lesions on the basis of radiographic characteristics.

Microscopic Features: The microscopic features vary according to the specific disease actually represented. Refer to the chapters on radiolucent and radiopaque lesions in which descriptions of fibro-osseous lesions and central jaw neoplasms are presented.

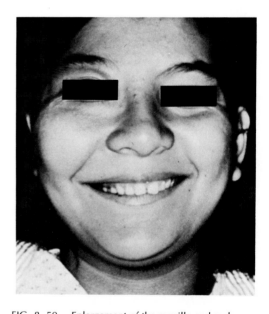

FIG. 8–50. Enlargement of the maxilla and malar eminence in fibrous dysplasia of bone. (Courtesy of Drs. R. Hecker and H. Kramer.)

Differential Diagnosis: Osseous enlargements are differentiated from one another on the basis of clinical, radiologic, and microscopic features. Osseous enlargements may simulate other diffuse facial swellings included here. By merely palpating the area, the clinician can determine the osseous nature of the enlargement and essentially rule out enlargements of soft tissue origin.

Treatment: The treatment varies considerably, based upon the final diagnosis.

References

1. Gardner, A. F. and Halpert, L.: Fibrous dysplasia of the skull with special reference to the oral regions. Dent. Prac. Dent. Rec. *13*:337, 1963.
2. Lewin, M. L.: Nonmalignant maxillofacial tumors in children. Plast. Reconstr. Surg. *38*:186, 1966.
3. Schmaman, A., Smith, I., and Ackerman, L. V.: Benign fibro-osseous lesions of the mandible and maxilla; A review of 35 cases. Cancer *26*:303, 1971.
4. Waldron, C. A. and Giansanti, J. S.: Benign fibro-osseous lesions of the jaws: a clinical-radiologic-histologic review of sixty-five cases. I. Fibrous dysplasia of the jaws. Oral Surg. *35*:190, 1973.

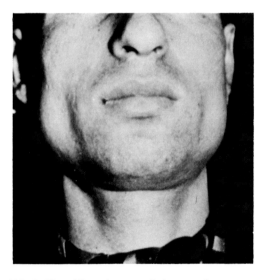

FIG. 8–51.   Bilateral masseteric hypertrophy.

Masseteric Hypertrophy

Age: Onset in young adulthood
Sex: No predilection

Clinical Features: Bilateral swellings located over the ascending ramus of the mandible characterize benign muscular hypertrophy of the masseters. The enlargement may be confused with parotid disease; however, if the patient is asked to clench his teeth, the enlargements increase in size and become firm as the result of muscular contraction. Pain is not a feature. The cause for this condition is not always apparent. Some instances appear to represent congenital disease, whereas others may be related to physiologic hypertrophy of muscle fibers from overuse of the jaws, as in bruxism.

Microscopic Features: Normal skeletal muscle fibers are present; some may show enlarged diameters.

Differential Diagnosis: The bilateral distribution differentiates masseteric hypertrophy from other facial swellings such as cellulitis, emphysema, or facial hemihypertrophy. Since the location is such that parotid disease may be confused with this entity, such disorders as Sjögren's syndrome, Mikulicz's disease, and Heerfordt's syndrome should be considered in the differential diagnosis. These can generally be eliminated on the basis of other clinical findings (a lack of xerostomia and increase in induration upon clenching), which are features of masseteric hypertrophy.

Treatment: No treatment is necessary.

References

1. Lash, H.: Benign masseteric hypertrophy. Surg. Clin. North Am. *43*:1357, 1963.
2. Bloem, J. J. and Van Hoof, R. F.: Hypertrophy of the masseter muscles. Plast. Reconstr. Surg. *47*:138, 1971.
3. Ginwalla, M. S. N.: Bilateral benign hypertrophy of the masseter muscle. J. Oral Surg. *19*:482, 1971.
4. Wade, W. M. and Roy, E. W.: Idiopathic masseter muscle hypertrophy: report of cases. J. Oral Surg. *29*:196, 1971.
5. Buchner, A., David, R., and Temkin, D.: Unilateral enlargement of the masseter muscle. Int. J. Oral Surg. *8*:140, 1979.

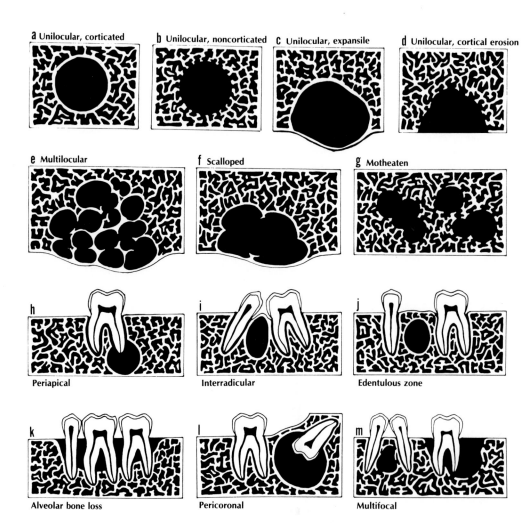

a Unilocular, corticated

b Unilocular, noncorticated

c Unilocular, expansile

d Unilocular, cortical erosion

e Multilocular

f Scalloped

g Motheaten

h Periapical

i Interradicular

j Edentulous zone

k Alveolar bone loss

l Pericoronal

m Multifocal

Radiolucent Lesions

9
Radiolucent Lesions of the Jaws

PERIAPICAL RADIOLUCENCIES

Apical Periodontitis
Periapical Cemental Dysplasia
Focal Sclerosing Osteomyelitis
Benign Cementoblastoma
Incisive Canal Cyst
Median Mandibular Cyst
Traumatic Cyst
Static Bone Cyst
Sublingual Gland Depression
Central Giant Cell Granuloma

INTER-RADICULAR RADIOLUCENCIES

Lateral Periodontal Cyst
Residual Cyst
Odontogenic Keratocyst
Primordial Cyst
Calcifying and Keratinizing Epithelial Odontogenic
   Cyst
Globulomaxillary Cyst
Surgical Ciliated Cyst
Osteoporotic Bone Marrow Defect
Central Ossifying Fibroma

PERIODONTAL (ALVEOLAR) BONE LOSS

Chronic Periodontitis
Diabetic Periodontitis
Periodontosis and Papillon-Lefevre Syndrome
Vanishing Bone Disease
Histiocytosis X
Cyclic Neutropenia
Squamous Odontogenic Tumor
Leukemia

WIDENED PERIODONTAL LIGAMENT SPACE

Periodontic/Endodontic Inflammation
Scleroderma
Osteogenic Sarcoma

PERICORONAL RADIOLUCENCIES

Dentigerous Cyst
Odontogenic Keratocyst
Cystogenic Ameloblastoma
Calcifying Epithelial Odontogenic Tumor
Odontogenic Adenomatoid Tumor
Ameloblastic Fibroma

Odontogenic Fibroma
Central Mucoepidermoid Carcinoma

MULTILOCULAR RADIOLUCENCIES

Odontogenic Keratocyst
Botryoid Odontogenic Cyst
Cherubism
Central Giant Cell Granuloma
Aneurysmal Bone Cyst
Hyperparathyroidism
Ameloblastoma
Myxoma
Odontogenic Fibroma*
Central Neurogenic Neoplasms
Central Arteriovenous Malformation
Pseudotumor of Hemophilia
Central Fibromatosis
Fibrous Dysplasia

MOTH-EATEN RADIOLUCENCIES

Osteomyelitis
Primary Intraosseous Carcinoma
Cystogenic Carcinoma
Metastatic Carcinoma
Osteosarcoma and Chondrosarcoma
Ewing's Sarcoma
Primary Lymphoma of Bone
Burkitt's Lymphoma
Fibrogenic and Neurogenic Sarcoma
Melanotic Neuroectodermal Tumor of Infancy

MULTIFOCAL RADIOLUCENCIES

Basal Cell Nevus Syndrome
Histiocytosis X
Multiple Myeloma
Cherubism†
Periapical Cemental Dysplasia‡

GENERALIZED OSTEOPOROTIC LESIONS

Osteomalacia
Senile Osteoporosis
Steroid Osteoporosis
Sickle Cell Anemia
Thalassemia Major

---

*See Pericoronal Radiolucencies.
†See Multiocular Radiolucencies.
‡See Periapical Radiolucencies.

The diseases that affect the osseous marrow and cortex of the jaw bones are included both in this chapter and in the succeeding chapter dealing with radiopaque lesions. Central lesions of the jaws may manifest signs and symptoms such as pain, discomfort, paresthesia, and swelling, or they may be discovered serendipitously when full-mouth radiographs or panographic surveys are procured.

It should be stressed from the onset that a definitive diagnosis can rarely be secured on the basis of radiologic features alone; a thorough case history and a bone biopsy will be required in most instances. The radiolucent lesions are grouped according to location and configuration. It is axiomatic that this categorization is not all-inclusive; the entities listed in a given category are not always represented by the radiographic headings under which they are listed. Rather, the diseases have been placed under a given pattern heading because it is that particular configuration that the disease most often assumes.

Some generalizations can be put forward with regard to radiolucent lesions of the jaws. A unilocular radiolucency with well-demarcated boundaries or cortication is usually indicative of a benign, slow-growing process. Radiolucencies with ill-defined or irregular margins may be either benign or malignant.

Radiolucencies surrounding the crown of a tooth are, as a rule, cystic or neoplastic lesions of odontogenic origin. Multilocular radiolucencies with well-defined margins frequently show cortical expansion. Lesions with this configuration are generally benign yet aggressive reactive or neoplastic disorders. When evaluating unilocular radiolucencies, one should remember that those diseases categorized as *multilocular radiolucencies* must initially appear as unilocular lesions, with or without expansion depending upon the size of the growth.

Since arteriovenous malformations are radiolucent, surgical biopsy should not be performed on radiolucent lesions of the jaws before needle aspiration of the defect is attempted.

The most common periapical radiolucency is apical periodontitis secondary to pulp necrosis. Periapical cemental dysplasia and traumatic cyst are less common yet are by no means rare. The lateral periodontal cyst and odontogenic keratocyst are the most common inter-radicular radiolucent lesions.

Alveolar bone loss is the hallmark of periodontal disease and is seen in nearly half of the adult population. Nevertheless, the clinician should be aware of the fact that many life-threatening diseases (diabetes, histiocytosis X, leukemia, and malignant neoplasms) can manifest identical radiographic features.

The most common multilocular radiolucencies are the odontogenic keratocyst, central giant cell granuloma, and ameloblastoma. Central arteriovenous malformations are potentially lethal if traumatized or tampered with surgically. Osteomyelitis is the most common disease showing a moth-eaten pattern. A variety of sarcomas and metastatic carcinoma show similar radiologic features; however, these malignancies, as opposed to osteomyelitis, are represented by expansion of the cortical plates.

The most common multifocal radiolucency is periapical cemental dysplasia; this is included among the periapical radiolucencies. The acute disseminated form of histiocytosis X and multiple myeloma, both manifesting multiple radiolucent lesions, are potentially lethal diseases. Generalized rarefaction or osteoporotic lesions involving the entire skeleton will usually exhibit jawbone changes. Senile osteoporosis is the most common condition, while the genetic hemolytic anemias are potentially, yet rarely, lethal.

PERIAPICAL RADIOLUCENCIES

Apical Periodontitis (Abscess, Granuloma, and Cyst)

Age: Adults
Sex: No predilection
Clinical and Radiographic Features: Inflammatory lesions of bone resulting from apical progression of dental pulp inflammation evolve subsequent to dental caries or trauma to the teeth. Radiographically the lesions are usually well circumscribed and are located directly below the apex of the involved teeth. If the source of infec-

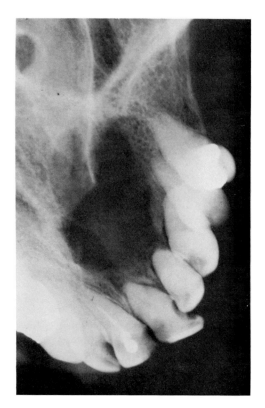

FIG. 9–1. Large apical periodontal cyst associated with a nonvital lateral incisor.

tion emanates from an accessory root canal, the radiolucency may be laterally displaced. Any tooth with a carious pulp exposure can develop periapical disease; however, incisors and first molars are most frequently involved. Radiographically, abscesses, granulomas, or cysts present the same features and cannot be differentiated without microscopic examination. Acute periapical abscess is accompanied by severe pain which often interferes with sleep. Pain on percussion is a feature. Granulomas and cysts may be asymptomatic or associated with a dull ache or occasionally, severe pain. If the periapical lesion resolves with treatment yet is not replaced by bone, a residual periapical fibrous scar may persist. Even after extraction of the necrotic tooth, a through-and-through fibrous defect may persist and be radiographically demonstrable as an ill-defined radiolucency. Infection may spread, with intraoral fistulation and parulis formation. Infected maxillary teeth may drain into the maxillary sinus, into tissues of the face, producing a cellulitis, or, rarely, inflammation may spread via the facial

veins and progress to cavernous sinus thrombosis. Mandibular teeth may drain buccally, causing space infections or Ludwig's angina, which, if left untreated, may progress into the parapharyngeal spaces and ultimately into the mediastinum. This in turn may be fatal, since constriction is caused by edema of the airway.

Microscopic Features: Periapical abscess shows loose areolar granulation tissue and diffuse sheets of neutrophils with scattered macrophages. Granulomas are composed of fibrous and granulation tissue with a diffuse or patchy subacute or chronic inflammatory cell infiltrate. The apical periodontal cyst is lined by nonkeratinizing squamous epithelium, often fragmented and with elongated anastomosing rete ridges. Hyaline bodies are often present within the spinous layer. Transmigration of neutrophils into the spinous cell layer is common. The fibrous and granulation tissue wall is infiltrated with inflammatory cells and often contains cholesterol clefts.

Differential Diagnosis: Apical periodontitis may be radiographically identical to immature periapical cemental dysplasia, focal condensing osteitis, benign cementoblastoma, and traumatic cyst. The presence of deep carious lesions or a history of a traumatic episode implicates an infectious or inflammatory lesion of pulpal origin. The diagnosis is confirmed by a negative response to vitalometer testing. Many other primary cysts and tumors of the jaws will often lie in juxtaposition to tooth roots; however, the teeth are vital.

Treatment: Teeth with periapical inflammation are nonvital and require endodontic therapy or extraction. Should the periapical radiolucency fail to resolve within 6 to 12 months, apical curettage with apicoectomy is indicated.

References

1. Bhaskar, S. N.: Periapical lesions—types, incidence, and clinical features. Oral Surg. 21:657, 1966.
2. Lalonde, E. R. and Luebke, R. G.: The frequency and distribution of periapical cysts and granulomas, an evaluation of 800 specimens. Oral Surg. 25:861, 1968.
3. Lineberg, W. B., Waldron, C. A., and Delanne, G. F.: A clinical, roentgenographic and histopathologic evaluation of periapical lesions. Oral Surg. 17:467, 1972.
4. Patterson, S. S. and Hillis, P. D.: Scar tissue associated with the apices of pulpless teeth prior to endodontic therapy. Oral Surg. 33:450, 1972.
5. Brynolf, I.: Radiography of the periapical region as a diagnostic aid. I. Diagnosis of marginal changes. Dent. Radiogr. Photogr. 51:21, 1978.

Periapical Cemental Dysplasia

Age: Middle-aged adults
Sex: Female predilection

Clinical and Radiographic Features: More common among Negroes than Caucasians, periapical cemental dysplasia or cementoma appears radiographically as a nonexpansile radiolucency in its early or immature stage. The lesion may be single or multiple and is considerably more common in the anterior mandible. Incisors and premolars are more often associated with the periapical radiolucencies, and periapical cemental dysplasia does not involve molar teeth unless multiple lesions are present. The radiolucency is usually but not invariably circumscribed and located subjacent to an intact apical periodontal ligament space. The overlying teeth are vital, clinical evidence of expansion is lacking, and pain is not a feature. The etiology is unknown.

Microscopic Features: The early stage of periapical cemental dysplasia is characterized by the presence of hypercellular fibrous tissue with irregular, small osseous trabeculae or curvilinear cemental trabeculae. Droplet calcifications are frequently observed.

Differential Diagnosis: Periapical cemental dysplasia can be differentiated from apical periodontitis on the basis of vitalometer testing, as the pulp is vital in the former disease. Focal condensing osteitis and cementoblastoma are usually associated with molars rather than with anterior teeth.

Treatment: Nonexpansile periapical radiolucencies associated with vital anterior teeth are clinically considered to represent periapical cemental dysplasia. No treatment is required. The patient should be recalled for periodic radiographic evaluation, to assure that the lesion follows the usual progression into mature stages with opacification. If the lesion progressively enlarges or causes expansion, it probably represents another disease and biopsy is indicated.

References

1. Chaudhry, A. P., et al.: Periapical fibrous dysplasia (cementoma). J. Oral Surg. 16:483, 1958.
2. Zegarelli, E. V., et al.: The cementoma, a study of 230 patients with 435 cementomas. Oral Surg. 17:219, 1964.
3. Hamner, J. E., Scofield, H. J., and Cornyn, J.: Benign fibroosseous jaw lesions of periodontal membrane origin. Cancer 22:861, 1968.
4. Krausen, A. S., et al.: Cementomas—aggressive or innocuous neoplasms? Arch. Otolaryngol. 103:349, 1977.

Focal Sclerosing Osteomyelitis

Age: Teenagers and young adults
Sex: No predilection

Clinical and Radiographic Features: Whereas focal sclerosing osteomyelitis is most often observed as a radiopaque lesion, it may evolve from a radiolucent stage, which becomes progressively opacified. This rare form is characterized by a well-circumscribed periapical radiolucency in association with a carious mandibular molar. The caries are usually deep, and the crown may appear gutted. The pulp from the overlying tooth is vital with a chronic inflammatory cell infiltrate (i.e.,

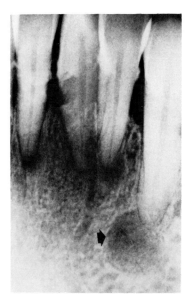

FIG. 9–2. Small periapical radiolucencies at the apices of the incisors and a larger one below the cuspid representing periapical cemental dysplasia.

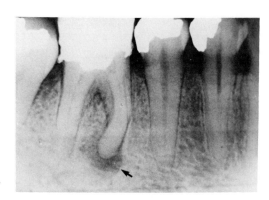

FIG. 9–3. Focal sclerosing osteomyelitis beginning as a radiolucent lesion in early stages.

chronic pulpitis). The area may be asymptomatic or a dull ache may be present. Response to vital-ometer testing is often altered; however, the over-lying tooth rarely tests nonvital since the pulp is inflamed rather than necrotic.

Microscopic Features: Hypercellular or mod-erately cellular fibrous connective tissue is stippled with small, irregular osseous trabeculae that are usually rimmed by osteoblasts. Curvilinear ce-mental trabeculae and ovoid calcifications may also be seen. The pulp from the overlying tooth is vital, with a chronic inflammatory cell infiltrate.

Differential Diagnosis: Focal osteitis is most frequently confused with periapical cemental dys-plasia. The two can be differentiated on clinical grounds. Focal osteitis arises in association with posterior teeth with a large carious lesion, whereas periapical cemental dysplasia involves noncarious vital anterior teeth. Benign cementoblastoma may show similar features in the radiolucent stage. This lesion is not associated with caries and pulpitis. In addition, cortical expansion is a feature of ce-mentoblastoma but is rarely seen in focal osteitis. The microscopic appearance may be indistin-guishable from that of other fibro-osseous lesions of the jaws, so that the diagnosis depends upon clinical features.

Treatment: Since the pulp is inflamed and may progress into an acute phase, with ultimate ne-crosis, endodontic therapy is indicated.

References
1. Eversole, L. R., Sabes, W. R., and Rovin, S.: Fibrous dysplasia: a nosologic problem in the diagnosis of fibro-osseous lesions of the jaws. J. Oral Pathol. *1*:189, 1972.
2. Fireman, S. M.: Osteosclerotic lesions of the jaws. Oral Health 66:27, 1976.

Benign Cementoblastoma

Age: Teenagers and young adults
Sex: No predilection

Clinical and Radiographic Features: A true neoplasm of cementoblastic origin, the benign ce-mentoblastoma is seen to arise in association with tooth roots. Molar teeth, particularly the mandib-ular first molar, are the predominant sites for this lesion, usually encountered in a radiopaque stage. Early lesions may be radiolucent. They are well circumscribed and envelop one or both roots, usu-ally extending midway up the root surface. They are well demarcated and may be totally lucent or contain calcific flecks. Expansion of the buccal and/or lingual cortical plates occurs and, if of sig-nificant magnitude, may be demonstrated on oc-

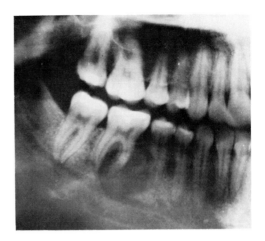

FIG. 9–4. Benign cementoblastoma in the early im-mature stage. (From Eversole, L. R., et al.: Benign ce-mentoblastoma. Oral Surg. 36:824, 1973.)

clusal radiographs. The tooth tests vital, pain is not a feature, and a dull, ankylosed sound is pro-duced when the tooth is percussed.

Microscopic Features: Linear-radiating trabec-ulae of osseous tissue are dispersed throughout a fibrous marrow and are intimately associated with and fused to the root cementum. These trabeculae generally show polarization patterns more con-sistent with osseous tissue than with cementum; rimming by osteoblasts is a prominent feature.

Differential Diagnosis: Cementoblastoma in its immature radiolucent stage must be differentiated from focal sclerosing osteomyelitis, apical perio-dontitis, and periapical cemental dysplasia. These latter entities do not produce an ankylosed sound when percussed and fail to expand the cortical plates. Periapical cemental dysplasia involves an-terior teeth, whereas cementoblastoma arises from the root area of posterior teeth.

Treatment: A vital posterior tooth with an ex-pansive periapical radiolucency probably repre-sents cementoblastoma in its early stage. Surgical exploration with biopsy is advisable. If a gritty or cartilage-like tissue is encountered during surgery and appears to be fused to the root surface, the tooth and accompanying fused tumor mass should be excised in toto. If left untreated, the lesion may progressively enlarge and expand the encasing bone.

References
1. Eversole, L. R., Sabes, W. R., and Dauchess, V. G.: Benign cementoblastoma. Oral Surg. 36:824, 1973.
2. Cherrick, H. M., et al.: Benign cementoblastoma;

a clinicopathologic evaluation. Oral Surg. *37*:54, 1974.

3. Corio, R. L., et al.: Benign cementoblastoma. Oral Surg. *41*:524, 1976.

4. Farman, A. G., et al.: Cementoblastoma: report of case. J. Oral Surg. *37*:198, 1979.

Incisive Canal Cyst

Age: Adults

Sex: No predilection

Clinical and Radiographic Features: The incisive canal cyst is a developmental nonodontogenic cyst derived from embryonic epithelial remnants of the nasopalatine duct or incisive canal. It is a well-delineated oval or heart-shaped radiolucency located between and apical to the two maxillary central incisors directly in the midline. It rarely causes facial expansion, yet palatal swelling is common. Occasionally, the incisors will evince root resorption. The cyst is asymptomatic and the teeth test vital. It is sometimes difficult to ascertain radiographically whether or not the radiolucency is truly pathologic or merely represents a large incisive foramen. Cystic unilocular lesions of the palatal midline (median palatal cyst) may represent true fissural cysts from epithelial entrapment of the fusing secondary palatal processes. Alternatively, these lesions may represent posterior extension of an incisive canal cyst.

Microscopic Features: The cyst may be lined

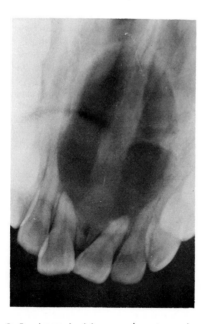

FIG. 9–5.   Large incisive canal cyst causing root divergence.

by stratified squamous epithelium, respiratory epithelium, or both. When respiratory epithelium is present, mucous goblet cells may be seen. The fibrous wall characteristically is traversed by large neurovascular bundles.

Differential Diagnosis: A midline radiolucency of the maxilla almost invariably represents incisive canal cyst. Rarely, lateral periodontal cysts, primordial cysts, and odontogenic keratocysts arise in this location.

Treatment: When a radiologic diagnosis of incisive canal cyst is made, treatment may consist of surgical enucleation or periodic radiographic follow-up. Progressive enlargement warrants surgical intervention.

References

1. Stafne, E. C., et al.: Median anterior maxillary cysts. J. Am. Dent. Assoc. *23*:801, 1936.

2. Abrams, A. M., et al.: Nasopalatine cysts. Oral Surg. *16*:306, 1963.

3. Schiff, B. A., Kringstein, G., and Stoopack, J. C.: An extremely large and facially distorting nasopalatine duct cyst. Oral Surg. *27*:590, 1969.

4. Campbell, J. J., Baden, E., and Williams, A. C.: Nasopalatine cyst of unusual size: report of case. J. Oral Surg. *31*:776, 1973.

5. Taintor, J. F. and Fahid, A.: Case report: median palatine cyst. Dent. Survey *53*:33, 1977.

Median Mandibular Cyst

Age: Adults

Sex: No known predilection

Clinical and Radiographic Features: The median mandibular cyst is theoretically a fissural cyst that evolves from entrapped epithelial remnants enclaved in the mandibular symphysis region subsequent to fusion of the mandibular processes. Some authors dispute this theory and ascribe the cystic lesion to various other pathogenetic derivations from odontogenic sources (i.e., primordial cyst from a supernumerary bud, lateral periodontal cyst, odontogenic keratocyst). It appears as a unilocular, often expansile radiolucency underlying vital mandibular incisors.

Microscopic Features: Some cases represent odontogenic keratocyst. Others are lined by nonkeratinizing stratified squamous epithelium, whereas others have been reported with a respiratory lining. This feature does not necessarily support a fissural origin, since other odontogenic cysts may exhibit respiratory metaplasia. Furthermore, this region does not typically harbor respiratory epithelium during the embryonic morphogenetic period.

Differential Diagnosis: Traumatic cyst may

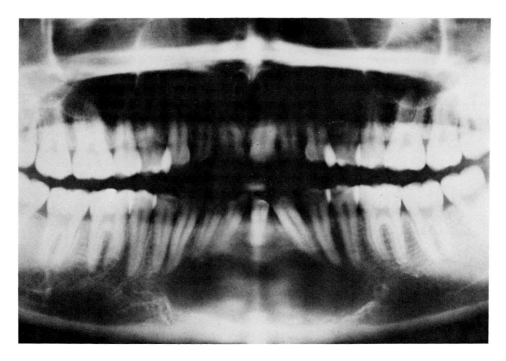

FIG. 9–6. Median mandibular cyst underlying vital teeth.

occur in this location, yet rarely expands bone. Likewise, the sublingual salivary gland depression, also nonexpansile, is characterized by a radiolucency in the anterior mandible. Apical cysts and granulomas can be ruled out when pulp vitality is documented.

Treatment: Surgical enucleation or curettage is the treatment of choice.

References

1. Blair, A. E. and Wadsworth, W.: Median mandibular developmental cyst. J. Oral Surg. 26:735, 1968.
2. Tilson, H. B. and Bauerle, J. E.: Median mandibular cyst: report of case. J. Oral Surg. 28:519, 1970.
3. Albers, D. D.: Median mandibular cyst partially lined with pseudostratified columnar epithelium. Oral Surg. 36:11, 1973.
4. Buchner, A. and Ramon, Y.: Median mandibular cyst—a rare lesion of debatable origin. Oral Surg. 37:431, 1974.
5. Soskolne, W. A. and Sheteyer, A.: Median mandibular cyst. Oral Surg. 44:84, 1977.

Traumatic (Hemorrhagic) Cyst

Age: Young adults

Sex: Slight male predilection

Clinical and Radiographic Features: The traumatic cyst does not represent a true epithelial cyst; rather, it is an empty or fluid-filled cavity of bone

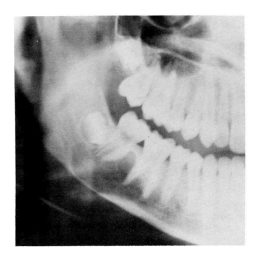

FIG. 9–7. Traumatic or hemorrhagic bone cyst appearing as a periapical radiolucency. The overlying molars tested vital.

lined with a fibrous or granulation tissue membrane. The term *traumatic* was used to implicate trauma as a causative factor; however, less than half of the instances are associated with any significant trauma to the jaw. The etiology remains unknown. Clinically, pain and expansion are unusual. The lesion is located most often in the body or anterior portion of the mandible, and radiographically it is radiolucent. A classic feature is its tendency to scallop between the tooth roots. Portions of the cystic lesion are well demarcated from the neighboring bone, whereas in other areas the margins are ill defined. The teeth that overlie the lesion test vital.

Microscopic Features: When biopsy is attempted, an empty space in the medullary bone is encountered. A thin membrane may line the cavity and is characterized microscopically by the presence of fibrous granulation tissue that usually shows mild to moderate inflammation.

Differential Diagnosis: Traumatic cysts must be differentiated from apical periodontitis on the basis of vitality testing. The teeth overlying traumatic cysts are vital. Since these lesions may be extensive and show peripheral scalloping, they could be mistaken for one of the lesions included as multilocular radiolucencies, e.g., keratocyst, central giant cell granuloma, and certain odontogenic tumors. These lesions are usually expansile, whereas traumatic cysts generally do not expand the cortex. Aspiration of a traumatic cyst may be negative or yield a blood-tinged fluid.

Treatment: Following aspiration, the area should be entered surgically. A portion of the lining membrane should be made to induce hemorrhage into the bone cavity. The clot organizes, ossifies, and remodels within 6 to 12 months.

References

1. Howe, G. L.: "Haemorrhagic cysts" of the mandible. Br. J. Oral Surg. 3:55, 1965.
2. Hansen, L. S., Sapone, J., and Sproat, R. C.: Traumatic bone cysts of the jaws. Oral Surg. 37:899, 1974.
3. Winer, R. A. and Doku, H. C.: Traumatic bone cyst in the maxilla. Oral Surg. 46:367, 1978.
4. Davis, W. M., Buchs, A. V., and Davis, W. M.: Extravasation cyst diagnostic curettement: a treatment. Report of 15 cases and suggested treatment. Oral Surg. 47:2, 1979.

Static Bone Cyst

Age: Onset in childhood
Sex: Female predilection

Clinical and Radiographic Features: The static bone cyst or submandibular salivary gland depression is usually discovered coincidentally on dental roentgenograms since no symptoms are associated with this benign developmental process. The lesion is a well-circumscribed corticated oval radiolucency situated periapical to the second or third mandibular molar. The defect is not in con-tinuity with root tips; rather, it is located below the inferior alveolar canal. It is often bilateral. The lesion reflects a lingual depression of the cortical plate in which normal salivary gland tissue rests. A sialogram may be obtained and will disclose the presence of ductal elements converging in the region of the radiolucent defect.

Microscopic Features: The contents of salivary depressions consist of normal submandibular salivary tissue, depending on the site of involvement.

Differential Diagnosis: The localization of submandibular gland depressions below the alveolar canal in the absence of expansion or pain is characteristic, allowing for a radiologic diagnosis.

Treatment: No treatment is required. Periodic radiographic follow-up is recommended to ensure that no growth is taking place.

References

1. Stafne, E. C.: Bone cavities situated near the angle of the mandible. J. Am. Dent. Assoc. 29:1969, 1942.
2. Choukas, N.C.: Developmental submandibular gland defect of the mandible. J. Oral Surg. 31:209, 1973.
3. Oikarinen, V. J., Wolf, J., and Julku, M.: A stereosialographic study of developmental mandibular bone defects (Stafne's idiopathic bone cavities). Int. J. Oral Surg. 4:51, 1975.

Sublingual Gland Depression

Age: Onset in childhood
Sex: No known predilection

Clinical and Radiographic Features: The sublingual glands may reside within a lingual bone depression, similar to the static bone cyst in relation to the submandibular glands. The lesion lies apical to the anterior mandibular teeth and is a well-circumscribed unilocular radiolucency. Bilateral defects may be witnessed. The lucent foci may show progressive enlargement, which arrests in the teenage years. There is no evidence of cortical expansion.

Microscopic Features: A biopsy will disclose the presence of normal-appearing sublingual gland tissue.

Differential Diagnosis: The teeth are vital, and periapical cemental dysplasia may be considered. Usually the radiolucent area encompasses the apical one-third of the root. There is no racial predilection. Because the disease is rare, an exploratory biopsy is usually performed to rule out some other disease process that may coincide in this location. In a youngster with no clinical evidence of expansion, sublingual gland depression should

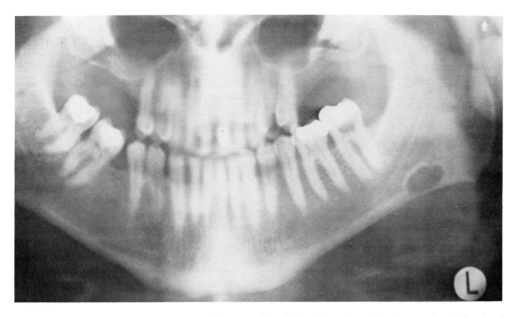

FIG. 9–8.   Unilocular, well-circumscribed radiolucency lying below the inferior alveolar canal and allowing for differentiation of the static bone cyst from periapical lesions in direct continuity with tooth roots.

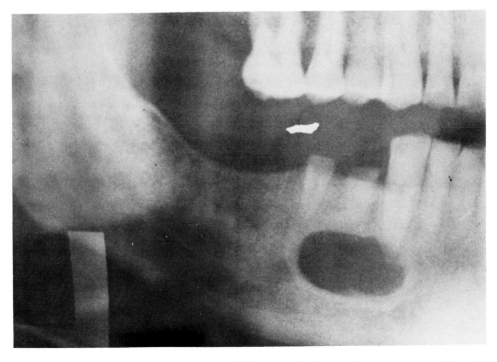

FIG. 9–9.   Periapical radiolucency underlying mandibular cuspid and premolars representing sublingual gland depression.

be considered; a lingual surgical approach can be used for exploratory purposes.

Treatment: Once a definitive diagnosis has been obtained by exploration and/or biopsy, no treatment is necessary.

References

1. Friedman, J.: Ectopic sublingual glands. Oral Surg. *18*:219, 1964.
2. Stene, T. and Pedersen, K. N.: Aberrant salivary gland tissue in the anterior mandible. Oral Surg. *44*:72, 1977.

Central Giant Cell Granuloma

Age: Young adults
Sex: Female predilection

Clinical and Radiographic Features: Central giant cell granuloma is a neoplastic-like reactive proliferation of the jaws that usually exhibits a multilocular pattern as observed radiographically. Early smaller lesions are usually unilocular and frequently lie apical to vital teeth. The lesion is more common in the mandible than in the maxilla underlying anterior or premolar teeth. Buccal or lingual cortical expansion can often be detected both clinically and radiographically; expansile lesions can cause root divergence or resorption.

Microscopic Features: Multinucleated giant

cells, dispersed throughout a hypercellular fibro-vascular stroma, possess randomly arranged nuclei that are either pyknotic and hyperchromatic or oval and stippled with prominent nucleoli. Erythrocyte engorgement of vessels and extravascular hemosiderin pigment are frequently observed as are occasional osseous trabeculae.

Differential Diagnosis: The overlying teeth are generally vital, a feature that eliminates apical periodontitis. When expansion is present most of the other lesions listed here can be eliminated with exception of cementoblastoma, which is rarely encountered in the incisor-premolar region. Other neoplastic processes and keratocysts can coincidentally arise in periapical location and expand bone. Biopsy is required to make the diagnosis.

Treatment: Thorough curettage is the treatment of choice. When the diagnosis has been established, appropriate laboratory tests should be performed to rule out brown tumor of hyperparathyroidism.

References

1. Austin, L. T., Jr., Dahlin, D. C., and Royer, R. A.: Giant-cell reparative granuloma and related conditions affecting the jawbones. Oral Surg. *12*:1285, 1959.
2. Waldron, C. A. and Shafer, W. G.: The central giant cell reparative granuloma of the jaws; an analysis of 38 cases. Am. J. Clin. Pathol. *45*:437, 1966.

INTER-RADICULAR RADIOLUCENCIES

Lateral Periodontal Cyst

Age: Adults
Sex: Slight female predilection

Clinical and Radiographic Features: The lateral periodontal cyst may arise from epithelial rests in

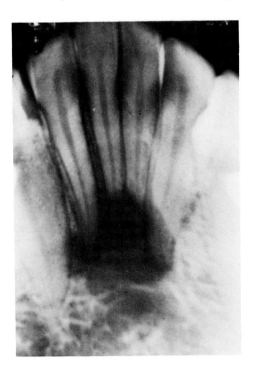

FIG. 9–10.   Central giant cell granuloma appearing as a periapical radiolucency with root resorption.

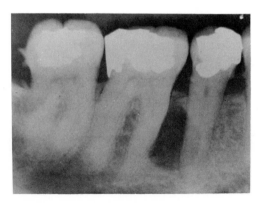

FIG. 9–11.   Lateral periodontal cyst interposed between two vital mandibular teeth.

the periodontal ligament or may represent a primordial cyst originating from a supernumerary tooth bud. The fact that this cyst is most frequently encountered in the mandibular premolar region, a common location for supernumerary teeth, lends credence to this latter hypothesis. Radiographically, the lateral periodontal cyst is an interradicular radiolucency with well-defined or corticated margins. The adjacent teeth usually show some degree of root divergence, and they are vital when evaluated with an electric pulp tester. The buccal cortical plate may or may not show moderate bulging when examined clinically. Pain is not a feature.

Microscopic Features: The cyst lining is either nonkeratinizing stratified squamous or stratified cuboidal epithelium that shows a tendency for convolution and irregularity. The fibrous wall manifests minimal inflammation.

Differential Diagnosis: Lateral periodontal cyst may be differentiated from a laterally displaced apical periodontal cyst on the basis of vitalometer testing since the former arise developmentally, having no relationship to pulpal disease. The radiographic features may be identical to those of keratocyst, primordial cyst, globulomaxillary cyst, incisive canal cyst, and calcifying epithelial odontogenic (Gorlin) cyst. Biopsy is required to differentiate among most of these entities.

Treatment: Surgical enucleation or curettage with preservation of adjoining teeth is the treatment of choice.

References

1. Standish, S. M. and Shafer, W. G.: The lateral periodontal cyst. J. Periodontol. 29:27, 1958.
2. Moskow, B. S., et al.: Gingival and lateral periodontal cysts. J. Periodontol. 41:9, 1970.
3. Fantasia, J. E.: Lateral periodontal cyst. Oral Surg. 48:237, 1979.
4. Wysocki, G. P., et al.: Histogenesis of the lateral periodontal cyst and the gingival cyst of the adult. Oral Surg. 50:327, 1980.

Residual Cyst

Age: Adults

Sex: Male predilection

Clinical and Radiographic Features: A residual cyst is any type of odontogenic cyst that persists in bone after the tooth with which it was associated has been removed. Therefore, a residual cyst may represent an apical periodontal cyst if a necrotic tooth overlying the lesion was extracted, or it may represent a dentigerous cyst if an impacted tooth was removed. Radiographically, the lesion is a

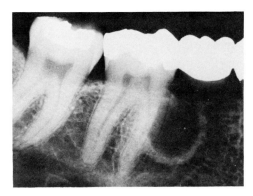

FIG. 9–12. Residual periapical cyst located in a site previously occupied by a carious nonvital tooth.

well-circumscribed, often corticated radiolucency located in an edentulous region once occupied by a tooth.

Microscopic Features: Residual cysts are lined by noncornified stratified squamous epithelium that may contain hyaline bodies within the spinous cell layer. The fibrous wall generally shows an inflammatory cell infiltrate.

Differential Diagnosis: The residual cyst is easily confused radiographically with primordial cyst. The latter arises in lieu of a tooth, whereas the former arises in relation to an extracted tooth. Residual cyst may also be confused radiographically with keratocyst, lateral periodontal cyst, and calcifying epithelial odontogenic cyst. Biopsy is required to arrive at a definitive diagnosis.

Treatment: Surgical enucleation or curettage is the treatment of choice.

References

1. Ahlstrom, U., Johnson, C. C., and Lautz, B.: Radicular and residual cysts of the jaws: a long term roentgenographic study following cystectomies. Odontol. Rev. 20:11, 1969
2. Cabrini, R. L., Barros, R. E., and Albano, H.: Cysts of the jaws: a statistical analysis. J. Oral Surg. 28:485, 1970.

Odontogenic Keratocyst

Age: Adults

Sex: No predilection

Clinical and Radiographic Features: The odontogenic keratocyst is a specific form of odontogenic cyst that is microscopically distinct. It may assume the character of any of the odontogenic cysts and therefore may represent a keratinizing variant of the lateral periodontal cyst. Radiographically, when inter-radicular it is a well-marginated radiolucency with a propensity for root divergence

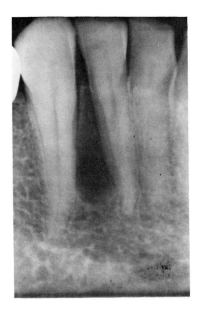

FIG. 9–13.   Inter-radicular radiolucency with mild root divergence, representing an odontogenic keratocyst.

and cortical expansion. It is not found in relation to nonvital teeth; pain is not a symptom. When multiple keratocysts of the jaws are observed, the nevoid basal cell carcinoma syndrome should be investigated.

Microscopic Features: The lumen is often filled with desquamated keratin. The lining, stratified squamous epithelium, possesses a corrugated parakeratin layer, an attenuated spinous cell layer, and a polarized basal cell layer. In general, the fibrous wall is free from inflammation.

Differential Diagnosis: Lateral odontogenic keratocyst must be differentiated by biopsy from lateral periodontal cyst, primordial cyst, residual cyst, globulomaxillary cyst, incisive canal cyst, and calcifying epithelial odontogenic cyst. In addition, the odontogenic adenomatoid tumor and any of those lesions classified with the multilocular radiolucencies may begin as unilocular radiolucencies in an inter-radicular location.

Treatment: Surgical enucleation is indicated. At surgery, the keratocyst is represented by a thin delicate membrane. Small cysts have a low recurrence rate, probably under 20 percent, whereas large expansile lesions commonly recur following curettage.

References
1. Hansen, J.: Keratocysts in the jaws. In *Second International Conference on Oral Surgery.* Copenhagen, Munksgaard, 1967, pp. 128–134.
2. Browne, R. M.: The odontogenic keratocyst. Br. Dent. J. *128*:225, 1970.
3. Brannon, R. B.: The odontogenic keratocyst. A clinicopathologic study of 312 cases. Part I. Clinical features. Oral Surg. *42*:54, 1976.
4. Brannon, R. B.: The odontogenic keratocyst: a clinicopathologic study of 312 cases. II. Histologic features. Oral Surg. *43*:233, 1977.
5. Wright, J. M.: The odontogenic keratocyst: orthokeratinized variant. Oral Surg. *51*:609,1981.

Primordial Cyst

Age: Onset in young adulthood
Sex: No predilection

Clinical and Radiographic Features: Primordial cysts arise from a developing tooth that fails to differentiate; rather, the odontogenic epithelium becomes cystic prior to the formation of dental hard tissues. Radiographically, the primordial cyst is unilocular, radiolucent, and well demarcated. The lesion is inter-radicular or adjacent to teeth and is always present in an area where a tooth would normally have developed. The most common locations are third molar regions and the midline of the maxilla, apparently from the tooth germ of a mesiodens.

Microscopic Features: Primordial cysts are lined by stratified squamous epithelium, and most of them represent keratocysts. The fibrous wall usually lacks an inflammatory cell infiltrate.

Differential Diagnosis: The primordial cyst may be radiographically differentiated from the residual cyst because the former arises in lieu of a tooth, whereas the latter is seen after tooth extraction. The primordial cyst must also be differentiated from lateral periodontal cyst and calcifying epithelial odontogenic cyst.

Treatment: Surgical enucleation is the treatment of choice.

References
1. Robinson, H. B. G.: Classification of cysts of the jaws. Am. J. Orthod. Oral Surg. *31*:370, 1945.
2. Shear, M.: Primordial cysts. J. Dent. Assoc. S. Afr. *15*:211, 1960.
3. Soskolne, W. A. and Shear, M.: Observations on the pathogenesis of primordial cysts. Br. Dent. J. *123*:321, 1967.
4. Forssell, K., Kallioniemi, H., and Sainio, P.: Microcysts and epithelial islands in primordial cysts. Proc. Finn. Dent. Soc. *75*:99, 1979.

Calcifying and Keratinizing Epithelial Odontogenic Cyst

Age: No predilection
Sex: No predilection

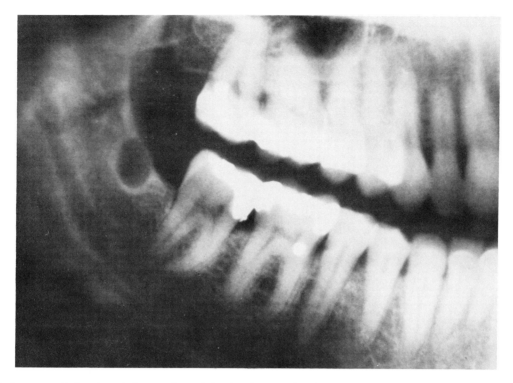

FIG. 9–14. Unilocular radiolucency located distal to the second molar representing a primordial cyst.

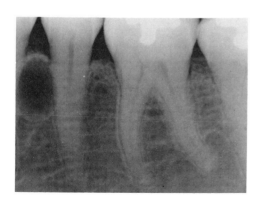

FIG. 9–15. The calcifying epithelial odontogenic cyst is usually a well-circumscribed radiolucency located in the premolar region.

Clinical and Radiographic Features: The calcifying and keratinizing epithelial odontogenic cyst, or Gorlin cyst, arises most often in the premolar region of the mandible, appearing as a well-demarcated unilocular radiolucency located interproximally. The lesion may be entirely radiolucent or may contain radiopaque calcific flecks. Divergence of the juxtaposed roots is a common finding. Nearly one-fourth of these cysts are located pe-ripheral to bone on the attached gingiva. The teeth test vital, and pain is not a feature.

Microscopic Features: The lining epithelium shows distinct pathognomonic features. The basal cell layer is polarized, assuming the posture of ameloblasts. The spinous cell layer resembles that of stratified squamous epithelium or may acquire the features of stellate reticulum. Melanin pigment has been reported to occur in these lesions. The spinous cells undergo keratinization toward the luminal surface; large eosinophilic cells with vacuoles replacing nuclei are apparent, termed *ghost cells.* An eosinophilic dentinoid material is often found within the fibrous wall in juxtaposition to the basal cells. Occasionally, the epithelium proliferates along the differentiated lines just enumerated yet fails to form a true cyst. Many Gorlin cysts are therefore benign neoplastic proliferations rather than true cysts.

Differential Diagnosis: Calcifying epithelial odontogenic cysts in the entirely radiolucent stage may be confused radiographically with lateral periodontal cyst, odontogenic keratocyst, primordial cyst, residual cyst, or one of the nonodontogenic developmental cysts if located in specific areas in which confusion may occur. Apical periodontal cysts arising from a necrotic lateral pulp canal can be ruled out on the basis of vitalometry.

Treatment: Surgical excision or curettage is the treatment of choice. Recurrence is rare.

References

1. Abrams, A. M. and Howell, F. W.: The calcifying odontogenic cyst. Oral Surg. 25:594, 1968
2. Gorlin,R. J., et al.: The calcifying odontogenic cyst—a possible analogue of the cutaneous calcifying epithelioma of Malherbe. Oral Surg. 15:1235, 1962.
3. Freedman, P. D., Lumerman, H., and Gee, J. K.: Calcifying odontogenic cysts: A review and analysis of seventy cases. Oral Surg. 40:93, 1975.
4. Altini, M. and Farman, A. G.: The calcifying odontogenic cyst: Eight new cases and a review of the literature. Oral Surg. 40:751,1975.
5. Soames, J. V.: A pigmented calcifying odontogenic cyst. Oral Surg. 53:395, 1982.

Globulomaxillary Cyst

Age: Young adults
Sex: No predilection

Clinical and Radiographic Features: The globulomaxillary cyst is believed to develop from epithelium that becomes enclosed at the time of fusion of the fissure, separating the globular portion of the maxillary process from the median nasal

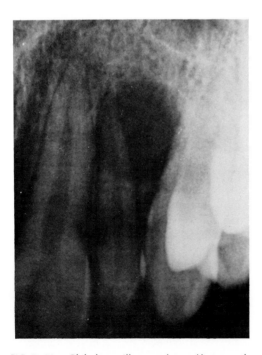

FIG. 9–16.   Globulomaxillary cyst located between the maxillary lateral incisor and cuspid.

process. Since embryologic processes do not fuse per se, it has been suggested that this cyst is not a true fissural cyst but perhaps represents an odontogenic cyst. Regardless of its origin, the globulomaxillary cyst is characteristically located between the maxillary lateral incisor and cuspid, manifesting a unilocular radiolucency that is usually, but not invariably, well circumscribed. Root divergence is a constant finding.

Microscopic Features: The cyst lining is usually composed of stratified squamous epithelium. Respiratory epithelium may be present as well. The fibrous wall is generally devoid of inflammation.

Differential Diagnosis: Globulomaxillary cyst may be confused radiographically with a laterally displaced apical periodontal cyst. The latter can be eliminated when the teeth test vital. Odontogenic keratocyst, lateral periodontal cyst, and calcifying epithelial odontogenic cyst should be considered in the differential diagnosis. Certain odontogenic tumors, the odontogenic adenomatoid tumor in particular, should also be included, based upon location and radiography. Aspiration will usually yield a straw-colored fluid if the lesion represents a cyst. Biopsy is required to arrive at a definitive diagnosis.

Treatment: Surgical enucleation should be performed because the cyst enlarges slowly yet progressively, causing displacement of teeth. Recurrence is unusual, provided the entire cyst is removed.

References

1. Ferenczy, K.: The relationship of globulomaxillary cysts to the fusion of embryonal processes and to cleft palate. Oral Surg. 11:1388, 1958.
2. Christ, T. F.: The globulomaxillary cyst: an embryologic misconception. Oral Surg. 30:515, 1970.
3. Little, J. W. and Jakobsen, J.: Origin of the globulomaxillary cyst. J. Oral Surg. 31:188, 1973.
4. Taicher, S. and Azaz, B.: Lesions resembling globulomaxillary cysts. Oral Surg. 44:25, 1977.
5. Wysocki, G. P.: The differential diagnosis of globulomaxillary radiolucencies. Oral Surg. 51:281, 1981.

Surgical Ciliated Cyst

Age: Adults
Sex: Male predilection

Clinical and Radiographic Features: Following a Caldwell-Luc operation, fragments of sinus epithelial lining may become entrapped in the maxillary surgical site. If this epithelium undergoes benign cystic proliferation, a unilocular well-delineated radiolucency will become discernible in the maxilla. The lesion lies within the alveolar

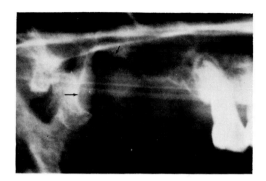

FIG. 9–17. Well-circumscribed radiolucency in the tuberosity subsequent to a Caldwell-Luc procedure, typical for surgical ciliated cysts.

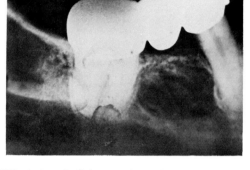

FIG. 9–18. Radiolucency in previous extraction site representing an osteoporotic bone marrow defect. (Courtesy of Dr. H. M. Cherrick.)

bone subjacent to the antral floor and is generally confined to an edentulous or inter-radicular area in the posterior maxilla. Pain or discomfort may be present.

Microscopic Features: The cyst is lined by pseudostratified columnar ciliated epithelium. The connective tissue wall may display an inflammatory cell infiltrate.

Differential Diagnosis: By virtue of its location, the surgical ciliated cyst may radiographically resemble an apical periodontal cyst, residual odontogenic cyst, or low sinus extension. A history of previous sinus surgery coupled with biopsy will allow for a definitive diagnosis.

Treatment. Surgical enucleation is the treatment of choice.

References

1. Gregory, G. T. and Shafer, W. G.: Surgical ciliated cysts of the maxilla: report of cases. J. Oral Surg. 16:251, 1958.
2. Shafer, W. G., Hine, M. K., and Levy, B. M.: A Textbook of Oral Pathology, 4th Ed. Philadelphia, W. B. Saunders Co., 1983, p. 545.
3. Kaneshiro, S., et al.: The postoperative maxillary cyst: report of 71 cases. J. Oral Surg. 39:191, 1981.

Osteoporotic Bone Marrow Defect

Age: Middle-aged adults

Sex: Female predilection

Clinical and Radiographic Features: Following tooth extraction, the socket may heal by formation of hematopoietic marrow rather than cancellous bone. This results in a radiolucency located in the edentulous region previously occupied by a tooth. The radiolucency characteristically shows ill-defined ragged margins that blend into the normal adjacent cancellous bone. Cortical expansion does not occur, and pain is not a feature.

Microscopic Features: Adipose tissue is seen with multiple foci of hematopoietic blast cells of myeloid, erythroid, lymphoid, and megakaryocytic cell lines. Thin osseous trabeculae are also encountered.

Differential Diagnosis: A nonexpansile poorly marginated radiolucency in an edentulous or interproximal area is probably an osteoporotic bone marrow defect. The other inter-radicular radiolucencies listed in this chapter show well-defined borders. Other nonexpansile poorly demarcated radiolucencies include multiple myeloma, histiocytosis X, and metastatic cancer. For this reason, even though suspicion is high for bone marrow defect, a biopsy should be performed.

Treatment: Once the diagnosis has been confirmed by biopsy, no further treatment is needed.

References

1. Standish, S. M. and Shafer, W. G.: Focal osteoporotic bone marrow defects of the jaws. J. Oral Surg. 20:123, 1962.
2. Crawford, B. E. and Weathers, D. R.: Osteoporotic marrow defects of the jaws. J. Oral Surg. 28:600, 1970.

Central Ossifying (Cementifying) Fibroma

Age: Children and young adults

Sex: Female predilection

Clinical and Radiographic Features: Ossifying fibroma of bone is a neoplasm representing one of the benign fibro-osseous lesions of the jaws. When the tumor synthesizes cementum rather than osteoid, the lesion is referred to as a cementifying fibroma. Clinically, the lesion manifests as a painless enlargement with cortical expansion, and the mandible is affected far more frequently than the maxilla. Radiographically, the lesion is unilocular, although multilocular patterns are also

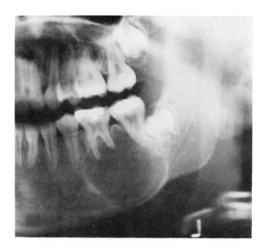

FIG. 9–19. Radiolucency with expansion of inferior border of mandible extending between molar roots, representing a central ossifying fibroma. (Courtesy of Dr. C. Parks.)

encountered. Expansion with clearly demarcated borders is typical; in the mandible, a smooth bowing expansion of the inferior border is commonly observed. The lesion usually extends between teeth and causes root divergence. In the early growth stage, the lesion may appear entirely radiolucent; with time, the center becomes progressively radiopaque as more calcified product is elaborated. If left untreated, the tumor may reach massive proportions and result in marked facial disfigurement.

Microscopic Features: A highly cellular fibroblastic stroma prevails, with the presence of delicate collagen fibers. Capillaries course throughout this stroma, and foci of osteoid trabeculae are observed. In radiolucent lesions, the fibrous element is predominant and the osteoid matrix is poorly calcified. When ovoid or curvilinear trabeculae prevail and show polarization patterns consistent with cementum, then the lesion is differentiating along periodontal ligament progenitor cell lines. These cementifying patterns are more often seen in Negro than white patients.

Differential Diagnosis: Ossifying and cementifying fibromas in the early radiolucent stage must be differentiated from various cysts appearing as inter-radicular radiolucencies and from other fibro-osseous and central neoplasms included in the section on multilocular radiolucencies, since any of those lesions may begin as a unilocular radiolucency. Differentiation from fibrous dysplasia is not difficult when microscopic and radio-

logic features are considered together. Fibrous dysplasia evinces poorly demarcated borders radiographically, whereas ossifying and cementifying fibromas show well-marginated borders.

Treatment: Surgical enucleation is rarely followed by recurrence. Nevertheless, aggressive behavior is encountered, and some cases manifest multiple recurrences. In these instances, en bloc resection may be required to eradicate the disease.

References

1. Waldron, C. A.: Fibro-osseous lesions of the jaws. J. Oral Surg. *28*:58, 1970.
2. Eversole, L. R., Sabes, W. R. and Rovin, S.: Fibrous dysplasia: A nosologic problem in the diagnosis of fibro-osseous lesions of the jaws. J. Oral Pathol. *1*:189, 1972.
3. Waldron, C. A. and Giansanti, J. S.: Benign fibro-osseous lesions of the jaws: A clinical-radiologic-histologic review of sixty-five cases. Part II. Benign fibro-osseous lesions of periodontal ligament origin. Oral Surg. *35*:340, 1973.
4. Carlisle, J. E. and Hammer, W. B.: Giant central ossifying fibroma of the mandible: report of case. J. Oral Surg. *37*:206, 1979.
5. Walter, J. M., Jr., et al.: Aggressive ossifying fibroma of the maxilla: review of the literature and report of case. J. Oral Surg. *37*:276, 1979.

PERIODONTAL (ALVEOLAR) BONE LOSS

Chronic Periodontitis

Age: Middle-aged adults

Sex: No predilection

Clinical and Radiographic Features: The most common cause of alveolar bone loss, as evidenced radiographically, is chronic periodontitis. Indeed, it is the most common oral disease of adulthood. Whereas overt manifestations are encountered during middle age, early features of the disease are often apparent in teenagers and young adults. Periodontal pockets in excess of 3 mm are indicative of early periodontitis. Radiographically, the alveolar bone evinces either a uniform apical migration (horizontal bone loss) or multifocal sharply demarcated trenching (vertical bone loss). The earliest stage is a V-shaped wedge seen on the alveolar process in the interproximal region. The gingiva may be edematous and hyperemic. Itching is often a symptom; however, the disease may become severe without any symptoms of pain. The precise etiology is unknown, but the severity of inflammation and bone loss is proportional to the amount of accumulated plaque and calculus.

Microscopic Features: The crevicular epithelium lacks a cornified layer and shows elongation of rete ridges with transmigration of neutrophils

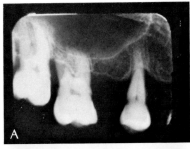

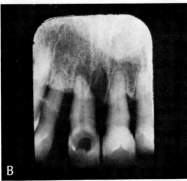

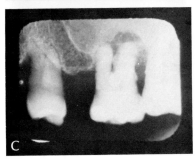

FIG. 9–20.   Alveolar bone loss in chronic periodontitis.

into the spinous layer. The subjacent fibrous and granulation tissues are avidly infiltrated with plasma cells and lymphocytes.

Differential Diagnosis: Rapid alveolar bone loss may occur in conjunction with juvenile diabetes, cyclic neutropenia, histiocytosis X, and leukemia. These diseases should be strongly considered in the differential diagnosis of alveolar bone loss in young adults and teenagers. Periodontosis must be included in the differential diagnosis yet shows a specific distribution of bone loss.

Treatment: Prevention is the key to control of periodontal disease. This is accomplished by instituting periodic dental prophylaxis in conjunction with daily toothbrushing and flossing. Diets low in refined sugar and carbohydrate also aid in minimizing plaque accumulation. Once alveolar

bone loss with pocket formation develops, root planing, curettage, or periodontal surgery is indicated.

References

1. Marshall-Day, C. D., Stephens, R. G., and Quigley, L. F. Jr.: Periodontal disease; prevalence and incidence. J. Periodontol. 26:185, 1955.
2. Goldman, H. M. and Cohen, D. W.: The infrabony pocket: classification and treatment. J. Periodontol. 29:272,1958.
3. Theilade, J.: An evaluation of the reliability of radiographs in the measurement of bone loss in periodontal disease. J. Periodont. 31:143, 1960.
4. Prichard, J. F.: The role of the roentgenogram in the diagnosis and prognosis of periodontal disease. Oral Surg. 14:182, 1961.
5. Sheridan, P. J. and Reeve, C. M.: Periodontal Disease. In Oral Roentgenographic Diagnosis, edited by E. C. Stafne and J. A. Gibilisco. Philadelphia, W. B. Saunders Co., 1975, ch. 8.

Diabetic Periodontitis

Age: Young and middle-aged adults

Sex   No predilection

Clinical and Radiographic Features: Nonspecific chronic periodontitis develops at an early age in diabetics, particularly in those with hyperglycemia of childhood onset. As a result of microangiopathic lesions throughout the body, including the periodontium, in conjunction with deficient fibroblastic energy metabolism due to decreased intracellular glucose utilization, wound healing is impaired. Periodontal disease progresses rapidly with widespread horizontal or vertical alveolar bone loss. Multiple foci of periodontal abscess formation often accompany the chronic disease process. Diabetes accompanied by premature periodontal disease is usually overt, and patients show elevated fasting blood glucose and glycosuria.

Microscopic Features: The microscopic features of diabetic periodontitis are the same as those described for uncomplicated chronic periodontitis. Occasionally, hyaline arteriolosclerosis can be demonstrated.

Differential Diagnosis: Premature alveolar bone loss is occasionally seen in uncomplicated periodontitis yet is also a feature of periodontosis, histiocytosis X, cyclic neutropenia, and leukemia. When severe or premature bone loss is encountered, a fasting blood glucose test and urinalysis should be performed. If the blood glucose is within normal limits, a 5-hour glucose tolerance test can be performed.

Treatment: Once diabetes is diagnosed, the

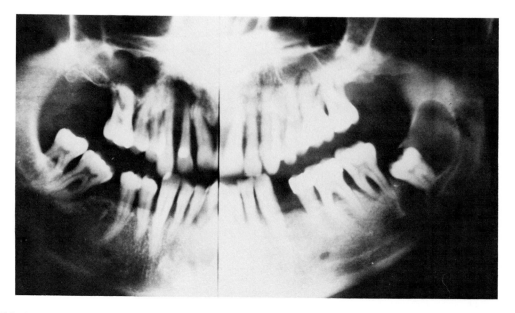

FIG. 9–21.   Premature horizontal and vertical bone loss in a diabetic. Also note coincidental dentigerous cyst around mandibular third molar.

patient requires medication in the form of oral hypoglycemic drugs or parenteral insulin. Referral to a physician is indicated. The periodontal disease should be managed the same as that uncomplicated by diabetes; however, if arteriolar vascular disease is widespread, the prognosis for controlling or preventing continuation of the periodontal lesions is not particularly good.

References

1. McMullen, J. A., et al.: Microangiopathy within gingival tissues of diabetic subjects with special reference to the prediabetic state. Periodontics 5:61,1967.
2. Hirshfeld, I.: Periodontal symptoms associated with diabetes. J. Periodontol. 21:211, 1950.
3. Benvetiste, R., Bixler, D., and Conneally, P. M.: Periodontal disease in diabetics. J. Periodontol. 38:271, 1967.
4. Finestone, A. J. and Boorujy, S. R.: Diabetes mellitus and periodontal disease. Diabetes 16:336, 1967.
5. Bartolucci, E. G. and Parkes, R. B.: Accelerated periodontal breakdown in uncontrolled diabetes. Pathogenesis and treatment. Oral Surg. 52:387, 1981.

Periodontosis and Papillon-Lefevre Syndrome

Age: Childhood onset
Sex: No predilection

Clinical and Radiographic Features: A disease of obscure etiology, periodontosis or juvenile per-

iodontitis represents an inflammatory lesion of the perodontium with the formation of periodontal pockets, loosening of teeth, and rapidly progressive alveolar bone loss. Local factors such as tooth-accumulated material and calculus are not significant etiologically. Immunopathic mechanisms, a granulocyte disorder, and anaerobic bacteria have been implicated as etiologic factors. The subgingival gram negative anaerobic flora is specific and unique to juvenile periodontosis and differs considerably from the flora isolated from the pockets of adult chronic inflammatory periodontal disease. Whether or not these organisms are pathogens and play a causative role is unknown. Radiographically, a classic topography of alveolar osseous recession is encountered. The periodontal tissues around the molars and incisors are selectively lost and replaced by granulation tissue, whereas the cuspids and premolars are spared or involved only to a minimal degree. However, not all instances of childhood-onset periodontal disease manifest this pattern. When this pattern of bone loss is accompanied by hyperkeratosis of the palms and soles, the condition is termed the Papillon-Lefevre syndrome. The disease has an autosomal recessive genetic pattern.

Microscopic Features: Biopsy specimens of pocket tissue show granulation tissue with non-specific chronic inflammation composed chiefly of lymphocytes and plasma cells.

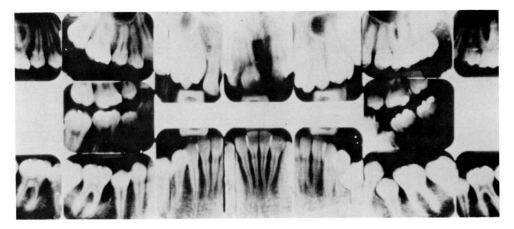

FIG. 9–22. Alveolar bone loss confined to incisor and molar regions in periodontosis. (Courtesy of Dr. W. Hall.)

Differential Diagnosis: Periodontitis, diabetic periodontitis, cyclic neutropenia, histiocytosis X, and leukemia must all be considered in the differential diagnosis. Onset at a young age and classic incisor-molar alveolar bone loss in conjunction with nonspecific chronic inflammation as evidenced microscopically lead to a diagnosis of periodontosis.

Treatment: The dental prognosis is poor. Teeth will lose periodontal support despite efforts directed toward plaque control. The teeth involved in alveolar bone degeneration should be maintained without resorting to heroic surgical procedures; when they are no longer functional, extraction and fabrication of a dental prosthesis are indicated.

References

1. Ingle, J.I.: Papillon-Lefevre syndrome; precocious periodontosis with associated epidermal lesions. J. Periodontol. *30*:230, 1959.
2. Gorlin, R. J., Sedano, H., and Anderson, J. E.: The syndrome of palmar-plantar hyperkeratosis and premature periodontal destruction of the teeth. J. Pediatr. *65*:895, 1964.
3. Newman, M. G. and Socransky, S. S.: Predominant cultivable microbiota in periodontosis. J. Periodont. Res. *12*:120, 1977.
4. Prabhu, S. R., Daftary, D. K., and Dholakia, H. M.: Hyperkeratosis palmoplantaris with periodontosis (Papillon-Lefevre syndrome): report of three cases; two occurring in siblings. J. Oral Surg. *37*:262, 1979.
5. Manouchehr-Pour, M. and Bissada, N.F.: Juvenile periodontitis (periodontosis): A review of the literature. J. West. Soc. Periodontol. *27*:86, 1979.

Vanishing Bone Disease (Massive Osteolysis)

Age: Teenagers and young adults
Sex: No predilection

Clinical and Radiographic Features: Vanishing bone disease (also known as massive osteolysis, phantom bone disease, and Gorham disease) is one of the most enigmatic processes in medicine and dentistry. Entire bones, for no apparent reason, undergo massive resorption until the entire osseous membrane has completely disappeared radiographically, grossly, and histologically. Virtually any bone may be affected by this idiopathic resorptive process, including the jaws. Symptoms are lacking until resorption proceeds to the extent that pathologic fracture becomes a complication. Normal osseous tissues are replaced by fibrous connective tissue. The process pursues a protracted course, with disappearance of the affected bone after many years. Radiographically, the lesions begin as localized, ill-defined osteoporotic foci, which coalesce to yield massive zones of osteolysis with noncorticated borders. The loss of bone may begin at the alveolar crest, with an appearance resembling progressive advanced periodontitis. Often, more than one jaw quadrant is involved. Eventually, the entire mandible, hemimandible, or maxilla may virtually disappear from view radiographically. Serum calcium and phosphorus are within normal limits.

Microscopic Features: Normal osseous trabeculae are present and show foci of resorption. In the resorbed zones, fibrous tissue predominates with proliferation of capillaries. A chronic inflammatory cell infiltrate is often encountered. Pronounced osteoclastic activity is not a feature.

Differential Diagnosis: The radiographic appearance of massive osteolysis may resemble that seen in periodontitis, histiocytosis X, malignancy,

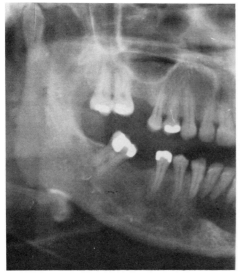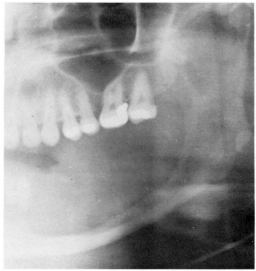

FIG. 9–23. Widespread alveolar bone loss in the absence of tumor or any identifiable etiologic agent, representing massive osteolysis.

and diabetes. The diagnosis is generally made when cultures are negative and the aforementioned entities are excluded on the basis of histologic examination. Thus the diagnosis rests on the process of exclusion. Often long-term follow-up is required before a definitive diagnosis can be rendered.

Treatment: Bone grafts are usually unsuccessful, as they too become involved in the resorptive process. Since the etiology remains unknown, no successful treatment has been realized.

References

1. Gorham, L. W. and Stout, A. P.: Massive osteolysis (acute spontaneous absorptiion of bone, phantom bone, disappearing bone). J. Bone Joint Surg. *37A*:985, 1955.
2. El-Mofty, S.: Atrophy of the mandible (massive osteolysis). Oral Surg. *31*:690, 1971.
3. Cherrick, H. M., King, O. H., Jr., and Dorsey, J. N., Jr.: Massive osteolysis (disappearing bone, phantom bone, acute absorption of bone) of the mandible and maxilla. J. Oral Med. *27*:67, 1972.
4. Phillips, R. M., Bush, O. B., and Hall, D. H.: Massive osteolysis (phantom bone, disappearing bone): report of case with mandibular involvement. Oral Surg. *34*:886, 1972.
5. Murphy, J. B., Doku, H. C., and Carter, B. L.: Massive osteolysis: phantom bone diseae. J. Oral Surg. *36*:318, 1978.

Histiocytosis X (Nonlipid Reticuloendotheliosis)

Age: Children and teenagers
Sex: Male predilection

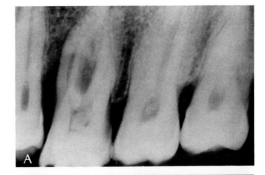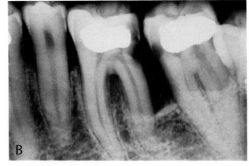

FIG. 9–24. Localized vertical alveolar bone loss in histiocytosis X.

Clinical and Radiographic Features: Histiocytosis X is a disease process with a wide spectrum of severity. The basic pathologic process is a neoplasia-like disorder whereby normal tissues are infiltrated with histiocytes. The younger the patient, the worse the prognosis. Infants show soft tissue histiocytic infiltrates of the skin, spleen, liver, and lymph nodes. This form, known as acute disseminated histiocytosis or Letterer-Siwe disease, is usually fatal. Older children develop the chronic disseminated form, also known as Hand-Schuller-Christian disease. Histiocytic infiltration of the pituitary and retrorbital soft tissue leads to diabetes insipidus and exophthalmos respectively. Intraosseous lesions and otitis media are also features of the chronic disseminated form. The chronic limited form is more common among teenagers and young adults, is restricted to bone, and is termed *eosinophilic granuloma of bone.* Pulmonary infiltration by histiocytes may occur in all three forms and can be detected radiographically. Radiographically, the lesions of histiocytosis X appear as well-demarcated yet noncorticated radiolucencies. Importantly, the lesions often simulate periodontal disease. Multifocal zones of vertical alveolar bone loss are encountered and may actually completely engulf the apices, giving the impression that the involved teeth are floating in space.

Microscopic Features: Bone defects contain diffuse sheets of histiocytes that possess voluminous amphophilic cytoplasm with an oval or kidney-shaped vesicular nucleus. Multinucleated giant cells are often seen; in the chronic forms, foam cells may predominate, yielding a lipogranulomatous picture. Scattered or clustered eosinophils are more numerous in the chronic limited form (eosinophilic granuloma).

Differential Diagnosis: When histiocytosis X manifests multifocal zones of periodontal destruction, periodontitis, diabetic periodontitis, cyclic neutropenia, and leukemia must be considered. Signs and symptoms of extraosseous disease are encountered in the disseminated forms, and biopsy will disclose the characteristic microscopy of histiocytosis X. When the diagnosis has been rendered, a skeletal survey and physical examination should be performed to determine the extent of disease.

Treatment: Teeth may be saved if the osseous lesions are not too extensive. When alveolar bone is resorbed significantly, it will not regenerate after treatment. Treatment of choice is thorough curettage.

References

1. Sedano, H. O., et al.: Histiocytosis X. Oral Surg. 27:760, 1969.
2. Chase, D. C., Eversole, L. R., and Hall, H. D.: Histocytosis X with jaw involvement. J. Oral Surg. 32:494, 1974.
3. Ragab, R. R. and Rake, O.: Eosinophilic granuloma with bilateral involvement of both jaws. Int. J. Oral Surg. 4:73, 1975.
4. Soskolne, W. A., Lustman, J., and Azaz, B.: Histiocytosis X: report of six cases initially in the jaws. J. Oral Surg. 35:30, 1977.
5. Hartmen, K. S.: Histiocytosis X: A review of 114 cases with oral involvement. Oral Surg. 49:38, 1980.

Cyclic Neutropenia

Age: Teenagers and young adults
Sex: No predilection

Clinical and Radiographic Features: Cyclic neutropenia is a blood dyscrasia in which a selective diminution in neutrophilic granulocytes develops on a predictably recurrent periodic basis. The neutrophils disappear from the circulation as

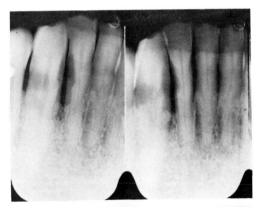

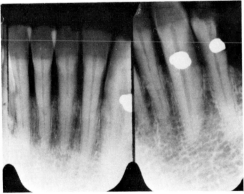

FIG. 9–25. Horizontal alveolar bone loss in cyclic neutropenia.

a result of a bone marrow maturation defect of unknown etiology. The leukocyte count drops for 5 to 7 days at regular 21-day intervals. In the interim, the white and differential counts are virtually normal; however, neutrophils rarely are present in numbers exceeding 50 percent of the total leukocyte population. During neutropenia, ragged oral aphthous-like ulcerations appear; when the white count returns to normal, the ulcers heal. The other chief oral manifestation is premature, or precocious, alveolar bone loss with classic clinical manifestations of periodontitis.

Microscopic Features: Curettage from periodontal pockets shows granulation tissue with a mononuclear inflammatory cell infiltrate. The oral ulcers are notably devoid of neutrophils.

Differential Diagnosis: Precocious periodontal bone loss may be seen in diabetic periodontitis, periodontosis, histiocytosis X, and leukemia as well as in cyclic neutropenia. Regularly recurring ulcerations of the mucosa should arouse suspicion. The diagnosis can be secured by obtaining complete blood counts every 4 days for a 3-week period in order to demonstrate the neutropenic phase.

Treatment: Efforts to control plaque, to institute home-care oral hygiene, and to palliate the oral ulcerations with an antihistamine/Kaopectate oral rinse should be made. The patient should be referred to a hematologist to manage the blood dyscrasia and watch for complications such as recurrent infection.

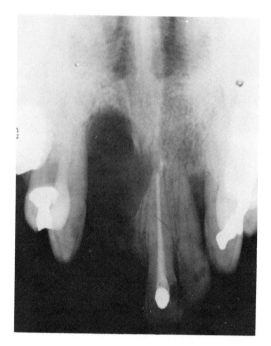

FIG. 9–26.   Periodontal defect in squamous odontogenic tumor. (Courtesy of Dr. A. Jonker.)

References

1. Gorlin, R. J. and Chaudhry, A. P.: The oral manifestations of cyclic (periodic) neutropenia. Arch. Dermatol. *82*:344, 1960.
2. Smith, J. F.: Cyclic neutropenia. Oral Surg. *18*:312, 1964.
3. Gates, G. F.: Chronic neutropenia presenting with oral lesions. Oral Surg. *27*:563, 1969.
4. Binon, P. and Dykema, R.: Rehabilitative management of cyclic neutropenia. J. Prosth. Dent. *31*:52, 1974.
5. Rylander, H. and Ericsson, I.: Manifestations and treatment of periodontal disease in a patient suffering from cyclic neutropenia. J. Clin. Periodontol. *8*:77, 1981.

Squamous Odontogenic Tumor

Age: Young adults

Sex: Female predilection

Clinical and Radiographic Features: Squamous odontogenic tumor is a hamartomatous proliferation of odontogenic epithelium, probably arising from the rests of Malassez. The maxillary incisor-canine area and mandibular molar area are the primary sites of involvement. Whereas most cases are unifocal, multicentric lesions are occasionally witnessed. Tooth mobility is the chief presenting sign; radiographically, a localized radiolucency interposed between contiguous teeth appears as a well-circumscribed periodontal defect. Most cases are either triangular or semicircular in configuration. Some lesions exhibit an intact overlying alveolar crest; most, however, extend coronally with loss of crestal bone.

Microscopic Features: Oval, round, and curvilinear nests of squamous epithelial cells are dispersed throughout a mature collagenous stroma. The basilar stratum fails to show polarization. Cystic degeneration is commonly seen, and some of the squamous nests exhibit ovoid crystalloid structures.

Differential Diagnosis: The radiographic features simulate a localized periodontal defect enveloping roots. Histiocytosis X should also be considered in the differential diagnosis.

Treatment: Most cases fail to recur following extraction of the involved tooth and thorough curettage of the lesional tissue. Maxillary lesions may be more extensive, involving the sinus; resection may be required to prevent recurrence.

References

1. Pullon, P. A., et al.: Squamous odontogenic tumor. Report of six cases of a previously undescribed lesion. Oral Surg. 40:616, 1975.
2. Doyle, J. L., et al.: Squamous odontogenic tumor: Report of three cases. J. Oral Surg. 35:994, 1977.
3. McNeill, J., Price, H. M., and Stoker, N. G.: Squamous odontogenic tumor: Report of case with long-term history. J. Oral Surg. 38:466, 1980.
4. Carr, R. F., Calton, D. M., Jr., and Marks, R. B.: Squamous odontogenic tumor: Report of case. J. Oral Surg. 39:297, 1981.
5. Goldblatt, L. I., Brannon, R. B., and Ellis, G. L.: Squamous odontogenic tumor. Report of five cases and review of the literature. Oral Surg. 54:187, 1982.

Leukemia

Age: Childhood and adult forms
Sex: No predilection

Clinical and Radiographic Features: Leukemias are classified according to the leukocyte blast cell of origin. The more common forms are myelogenous (granulocyte precursors) and lymphocytic. Furthermore, both acute and chronic forms exist. The former pursues a rapid, often fatal course; however, cures can be achieved with combination drug chemotherapy. The chief clinical signs and symptoms include malaise, low-grade fever, pallor, and dyspnea. Gingival hemorrhage, petechiae, and ecchymoses develop when the platelet count drops subsequent to bone marrow replacement by malignant leukocytes. Gingival enlargement is a feature, with boggy erythematous swellings beginning in the interdental papilla area; these oral manifestations do not often occur, however. Nevertheless, it is important to recognize the fact that leukemic infiltration may involve the periodontium, producing a radiographic picture not unlike that of periodontal disease with vertical pocket formation.

Microscopic Features: Curettage or an incisional biopsy will disclose the presence of diffuse sheets of poorly differentiated leukocyte blast cells. Regardless of whether the leukemia is myeloid, erythroid, or lymphoid, the blast cells are mononuclear and usually monomorphic. Zones of necrosis may be encountered.

Differential Diagnosis. Radiographic evidence of alveolar bone loss in leukemia may be identical to that seen in nonspecific periodontitis, diabetic periodontitis, periodontosis, histiocytosis X, or cyclic neutropenia. Other symptoms, such as fatigue, malaise, petechia, ecchymosis, and gingival hemorrhage, warrant workup for leukemia. A complete blood count should be obtained.

Treatment: Chemotherapeutic control should be instituted as soon as possible by an oncologist or hematologist. Oral lesions will respond to systemic medications used for control of leukemia.

References

1. Burket, L. W.: A histopathologic explanation for the oral lesions in acute leukemias. Am. J. Orthod. Oral Surg. 30:516, 1944.
2. Curtis, A. B.: Childhood leukemias: osseous changes in jaws on panoramic dental radiographs. J. Am. Dent. Assoc. 83:844, 1971.
3. Segelman, A. E. and Doku, H. C.: Treatment of the oral complications of leukemia. J. Oral Surg. 35:469, 1977.
4. Michand, M., et al.: Oral manifestations of acute leukemia in children. J. Am. Dent. Assoc. 95:1145, 1977.
5. Bressman, E., et al.: Acute myeloblastic leukemia with oral manifestations: Report of a case. Oral Surg. 54:401, 1982.

WIDENED PERIODONTAL LIGAMENT SPACE

Periodontic/Endodontic Inflammation

Age: Adults
Sex: No predilection

Clinical and Radiographic Features: Infection of periodontal origin may spread down the entire periodontal ligament, producing a localized widening of the periodontal ligament space. This may be circumradicular or localized to only the mesial or only the distal root region. The periodontal defect can be probed and will often induce exudation through the gingival sulcus. The infection can progress through lateral accessory canals or proceed in retrograde fashion through the apical for-

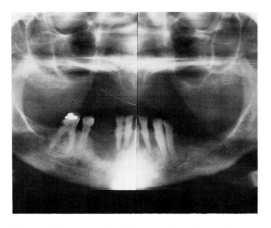

FIG. 9–27. Leukemic infiltrate with advanced periodontal bone loss in the anterior mandible.

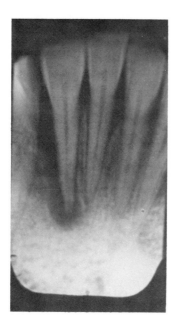

FIG. 9–28. Widened PDL space involving nonvital lateral incisor representing combined periodontic-endodontic inflammation.

amen to initiate pulp necrosis. Alternatively, pulpal infection may progress both apically and laterally via accessory canals to involve the lateral periodontal ligament, and the infection may spread coronally with sulcular drainage.

Microscopic Features: Tissue removed from the widened periodontal ligament is granulation tissue, usually exhibiting a subacute inflammatory cell infiltrate.

Differential Diagnosis: The localized widening of the periodontal ligament space in endodontic/periodontic infection may radiographically resemble incipient osteogenic sarcoma. Periodontal probing and pulp vitality testing will usually allow for a clinical diagnosis. More advanced cases may radiographically resemble histiocytosis X. When no exudate appears after probing or when the defect resists insertion of the periodontal probe, a biopsy should be procured.

Treatment: Advanced cases with pulp necrosis and excessive mobility usually require extraction. In some instances, endodontic therapy with splinting to adjacent teeth will be successful, thus avoiding extraction.

References

1. Seltzer, S., Bender, I. B., and Ziontz, M.: The interrelationship of pulp and periodontal disease. Oral Surg. *16*:1474, 1963.

2. Rubach, W. C. and Mitchell, D. F.: Periodontal disease, accessory canals, and pulp pathosis. J. Periodontol. *36*:34, 1965.

Scleroderma

Age: Middle-aged adults
Sex: Female predilection

Clinical and Radiographic Features: The systemic form of scleroderma is a collagen-immune disease affecting fibrous tissues of the dermis, submucosa of the gastrointestinal tract, and various internal organs. The skin becomes stiff and board-like, losing its flexibility. This change is most obvious on the face, which becomes wrinkle-free and expressionless. As the disease progresses, virtually all body surfaces become involved. The periodontium is affected in a limited number of instances. The crestal alveolar bone is not compromised; rather, a uniform generalized widening of the periodontal ligament space is observed. A pronounced notching of the inferior border of the mandible just anterior to the angle region is also a feature in scleroderma and resorption of the mandibular condyle has been reported to occur.

Microscopic Features: The periodontal ligament contains dense collagen fibers not unlike those seen in the normal ligament.

Differential Diagnosis: Uniform widening of the periodontal ligament space is seen when a tooth is in severe traumatic occlusion or partially avulsed or, rarely, in periodontitis. If the condition is localized to one or two teeth, early osteogenic sarcoma must be considered in the differential diagnosis. When uniform widening involves the entire dentition, the classic skin changes of scleroderma are invariably encountered.

Treatment: The involved teeth are generally secure and not prone to exfoliation. The disease

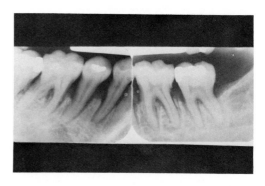

FIG. 9–29. Generalized widening of PDL spaces in scleroderma.

is treated with steroids or immunosuppressive drugs and should be managed by a dermatologist.

References

1. Stafne, E. C. and Austin, L. T.: Characteristic dental findings in acrosclerosis and diffuse scleroderma. Am. J. Orthod. Oral Surg. *30*:25, 1944.
2. Green, D.: Scleroderma and its oral manifestations. Oral Surg. *15*:1313, 1962.
3. White, S. C., et al.: Oral radiographic changes in patients with progressive systemic sclerosis (scleroderma). J. Am. Dent. Assoc. *94*:1178, 1977.
4. Caplan, H. I. and Benny, R. A.: Total osteolysis of the mandibular condyle in progressive systemic sclerosis. Oral Surg. *46*:362, 1978.
5. Marmary, Y., Glaiss, R., and Pisanty, S.: Scleroderma: Oral manifestations. Oral Surg. *52*:32, 1981.

Osteogenic Sarcoma

Age: Adults
Sex: Slight male predilection

Clinical and Radiographic Features: Primary osteogenic sarcoma of the jaws may manifest a variety of radiographic alterations ranging from radiolucent to radiopaque. It is included in this section because of its tendency to manifest localized symmetrical widening of the periodontal ligament space when the lesion is incipient. At this stage, mild cortical expansion may be observed.

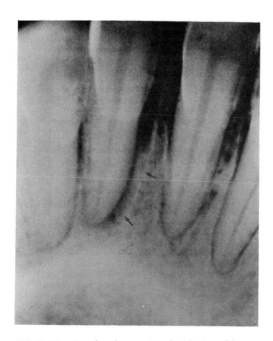

FIG. 9–30. Localized symmetrical widening of the periodontal ligament space in a patient with incipient osteogenic sarcoma. (Courtesy of Dr. B. A. Levy.)

The medullary bone adjacent to the widened ligament spaces may be normal or show a ragged moth-eaten pattern. There is usually no pain.

Microscopic Features: Osteogenic sarcoma may be predominantly fibroblastic, chondroblastic, or osteoblastic. The cellular elements display hypercellularity, hyperchromatism and pleomorphism. Osteoid is elaborated in irregular fashion and is profusely endowed with lacunar spaces containing pleomorphic nuclei. The trabecular are similarly rimmed by angular malignant osteoblasts. When cartilage is present, lacunae are numerous and often encase multiple nuclei.

Differential Diagnosis: Localized widening of the periodontal ligament space should always arouse suspicion of osteogenic sarcoma. Similar changes are seen in localized traumatic occlusion and traumatically avulsed teeth. When clinical features of these latter two conditions are not apparent, biopsy is indicated.

Treatment: Osteogenic sarcoma requires resection of the jaw, hemimandibulectomy, or partial maxillectomy and should be managed by a head and neck tumor surgeon. Metastases are usually hematogenous; nodal spread is uncommon. The 5-year survival is less than 35 percent.

References

1. Kragh, L. V., Dahlin, D. C., and Erich, J. B.: Osteogenic sarcoma of the jaws and facial bones. Am. J. Surg. 96:496, 1958.
2. Garrington, G. E., et al.: Osteosarcoma of the jaws. Cancer 20:377, 1967.
3. Gardner, D. G. and Mills, D. M.: The widened periodontal ligament of osteosarcoma of the jaws. Oral Surg. *41*:652, 1976.
4. Russ, J. E. and Jesse, R. H.: Management of osteosarcoma of the maxilla and mandible. Am. J. Surg. *140*:572, 1980.

PERICORONAL RADIOLUCENCIES

Dentigerous Cyst

Age: Young adults
Sex: No predilection

Clinical and Radiographic Features: The follicular or dentigerous cyst is the most common type of developmental odontogenic cyst. By definition it is a cystic lesion derived from the reduced enamel epithelium encompassing the crown of an impacted tooth. The pericoronal radiolucency is typically well demarcated and may be extensive. The third molars and cuspids are most frequently involved. Cortical expansion and multilocularity may occasionally occur with simple dentigerous cysts; however, these features are more often in-

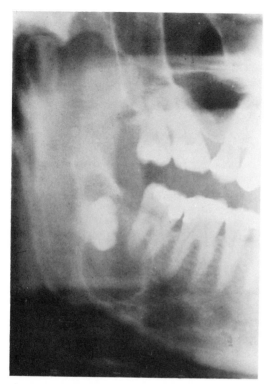

FIG. 9–31.   Dentigerous cyst around third molar.

moved if it cannot be orthodontically erupted, and the cyst should be thoroughly curetted.

References

1. Gorlin, R. J.: Potentialities of oral epithelium manifest by mandibular dentigerous cysts. Oral Surg. *10*:271, 1957.
2. Dachi, S. F. and Howell, F. V.: A survey of 3,874 routine full-mouth radiographs. II. A study of impacted teeth. Oral Surg. *14*:1165, 1961.
3. Mourshed, F.: A roentgenographic study of dentigerous cysts. I. Incidence in a population sample. Oral Surg. *18*:47, 1964.
4. Szerlip, L.: Displaced third molar with dentigerous cyst—an unusual case. J. Oral Surg. *36*:551, 1978.
5. Hettwer, K.J.: Large cyst of the mandible partially lined by ciliated epithelium. J. Oral & Maxillofacial Surg. *40*:185, 1982.

Odontogenic Keratocyst

Age: Adults
Sex: No predilection

Clinical and Radiographic Features: Because of its protean radiographic manifestations, the odontogenic keratocyst is included under many categories in this chapter. Perhaps its most common radiographic presentation is that of a pericoronal radiolucency. The cyst is often encountered when it has reached a size sufficient to

dicative of neoplastic transformation or keratinizing metaplasia within the cyst lining.

Microscopic Features: A lining composed of eosinophilic columnar (reduced enamel) epithelium is encountered in dentigerous cysts removed from younger patients. In older individuals, the lining is composed of stratified squamous epithelium, which is devoid of a cornified layer and fails to display significant rete-ridge formation. Mucous metaplasia, surface cilia, and hyaline bodies are often present within the lining epithelium. The fibrous wall may be devoid of inflammation or may possess a chronic inflammatory cell infiltrate. Varying numbers of oval or elongated odontogenic cell rests are usually seen, and cholesterol clefts may occupy focal regions of the fibrous wall.

Differential Diagnosis: A nonexpansile pericoronal radiolucency is usually a simple dentigerous cyst. Since many odontogenic tumors, keratocysts, and even malignant neoplasms can arise from the epithelial lining, all dentigerous cysts should be removed and examined microscopically.

Treatment: The impacted tooth should be re-

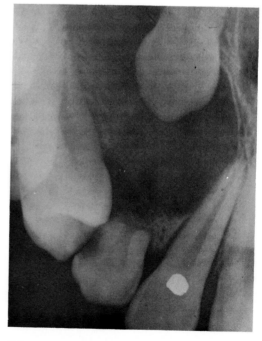

FIG. 9–32.   Odontogenic keratocyst appearing as a pericoronal radiolucency.

produce cortical expansion with noticeable deformity. The impacted tooth is often displaced to the outer margin of the radiolucency, and root development is usually incomplete. The mandibular third molar area is the most common location. Large cysts tend to be multilocular. If multiple pericoronal radiolucencies are present and are microscopically keratinizing, the nevoid–basal cell carcinoma syndrome should be considered.

Microscopic Features: The lining epithelium is attenuated, displaying a corrugated parakeratin or keratin surface, and the basal cell layer is polarized without manifestations of rete-ridge formation. The fibrous wall rarely contains significant inflammation. Epithelial cell rests are present within the fibrous wall and satellite or daughter cysts are frequently observed.

Differential Diagnosis: Expansile or loculated pericoronal radiolucencies typical of keratocysts are also featured when neoplastic transformation develops in a dentigerous cyst. Biopsy is required to differentiate among the various lesions presenting this radiographic pattern.

Treatment: Thorough curettage should be instituted, along with extraction. Neighboring teeth may need to be sacrificed if significant root resorption has developed. Odontogenic keratocysts are aggressive lesions and may be difficult to eradicate. Recurrence rates in excess of 30 percent have been recorded. Recurrent lesions may require en bloc resection. Cysts that are characterized histologically by orthokeratin as opposed to parakeratin show a better prognosis with a significantly lower rate of recurrence.

References

1. Pindborg, J. J. and Hansen, J.: Studies on odontogenic cyst epithelium. II. Clinical and roentgenographic aspects of odontogenic keratocysts. Acta Pathol. Microbiol. Scand. 58:283, 1963.
2. Payne, T. F.: An analysis of the clinical and histopathologic parameters of the odontogenic keratocyst. Oral Surg. 33:538, 1972.
3. Brannon, R. B.: The odontogenic keratocyst. A clinicopathologic study of 312 cases. Part I. Clinical features. Oral Surg. 42:54, 1976.
4. Brannon, R. B.: The odontogenic keratocyst: a clinicopathologic study of 312 cases. II. Histologic features. Oral Surg. 43:233, 1977.
5. Wright, J. M.: The odontogenic keratocyst, orthokeratinized variant. Oral Surg. 51:609, 1981.

Cystogenic Ameloblastoma

Age: Young adults

Sex: No predilection

Clinical and Radiographic Features: Amelo-

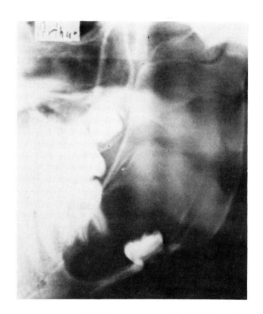

FIG. 9–33. Ameloblastoma arising from a large dentigerous cyst. (Courtesy of Dr. Bernard Karian.)

blastomas may arise from any source of odontogenic epithelium. Approximately 20 percent are associated with the crown of an impacted tooth, usually a mandibular third molar. While invasive ameloblastomas usually affect middle-aged adults, those that arise from the linings of dentigerous cysts are typically encountered during the second or third decades. Whereas the pericoronal radiolucency may be small, most cystogenic ameloblastomas exhibit a classic radiographic pattern characterized by a large unilocular radiolucency involving the entire ramus, extending to the coronoid process. They are most frequently associated with an impacted, displaced third molar showing incomplete root formation. Occasionally, these tumors are multilocular or evince scalloped margins. When expansion occurs, clinically observable deformity or facial asymmetry may be apparent. Pain and paresthesia are generally not evident.

Microscopic Features: Most pericoronal ameloblastomas arise from the odontogenic epithelial lining of dentigerous cysts. The earliest evidence of transformation is characterized by polarization of basal cells, superior displacement of nuclei, hyperchromatism, and cytoplasmic vacuolization. Slender tube-like rete ridges extend into the fibrous wall, and the overlying spinous layer resembles stellate reticulum. When the bulk of the tumor protrudes luminally, the designation *luminal ame-*

loblastoma is used; when the majority of tumor cells invade the fibrous wall, *mural ameloblastoma* is the designation. The term *unicystic ameloblastoma* has been applied to those lesions in which ameloblasts line the entire cyst. The later stages of oncogenesis manifest typical histomorphologic features of ameloblastoma.

Differential Diagnosis: Ameloblastomas arising from dentigerous cysts are radiographically indistinguishable from odontogenic keratocysts, other odontogenic tumors included in this section, and carcinoma arising in a dentigerous cyst. Biopsy is required for a definitive diagnosis.

Treatment: Luminal and early mural ameloblastomas do not invade the encasing bony crypt. The initial therapy should be curettage when lesions arise in the mandible. Maxillary tumors that have perforated the antrum are extremely difficult to control with curettage. A partial maxillary resection is recommended in these instances.

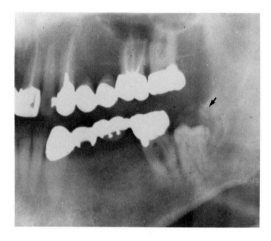

FIG. 9–34.   Calcifying epithelial odontogenic tumor associated with impacted third molar.

References

1. Stanley, H. R. and Diehl, D. L.: Ameloblastoma potential of follicular cysts. Oral Surg. 20:260, 1965.
2. Vickers, R. A. and Gorlin, R. J.: Ameloblastoma: delineation of early histopathologic features of neoplasia. Cancer 26:699, 1970.
3. Robinson, L. and Martinez, M. G.: Unicystic ameloblastoma. A prognostically distinct entity. Cancer 40:2278, 1977.
4. Shteyer, A., Lustmann, J., and Lewin-Epstein, J.: The mural ameloblastoma: review of the literature. J. Oral Surg. 36:866, 1978.
5. Eversole, L.R., Leider, A. S., and Strub, D.: Radiographic characteristics of cystogenic ameloblastoma. Oral Surg. 57:572, 1984.

Calcifying Epithelial Odontogenic Tumor

Age: Young and middle-aged adults
Sex: No predilection

Clinical and Radiographic Features: The calcifying epithelial odontogenic (Pindborg) tumor is rare: when it occurs, it is usually found in association with an impacted tooth. Because the tumor contains foci of calcification, it may show radiopaque flecks, powder-like opacities, or irregular confluent calcific globules. Many tumors, however, are predominantly or entirely radiolucent. Cortical expansion is a regular feature, and the radiolucency may be traversed by thin opaque septae. The margins are generally well demarcated, although it is not uncommon to encounter radiographic zones of poor margination where the lesion tends to blend imperceptibly into the adjacent normal medullary bone.

Microscopic Features: The neoplastic epithelial cells grow in a variety of patterns, ranging from diffuse sheet-like arrangements to islands and invasive cords. The individual cells bear very little resemblance to components of the tooth germ. They are polygonal, eosinophilic, and contain large nuclei that are often hyperchromatic; significant pleomorphism may be present despite the benignity of the tumor. A clear cell variant exists and is distinguished by sheets and islands of tumor cells that are devoid of stainable cytoplasm. Eosinophilic hyaline is associated with epithelium, and stains are positive for amyloid. Both dystrophic and concentrically laminated Leisegang calcifications are encountered. The radiolucent lesions contain less calcification than the tumors with opacities.

Differential Diagnosis: Calcifying epithelial odontogenic tumors with irregular, poorly demarcated expansile borders may give the radiographic appearance of osteogenic and chondrogenic sarcoma or osteolytic metastatic tumor. Identification of an impacted tooth in association with such a lesion is more suggestive of odontogenic neoplasm. More clearly demarcated tumors must, by biopsy, be differentiated from keratocyst, ameloblastoma, mixed odontogenic tumor, and dentigerous cyst with carcinomatous transformation.

Treatment: The Pindborg tumor is aggressive and requires total or en bloc resection. Simple enucleation or curettage is generally inadequate, and the tumor recurs.

References

1. Pindborg, J. J.: The calcifying epithelial odontogenic tumor; review of literature and report of an extra-osseous case. Acta Odontol. Scand. 24:419, 1966.
2. Chaudhry, A. P., et al.: Calcifying epithelial odontogenic tumor; A histochemical and ultrastructural study. Cancer 30:519, 1972.
3. Krolls, S. O. and Pindborg, J. J.: Calcifying epithelial odontogenic tumor. A survey of 23 cases and discussion of histomorphologic variations. Arch. Pathol. 98:206, 1974.
4. Franklin, C. D. and Pindborg, J. J.: The calcifying epithelial odontogenic tumor. Oral Surg. 42:753, 1976.
5. Sadeghi, E. M. and Hopper, T. L.: Calcifying epithelial odontogenic tumor. J. Oral Surg. 40:225, 1982.

Odontogenic Adenomatoid Tumor

Age: Teenagers
Sex: Female predilection

Clinical and Radiographic Features: While the odontogenic adenomatoid tumor may arise between teeth, over 75 percent are associated with the crown of an impacted tooth. The maxilla is more often affected, with a pericoronal radiolu-

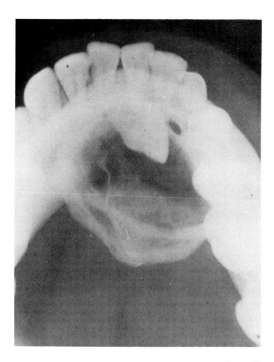

FIG. 9–35. Impacted cuspid with an expansile well-circumscribed pericoronal radiolucency, representing an odontogenic adenomatoid tumor.

cency enveloping the crown of a cuspid. The radiolucency often contains radiopaque flecks because portions of the tumor can calcify. Whereas simple dentigerous cysts emanate from the cervix of the tooth, the odontogenic adenomatoid tumor often manifests a pericoronal radiolucency that almost completely engulfs the entire tooth, including the root. It is almost invariably unilocular and is well demarcated or corticated. Painless cortical expansion is often the presenting sign.

Microscopic Features: The tumor is surrounded by a dense fibrous capsule. The epithelial neoplastic tissue often assumes the appearance of a cyst with luminal proliferation. The epithelial cells are elongated and arrange themselves in swirls. This growth pattern yields a granuloma-like configuration. Admixed with the spindle cell component are oval nests of columnar epithelial cells with ameloblastic cytologic features. These cells are oriented about an eosinophilic secretion product and in classic examples assume ductal patterns with a central lumen. Hyaline eosinophilic elements are also present, and in many areas these cell products undergo a dystrophic type of calcification.

Differential Diagnosis: Odontogenic adenomatoid tumors seen as pericoronal radiolucencies must be differentiated from ordinary dentigerous cysts, keratocysts, and other odontogenic tumors that may arise from cyst lining. The young age, anterior location, and tendency for the radiolucency to envelop the lower root region of the impacted tooth are highly suggestive of odontogenic adenomatoid tumor. Biopsy is required to obtain a definitive diagnosis.

Treatment: Extraction with simple enucleation of the neoplasm is adequate treatment. The tumor almost never recurs.

References

1. Abrams, A. M., et al.: Adenoameloblastoma; a clinical pathologic study of ten new cases. Cancer 22:175, 1968.
2. Giansanti, J. S., Someren, A., and Waldron, C. A.: Odontogenic adenomatoid tumor (adenoameloblastoma). Oral Surg. 30:69, 1970.
3. Courtney, R. M. and Kerr, D. A.: The odontogenic adenomatoid tumor. Oral Surg. 39:424, 1975.
4. Tsaknis, P. J., Carpenter, W. M., and Shade, N. L.: Odontogenic adenomatoid tumor: report of case and review of the literature. J. Oral Surg. 35:146, 1977.

Ameloblastic Fibroma

Age: Children and teenagers
Sex: No predilection

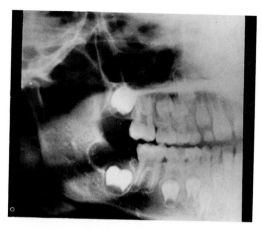

FIG. 9–36. Ameloblastic fibroma, a mixed odontogenic tumor appearing as a pericoronal radiolucency surrounding the crown of an unerupted molar.

Clinical and Radiographic Features: The mixed odontogenic tumors include ameloblastic fibroma, ameloblastic fibrodentinoma, ameloblastic fibro-odontoma, and odontoma. Only ameloblastic fibroma is entirely radiolucent. While all of the mixed odontogenic tumors may begin as radiolucent lesions, the remainder will eventually develop radiopaque foci. Over 90 percent of ameloblastic fibromas are associated with an impacted tooth and therefore appear as pericoronal radiolucencies. They may be unilocular or multilocular, expansile or nonexpansile, and when initially detected they may be either large or quite small. The ameloblastic fibroma grows slowly, yet if left untreated has a significant growth potential. A microscopically malignant clinically aggressive mixed odontogenic tumor has been described as ameloblastic fibrosarcoma.

Microscopic Features: The mixed odontogenic tumors possess both epithelial and mesenchymal tumor elements, and they mimic the histiogenic differentiation of the developing tooth germ. The least differentiated is the ameloblastic fibroma. It is composed of a diffuse mass of embryonic mesenchyme, which is traversed by elongated cords of cuboidal or columnar odontogenic epithelial cells that resemble the dental lamina. These cords terminate in bulbous projections that contain a central stellate reticulum. Ameloblastic fibrodentinomas are similar, yet a dense eosinophilic dentinoid material lies in juxtaposition to the epithelial element. Ameloblastic fibro-odontomas are further differentiated in that both dentin and enamel matrix are formed and are admixed with zones

identical to simple ameloblastic fibroma. The odontoma contains all elements of the mature tooth germ yet does not evince a significant soft tissue cellular overgrowth.

Ameloblastic fibrosarcoma exhibits a sarcomatoid mesenchymal element that is hypercellular; the individual fibroblasts are pleomorphic and hyperchromatic with discernible mitotic figures.

Differential Diagnosis: Pericoronal radiolucencies representing ameloblastic fibroma may be radiographically identical to simple dentigerous cyst, odontogenic keratocyst, ameloblastoma, Pindborg tumor, or carcinoma arising from a dentigerous cyst. These latter lesions tend to arise in adults rather than youngsters. Biopsy is required to obtain a definitive diagnosis.

Treatment: Enucleation with extraction of the impacted tooth is recommended. The ameloblastic fibroma has a limited tendency to recur. Whereas ameloblastic fibrosarcomas are apparently nonmetastasizing, they are aggressive and recurrence after curettage is commonplace. These tumors should be treated by en bloc resection.

References

1. Gorlin, R. J., et al.: Odontogenic tumors. Cancer *14*:73, 1961.
2. Trodahl, J. N.: Ameloblastic fibroma: A survey of cases from the Armed Forces Institute of Pathology. Oral Surg. *33*:547, 1972.
3. Leider, A. S., Nelson, J. F., and Trodahl, J. N.: Ameloblastic fibrosarcoma of the jaws. Oral Surg. *33*:559, 1972.
4. Regezi, J. A., Kerr, D. A., and Courtney, R. M.: Odontogenic tumors: an analysis of 706 cases. J. Oral Surg. *36*:771, 1978.
5. Zallen, R. D., Preskar, M. H., and McClary, S. A.: Ameloblastic fibroma. J. Oral Surg. *40*:513, 1982.

Odontogenic Fibroma

Age: Teenagers and young adults

Sex: No known predilection

Clinical and Radiographic Features: The odontogenic fibroma is a benign neoplasm derived from the mesenchymal tissues of the odontogenic apparatus. Clinically, a painless expansion of the cortical plates is observed, and larger lesions will disclose an obvious facial swelling. The tumor is rare and probably occurs as frequently in the maxilla as it does in the mandible. Whereas a well-delineated multilocular expansile lesion is often observed, this tumor is also likely to exhibit a unilocular radiolucent configuration. Root resorption or divergence is common; association with an impacted tooth is rare.

Microscopic Features: Two histologic variants

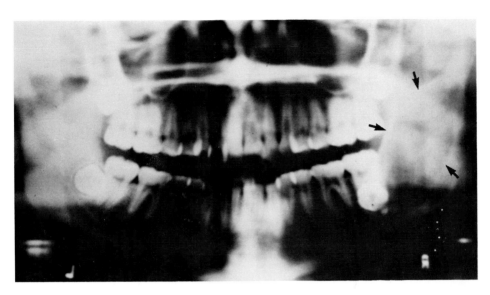

FIG. 9–37.   Impacted third molar with pericoronal radiolucency extending into ramus, representing an odontogenic fibroma.

are encountered. The more common appearance is that of a mature fibrous proliferation without pronounced fibroblastic hypercellularity. Scattered throughout the fibrous growth are round or oval quiescent-appearing odontogenic epithelial rests. The less common classic form fails to show epithelial rests. The fibrous proliferation is more embryonal with stellate-appearing cells that resemble the developing dental papilla.

Differential Diagnosis: Odontogenic fibroma clinically and radiographically resembles many of the other disease processes included here. The loculations are, however, generally macrolocular as opposed to the microlocules seen in arteriovenous malformation. Aspiration is still essential, and biopsy is required to secure a definitive diagnosis.

Treatment: Enucleation is the treatment of choice. Behavior and recurrence tendencies are not well known; insufficient data have been published.

References

1. Knight, W. O. and Caulfield, J. J.: Abbreviated case report. Odontogenic fibroma. Oral Surg. 34:381, 1972.
2. Wesley, R. K., Wysocki, G. P., and Mintz, S. M.: The central odontogenic fibroma. Oral Surg. 40:235, 1975.
3. Gardner, D. G.: The central odontogenic fibroma: An attempt at clarification. Oral Surg. 50:425, 1980.
4. Dahl, E. C., Wolfson, S. H., and Hangen, J. C.: Central odontogenic fibroma: review of literature and report of cases. J. Oral Surg. 39:120, 1981.
5. Schofield, I. O. F.: Central odontogenic fibroma: report of case. J. Oral Surg. 39:218, 1981.

Central Mucoepidermoid Carcinoma

Age: Young adults
Sex: No predilection

Clinical and Radiographic Features: Mucoepidermoid carcinoma arising centrally in bone is rare. When it does it is often, but not always, associated with an impacted tooth. Many instances have been reported in which the neoplasm could be demonstrated to arise from the epithelial lining of a dentigerous cyst. The pericoronal radiolucency is well demarcated and tends to be multilocular. The posterior mandible is the most frequent location. Expansion is encountered. Pain is generally not a feature, but paresthesia may develop with large lesions. Squamous cell carcinoma has also been reported to arise from the lining of odontogenic cysts.

Microscopic Features: Evidence of a dentigerous cyst lining may be encountered or the neoplastic tissue may be so dominant that demonstrable origin from a cyst is obscured. The tumors are usually low grade with cystic spaces lined by columnar and mucus-secreting cells admixed with epidermal spinous cells. Squamous cell carcino-

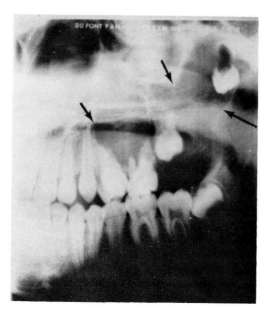

FIG. 9–38. Impacted third molar with associated radiolucency filling the sinus, representing a central mucoepidermoid carcinoma arising from the lining of a dentigerous cyst. (Courtesy of Dr. H. Cherrick.)

mas show the same features as those derived from surface mucosa.

Differential Diagnosis: Pericoronal radiolucencies representing central mucoepidermoid carcinoma may show radiographic features in common with dentigerous cysts, keratocysts, or odontogenic neoplasms. The true nature of the disease can be ascertained only after microscopic evaluation.

Treatment: Central mucoepidermoid carcinoma of the jaws is usually of the low-grade variety. High-grade tumors in this location are unusual. When the tumor is low grade, the disease can be cured by resection. Lymph node dissection should be performed when clinically palpable nodes are encountered.

References

1. Smith, R. L., Dahlin, D. C., and Waite, D. E.: Mucoepidermoid carcinomas of the jaw bones. J. Oral Surg. 26:387, 1968.
2. Schultz, W. and Whitten, J. B.: Mucoepidermoid carcinoma in the mandible: report of case. J. Oral Surg. 27:337, 1969.
3. Eversole, L. R., Sabes, W. R., and Rovin, S.: Aggressive growth and neoplastic potential of odontogenic cysts; with special reference to central epidermoid and mucoepidermoid carcinoma. Cancer 35:270, 1975.
4. Fredrickson, C. and Cherrick, H. M.: Central mu-

coepidermoid carcinoma of the jaws. J. Oral Med. 33:80, 1978.

MULTILOCULAR RADIOLUCENCIES

Odontogenic Keratocyst

Age: Adults
Sex: No predilection

Clinical and Radiographic Features: The odontogenic keratocyst is probably the most common lesion to produce an expansile multilocular radiolucency of the jaws. It has been included in the differential diagnosis of pericoronal and interradicular radiolucencies because it is commonly seen in those relationships as well. When the keratocyst is multilocular, it generally manifests clinically obvious expansion. The posterior body and ramus of the mandible are the most frequent areas of involvement. The lesion is aggressive and if left untreated may destroy large areas of bone. Cortical expansion is usually seen; however, the cortex may actually be perforated. When multiple keratocysts are detected, examination of the skin for basal cell nevi and a radiograph of the chest or demonstration of a bifid rib should be undertaken.

Microscopic Features: The cyst lumen is usually filled with keratin. The stratified squamous epithelial lining possesses a corrugated parakeratin layer, an attenuated spinous layer, and a polarized basal cell layer with no rete-ridge forma-

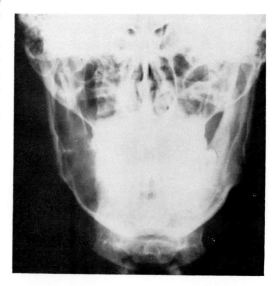

FIG. 9–39. Multilocular keratocyst of posterior mandible and ramus.

tion. Occasionally, however, bulbous epithelial extensions invaginate into the fibrous wall where they proliferate and give rise to satellite (daughter) cysts. Some keratocysts are lined by epithelium synthesizing orthokeratin.

Differential Diagnosis: A multilocular radiolucency representing keratocyst must be differentiated from all of the other lesions listed in this section. If an impacted tooth is present in association with the radiolucency, the lesion is odontogenic and the entities listed as pericoronal radiolucencies must be included in the differential diagnosis. Aspiration is usually negative with keratocysts because they are filled with caseous keratin rather than fluid.

Treatment: Initial therapy should consist of thorough enucleation and curettage. Recurrence rates for large multilocular keratocysts are greater than 50 percent, while recurrence for lesions under 2 cm is less than 30 percent. The orthokeratinized variety rarely recurs following curettage. Recurrent cysts can be recuretted or excised en bloc.

References

1. Brown, R. M.: The odontogenic keratocyst. Br. Dent. J. *128*:225,1970.
2. Payne, T. G.: An analysis of the clinical and histopathologic parameters of the odontogenic keratocyst. Oral Surg. *33*:538, 1972.
3. Forssell, K., Sorvari, T. E., and Oksala, E.: A clinical and radiographic study of odontogenic keratocysts in jaws. Proc. Finn. Dent. Soc. *70*:121, 1974.
4. Brannon, R. B.: The odontogenic keratocyst: a clinicopathologic study of 312 cases. I. Clinical features. Oral Surg. *42*:54, 1976.
5. Wright, J. M.: The odontogenic keratocyst: orthokeratinized variant. Oral Surg. *51*:609, 1981.

Botryoid Odontogenic Cyst

Age: Predilection unknown
Sex: Predilection unknown

Clinical and Radiographic Features: The botryoid odontogenic cyst is a rare lesion that grossly resembles a cluster of grapes. It is found central in bone and may appear unilocular or multilocular radiographically. A soft tissue location for this lesion has been observed as well. Expansion is observed in central lesions. The origin of this cyst is unknown yet is probably odontogenic. Microscopically, it closely resembles gingival and lateral periodontal cysts.

Microscopic Features: The lesion is multicystic, and each cystic cavity is separated from others by fibrous septae. The lining epithelium is low cuboidal or squamous, being only 1 or 2 cells

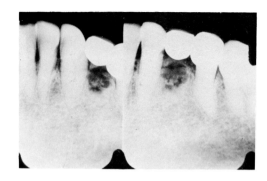

FIG. 9–40.   Botryoid odontogenic cyst underlying bridge pontic.

thick. Focal acanthotic clear cell clusters are randomly scattered along the lining.

Differential Diagnosis: This unusual cyst may radiographically resemble lateral periodontal cyst or when multilocular or scalloped it cannot be differentiated from the other lesions listed in this section.

Treatment: Enucleation is the treatment of choice. Too few cases have been reported to yield any information on behavior or rate of recurrence.

References

1. Weathers, D. R. and Waldron, C. A.: Unusual multilocular cysts of the jaws (botryoid odontogenic cysts). Oral Surg. *36*:235, 1973.
2. Wysocki, G. P., et al.: Histogenesis of the lateral periodontal cyst and the gingival cyst of the adult. Oral Surg. *50*:327, 1980.

Cherubism (Familial Fibrous Dysplasia)

Age: Childhood onset
Sex: Slight male predilection

Clinical and Radiographic Features: Cherubism is familial and there is evidence that it represents an autosomal dominant trait with variable expressivity. The term is descriptive of the clinical appearance. The posterior mandible is expanded bilaterally, yielding a cherubic facies. Radiographically, extensive multilocular radiolucencies occupy the entire ramus and posterior body of the mandible on both sides. Delicate septae course throughout the radiolucent lesion, and the anterior limits are generally ill defined. The maxillary tuberosity regions often contain expansile multilocular radiolucencies as well. Premature exfoliation of deciduous teeth or impaction and displacement may be features. The progressive expansion begins in early childhood and eventually the growth becomes static, usually shortly after puberty.

Microscopic Features: Loose areolar fibrous

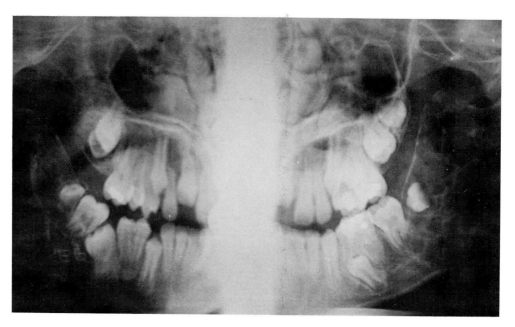

FIG. 9–41.   Bilateral multilocular radiolucencies of the posterior mandible in a patient with familial fibrous dysplasia.

connective tissue or even hypercellular fibrous tissue is present and contains isolated, poorly formed osseous tissue and multinucleated giant cells. Vascular channels evince perivascular collagenous condensation or cuffing.

Differential Diagnosis: The clinicoradiologic features are pathognomonic when a familial tendency can be demonstrated. A biopsy should be performed because multiple keratocysts or brown tumors of hyperparathyroidism could show similar characteristics, particularly if no familial tendency can be ascertained.

Treatment: Surgical intervention during childhood is not recommended. The lesion will recur and may actually be activated by the procedure. When growth has ceased, cosmetic osseous contouring may be instituted.

References

1. Topazian, R. G. and Costich, E. R.: Familial fibrous dysplasia of the jaws (cherubism). J. Oral Surg. 23:559, 1965.
2. Hamner, J. E., III, and Ketcham, A. S.: Cherubism: an analysis of treatment. Cancer 23:1133, 1969.
3. Grunebaum, M.: Nonfamilial cherubism: report of two cases. J. Oral Surg. 31:632, 1973.
4. Kuepper R. C. and Harrigan, W. F.: Treatment of mandibular cherubism. J. Oral Surg. 36:638, 1978.

Central Giant Cell Granuloma

Age: Young adults
Sex: Female predilection

Clinical and Radiographic Features: The central giant cell granuloma is an aggressive reactive process of the jaw bones that arises most often in the mandible anterior to the first molars. Indeed, it is the most common anteriorly located multilocular expansile radiolucency. Smaller lesions may be unilocular, and most are detected when clinical expansion alerts the patient to the disease. When roentgenograms are obtained, a soap-bubble loculated radiolucency is encountered. Cortical expansion is seen radiographically, and the margins of the radiolucency are well demarcated. Root divergence and resorption are frequent findings. The overlying teeth remain vital, and pain or paresthesia is generally not present. The lesion is capable of rapid growth.

Microscopic Features: A highly cellular fibrovascular stroma prevails. Dispersed throughout are multinucleated giant cells that tend to lie in juxtaposition to vascular channels. Osteoid or osseous trabeculae are present in most lesions, and hemosiderin granules may be deposited in profusion.

Differential Diagnosis: Brown tumor of hyperparathyroidism is clinically, radiographically, and microscopically indistinguishable from giant cell granuloma. A serum calcium determination should be obtained to check for parathyroid ad-

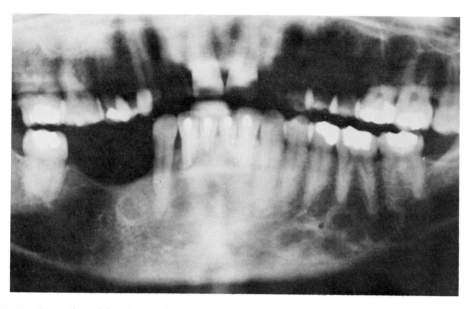

FIG. 9–42. Expansile multilocular radiolucency of the anterior mandible representing a central giant cell granuloma.

enoma. Radiographically, giant cell granuloma may be confused with the other lesions listed in this section. Aspiration may be negative or, because of the vascularity of the lesion, small amounts of blood may be obtained.

Treatment: Surgical enucleation is the treatment of choice. Teeth may need to be sacrificed to completely eradicate the disease. If the lesion is not totally excised, it may recur.

References

1. Shklar, G. and Meyer, I.: Giant cell tumors of the mandible and maxilla. Oral Surg. *14*:809, 1961.
2. Waldron, C. A. and Shafer, W. G.: The central giant cell reparative granuloma of the jaws; an analysis of 38 cases. Am. J. Clin. Pathol. *45*:437, 1966.
3. Leban, S. G., et al.: The giant cell lesion of jaws: neoplastic or reparative? J. Oral Surg. *29*:398, 1971.
4. Curtis, M. L., Hatfield, C. G., and Pierce, J. M.: A destructive giant cell lesion of the mandible. J. Oral Surg. *31*:705, 1973.
5. Granite, E. L., Aronoff, K., and Gold, L.: Central giant cell granuloma of the mandible: A case report. Oral Surg. *53*:241, 1982.

Aneurysmal Bone Cyst

Age: Young adults

Sex: No predilection

Clinical and Radiographic Features: The aneurysmal bone cyst is not a true cyst. It is closely related pathogenically to the giant cell granuloma,

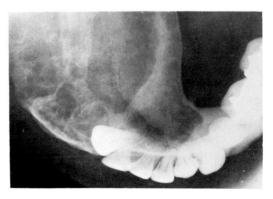

FIG. 9–43. Multilocular radiolucency with marked expansion due to aneurysmal bone cyst. (From Oliver, L. P.: Aneurysmal bone cyst. Oral Surg. *35*:67, 1973.)

being an aggressive reactive process. Since the lesion is composed of large vascular sinusoids, blood can be aspirated with a syringe. The blood coursing through the lesion is under low pressure so that a bruit cannot be auscultated. The lesion has a great potential for growth and may produce marked expansion and deformity. The multilocular radiolucency is traversed by thin septae, and cortical expansion is radiographically demonstrable. The mandibular body is the most frequent site for this lesion and, when it is large, the inferior border shows a significant blowout expansile bulge. Aneurysmal bone cyst is occasionally encountered in association with other fibro-osseous lesions of the jaws such as giant cell granuloma and fibrous dysplasia.

Microscopic Features: Large tortuous blood-filled sinusoidal channels are lined by a flat endothelial layer. The surrounding tissue is fibroblastic and hypercellular. Multinucleated giant cells lie adjacent to the sinusoids, and osteoid trabeculae tend to orient themselves in close proximity to the vascular spaces.

Differential Diagnosis: Radiographically, the aneurysmal bone cyst may demonstrate features indistinguishable from the other multilocular radiolucencies included in this section. Aspiration of blood will allow for limitation of the differential diagnosis; however, central arteriovenous malformation or hemangioma of bone also yields a bloody aspirate. A bruit is usually present in the latter, but not in aneurysmal bone cyst. Carotid time-lapse angiography may be of aid when attempting to differentiate aneurysmal bone cyst from arteriovenous malformation, since blood traverses the former slowly while it progresses through the latter at a rapid rate.

Treatment: Despite the rapid growth and aggressiveness of the aneurysmal bone cyst, simple enucleation rarely results in recurrence. At surgery, the lesion may hemorrhage profusely; however, the blood is not under a great degree of pressure.

References
1. Bhaskar, S. N., et al.: Aneurysmal bone cyst and other giant cell lesions of the jaws; report of 104 cases. J. Oral Surg. 17:30, 1959.
2. Daugherty, J. W. and Eversole, L. R.: Aneurysmal bone cyst of the mandible: report of case. J. Oral Surg. 29:737, 1971.
3. Biesecker, J. L., et al.: Aneurysmal bone cysts: a clinicopathologic study of 66 cases. Cancer 26:615, 1970.
4. Reyneke, J. P.: Aneurysmal bone cyst of the maxilla. Oral Surg. 45:441, 1978.
5. Steidler, N. W., Cook, R.M., and Reade, P. C.: Aneurysmal bone cysts of the jaws: a case report and review of the literature. Br. J. Oral Surg. 16:254, 1979.

Hyperparathyroidism

Age: Middle-aged adults

Sex: Female predilection

Clinical and Radiographic Features: A parathyroid adenoma secretes excessive amounts of parathormone, which mobilizes calcium into the serum and leads to osteoporosis with elevated serum calcium. The poorly mineralized bone is

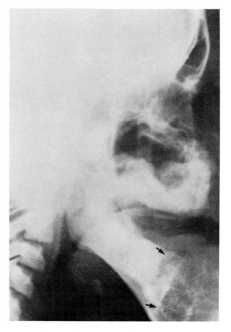

FIG. 9–44. Massive expansile multilocular radiolucency of anterior mandible representing a brown tumor of hyperparathyroidism. (Courtesy of Drs. S. Dachi and S. Rovin.)

replaced by fibrous tissue, resulting in the condition known as *osteitis fibrosa cystica*. Calcium salts precipitate in the kidneys with urolithiasis, which in turn contributes to pyelonephritis. Secondary hyperparathyroidism may occur in renal disease where calcium is lost in the urine, causing a compensatory parathyroid hyperplasia. In addition to parathyroid adenoma and renal secondary hyperparathyroidism, certain malignant neoplasms, such as oat cell carcinomas of the lung, secrete excess parathormone with the development of hyperparathyroidism. Late in the course of the disease, lesions may develop in any bone, including the jaws. These are giant cell tumors known as brown tumors. In the jaws, they appear as expansile multilocular radiolucencies.

Microscopic Features: The microscopic features of brown tumor are indistinguishable from those of central giant cell granuloma. Fibrovascular tissue is admixed with numerous multinucleated giant cells. Trabeculae of bone may be present.

Differential Diagnosis: The brown tumor of hyperparathyroidism is clinically, radiographically, and microscopically indistinguishable from central giant cell granuloma. For this reason a bone chemistry panel must be evaluated. Serum calcium is elevated, phosphorus is low, and alkaline phosphatase is within normal limits. Radiographically, brown tumor may resemble the other radiolucencies included in this section.

Treatment: After the diagnosis has been established, the patient should be referred to a surgeon for excision of the parathyroid adenoma or for evaluation of renal function when secondary hyperparathyroidism is suspected. When this workup is negative, an endocrine-secreting carcinoma should be ruled out. The jaw lesions will resolve after treatment; however, expansion may be maintained. Elective cosmetic osseous contouring may then be performed.

References

1. Silverman, S., Jr., et al.: Dental aspects of hyperparathyroidism. Oral Surg. 15(Suppl. 2):84, 1962.
2. Carlotti, A. E., Camitta, F. D., and Connor, T. B.: Primary hyperparathyroidism with giant cell tumors of the maxilla: report of case. J. Oral Surg. 27:722, 1969.
3. Chapnick, P.: A review of hyperparathyroidism and an interesting case presenting with a giant cell lesion. Trans. Congr. Int. Assoc. Oral Surg. 4:44, 1973.

Ameloblastoma

Age: Middle-aged adults

Sex: No predilection

Clinical and Radiographic Features: The ameloblastoma is classically a multilocular radiolucency with a predilection for the posterior mandible. The roentgenogram shows a well-circumscribed, expansile soap-bubble radiolucency with clearly demarcated borders. The neoplasm may arise from the lining of a dentigerous cyst but more often arises independent of any association with impacted teeth. It shows a progressive moderate growth rate and, if left untreated, may reach enormous proportions. Expansion is seen clinically and radiographically. Pain is generally not a symptom. Maxillary tumors frequently perforate into the antrum and may grow freely, with extension into the nasal cavity, ethmoid sinuses, and cranial base. A small number of microscopically benign ameloblastomas have been reported to undergo distant metastases.

Microscopic Features: Ameloblastomas show various growth patterns; however, none of these histomorphologic variations has any bearing on predicting growth potential, metastatic potential, or prognosis. The classic microscopic features of ameloblastoma are represented by sheets and islands of tumor cells showing an outer rim of col-

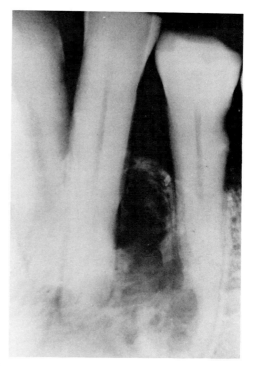

FIG. 9–45. Multilocular radiolucency with root divergence and resorption in ameloblastoma. (Courtesy of Dr. Sheldon Rovin.)

umnar ameloblasts with nuclei polarized away from the basement membrane. The center of these nests is composed of stellate-shaped epithelial cells that mimic the stellate reticulum. Occasionally, these cells show squamous metaplasia or contain eosinophilic granular cells. Plexiform, cystic, and basaloid patterns are often dominant. Rarely, an ameloblastoma exhibits cytologic features of malignancy. Tumors of this nature maintain histologic resemblance to benign ameloblastoma with an outer columnar stratum and a central stellate reticulum zone with squamous differentiation. These tumors are diagnosed as ameloblastic carcinoma.

Differential Diagnosis: The expansile multilocular pattern of ameloblastoma is also encountered in other odontogenic and nonodontogenic lesions listed in this section. Aspiration is negative, and biopsy is required to obtain a definitive diagnosis.

Treatment: Curettage may be attempted for small mandibular ameloblastomas. Recurrence rates are high. Larger lesions, particularly those extending to the inferior border, require en bloc resection or hemimandibulectomy. Maxillary ameloblastomas require resection because they tend to invade the antrum; any attempt to eradicate tumor by curettage will fail and, importantly, recurrences may not be controlled by subsequent surgical resection. Less than 1 percent of benign-appearing ameloblastomas will metastasize to distant sites. These metastatic tumors are frequently the granular cell type.

References

1. Small, I. A. and Waldron, C. A.: Ameloblastoma of the jaws. Oral Surg. 8:281, 1955.
2. Carr, R. G. and Halperin, V.: Malignant ameloblastomas from 1953 to 1966. Review of the literature and report of a case. Oral Surg. 26:514, 1968.
3. Sehdev, M. K., et al.: Ameloblastoma of maxilla and mandible. Cancer 33:324, 1974.
4. Hartman, K. H.: Granular cell ameloblastoma. A survey of twenty cases from the Armed Forces Institute of Pathology. Oral Surg. 38:241, 1974.
5. Tsaknis, P. J. and Nelson, J. F.: The maxillary ameloblastoma: an analysis of 24 cases. J. Oral Surg. 38:336, 1980.

Myxoma

Age: Young and middle-aged adults

Sex: No predilection

Clinical and Radiographic Features: The myxoma, because of its limitation to jaw bones, is included as an odontogenic neoplasm, which probably originates from the dental papilla or follicular mesenchyme. It is typically multilocular and expansile, and some cases are associated with impacted teeth. The septae coursing through the radiolucency are extremely delicate and look like a finely reticulated spiderweb. The border may be clearly delineated, but occasionally the marginal limits of the tumor are indiscrete. Myxomas are slow growing but are aggressively invasive; if left untreated, they may become huge. The body of the mandible is the favored site. Maxillary myxomas may perforate and invade the antrum.

Microscopic Features: The microscopic pattern is distinctive. Spindle and stellate fibroblasts are associated with basophilic ground substance and delicate immature collagen fibers representing myxomatous tissue. Oval odontogenic epithelial cell rests may or may not be present.

Differential Diagnosis: A delicate reticulated pattern of septae, as seen radiographically in a multilocular radiolucency, is highly suggestive of myxoma. Regardless, the other lesions in this section must be included in the differential radiographic diagnosis. Aspiration is negative, and biopsy is indicated.

Treatment: Myxomas are grossly gelatinous or mucoid, so curettage is untenable in most instances. Occasionally, myxomas are more fibrous and can be managed by curettage with less chance for recurrence than those with a mucoid consistency. En bloc resection should be performed, particularly in larger gelatinous lesions, to circumvent recurrence.

References

1. Barros, R. E. and Cabrini, R. L.: Myxoma of the jaws. Oral Surg. 27:225, 1969.
2. Ghosh, B. C., et al.: Myxoma of the jaws. Cancer 31:237, 1973.
3. White, D. K., et al.: Odontogenic myxoma: a clinical and ultrastructural study. Oral Surg. 39:901, 1975.
4. Harder, F.: Myxoma of the jaws. Int. J. Oral Surg. 7:148, 1978.
5. Gandra, Y. R., et al.: Central myxoma of the mandible in a child: report of case. J. Oral Surg. 39:769, 1981.

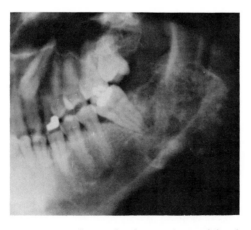

FIG. 9–46. Finely reticulated pattern in a multilocular radiolucency representing odontogenic myxoma. (Courtesy of Dr. James Shemke.)

Central Neurogenic Neoplasms

Age: No predilection

Sex: No predilection

Clinical and Radiographic Features: Neurilemmomas and neurofibromas arising from the sheath cells of the inferior alveolar nerve appear as unilocular or multilocular radiolucencies along the course of the nerve. Of all bones in the body, excluding the temporal bone, the mandible is the most common site for central nerve sheath neoplasms. This is probably because no other bone transports a nerve for such a distance. Expansion of the buccal plate is common, yet pain is not a feature. Paresthesia may or may not be present. Central neurofibromas are more likely to be soli-

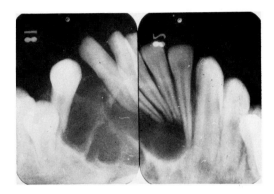

FIG. 9–47. Multilocular radiolucency due to a central neural sheath neoplasm. (From Sugimura, et al.: A case of neurilemmoma in the mandible. Int. J. Oral Surg. 3:194, 1974.)

tary than to represent stigmata of von Recklinghausen's neurofibromatosis.

Microscopic Features: Nerve sheath tumors of bone display the same microscopic features as their soft tissue counterparts. Neurilemmomas are composed of spindle cells arranged in palisading columns and swirls separated by finely fibrillar vacuolated connective tissue. Neurofibromas contain fibroblastic nuclei haphazardly arranged and admixed with wavy delicate collagen fibers with myxomatous regions. Plexiform or organoid patterns are commonly observed.

Differential Diagnosis: Multilocular central neural tumors must be differentiated from the other lesions included here. They often show widening of the inferior alveolar canal with scalloped margins that make radiographic distinction from the traumatic cyst impossible. Biopsy is required to arrive at a definitive diagnosis.

Treatment: Simple surgical nucleation is the treatment of choice. Recurrence is uncommon.

References

1. Sampter, T. G., Vellios, F., and Shafer, W. G.: Neurilemmoma of bone. Report of 3 cases with a review of the literature. Radiology 75:215, 1960.
2. Eversole, L. R.: Central benign and malignant neural neoplasms of the jaws. J. Oral Surg. 27:716, 1969.
3. Ellis, G. L., Abrams, A. M., and Melrose, R. J.: Intraosseous benign neural sheath neoplasms of the jaws. Report of seven new cases and review of the literature. Oral Surg. 44:731, 1977.
4. Wright, B. A. and Jackson, D.: Neural tumors of the oral cavity. A review of the spectrum of benign and malignant neural tumors of the oral cavity and jaws. Oral Surg. 49:509, 1980.
5. Satterfield, S. D., Elzay, R. P., and Mercuri, L.:

Mandibular central schwannoma: report of case. J. Oral Surg. 39:776, 1981.

Central Arteriovenous Malformation

Age: Children and teenagers
Sex: Female predilection

Clinical and Radiographic Features: An arteriovenous malformation of the mandible is potentially lethal and extremely dangerous when teeth are surrounded by the lesion, since they will become loose and, if extracted, uncontrollable hemorrhage will often result. Spontaneous gingival hemorrhage or seeping of blood from the gingival sulci is a common sign. The malformation develops from the central vessels of the mandible during early childhood. High arterial pressure is exerted within the vessels because of direct communication of arteries with veins (an interposed capillary bed fails to develop). This often causes compensatory expansion of the cortices and a bruit can be heard on auscultation. The overlying skin may be warmer than that on the uninvolved side. Radiographically, A-V malformations are microloculated. These tiny locules represent small arterial channels. Bright-red fresh blood is obtained on aspiration. Indeed, the plunger of the syringe may be forced out as a result of the pressure within the lesion. Feeder vessels are derived from the ipsilateral inferior alveolar artery; however, contralateral vascular communications are common. Unfortunately, cases have been demonstrated in which the vertebral vessels anastomose with the arterial channels of the jaw lesion. Angiography will clearly demonstrate these anastomoses. Occasionally, central vascular anomalies are under low pressure. In these instances, they are perhaps more aptly termed *central hemangiomas*.

Microscopic Features: Biopsy should not be performed when aspiration is positive and a bruit is detected. Resected mandibles show large-caliber muscular vascular channels, which course profusely throughout the medullary bone.

Differential Diagnosis: Central A-V malformations show radiographic features in common with the other multilocular radiolucencies included here. A blood aspirate and detectable bruit allow for a clinical diagnosis. A central A-V malformation may exist in the absence of a bruit or cortical expansion. In these cases, since aspiration is positive, differentiation from an aneurysmal bone cyst is critical. Time-lapse angiography is indicated as blood passes through an A-V malformation rapidly, whereas the time phase of aneu-

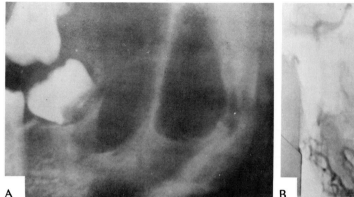
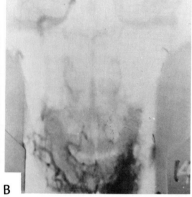

FIG. 9–48. *A:* Multilocular radiolucency in ramus of mandible, an arteriovenous malformation. *B:* Ipsilateral carotid subtraction angiogram showing filling of the central vascular defect on the opposite side.

rysmal bone cysts is not much different from that of a normal arterial-capillary-venous clearance.

Treatment: Iatrogenic embolization with autologous muscle chips or other materials is contraindicated, as pulmonary embolism may occur (the vascular lumina may remain patent and equal in size through the course of the defect). The external carotids should be ligated bilaterally with resection of the involved portion of mandible. Even then hemorrhage may be profuse. Ten units of donor blood should be available if needed.

References

1. Lund, B. A. and Dahlin, D. C.: Hemangiomas of the mandible and maxilla. J. Oral Surg. *22:*234, 1964.
2. McComb, R. J. and Traut, J. R.: Spontaneous oral hemorrhage; arteriovenous aneurysm. Br. Dent. J. *128:*239, 1970.
3. Hartley, J. H. and Shatten, W. E.: Cavernous hemangioma of the mandible. Plast. Reconstr. Surg. *50:*287, 1972.
4. Worth, H. M. and Stoneman, D. W.: Radiology of vascular abnormalities in and about the jaws. Dent. Radiogr. Photog. *52:*1, 1979.
5. Halzonitis, J. A., Kountouris, J., and Halzonitis, N. A.: Arteriovenous aneurysm of the mandible. Oral Surg. *53:*454, 1982.

Pseudotumor of Hemophilia

Age: Children
Sex: Males

Clinical and Radiographic Features: Hemophilia, an X-linked recessive disease, affects males primarily and results in a deficiency of coagulation factor VIII. Gingival bleeding, ecchymosis, and hemarthrosis are the major findings. Two percent of the patients will experience subperiosteal hemorrhage following trauma. Patients with factor IX deficiency may experience similar problems. The

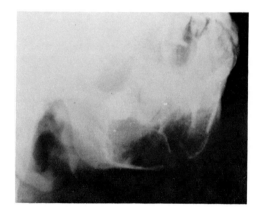

FIG. 9–49. Hemophilic pseudotumor involving the mandible.

subperiosteal focus of hemorrhage may progress to involve medullary bone. Clinically, a firm expansile mass is observed over the body and angle of the mandible. Radiographically, a multilocular radiolucency is observed and is expansile.

Microscopic Features: The lesion shows foci of granulation tissue, fibrous tissue, hematoma with extravasated erythrocytes, and reactive new bone formation. Cystic spaces without an epithelial lining are also frequently encountered.

Differential Diagnosis: A multicystic expansile mass in the mandible of a patient with a genetic coagulation disorder and a history of trauma will suggest the diagnosis of hemophilic pseudotumor. Alternatively, a hemophiliac could, of course, develop any of the other lesions included here. A biopsy is recommended for securing a definitive diagnosis.

Treatment: Biopsy and definitive surgery must be performed following administration of the appropriate factor cryoprecipitate. Curettage is the treatment of choice. The mandible may heal yet remain expanded.

References:

1. Abell, J. M., Jr., and Bayley, R. W.: Hemophilic pseudotumors of the mandible. Arch. Surg. *81*:569, 1960.
2. Stoneman, D. W., Beierl, C., and Douglas, C.: Pseudotumor of hemophilia in the mandible. Oral Surg. *40*:811, 1975.
3. Mulkey, T. F.: Hemophilic pseudotumors of the mandible. J. Oral Surg. *35*:561, 1977.
4. Marquez, J. L., et al.: Hemophilic pseudotumor of the inferior maxilla. Report of a case. Oral Surg. *53*:347, 1982.

Central Fibromatosis (Desmoplastic Fibroma)

Age: Teenagers and young adults

Sex: No predilection

Clinical and Radiographic Features: Aggressive juvenile fibromatosis is a reactive fibroblastic proliferation of the soft tissues. Rarely, histologically similar lesions arise centrally in the jawbones and are reminiscent of central desmoplastic fibromas that arise in the long bones. Rapid expansion with facial asymmetry is the usual presenting sign, and the mandible is more often the site of origin. Radiographically, a well-delineated multilocular or unilocular pattern is encountered with concomitant root resorption or divergence. Perforation of the cortex is by no means rare, and when large lesions occur it may be difficult to determine whether the lesion arose centrally with perforation or peripherally with bony invasion.

Microscopic Features: The lesion is hypercellular, being composed of fibroblasts and varying amounts of collagen. The collagen fibers are usually thin and delicate with fasciculations and her-

ringbone, chevron, or storiform configurations. In keeping with desmoplastic fibroma of long bones, some of these fibroblastic proliferations synthesize more mature, dense collagen bundles. Osseous trabeculae are either lacking or are a minor element.

Differential Diagnosis: Fibromatosis central in bone cannot be differentiated with certainty from the other aggressive neoplasms included here. A history of rapid expansion and ability to clinically and radiographically detect cortical perforation in a teenage patient should arouse suspicion of fibromatosis.

Treatment: Fibromatosis is aggressive with significant potential for growth despite its benignity. Indeed, some pathologists prefer to refer to these lesions as nonmetastasizing fibrosarcomas. Small lesions with total osseous confinement may be successfully managed by thorough enucleation and curettage. Large or massive tumors with cortical perforation will usually require marginal or en bloc resection.

References

1. Fisher, A. V. and Philipsen, H. P.: Desmoplastic fibroma of the jawbones. Int. J. Oral Surg. *5*:285, 1976.
2. Peed, L. F. and Epker, B. N.: Aggressive juvenile fibromatosis involving the mandible: surgical excision with immediate reconstruction. Oral Surg. *43*:651, 1977.
3. Henefer, E. P., Bishop, H. C., and Brown, A.: Juvenile fibromatosis with invasion of the mandible: report of two cases. J. Oral Surg. *36*:965, 1978.
4. Freedman, P. D., Cardo, V. A., and Kerpel, S. M.: Desmoplastic fibroma (fibromatosis) of the jawbones. Oral Surg. *46*:386, 1978.
5. Melrose, R. J. and Abrams, A. M.: Juvenile fibromatosis affecting the jaws. Report of three cases. Oral Surg. *49*:317, 1980.

Fibrous Dysplasia

Age: Teenagers

Sex: No predilection

Clinical and Radiographic Features: Whereas fibrous dysplasia of the jaws is more frequently encountered in the maxilla as a ground-glass radiopacity, when the mandible is involved the lesion often assumes a multilocular radiolucent pattern. Characteristically, expansion is evident and the radiographic margins of the growth are indiscrete. The expansion develops insidiously during the early teenage years with progressive slow growth. The growth potential begins to wane as skeletal maturity ensues. In rare instances, fibrous dysplasia shows a rapid enlargement with an ag-

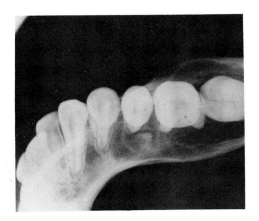

FIG. 9–50. Central fibromatosis.

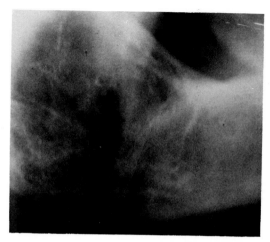

FIG. 9–51. Diffuse, poorly marginated multicystic lesion of posterior mandible in monostotic fibrous dysplasia.

gressive clinical course. Polyostotic lesions should be searched for by means of skull films and a skeletal survey.

Microscopic Features: A hypercellular proliferative fibrous tissue element predominates the sections. Dispersed throughout are irregular, poorly formed osseous trabeculae that are usually but not invariably fetal or woven. These trabeculae are often devoid of any osteoblastic rimming.

Differential Diagnosis: When fibrous dysplasia appears as a multilocular radiolucency, it must be differentiated from the other diseases included here as multilocular lesions. The lack of definition at the lesional borders is highly suggestive of fibrous dysplasia, yet biopsy must be performed to confirm the clinicoradiologic impression.

Treatment: Treatment should be postponed until growth of the lesion subsides. Surgical intervention before cessation of growth may actually result in activation of the lesion. In those lesions showing a rapidly proliferative course, close follow-up should be instituted. If the lesion begins to manifest massive growth potential, resection should be considered. In the ordinary, less aggressive and common form of the disease, cosmetic osseous contouring can be undertaken when growth ceases. Radiation therapy has been shown to predispose to postradiation sarcoma.

References
1. Zimmerman, D. C., Dahlin, D. C., and Stafne, E. C.: Fibrous dysplasia of the maxilla and mandible. Oral Surg. *11*:55, 1958.
2. Eversole, L. R., Sabes, W. R., and Rovin, S.: Fibrous dysplasia; a nosologic problem in the diagnosis of fibro-osseous lesions of the jaws. J. Oral Pathol. *1*:189, 1972.
3. Waldron, C. A. and Giansanti, J. S.: Benign fibro-osseous lesions of the jaws: a clinical-radiologic-histologic review of sixty-five cases. I. Fibrous dysplasia of the jaws. Oral Surg. *35*:190, 1973.

MOTH-EATEN RADIOLUCENCIES

Osteomyelitis

Age: No predilection
Sex: No predilection

Clinical and Radiographic Features: Osteomyelitis of the jaws usually originates from odontogenic infection. It may be acute, subacute, or chronic, the first being most painful. The patient is usually only slightly febrile, and cervical lymphadenopathy is a frequent finding. Staphylococci and streptococci are the predominant causative organisms; however, actinomycetes and anaerobic gram-negative bacilli are cultured in many instances. Clinically, in acute and subacute stages, multiple fistulae with draining purulent exudate are encountered. Paresthesia and pain are associated with acute infections. Radiographically, the cortices rarely show expansion. The lesion may be multilocular or show approximating multifocal radiolucencies with ill-defined, moth-eaten margins. Radiopaque sequestrae are frequently seen to "float" within radiolucent crypts. Specific forms of chronic osteomyelitis (phosphorus poisoning, syphilis, and tuberculosis) may involve the jaws. Another specific osseous inflammation, osteoradionecrosis, develops in jaws of patients undergoing radiation therapy for oral carcinoma. Patients with Paget's disease of bone and osteopetrosis are

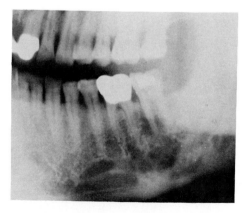

FIG. 9–52. Osteomyelitis showing a diffuse moth-eaten radiolucent pattern.

prone to develop widespread osteomyelitis of the jaws from odontogenic infection.

Microscopic Features: Osseous trabeculae and necrotic bone are surrounded by granulation tissue, necrotic debris, and inflammatory cells. The inflammatory cell infiltrate varies depending upon whether the process is acute, subacute, or chronic. Syphilitic osteomyelitis may display foci of gummatous necrosis. Tuberculous osteomyelitis is characterized by the presence of specific granulomatous inflammation with Langhans' giant cells.

Differential Diagnosis: When an offending necrotic tooth overlies the radiographic defect, when pain is present and the patient is febrile, a clinical diagnosis can usually be made. Nevertheless, moth-eaten radiolucencies occur in metastatic and primary epithelial and mesenchymal malignant neoplasms. Failure to respond within 2 weeks to therapeutic measures to control infection necessitates biopsy.

Treatment: Nonspecific osteomyelitis requires elimination of the source of infection (tooth extraction), incision and drainage if spaces are involved, and antibiotic therapy. Penicillin is the drug of choice. Before antibiotic therapy is instituted, a sterile aspirate should be obtained and submitted for both routine and anaerobic culture and sensitivity tests. In patients with high fever, space infection, or accompanying cellulitis, hospitalization with intravenous antibiotic therapy and supportive care may be required. Surgical debridement with removal of sequestra is indicated when widespread osseous involvement is seen.

References

1. Mowlem, R.: Osteomyelitis of the jaw. Proc. R. Soc. Med. 38:452, 1945.
2. Kinnmann, J. E. G. and Lee, H. S.: Chronic osteomyelitis of the mandible; clinical study of thirteen cases. Oral Surg. 25:6, 1968.
3. Musser, L. M., Tulumello, T. N., and Hiatt, W. R.: Actinomycosis of the anterior maxilla. Oral Surg. 44:21, 1977.
4. Yakata, H., et al.: Actinomycotic osteomyelitis of the mandible. J. Oral Surg. 36:720, 1975.
5. Saunders, B.: Current concepts in the management of osteomyelitis of the mandible. J. Oral Med. 33:40, 1978.

Primary Intraosseous Carcinoma

Age: Middle-aged adults
Sex: Male predilection

Clinical and Radiographic Features: Primary malignant epithelial tumors central in bone are extremely rare, but may arise from odontogenic epithelium enclosed within the periodontal ligament or other intraosseous locations. The chief clinical manifestations are the same as those for metastatic carcinomas of the jaws. Clinically demonstrable expansion, paresthesia, pain, and, occasionally, unexplained loosening of teeth occur. Radiographically, the lesion is multilocular with poorly defined borders. Expansion or cortical perforation is encountered. Primary squamous cell carcinomas of the jaws may also arise from the linings of odontogenic cysts, usually residual cysts.

Microscopic Features: Intraosseous carcinoma shows sheets and islands of neoplastic epithelium manifesting the cardinal signs of malignancy— hyperchromatism, pleomorphism, and mitoses. Acanthotic regions resembling pearl formation are occasionally present. Thus, the tumor closely resembles squamous cell carcinoma. A distinctive feature is the odontogenic nature of the tumor cells. An outer rim of ameloblastic cells occupies the position usually assumed by basal cells in an ordinary squamous cell carcinoma. Carcinomas arising from odontogenic cysts usually do not show odontogenic features; rather, they represent typical squamous cell carcinoma.

Differential Diagnosis: The moth-eaten radiolucent pattern of intraosseous carcinoma is similar to that of osteomyelitis; however, cortical expansion is not common in infectious processes. Primary malignant mesenchymal tumors must also be included in the differential diagnosis. Metastatic carcinoma must be ruled out even after biopsy by thorough physical examination and diagnostic radiologic surveys. Only then may the tumor be considered a primary carcinoma of the jaws.

Treatment: Resection of the involved segment with regional node dissection is recommended. Chest films should be evaluated for distant spread. Survival rates are under 30 percent for 5 years.

References

1. Shear, M.: Primary intra-alveolar epidermoid carcinoma of the jaw. J. Pathol. 97:645, 1969.
2. Sirsat, M. V., Sampat, M. B., and Shrikhande, S. E.: Primary intra-alveolar squamous cell carcinoma of the mandible. Oral Surg. 35:366, 1973.
3. Coonar, H.: Primary intraosseous carcinoma of maxilla. Br. Dent. J. 147:47, 1979.

Cystogenic Carcinoma

Age: Elderly
Sex: Male predilection

Clinical and Radiographic Features: Squamous

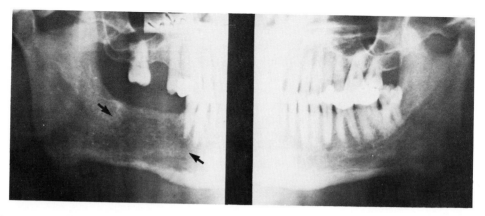

FIG. 9–53.   Nondiscrete diffuse radiolucency of mandible in primary intraosseous carcinoma.

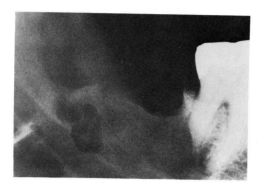

FIG. 9–54.   Cystogenic carcinoma of the jaw showing root resorption.

cell carcinoma may, on rare occasions, arise from the lining of odontogenic cysts. Central mucoepidermoid carcinoma, a malignant salivary neoplasm, may also evolve from odontogenic cyst linings. Whereas squamous cancers are more often associated with residual cysts of the mandibular body, mucoepidermoid tumors are generally observed in the posterior mandible, and tumorigenesis from a dentigerous cyst can often be speculated or even documented. Maxillary cases have also been reported; however, documented origin from cyst lining is problemmatic when antral involvement exists. Clinically, paresthesia is a frequent yet certainly not invariable symptom. Radiographically, a poorly marginated unilocular or moth-eaten pattern is observed.

Microscopic Features: Remnants of ordinary stratified squamous epithelial lining are seen with both mural and luminal proliferation of squamous cell carcinoma exhibiting nuclear hyperchroma-

tism, pleomorphism, increased mitotic activity, and keratin pearl formation. Cystogenic mucoepidermoid tumors are usually of the low-grade variety with solid and cystic islands comprised of mucous, epidermoid, and intermediate cells.

Differential Diagnosis: Cystogenic cancers, especially when paresthesia is present, radiographically and clinically simulate other malignant bone tumors including metastatic carcinoma, intraosseous carcinoma, and primary sarcomas. Biopsy with documented evidence of typical cyst lining is required for the diagnosis.

Treatment: Complete block resection is required; should any palpable nodes be discovered, a neck dissection is indicated. Because of insufficient data on these lesions, the prognosis remains unknown.

References

1. Gardner, A. G.: The odontogenic cyst as a potential carcinoma, a clinicopathologic appraisal. J. Am. Dent. Assoc. *78*:746, 1969.
2. Hampl, P. F. and Harrigan, W. F.: Squamous cell carcinoma probably arising from an odontogenic cyst: report of case. J. Oral Surg. *31*:359, 1973.
3. Lapin, R.: Squamous cell carcinoma arising in a dentigerous cyst. J. Oral Surg. *31*:354, 1973.
4. Eversole, L. R., Sabes, W. R., and Rovin, S.: Aggressive growth and neoplastic potential of odontogenic cysts, with special reference to central epidermoid and central mucoepidermoid carcinoma. Cancer *35*:270, 1975.

Metastatic Carcinoma

Age: Adult predilection
Sex: Male predilection

Clinical and Radiographic Features: Metastasis to the jaws from primary carcinoma located in visceral or parenchymal organs (usually the lung,

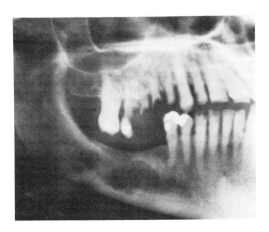

FIG. 9–55. Diffuse irregular radiolucency of the mandibular body representing a metastatic carcinoma from the lung.

breast, colon, or prostate) may reach the medullary bone by hematogenous spread via arterial dissemination from tumor foci located in the lungs or via retrograde migration of tumor emboli through Batson's paravertebral plexus, thereby bypassing the lungs. Metastatic cancer is the most common malignancy of the jawbones. Whereas most instances of osseous metastasis to the jaws appear as irregular moth-eaten expansile radiolucencies, some metastatic carcinomas may induce ossification so that areas of radiolucency are admixed with irregular radiopaque foci. Prostatic and thyroid tumors are more prone to demonstrate osteoblastic foci. Juxtaposed teeth may show root resorption; however, large areas of osseous destruction with no resorptive changes of the teeth are more common. The angle and body of the mandible are the favored sites of deposition, probably because of the rich intraosseous vascularity in these areas. The most important and consistent clinical findings include swelling, paresthesia of the lip, and deeply situated bone pain. Loosening of teeth is also a frequent finding.

Microscopic Features: Nests, islands, and cords of neoplastic epithelium are supported by a fibrous stroma. In the case of osteoblastic metastasis, extensive osteoplasia may be demonstrated microscopically. The individual tumor cells may show a keratinizing, adenoid, or anaplastic morphology depending upon the site of origin of the primary tumor.

Differential Diagnosis: The irregular poorly margined expansile radiolucencies encountered in metastatic carcinoma may also be seen in other malignant tumors of the jaws: reticulum cell sarcoma, Ewing's sarcoma, Burkitt's lymphoma, and osteogenic, chondrogenic, or fibrogenic sarcomata. Osteomyelitis rarely shows expansion. A history of cancer elsewhere or the presence of paresthesia is highly suggestive of metastatic cancer. Primary intra-alveolar carcinoma shows microscopic features that are somewhat unusual; however, the diagnosis should be reserved for those patients in whom exhaustive examination procedures fail to disclose the presence of a primary carcinoma located elsewhere.

Treatment: The discovery of a metastatic deposit in the jaws carries an extremely poor prognosis. Once the diagnosis is rendered, a complete workup is indicated to locate the primary tumor, as is a metastatic radiographic series to search for other sites of osseous metastasis. In most cases the disease is treated palliatively, and radiation therapy may be indicated to relieve pain. Rarely, the jaw lesion may represent a single focus of metastasis and the disease may be treatable by surgical and/or radiation therapy to both the primary tumor and jaw metastasis.

References

1. Castigliano, S. G. and Rominger, C. J.: Metastatic malignancy of jaws. Am. J. Surg. *87:*496, 1954.
2. Cash, C. D., et al.: Metastatic tumors of the jaws. Oral Surg. *14:*897, 1961.
3. Carter, D. G., Anderson, E. E., and Currie, D. P.: Renal cell carcinoma metastatic to the mandible. J. Oral Surg. *35:*992, 1977.
4. Perriman, A. O. and Figures, K. H.: Metastatic retinoblastoma of the mandible. Oral Surg. *45:*741, 1978.
5. Goveia, G. and Bahn, S.: Asymptomatic hepatocellular carcinoma metastatic to the mandible. Oral Surg. *45:*424, 1978.

Osteosarcoma and Chondrosarcoma

Age: Adults
Sex: No predilection (female predilection in mandibular tumors)

Clinical and Radiographic Features: Whereas both osteogenic and chondrogenic sarcomas are capable of calcification, with resultant opacification on radiographs, many forms fail to show significant calcification and appear as irregular, poorly delineated expansile radiolucencies. Both tumors are rare in the jaws; as opposed to osteosarcoma of other bones, jaw lesions tend to occur in older individuals as well as in teenagers. The mandible is affected more often than the maxilla. Both osteo- and chondrosarcomas are rapidly growing neoplasms with a propensity for distant

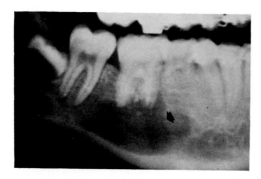

FIG. 9–56. Poorly marginated radiolucency in the mandibular body in osteogenic sarcoma.

rather than nodal metastasis. Expansion, pain, and paresthesia are common features.

Microscopic Features: Osteogenic sarcoma exists in three histomorphologic variations: osteoblastic, chondroblastic, and fibroblastic. The latter is most often radiolucent. The histology cannot be correlated with prognostic predictability. Chondrosarcomas generally contain hyaline cartilage with pleomorphic chondroblasts. A specific histologic variant, the mesenchymal chondrosarcoma, has a predilection for the jaws. These tumors contain very little identifiable hyaline cartilage, but are composed of immature hypercellular spindle and stellate cells with intervening basophilic ground substance. Focal areas are traversed by cleft-like channels reminiscent of hemangioendothelioma.

Differential Diagnosis: Osteo- and chondrosarcomas of moth-eaten radiolucent pattern resemble metastatic carcinoma, intra-alveolar carcinoma, and other mesenchymal malignancies such as reticulum cell sarcoma, Ewing's sarcoma, neurosarcoma, and fibrosarcoma of bone. Biopsy is required to obtain a definitive diagnosis.

Treatment: Hemimandibulectomy or maxillectomy is required. Radium needle implants, followed by resection, have also been employed. The 5-year survival for osteogenic sarcoma of the jaws is under 50 percent. Mandibular tumors show a better prognosis than those arising in the maxilla. Since regional metastases are extremely rare, prophylactic neck dissection is not indicated.

References
1. Chaudhry, A. P., et al.: Chondrogenic tumors of the jaws. Am. J. Surg. 102:403, 1961.
2. Garrington, G. E., et al.: Osteosarcoma of the jaws. Cancer 20:377, 1967.
3. Chambers, R. G. and Mahoney, W. D.: Osteogenic sarcoma of the mandible: current management. Am. J. Surg. 36:463, 1970.
4. High, C. L. and Glass, R. T.: Osteosarcoma of the mandible. Oral Surg. 45:678, 1978.
5. Christensen, R. E.: Mesenchymal chondrosarcoma of the jaws. Oral Surg. 54:197, 1982.

Ewing's Sarcoma

Age: Teenagers
Sex: Male predilection

Clinical and Radiographic Features: Ewing's sarcoma is a rare primary malignant mesenchymal neoplasm of bone. The true cell of origin is unknown, but is probably an undifferentiated osseous mesenchymal cell. The disease is most frequently encountered in the long bones of the lower extremities, but may appear initially in the jaws, usually the mandible. Expansion with pain, paresthesia, or anesthesia usually constitutes the chief complaint. Unexplained loosening of teeth may also be a feature, and leukocytosis with elevated temperature is often encountered. Radiographically, the tumor is radiolucent with ill-defined margins. Expansion or erosion of the cortex is observed, and occasionally an osteophyte reaction or cortical redundancy (onion skinning) is demonstrable. If left untreated, widespread metastasis to other bones and visceral organs ensues rapidly.

Microscopic Features: The tumor is composed of diffuse sheets of hyperchromatic round cells with virtually no fibrous stroma. Septae traverse the neoplastic element, and tumor cells tend to orient themselves about blood vessels. Multifocal zones of necrosis are commonly seen.

Differential Diagnosis: Ewing's sarcoma may radiographically and clinically resemble osteomyelitis. Particularly when onion skinning is pres-

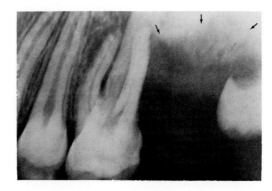

FIG. 9–57. Moth-eaten radiolucent lesion of tuberosity in a child with Ewing's sarcoma.

ent, confusion with Garre's periostitis may arise. The moth-eaten expansile radiographic appearance may also be seen in a variety of bone malignancies, including metastatic carcinoma, lymphoma, and other bone sarcomas. Biopsy is required to provide a definitive diagnosis.

Treatment: Ewing's sarcoma is a highly malignant neoplasm with a 5-year survival under 10 percent. The disease should be managed by an oncologist. Treatment is usually by radiation and chemotherapy. Surgical intervention is occasionally attempted. Teeth should be extracted before radiation therapy when they are embedded in tumor.

References

1. Crowe, W. W. and Harper, J. C.: Ewing's sarcoma with primary lesion in mandible. J. Oral Surg. 23:156, 1965.
2. Potdar, G. G.: Ewing's tumors of the jaws. Oral Surg. 29:505, 1970.
3. Carl, W., et al.: Ewing's sarcoma. J. Oral Surg. 31:472, 1971.
4. Rapaport, A., et al.: Ewing's sarcoma of the mandible. Oral Surg. 44:89, 1977.
5. Borghelli, R. F., Barros, R. E., and Zampieri, J.: Ewing's sarcoma of the mandible. Report of case. J. Oral Surg. 36:473, 1978.

Primary Lymphoma of Bone

Age: Young adults
Sex: Male predilection

Clinical and Radiographic Features: Primary lymphoma that originates from bone-marrow lymphoid precursor cells is generally of the non-Hodgkin's variety, lymphocytic and/or histiocytic type. This form was, in the past, referred to as reticulum cell sarcoma of bone. The pelvis and long bones of the lower extremities are the usual sites of origin, yet the jaws may be involved initially or jaw lesions may accompany tumor in other osseous sites. The clinical features include expansion, pain or paresthesia, and unexplained loosening of teeth. Radiographically, the medullary bone shows marked osseous destruction or merely a loss of trabeculation with ill-defined margins. Cortical expansion or perforation is often demonstrable radiographically.

Microscopic Features: The biopsy specimen shows diffuse sheets of oval to round nucleated cells separated by scant or often undiscernible stroma. The nuclei are larger than those of mature lymphocytes, and the nucleoplasm is moderately stained with stippling. Reticulum stains show a rich intercellular network of reticulum fibers. These tumors are usually classified as mixed histiocytic/lymphocytic lymphomas.

Differential Diagnosis: Ill-defined moth-eaten radiolucencies with pain, typical of primary lymphoma of bone, are also features of osteomyelitis. In the latter, an infectious source, usually odontogenic, is detectable; expansion of the cortex is unusual. These same radiographic features are seen with Ewing's sarcoma, other primary sarcomas of osteogenic mesenchymal tissue, and metastatic carcinoma. The diagnosis requires microscopic evaluation. Once the diagnosis has been secured, a complete blood count should be performed to rule out leukemia with infiltration into bone.

Treatment: Radiation therapy with or without chemotherapy is the treatment of choice and should be performed by an oncologist or radiation therapist. Teeth should be extracted from the radiation field before therapy. Five-year survival rates are good for this form of lymphoma, exceeding 70 percent.

References

1. Gerry, R. G. and Williams, S. F.: Primary reticulum cell sarcoma of the mandible. Oral Surg. 8:568, 1955.
2. Ivins, J. C. and Dahlin, D. C.: Malignant lymphoma (reticulum cell sarcoma) of bone. Mayo Clin. Proc. 38:375, 1963.
3. Lehrer, S., Roswit, B., and Federman, A.: The presentation of malignant lymphoma in the oral cavity and pharynx. Oral Surg. 41:441, 1976.
4. Cline, R. E. and Stenger, T. G.: Histiocytic lymphoma (reticulum-cell sarcoma). Report of five cases. Oral Surg. 43:422, 1977.

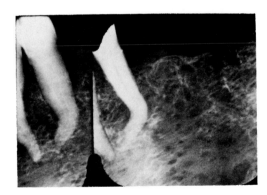

FIG. 9–58. Irregular, poorly defined radiolucencies representing primary lymphoma of bone. (From Melrose, R. J. and Abrams, A. M.: *Oral Tumors, A Visual Instruction Course.* Los Angeles, Eureka Press, 1974, p. 55.)

Burkitt's Lymphoma (African Lymphoma)

Age: Children
Sex: Male predilection

Clinical and Radiographic Features: Burkitt's (African) lymphoma is a unique form of lymphoma found primarily in Uganda and Kenya. Clinically similar cases have been discovered in the United States. The unique character of the disease rests with the predilection for tumor to involve certain organs and locations, namely the jaws, abdominal nodes, and ovaries. Other visceral tissues may be infiltrated as well. The disease occurs in a specific geographic locale and at specific ranges in altitude, implicating an insect vector of transmission. Accumulating evidence suggests that the Epstein-Barr virus may be causative (the same virus that causes the benign lymphoproliferative disorder infectious mononucleosis). Clinically, the tumor is capable of massive growth with marked expansion and facial disfigurement with loosening and displacement of teeth. Abdominal distension from node and visceral lesions is common. Radiographically, massive destruction of bone is observed with a moth-eaten, poorly marginated pattern. The cortex shows expansion or erosion and perforation.

Microscopic Features: There are diffuse sheets of mature lymphocytes, and the tumor is essentially devoid of fibrous stroma. Reticulum stains show a profuse network of reticulum around tumor cells. The pathognomonic microscopic pattern of Burkitt's lymphoma, referred to as the "starry-sky" appearance, is characterized by multiple foci of large pale-staining histiocytic cells with vesicular nuclei and generous amounts of cytoplasm dispersed randomly within a sea of darker staining lymphoid cells.

Differential Diagnosis: The combination of jaw lesions with abdominal masses in an African child is classic for Burkitt's lymphoma. In other geographic areas, the moth-eaten expansile radiolucency of Burkitt's lymphoma must be differentiated from other lesions occurring with equal or greater frequency. Osteomyelitis may show similar features, but expansion is uncommon. Other sarcomas of bone as well as metastatic childhood tumors (e.g., neuroblastoma, nephroblastoma) must be included in the differential diagnosis. Biopsy will disclose the characteristic histomorphology of Burkitt's lymphoma.

Treatment: This form of lymphoma is fatal, but chemotherapy effects remarkable tumor shrinkage and will account for extended remissions. The patient should be managed by a medical oncologist.

References

1. Burkitt, D.: A sarcoma involving the jaws in African children. Br. J. Surg. 48:218, 1958.
2. Lehner, T.: The jaws and teeth in Burkitt's tumor (African lymphoma). J. Pathol. Bacteriol. 88:581, 1964.
3. Terril, D. G., et al.: American Burkitt's lymphoma in Pittsburgh, Pennsylvania. Oral Surg. 44:411, 1977.
4. Adatia, A. K.: Significance of jaw lesions in Burkitt's lymphoma. Br. Dent. J. 145:263, 1978.
5. Ziegler, J. L.: Burkitt's lymphoma. CA 32:144, 1982.

Fibrogenic and Neurogenic Sarcoma

Age: Young and middle-aged adults
Sex: No predilection

Clinical and Radiographic Features: Sarcomas derived from fibroblasts or nerve sheath (Schwann cells, perineural fibroblasts) are occasionally encountered in bone. Indeed, central neurogenic sarcomas are encountered more frequently in the mandible than in any other bone, probably because of the unique anatomy by which the alveolar nerve traverses a long distance while encased in bone. The chief clinical findings include paresthesia, swelling, and loosening of teeth. Both fibrosarcomas and neurosarcomas will manifest as ill-defined radiolucencies, which may cause root resorption or divergence. Expansion may be obvious; however, large areas of osseous destruction may evolve in the absence of any expansion. Neurosarcomas often produce a fusiform widening of the inferior alveolar canal, tending to grow along the course of the nerve as high as the Gasserian ganglion.

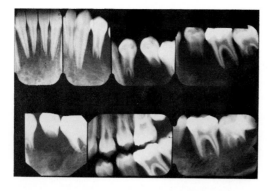

FIG. 9–59. Diffuse, destructive lesion in Burkitt's lymphoma. (From Sachs, R. L.: Burkitt's tumor (African lymphoma syndrome) in California. Oral Surg. 22:621, 1966.)

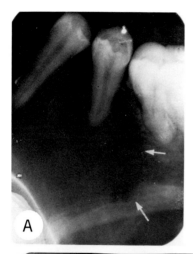

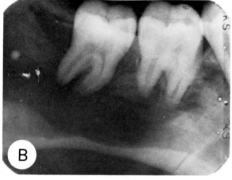

FIG. 9–60. Ill-defined radiolucency in mandible representing a central fibrosarcoma. (From Eversole, L. R., et al.: Central and peripheral fibrogenic and neurogenic sarcoma of the oral regions. Oral Surg. *36*:49, 1973.)

Microscopic Features: Both fibrogenic and neurogenic sarcomas are hypercellular spindle cell proliferations displaying very little or only moderate pleomorphism. Mitotic figures are usually numerous. The tumor cells grow in parallel fascicles, and palisading may be a feature of neural sheath malignancies. This is not a constant feature, however, and proof of origin from nerve sheath requires the demonstration of continuity between an intact nerve and the circumneural tumor mass.

Differential Diagnosis: An ill-defined enlargement of the inferior alveolar canal in conjunction with paresthesia is highly suggestive of central neurogenic sarcoma. Since both fibrosarcoma and neurosarcoma may show an expansile moth-eaten radiolucency with or without resorption of adjacent teeth, other malignant tumors including metastatic cancer and primary sarcomas of bone must be included in the differential diagnosis. Mi-

croscopic evaluation is necessary to secure a definitive diagnosis.

Treatment: Surgical resection, hemimandibulectomy, or partial maxillectomy, including at least 3 cm of tumor-free margin, is the treatment of choice. In the case of neurosarcoma, dissection of the inferior alveolar nerve, sampling for microscopic evidence of tumor, is advisable. Central fibrosarcoma has a better prognosis in the jaws than it does in other bones. The 5-year survival exceeds 50 percent.

References

1. Van Blarcom, C. W., Masson, J. K., and Dahlin, D. C.: Fibrosarcoma of the mandible; a clinicopathologic study. Oral Surg. *32*:428, 1972.
2. Eversole, L. R., Schwartz, W. D., and Sabes, W. R.: Central and peripheral fibrogenic and neurogenic sarcoma of the oral regions. Oral Surg. *36*:49, 1973.
3. Upton, L. G., Hayward, J. R., and Kerr, D. A.: Neurofibrosarcoma of the mandible. J. Oral Surg. *35*:504, 1977.
4. David, D. J., et al.: Malignant Schwannoma of the inferior dental nerve. Br. J. Plast. Surg. *31*:323, 1978.
5. Saw, D.: Fibrosarcoma of maxilla: report of a case with histochemical studies. Oral Surg. *47*:164, 1979.

Melanotic Neuroectodermal Tumor of Infancy

Age: Infancy
Sex: No predilection

Clinical and Radiographic Features: Melanotic neuroectodermal tumor of infancy is a benign neoplasm derived from neural crest cells with a propensity to involve tooth-bearing regions in the maxilla. The precise origin is controversial. At one time this neoplasm was classified with the odon-

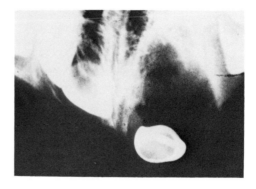

FIG. 9–61. Displaced developing incisor with underlying, poorly marginated radiolucency in melanotic neuroectodermal tumor of infancy. (Courtesy of Drs. D. Kerr, P. Pullon, and H. Hubinger.)

togenic tumors; however, cases have been reported in the skull, shoulder region, testes, and uterus. Some cells within the dental papillae have been shown to be derived from neural crest precursors, so the tumor may represent a neuroectodermal odontogenic lesion when it arises in the jaws. Early theories suggested origin from ectopic retinal tissues. These theories account for the various terms applied to this neoplasm (pigmented ameloblastoma, retinal anlage tumor, progonoma). The neoplasm is rarely encountered after 6 months of age and, as previously stated, is more often seen in the maxilla than the mandible. Clinically, the edentulous alveolus of the infant shows a smooth-surfaced bulging and is generally nonpigmented. Radiographically, the lesion is radiolucent with irregular, ill-defined margins. Developing teeth may lie within the radiolucent area or are significantly displaced by the neoplasm. As with other neoplasms of neuroblastic origin, vanillylmandelic acid may be detected in the urine. Apparently, some of these tumors, albeit few, are capable of metastasis.

Microscopic Features: The tumor is composed of alveolar nests of cells oriented about cleft-like spaces, with a surrounding dense fibrous stroma. Two cell types are encountered: An epithelioid polygonal cell with an oval vesicular nucleus is seen to contain melanin granules. The other cell type resembles a neuroblast having a round hyperchromatic nucleus with sparse or unidentifiable cytoplasm. These two types coexist in the alveolar clusters.

Differential Diagnosis: The poorly marginated borders of melanotic neuroectodermal tumor would appear to support a radiologic diagnosis of malignancy. Similar features may, of course, be seen in any of the malignant bone tumors included among the moth-eaten radiolucencies; however, none of the malignant osseous neoplasms shows a tendency to arise in infants. Therefore, a maxillary aggressive-appearing radiolucent lesion in a neonate should be considered to represent melanotic neuroectodermal tumor. Since sarcomas do occasionally arise in early childhood, biopsy confirmation is mandatory.

Treatment: Local curettage is the treatment of choice for this benign neoplasm. Recurrences have been recorded; however, most instances can be cured without resorting to en bloc resection. Since a few cases have metastasized, a complete radiologic evaluation should be performed, and close periodic follow-up is recommended.

References

1. Borello, E. D. and Gorlin, R. J.: Melanotic neuroectodermal tumor of infancy—a neoplasm of neural crest origin; report of a case associated with high urinary excretion of vanilmandelic acid. Cancer 19:196, 1966.
2. Allen, M. S., Jr., et al.: "Retinal anlage" tumors; melanotic progonoma, melanotic adamantinoma, pigmented epulis, melanotic neurectodermal tumor of infancy. Am. J. Clin. Pathol. 51:309, 1969.
3. Brekke, J. H. and Gorlin, R. J.: Melanotic neurectodermal tumor of infancy. J. Oral Surg. 33:858, 1975.
4. Block, J. C., et al.: Pigmented neuroectodermal tumor of infancy. An example of rarely expressed malignant behavior. Oral Surg. 49:279, 1980.
5. Gotcher, J. E., et al.: Recurrent melanotic neuroectodermal tumor of infancy: report of case and tumor heterotransplantation studies. J. Oral Surg. 38:702, 1980.

MULTIFOCAL RADIOLUCENCIES

Basal Cell Nevus Syndrome

Age: Teenagers
Sex: No predilection

Clinical and Radiographic Features: The basal cell nevus syndrome is an autosomal dominant genetic disease characterized by a primary triad with variable secondary anomalies. The chief features include nevoid basal cell carinomas, one or more bifid ribs, and multiple odontogenic keratocysts of the jaws. The basal cell lesions have limited growth potential, arise during childhood or early adulthood, and appear in regions of the skin not necessarily exposed to solar radiation. The keratocysts are multiple; they may be interradicular or pericoronal well-delineated unilocular radiolucencies; some may be multilocular. Cortical expansion in larger cysts is obvious clinically as well as radiographically. Other anomalies seen in the syndrome include frontal bossing, hypertelorism, calcified falx cerebri, prognathism, and palmar-plantar hyperkeratosis. Individuals with this disorder are also prone to develop medulloblastomas, malignant posterior fossa brain tumors.

Microscopic Features: The keratocysts of the basal cell nevus syndrome do not differ from those seen as solitary lesions. The lumen contains laminations of keratin. The lining epithelium displays a corrugated surface, attenuated spinous layer, and polarized basal cell layer.

Differential Diagnosis: The multifocal radiolucencies, particularly when many of them are pericoronal, in conjunction with bifid ribs and

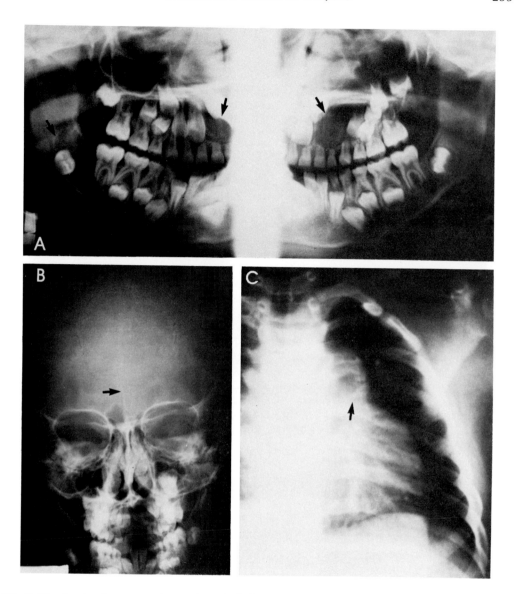

FIG. 9–62. Basal cell nevus syndrome. A: Multiple keratocysts of the jaws. B: Calcified falx cerebri. C: Rib anomalies. (Courtesy of Dr. John Kiesselbach.)

basal cell tumors are classic for the basal cell nevus syndrome. From the jaw films alone, the multifocal radiolucencies may resemble multiple keratocysts without other features of the syndrome, multiple dentigerous cysts, or even histiocytosis X. The latter rarely shows expansion.

Treatment: Thorough curettage of the jaw cysts is required. Chemical cautery of the bony crypt may be performed. Recurrences are common and will require repeated surgical intervention. The basal cell nevi may be too numerous to remove; however, they generally are not aggressive as are ordinary basal cell carcinomas. Since the condition is hereditary, siblings should be examined for features of the disease. A thorough neurologic workup with periodic examinations should be carried out to rule out medulloblastoma.

References

1. Gorlin, R. J., et al.: The multiple basal-cell nevi syndrome. Cancer 18:89, 1965.
2. Anderson, D. E. and Cook, W. A.: Jaw cysts and the basal cell nevus syndrome. J. Oral Surg. 24:15, 1966.
3. Ellis, D. J., Akin, R. K., and Bernhard, R.: Nevoid

basal cell carcinoma syndrome: report of case. J. Oral Surg. 30:851, 1972.

4. Giansanti, J. S. and Baker, G. O.: Nevoid basal cell carcinoma syndrome in Negroes: report of five cases. J. Oral Surg. 32:138, 1974.

5. Koutnick, A. W., et al.: Multiple nevoid basal cell epithelioma, cysts of the jaws, and bifid rib syndrome: report of case. J. Oral Surg. 33:686, 1975.

Histiocytosis X

Age: Children and young adults

Sex: Male predilection

Clinical and Radiographic Features: Histiocytosis X, a histiocytic proliferative disorder of the reticuloendothelial system and bone, exists in three forms: acute disseminated, chronic disseminated, and chronic limited variants. The latter two, previously termed Hand-Schuller-Christian disease and eosinophilic granuloma respectively, will be dealt with here because they are more apt to involve the jaws. Chronic disseminated histiocytosis manifest a classic triad of features: exophthalmos due to retro-orbital infiltration, diabetes insipidus due to posterior pituitary histiocytic infiltrates, and osseous lesions. Otitis media and lung infiltrations are also common. This form occurs in children and teenagers. Chronic limited histiocytosis is more often seen in young adults, is generally limited to bone with either solitary or multifocal osseous defects, and occasionally manifests pulmonary infiltrates. Jaw lesions in all forms of the disease show similar features. Pain and expansion are usually absent. Teeth may become loose for no apparent reason, and the gingiva may appear inflamed in involved areas. The lesions are more common in the mandible than maxilla and are often, yet not invariably, multifocal irregular radiolucencies lacking marginal cortication. When the alveolus is involved, the teeth may give the impression that they are floating in space, since they may be entirely encompassed by a radiolucent defect. The skull often contains punched-out radiolucencies.

Microscopic Features: Diffuse sheets of histiocytes with pale nuclei and abundant cytoplasm prevail. Occasionally, multinucleated histiocytes and foam cells are encountered. Multiple foci of eosinophilic abscesses are encountered. Fibrous stroma is scant.

Differential Diagnosis: Multifocal noncorticated radiolucencies of the jaws may occur in diseases other than the histiocytoses, including multiple myeloma, the basal cell nevus syndrome, and occasionally multifocal metastatic carcinoma and primary lymphoma of bone. Multiple early stage periapical cemental dysplasia must be considered in the differential diagnosis when lesions are located at the apex of teeth. Biopsy is required for definitive diagnosis. A skeletal radiographic survey should be obtained to check for disease in other bones.

Treatment: Chronic disseminated histiocytosis has a guarded prognosis. The disease responds to chemotherapy, particularly the Vinca alkaloids. The chronic limited form with jaw lesions can be treated by local curettage.

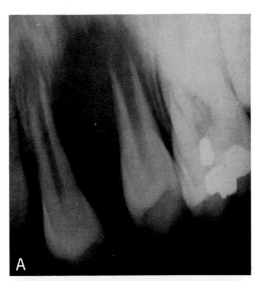
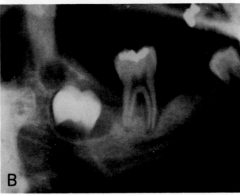

FIG. 9–63. Radiolucent lesions in both jaws in a patient with eosinophilic granuloma. (From Ragab, R. R. and Rake, O.: Eosinophilic granuloma with bilateral involvement of both jaws. Int. J. Oral Surg. 4:73, 1975.)

References

1. Sbarbaro, J. L., Jr., and Francis, K. C.: Eosinophilic granuloma of bone, JAMA 178:706, 1961.

2. Chase, D. C., Eversole, L. R. and Hall, H. D.: His-

tiocytosis X with jaw involvement. J. Oral Surg. 32:494, 1974.

3. Rapidis, A. D., et al.: Histiocytosis X. Analysis of 50 cases. Int. J. Oral Surg. 7:76, 1978.
4. Hartman, K. S.: Histiocytosis X: A review of 114 cases with oral involvement. Oral Surg. 49:38, 1980.
5. Granada, F. M. and McDaniel, R. K.: Multiple progressive eosinophilic granuloma of the jaws. J. Oral Maxillofacial Surg. 40:174, 1982.

Multiple Myeloma

Age: Middle-aged adults

Sex: No predilection

Clinical and Radiographic Features: Multiple myeloma is a malignant osseous neoplastic disorder of immunoglobulin-secreting plasma cells. It probably represents a multicentric malignancy, as multiple osseous foci of disease may be detected simultaneously. The jaws, usually the mandible, are involved in over one-fourth of the cases. Immunoglobulins, usually of a single class and allotype, are detected in serum. Bence-Jones protein, representing globulin fragments, is often detectable in the urine. When the jaw is involved, bone pain and paresthesia are common complaints. The tumor cells may perforate the cortex, causing a soft tissue bulge or antral invasion. Loosening of teeth may be observed. Radiographically, multiple oval well-demarcated but noncorticated radiolucencies are observed. Cortical expansion is rare, perforation being more common when the lesions extend to the periphery of bone. Root resorption may occur. A skeletal survey will disclose similar lesions in other bones, particularly the skull.

Microscopic Features: Monotonous sheets of relatively well-differentiated plasma cells prevail. Mitoses and multinucleated cells are frequent findings. As opposed to chronic inflammation with a predominance of plasma cells, myeloma infiltrates lack dense stroma or granulation tissue, and other inflammatory cells in virgin lesions are not encountered. Amyloid deposits are frequently present. Immunoperoxidase techniques can be performed on formalin fixed sections; the demonstration of monotypic antibody employing techniques for class immunoglobulin heavy chains, a single type of light chain, or the presence of J-protein are specific for myeloma.

Differential Diagnosis: The punched-out well-defined radiolucencies typical of myeloma may also occur in histiocytosis X, disseminated metastatic carcinoma, and primary lymphoma of bone. Multiple keratocysts should be included in the radiographic differential diagnosis. Microscopic examination is required for a definitive diagnosis.

Treatment. Multiple myeloma has a grave prognosis, with 5-year survival under 10 percent. The disease is treated by chemotherapy and should be managed by a medical oncologist.

References

1. Bruce, K. W. and Royer, R. Q.: Multiple myeloma occurring in the jaws. Oral Surg. 6:729, 1953.
2. Smith, D. B.: Multiple myeloma involving the jaws; review with report of an additional case. Oral Surg. 10:911, 1957.
3. Tabachnik, T. T. and Levine, B.: Multiple myeloma involving the jaws and oral soft tissues. Oral Surg. 34:931, 1976.
4. Wright, B. A., Wysocki, G. P., and Bannerjee, D.: Diagnostic use of immunoperoxidase techniques for plasma cell lesions of the jaws. Oral Surg. 52:615, 1981.
5. Matthews, J. B. and Basu, M. K.: Plasma cell lesions within the oral tissues: Immunoperoxidase staining of routinely fixed and processed tissue. Oral Surg. 54:414, 1982.

GENERALIZED OSTEOPOROTIC LESIONS

Osteomalacia

Age: Varies according to pathogenesis

Sex: No predilection

Clinical and Radiographic Features: Osteomalacia represents a collective of disorders, whereby osteoid is not thoroughly mineralized. Genetic and acquired deficiencies in calcium absorption and incorporation into bone matrix are responsible. Dietary vitamin D deficiency, or rickets, occurs in children as does the hereditary form of rickets, whereby an enzyme deficiency precludes the normal activation of vitamin D (hypophosphatemic or vitamin D refractory rickets). In both cases, lack of active vitamin D results in

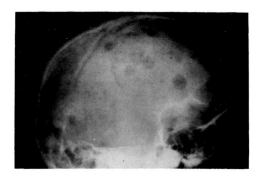

FIG. 9–64. Multifocal punched-out lesions of the skull, typically seen in multiple myeloma.

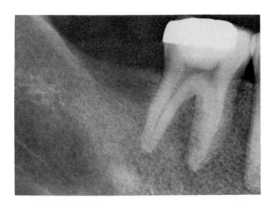

FIG. 9–65. Diffuse granular trabeculation in osteo-malacia secondary to advanced renal disease. (Courtesy of Dr. J. Campbell.)

deficient calcium absorption and incorporation into osteoid. Malabsorption syndromes such as biliary cirrhosis and various forms of steatorrhea encountered in adults are characterized by hypocalcemia. Renal osteodystrophy develops in late-stage glomerular disease as a consequence of renal calcium diuresis. Certain drugs, particularly anticonvulsants, interfere with enzymatic activation of vitamin D. Regardless of the mechanism, osteomalacia is the result of hypocalcemia. Radiographically, diffuse rarefaction is observed in both the maxilla and the mandible. The density of trabeculae per unit area is diminished, and the lamina dura may be quite thin. These radiographic alterations are often subtle and are not always observed. Pathologic fractures may also complicate the condition.

Microscopic Features: Routine histologic examination is not particularly revealing. During processing, decalcification occurs quickly. Otherwise, the histologic appearance of trabeculae in osteomalacia is usually unremarkable.

Differential Diagnosis: The diffuse rarefaction of osteomalacia is basically identical to that seen in osteoporosis and is similar to the changes observed in the other systemic diseases included here. Because many pathogenic mechanisms are involved, a complete medical evaluation is imperative. A biochemical bone panel to evaluate alkaline phosphatase, calcium, and phosphorus is necessary. The workup usually includes renal function tests, a renal panel, urinalysis, a liver panel, and a skeletal survey.

Treatment: Referral to an internist is recommended. Treatment consists of establishing an ap-propriate calcium balance and is based upon determining the underlying pathogenetic mechanism of the problem.

References

1. Stafne, E. C.: Dental roentgenologic manifestations of systemic disease. Radiology 58:507, 820, 1952.
2. Jaworski, Z. F. G.: Pathophysiology, diagnosis and treatment of osteomalacia: symposium on metabolic bone disease. Orthop. Clin. North Am. 3:623, 1972.
3. Reynolds, W. A. and Karo, J. J.: Radiologic diagnosis of metabolic bone disease: symposium on metabolic bone disease. Orthop. Clin. North Am. 3:521, 1972.

Senile Osteoporosis

Age: Elderly adults
Sex: Predominantly females

Clinical and Radiographic Features: Senile osteoporosis develops with ensuing age in conjunction with decreased anabolic hormones, particularly estrogen in postmenopausal women. Mineral content is not problemmatic as in osteomalacia; rather, the total bone matrix volume decreases. The axial skeleton is involved primarily, and a decrease in stature will become evident. Back pain may be a feature; as the appendicular skeleton becomes progressively involved, a minor fall may result in fracture. Jaw films in advanced cases will show thinning of the cortices, being most obvious in the mandible with a generalized loss of defined trabeculation. This loss of trabecular definition may yield a somewhat ground-glass or granular pattern with an overall general radiolucent appearance. The biochemical bone panel will generally be within normal limits.

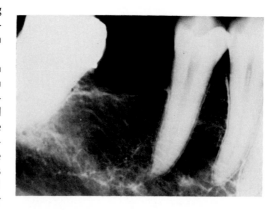

FIG. 9–66. Senile osteoporosis with loss of cortical prominence and altered trabeculation. (Courtesy of Dr. J. Campbell.)

Microscopic Features: In osteoporosis, low power assessment will disclose a thinning of the cortical bone with a decreased ratio of trabeculae to marrow. The medullary trabeculae are thin and atrophic without evidence of osteoblastic rimming.

Differential Diagnosis: Senile or postmenopausal osteoporosis is radiographically indistinguishable, in the jaws, from osteomalacia or steroid osteoporosis. The hemolytic anemias generally have a distinctive altered and unusual trabecular pattern.

Treatment: These elderly patients should limit their physical activities while maintaining proper and balanced nutrition. Referral to a physician is recommended.

References

1. Watson, L.: Endocrine bone disease. Practitioner *210*:376, 1973.
2. Conacher, W. D.: Metabolic bone disease in the elderly. Practitioner *210*:351, 1973.
3. Atkinson, P. J. and Woodhead, C.: The development of osteoporosis: a hypothesis based on a study of human bone structure. Clin. Orthop. *90*:217, 1973.
4. Keller, E. E. and Stafne, E. C.: Oral roentgenographic manifestations of systemic disease. In *Oral Roentgenographic Diagnosis,* edited by E. C. Stafne and J. A. Gibilisco. Philadelphia, W. B. Saunders Co., 1975, ch. 18.
5. Warren, R.: Osteoporosis. J. Oral Med. *32*:113, 1977.

Steroid Osteoporosis

Age: Varies according to pathogenesis
Sex: No predilection

Clinical and Radiographic Features: Osteoporotic changes develop in patients with elevated

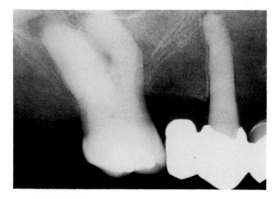

FIG. 9–67. Cushing's syndrome with loss of trabecular markings. (Courtesy of Dr. J. Campbell.)

blood corticosteroids. In Cushing's syndrome, either an adrenal cortical adenoma or a pituitary ACTH-secreting adenoma with adrenal cortical hyperplasia exists. Clinically, the facial tissues are edematous, yielding the so-called *moon facies;* other features include upper trunk adiposity, hypertension, and hyperglycemia. Elevated urine 17-ketosteroids and elevated serum cortisol can be detected. Treatment of immunopathic disorders such as lupus erythematosus, pemphigus, or mixed collagen diseases is usually effected by employing steroid medication. High doses over a prolonged period will result in cushingoid changes. Prolonged elevation of cortisone or steroid analogs will result in generalized osteoporosis affecting both the axial and appendicular skeleton, including the skull and jaws. Radiographically, the changes mimic those seen in senile osteoporosis with thin cortices, attenuated lamina dura, and generalized granular rarefaction.

Microscopic Features: The cortices are thin, and the medullary trabeculae are scant with abundant soft tissue marrow.

Differential Diagnosis: The diffuse rarefaction of steroid osteoporosis is essentially identical to that seen in senile osteoporosis. A history of systemic steroid medication or Cushing's syndrome will establish the diagnosis.

Treatment: Cushing's syndrome can be treated by surgical removal of the adrenal or pituitary tumor. Osteoporosis secondary to steroid administration can be minimized to some extent by prescribing the drug during early morning hours, which coincide with physiologic secretion peaks.

References

1. Stafne, E. C. and Lovestedt, S. A.: Osteoporosis of the jaws associated with hypercortisonism. Oral Surg. *13*:1445, 1960.
2. Duncan, H.: Osteoporosis in rheumatoid arthritis and corticosteroid-induced osteoporosis: symposium on metabolic bone disease. Orthop. Clin. North Amer. *3*:571, 1972.
3. Crilly, R. G., et al.: Post-menopausal and corticosteroid-induced osteoporosis. Front. Horm. Res. *5*:53, 1977.

Sickle Cell Anemia

Age: Childhood onset
Sex: No predilection

Clinical and Radiographic Features: Sickle cell anemia is an autosomal recessive inherited disease that affects less than 1 percent of the black population, in which a defective hemoglobin molecule is synthesized. This abnormal hemoglobin (HgS) can be detected with the use of hemoglobin

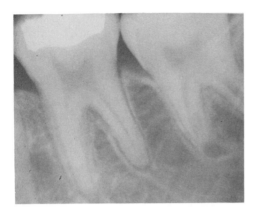

FIG. 9–68. Step-ladder trabeculation in sickle cell anemia. (Courtesy of Dr. R. Sanger.)

electrophoresis. Other abnormal hemoglobin molecules (e.g., HbC) may be encountered in sickle cell disease. Oxygen tension is low, and erythrocytes carrying this abnormal reduced hemoglobin assume altered morphology (sickled forms). During a crisis, sludging of cells occurs with formation of microthrombi. A severe crisis can be fatal. A compensatory bone marrow erythroblastic hyperplasia develops and leads to generalized osteoporotic changes radiographically. The clinical features include weakness, dyspnea, pallor, and generalized body pains. Jaw radiographs show a reduction in the number of trabeculae; those that remain are clearly defined and appear thickened. Some cases show a so-called *step-ladder* appearance with parallel horizontal trabeculation in the inter-radicular zone. The cortices are thin.

Microscopic Features: The microscopic features are not particularly diagnostic. Careful search for sickled erythrocytes within vessels should be undertaken.

Differential Diagnosis: The step-ladder effect and reduced trabeculation may be seen in normal patients. Similar radiographic changes may also be encountered in thalassemia. The other osteoporoses appear more granular on jaw radiographs. When the aforementioned radiographic features are encountered in black children, sickle cell anemia should be considered; a complete blood count, testing for sickle cell phenomenon, and hemoglobin electrophoresis should be ordered.

Treatment: There is no effective treatment. Parental genetic counseling is recommended.

References

1. Reynolds, J.: An evaluation of some roentgenographic signs in sickle -cell anemia and its variants. South. Med. J. 55:1123, 1962.
2. Mourshed, F. and Tuckson, C. R.: A study of the radiographic features of the jaws in sickle-cell anemia. Oral Surg. 37:812, 1974.
3. Sanger, R. O., Greer, R. O., and Auerbach, R. E.: Differential diagnosis of some simple osseous lesions associated with sickle cell anemia. Oral Surg. 43:538, 1977.
4. Sears, R. S.: The effects of sickle-cell disease on dental and skeletal maturation. ASDC J. Dent. Child. 48:275, 1981.

Thalassemia Major

Age: Childhood onset

Sex: No predilection

Clinical and Radiographic Features: Thalassemia, found predominantly among Italians and Greeks, is a hemoglobinopathy with resultant hemolytic anemia that represents a heritable defect in either the alpha or beta hemoglobin chain. Elevated fetal hemoglobin (HbF) is present in erythrocytes and can be quantitated, employing hemoglobin electrophoretic techniques. Major and minor beta (Cooley's anemia) and alpha forms

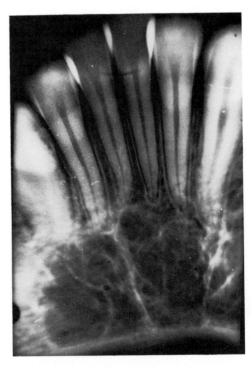

FIG. 9–69. Honeycomb trabeculation in thalassemia major. (Courtesy of Dr. H. Poyton.)

exist with full expression in the homozygous forms. Clinically, homozygotes are affected from birth or early childhood; pallor, malaise, and paroxysmal fever occur. Splenomegaly and appearance of mongoloid features with prominent malar region, incisor flaring, and depressed nasal bridge are common findings. Jaw and dental radiographic changes are not seen in every case; when present, the patient usually suffers from the beta major form of the disease. Various radiographic changes have been reported and include thinning of cortices, spiked roots, diffuse rarefaction with decreased yet prominent trabeculation, and in some instances, a diffuse and unmarginated honeycomb appearance. Skull films will often show vertical osteophytes emanating from the inner table of the calvarium producing the *hair-on-end* effect.

Microscopic Features: A biopsy that includes hematopoietic marrow or bone marrow aspiration smears will disclose hypochromic microcytes with poikilocytosis and anisocytosis. Large numbers of immature erythroblastoid cells are present, indicating a maturation arrest.

Differential Diagnosis: The radiographic features simulate, to some extent, those changes observed in sickle cell anemia. Elevated serum unconjugated bilirubin is present, and hemoglobin electrophoresis will disclose elevated amounts of fetal hemoglobin. The aforementioned bone marrow and peripheral blood changes are also of diagnostic importance.

Treatment: No effective treatment exists. Genetic counseling is recommended for parents.

References

1. Choremis, C., et al.: Pathogenesis of osseous lesions in thalassemia. J. Pediatr. 66:962, 1965.
2. Poyton, H. G. and Davey, K. W.: Thalassemia: changes visible in radiographs used in dentistry. Oral Surg. 25:564, 1968.
3. Logothetis, J., et al.: Cephalofacial deformities in thalassemia major (Cooley's anemia). Am. J. Dis. Child. 121:300, 1971.
4. Alexander, W. N. and Bechtold, W. A.: Alpha thalassemia minor trait accompanied by clinical oral signs. Oral Surg. 43:892, 1977.

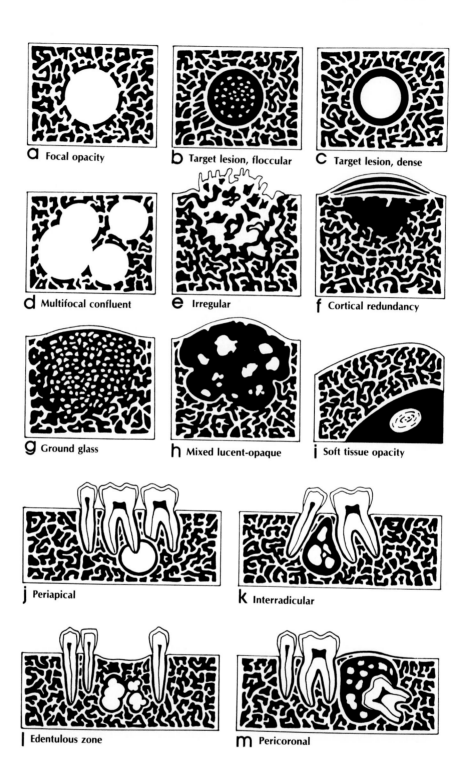

a Focal opacity

b Target lesion, floccular

c Target lesion, dense

d Multifocal confluent

e Irregular

f Cortical redundancy

g Ground glass

h Mixed lucent-opaque

i Soft tissue opacity

j Periapical

k Interradicular

l Edentulous zone

m Pericoronal

Radiopaque Lesions of the Jaws

10
Radiopaque Lesions of the Jaws

PERIAPICAL RADIOPACITIES

Periapical Cemental Dysplasia
Focal Sclerosing Osteomyelitis
Focal Periapical Osteopetrosis
Benign Cementoblastoma

INTER-RADICULAR RADIOPACITIES

Residual Focal Osteitis and Cementoma
Osteopetrotic Scar
Calcifying and Keratinizing Epithelial
    Odontogenic Cyst
Odontogenic Adenomatoid Tumor
Odontoma
Central Ossifying or Cementifying Fibroma
Benign Osteoblastoma

PERICORONAL RADIOPACITIES

Odontogenic Adenomatoid Tumor
Calcifying Epithelial Odontogenic Tumor
Ameloblastic Fibrodentinoma
Ameloblastic Fibro-odontoma
Odontoma
Odontoameloblastoma

TARGET LESIONS*

Periapical Cemental Dysplasia
Focal Sclerosing Osteomyelitis
Calcifying and Keratinizing Epithelial Odontogenic
    Cyst
Odontogenic Adenomatoid Tumor
Odontoma
Ameloblastic Fibro-odontoma
Odontoameloblastoma
Ossifying/Cementifying Fibroma
Benign Cementoblastoma
Osteoid Osteoma

GROUND-GLASS RADIOPACITIES

Fibrous Dysplasia
Osteitis Deformans
Hyperparathyroidism
Osteopetrosis

MULTIFOCAL CONFLUENT RADIOPACITIES

Osteitis Deformans
Florid Cemento-osseous Dysplasia
Gardner's Syndrome
Mandibular Tori and Exostoses

CORTICAL REDUNDANCIES

Garre's Periostitis
Infantile Cortical Hyperostosis
Generalized Cortical Hyperostosis
Juxtacortical Osteogenic Sarcoma

**IRREGULAR, ILL-DEFINED EXPANSILE
RADIOPACITIES**

Calcifying Epithelial Odontogenic Tumor
Osteogenic and Chondrogenic Sarcoma
Metastatic Carcinoma

SUPERIMPOSED SOFT TISSUE RADIOPACITIES

Sialolithiasis
Phlebolithiasis
Foreign Bodies
Calcified Lymph Nodes
Myositis Ossificans

ANTRAL OPACITIES

Maxillary Sinusitis
Antral Mucosal Cyst
Sinus Mucocele
Periapical Infection with Antral Polyps
Antral Mycoses
Displaced Teeth, Roots, and Foreign Bodies
Antrolith/Rhinolith
Odontoma
Osteomas and Exostoses
Benign Mesenchymal Neoplasms
Fibrous Dysplasia†
Inverted Papilloma
Antral Carcinoma
Antral Sarcoma

---

*Detailed descriptions of target lesions appear in the text
under the other headings included in this chapter.
†See Ground-glass Radiopacities.

Radiopacities portrayed on roentgeno-grams are a reflection of the potential for a disease to elaborate calcified products. They can also represent foreign objects lodged within bone or soft tissues superimposed on the normal osseous structures. The calcifiable matrices within the jaws include osseous tissue, cartilage, cementum, dentin, and enamel. Any lesions capable of forming these cell products may appear radiopaque. Since the matrix for calcification may be elaborated prior to any mineralization, many of the lesions with a radiopaque radiographic pattern may at an early stage in their development appear radiolucent. As mineralization of the matrices develops, the lesion will become progressively opaque. For this reason, many calcifying tumors or diseases will show a radiolucency with central opaque flecks or conglomerates. Many of the bone lesions presented in the previous chapter on radiolucencies will be included here since the later stages, for reasons just mentioned, will appear as radiopacities.

General radiologic considerations should be taken into account when one evaluates radiopaque lesions. Well-circumscribed corticated borders usually represent benign slow-growing diseases. Target lesions, opacities with a well-delineated radiolucent halo, are benign and are, as a rule, odontogenic in origin. Likewise, opacities associated with the crown of an impacted tooth are invariably odontogenic.

Diffuse radiopacities with ill-defined borders are difficult to interpret as they represent a wide range of both benign and malignant conditions. Multifocal radiopacities or those involving multiple quadrants of the jaws are generally benign fibro-osseous disorders.

Opacification of the antrum is usually, yet not invariably, the result of a soft tissue proliferation or represents the presence of fluid accumulation.

In some instances, a radiographic diagnosis can be made; however, a bone biopsy is generally necessary for definitive diagnosis or confirmation of the clinical impression.

The most common periapical radiopacities

are periapical cemental dysplasia, focal sclerosing osteomyelitis and focal periapical osteopetrosis.

The most common inter-radicular radiopacities include osteopetrotic scar and odontoma. Odontoma and odontogenic adenomatoid tumor are the more frequently encountered pericoronal radiopacities.

Fibrous dysplasia is the most common disease to manifest a ground-glass pattern, while tori and florid cemento-osseous dysplasia are the most common lesions yielding multifocal confluent radiopacities.

Garre's periostitis is the primary disease showing cortical layering. Potentially fatal diseases with an opaque radiographic appearance include the malignant bone neoplasms, Ewing's sarcoma, osteogenic and chondrogenic sarcomas, and metastatic carcinoma. Gardner's syndrome is accompanied by gastrointestinal tract malignancy.

Diffuse antral opacification is usually a radiographic sign of inflammatory allergic disease. Importantly, antral carcinoma will cause the antrum to appear clouded; this is potentially fatal.

PERIAPICAL RADIOPACITIES

Periapical Cemental Dysplasia

Age: Middle-aged adults
Sex: Female predilection

Clinical and Radiographic Features: Periapical cemental dysplasia or cementoma is most commonly encountered in Negroes. Solitary lesions

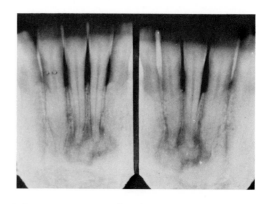

FIG. 10–1. Periapical radiopacity underlying vital teeth representing periapical cemental dysplasia.

are limited to anterior teeth. Multiple lesions are also located anteriorly, usually in the mandible but sometimes extending to the apices of first molars. Pain and expansion are lacking, and the teeth are vital. The etiology is unknown. Radiographically, single or multiple opacities are encountered apical to the incisors, cuspids, or premolars. They may appear with a target pattern or merely as well-delineated opacities. The apical lamina dura is often intact. Occasionally, the lesion is larger than the usual 0.5 to 1 cm, yet expansion will not be detectable. The lesion begins as a radiolucency; with ensuing time, calcification progresses so that a solid opaque mass becomes the dominant radiographic feature.

Microscopic Features: Mature lesions are composed of compact lamellar bone, quilted cementum, lamellar cementum, or a combination of these, with very little fibrous stroma. Those detected midway in development manifest a fibro-osseous pattern with a hypercellular fibrous element containing multiple ovoid or linear trabeculae of bone and cementum.

Differential Diagnosis: Periapical cemental dysplasia presents a radiopaque pattern similar to that encounterd with focal condensing osteitis, focal periapical osteopetrosis, and benign cementoblastoma. All these conditions tend to involve posterior teeth. Focal osteitis is associated with a deep carious lesion or restoration. and cementoblastomas are expansile. In the absence of expansion, a well-circumscribed opacity apical to anterior mandibular teeth can be considered to represent cementoma, and no biopsy is necessary.

Treatment: No treatment is necessary. When biopsy is deferred, the patient should be subjected to periodic radiographic follow-up to ensure that the lesion is not a proliferative one that coincidentally involves the periapical region. Biopsy is indicated if growth is observed.

References

1. Stafne, E. C.: Cementoma, a study of 35 cases. Dent. Surv. 9:27, 1933.
2. Fontaine, J.: Periapical fibro-osteoma or cementoma. J. Can. Dent. Assoc. 21:10, 1955.
3. Chaudhry, A. P., Spink, J. H., and Gorlin, R. J.: Periapical fibrous dysplasia (Cementoma). J. Oral Surg. 16:483, 1958.
4. Zegarelli, E. V., et al.: The cementoma, a study of 230 patients with 475 cementomas. Oral Surg. 17:219, 1964.
5. Hamner, J. E., Scofield, H. H., and Cornyn, J.: Benign fibro-osseous jaw lesions of periodontal membrane origin: An analysis of 249 cases. Cancer 22:861, 1968.

Focal Sclerosing Osteomyelitis

Age: Young adults
Sex: No predilection

Clinical and Radiographic Features: Low-grade pulpal inflammation, usually located in the first mandibular molar, will induce a reactive osteosclerotic response at the apex. The tooth tests vital since pulp necrosis is not present; rather, the pulp is vital yet inflamed. There is generally no pain; however, the patient sometimes complains of a dull ache. The most obvious clinical feature is the presence of gross caries or a large restoration with a deep pulpal floor. Radiographically, a well-demarcated radiopacity is located below the root apices, and occasionally extends up the root for a limited distance. The opacity does not merge with root cementum, so that a periodontal ligament space is usually discernible. The opacity may or may not be enveloped by a radiolucent halo. Cortices do not expand.

Microscopic Features: Depending upon the degree of calcification, the tissue may be composed of compact bone or cementum with scant stroma. In less calcified specimens, a fibro-osseous pattern with a hypercellular stroma prevails. Oval, linear, or curved trabeculae are dispersed throughout this stroma. The pulp may appear histologically unremarkable, or a vital pulp exhibiting a mild mononuclear inflammatory infiltrate may be encountered. Occasionally, pulpal necrosis is observed in teeth with periapical sclerotic foci.

Differential Diagnosis: The appearance of a well-circumscribed or target radiopacity at the apex of a first molar may be confused with per-

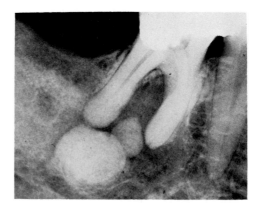

FIG. 10–2.   Molar tooth with deep restoration resulting in low-grade chronic pulpitis and manifesting radiodense circumscribed opacities representing focal sclerosing osteomyelitis.

iapical cemental dysplasia, focal periapical osteo-petrosis, or benign cementoblastoma. Focal os-teitis is the result of pulp disease with caries, whereas cementoma and focal osteopetrosis are not. Cementoblastoma shows fusion with the tooth root and expands bone, whereas neither of these features is encountered in focal sclerosing osteo-myelitis.

Treatment: Pulp extirpation with endodontic therapy is recommended.

References

1. Boyne, P. J.: Incidence of osteosclerotic areas in the mandible and maxilla. J. Oral Surg. *18*:486, 1960.
2. Eversole, L. R., Sabes, W. R., and Rovin, S.: Fibrous dysplasia; A nosologic problem in the diagnosis of fibro-osseous lesions of the jaws. J. Oral Pathol. *1*:189, 1972.
3. Fireman, S. M.: Osteosclerotic lesions of the jaws. Oral Health 66(7):27, 1976.
4. Farman, A. G., de V. Joubert, J. J., and Nortjé, C. J.: Focal osteosclerosis and apical periodontal pathoses in "European" and Cape coloured dental outpatients. Int. J. Oral Surg. 7:549, 1978.
5. Eversole, L. R., Stone, C. E., and Strub, D.: Focal sclerosing osteomyelitis and focal periapical osteo-petrosis: Radiographic patterns. Oral Surg. In press.

Focal Periapical Osteopetrosis

Age: Adults

Sex: No predilection

Clinical and Radiographic Features: Well-lo-calized radiopacities lying below the apices of vital, noncarious molar teeth represent focal os-teopetrosis. The etiology is obscure since no pulp inflammation is present; the teeth are asympto-matic and test vital with a vitalometer. Many oral radiologists prefer to include lesions of this nature with focal sclerosing osteomyelitis; because no clinical or radiologic evidence of pulpal insult can be detected, they have been arbitrarily segregated as a separate entity. The lesion is usually detected with routine periapical or panographic films. The opacity generally lacks a radiolucent halo, yet is well demarcated with respect to the surrounding bone. Any of the three mandibular molars may overlie the opacity.

Microscopic Features: Bone biopsy shows dense viable lamellar bone with fibrous marrow canals. Inflammatory cells are lacking.

Differential Diagnosis: Periapical osteopetrosis can be distinguished from cementoma by virtue of its posterior location and lack of racial, sex, or age predilection. Cementoblastoma can be elim-inated because no continuity with the root can be

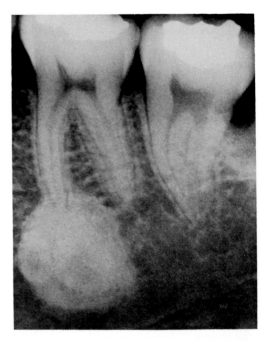

FIG. 10–3. Radiopaque nonexpansile mass on a vital noninflamed molar tooth, termed focal periapical osteo-petrosis.

demonstrated radiographically or by means of per-cussion. Expansion is also lacking. Focal con-densing osteitis must rank high in the differential diagnosis; however, neither deep caries, large res-torations, nor other sources of pulp inflammation can be demonstrated.

Treatment: The diagnosis is clinicoradiologic, and no treatment is required.

References

1. Boyne, P. J.: Incidence of osteosclerotic areas in the mandible and maxilla. J. Oral Surg. *18*:486, 1969.
2. Eversole, L. R., Stone, C. E., and Strub, D.: Focal sclerosing osteomyelitis and focal periapical osteo-petrosis: Radiographic patterns. Oral Surg. In press.

Benign Cementoblastoma

Age: Teenagers and young adults

Sex: No predilection

Clinical and Radiographic Features: A true neoplasm of cementoblasts, the benign cemen-toblastoma arises most often on the first mandib-ular molars. Other molar teeth and premolars are involved less frequently. Clinically, there is no pain; the cortex is slightly expanded both buccally and linguallly. The tooth is vital and usually non-carious. The involved tooth is ankylosed to the

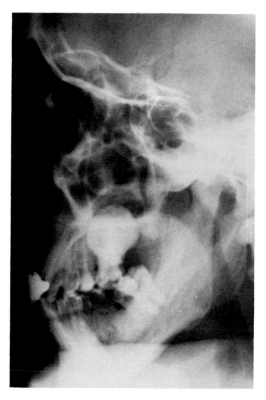

FIG. 10–4. Periapical opacity enveloping molar roots in benign cementoblastoma. (From Wiggins, H. E. and Karian, B. K.: Cementoblastoma of the maxilla: report of case. J. Oral Surg. 33:302, 1975. Copyright American Dental Association, reprinted by permission.)

tumor mass; upon percussion an audible difference between affected and unaffected teeth can be discerned. Radiographically, the apical mass may be lucent with either central opacities or a solid opacity. A thin radiolucent halo can be seen around densely calcified lesions. The tumor is expansile when visualized with occlusal radiographs, and on periapical films the mass extends occlusally to encompass and become confluent with the lower third of the molar roots.

Microscopic Features: Radially oriented trabeculae emanate from the attached root cementum. In most specimens, the trabeculae polarize like bone rather than cementum. Osteoblasts rim the trabeculae, often to the point of stratification. The marrow is fibrous.

Differential Diagnosis: Benign cementoblastoma must be differentiated from periapical cemental dysplasia, focal sclerosing osteomyelitis, and periapical osteopetrosis. Radiographic demonstration of confluency with tooth roots, the pres-

ence of expansion, a dull sound on percussion, and lack of pulp disease allow for a clinicoradiologic diagnosis.

Treatment: Since cementoblastomas are somewhat aggressive, they require excision. Removal cannot be achieved without sacrificing the ankylosed tooth.

References

1. Eversole, L. R., Sabes, W. R., and Dauchess, V. G.: Benign cementoblastoma. Oral Surg. 36:824, 1973.
2. Cherrick, H. M., et al.: Benign cementoblastoma. Oral Surg. 37:54, 1974.
3. Wiggins, H. E. and Karian, B. K.: Cementoblastoma of the maxilla: report of case. J. Oral Surg. 33:302, 1975.
4. Townes, T. M., Marks, R. B., and Carr, R. F.: Benign (true) cementoblastoma: report of cases. J. Oral Surg. 37:342, 1979.
5. Farman, A. G., et al.: Cementoblastoma: report of case. J. Oral Surg. 37:198, 1979.

INTER-RADICULAR RADIOPACITIES

Residual Focal Osteitis and Cementoma

Age: Adults

Sex: Osteitis—no predilection; Cementoma—female predilection

Clinical and Radiographic Features: When teeth overlying periapical cemental dysplasia (cementoma) or focal sclerosing osteomyelitis are extracted, the radiopaque mass often remains without undergoing resolution. As the alveolar bone resorbs, the lesion will appear to lie in an inter-radicular location in the edentulous zone. Radiographically, anterior focal opacities retain their features of periapical cemental dysplasia, whereas

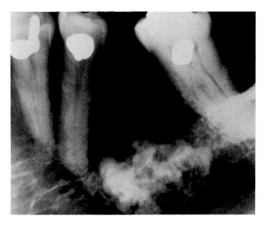

FIG. 10–5. Residual focal osteitis in edentulous space previously occupied by a molar tooth.

posterior opacities represent focal osteitis. In both instances, pain and expansion are lacking, and the lesion is well delineated with or without a circumferential radiolucent rim. As the alveolar bone atrophies, both lesions may sequestrate.

Microscopic Features: With both lesions dense lamellar bone or cementum is seen, with scant intervening fibrous marrow. When sequestration ensues, the calcified tissue is accompanied by in-flamed granulation tissue.

Differential Diagnosis: Residual osteitis or ce-mentoma is more regular, round, or oval than postextraction osteopetrotic scar. When a radio-lucent halo is present, the lesion cannot be dif-ferentiated radiographically from the calcifying odontogenic tumors included in this section. Bi-opsy is required to ascertain the true nature of the radiographically demonstrable process.

Treatment: Once the diagnosis has been es-tablished by trephinement or excisional bone bi-opsy, no further treatment is required.

References
1. Boyne, P. J.: Incidence of osteosclerotic areas in the mandible and maxilla. J. Oral Surg. *18*:486, 1969.
2. Eversole, L. R., Sabes, W. R., and Rovin, S.: Fibrous dysplasia; a nosologic problem in the diagnosis of fibro-osseous lesions of the jaws. J. Oral Pathol. *1*:189, 1972.

Osteopetrotic Scar

Age: Adults
Sex: No predilection

Clinical and Radiographic Features: Following tooth extraction or, occasionally, loss of decid-uous teeth, the socket heals with excessive ossi-fication. The result is a radiographically demon-strable opacity that lies within the edentulous space between contiguous teeth or is found in an inter-radicular location between permanent teeth when deciduous tooth loss elicited the reaction. The premolar and first molar regions are favored. Pain and expansion are lacking. Radiographically, the opaque lesion is elongated vertically or may assume an irregular yet well-delineated configu-ration.

Microscopic Features: Dense viable lamellar bone with scant fibrous marrow spaces is seen.

Differential Diagnosis: In the absence of ex-pansion or other symptoms, most lesions included in this section on inter-radicular radiopacities can be eliminated when the lesion assumes an elon-gated or irregular outline devoid of a radiolucent halo. If pain is present or if a fistula is observed,

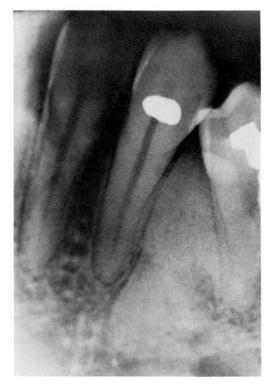

FIG. 10–6. Osteopetrotic scar between cuspid and premolar.

sequestration with osteomyelitis should be con-sidered.

Treatment: In the absence of pain or expansion with an elongated or irregular inter-radicular opacity, a clinicoradiologic diagnosis can be ren-dered. No treatment is required other than peri-odic radiographic follow-up.

References
1. Boyne, P. J.: Incidence of osteosclerotic areas in the mandible and maxilla. J. Oral Surg. *18*:486, 1960.
2. Brzovic, F. R., Belvederessi, M. E., and Faivovich, G. W.: Localized osteosclerosis in the jaws. Quin-tessence *3*:9, 1971.

Calcifying and Keratinizing Epithelial Odontogenic Cyst

Age: No predilection
Sex: No predilection

Clinical and Radiographic Features: The cal-cifying and keratinizing epithelial odontogenic or Gorlin cyst is a tumor-like cyst found predomi-nantly in the mandibular premolar region. Nearly one quarter of such cysts are peripheral, producing radiographically evident calcification above the

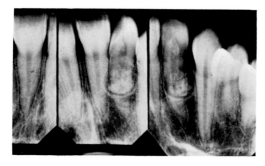

FIG. 10–7. Well-circumscribed target lesion representing a calcifying epithelial odontogenic cyst. (Courtesy of Dr. A. Leider.)

underlying cortex and manifesting a gingival swelling. Intrabony lesions may cause expansion. The teeth are vital, and pain is not a feature. Radiographically, the lesion begins as a radiolucency and progressively calcifies, yielding a target lesion (opaque, with a circumferential lucent halo). Midstage cysts may be predominantly lucent with centrally located calcific opaque flecks. Root divergence is a common finding.

Microscopic Features: The cyst lining is composed of stratified squamous epithelium with a rigidly polarized basal layer assuming ameloblastoid features. The spinous layer is often spongiotic, mimicking stellate reticulum. The luminal surface contains eosinophilic keratinized cells devoid of nuclei, so-called ghost cells. These cells undergo calcification. Melanin pigment may occasionally be encountered in these lesions. The fibrous wall often contains eosinophilic cell products resembling osteoid or dentinoid. When the cyst wall ruptures, an avid foreign-body reaction may ensue.

Differential Diagnosis: The intercellular target lesion seen with calcifying epithelial odontogenic cyst may be featured by other odontogenic tumors, including the odontogenic adenomatoid tumor, mixed odontogenic tumors, odontoma, and ossifying or cementifying fibroma. Microscopic evaluation is required to arrive at a definitive diagnosis.

Treatment: Enucleation with curettage is rarely complicated by recurrence.

References

1. Gorlin, R. J., et al.: The calcifying odontogenic cyst—a possible analogue of the cutaneous calcifying epithelioma of Malherbe. Oral Surg. 15:1235, 1962.
2. Ulmansky, M., et al.: Calcifying odontogenic cyst. J. Oral Surg. 27:415, 1969.
3. Freedman, P. D., Lumerman, H., and Gee, J. K.: Calcifying odontogenic cyst. Oral Surg. 40:93, 1975.
4. Seeliger, J. E. and Reyneke, J. P.: The calcifying odontogenic cyst: report of case. J. Oral Surg. 36:469, 1978.
5. Soames, J. V.: A pigmented calcifying odontogenic cyst. Oral Surg. 53:395, 1982.

Odontogenic Adenomatoid Tumor

Age: Teenagers
Sex: Female predilection

Clinical and Radiographic Features: While usually associated with the crown of an impacted anterior tooth, the odontogenic adenomatoid tumor may arise between tooth roots as well. Painless expansion is often the chief complaint. The maxillary incisor-cuspid region is the site of predilection. Radiographically, the tumor is well delineated, expansile with root divergence, and radiolucent with calcific flecks (target appearance).

Microscopic Features: The odontogenic adenomatoid tumor displays a thick fibrous capsule with an inner epithelial neoplastic component composed of organoid clusters of spindle cells. Columnar cells are arranged in rosettes or ductal patterns dispersed throughout the organoid cell

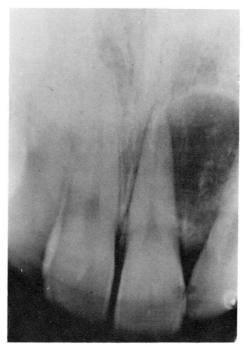

FIG. 10–8. Radiolucency with central opaque flecks in odontogenic adenomatoid tumor.

proliferation. Dystrophic calcifications are deposited throughout.

Differential Diagnosis: The expansile radiolucent lesion with central opacities or target appearance assumed by the odontogenic adenomatoid tumor is similar to or indistinguishable from that of the calcifying epithelial odontogenic cyst, other mixed odontogenic tumors, odontomas, and central ossifying or cementifying fibroma. The age, sex, and location favor a radiologic diagnosis of odontogenic adenomatoid tumor; however, microscopic confirmation is mandatory.

Treatment: Simple surgical enucleation is recommended. Recurrence is extremely rare.

References

1. Bhaskar, S. N.: Adenoameloblastoma; its histogenesis and report of 15 new cases. J. Oral Surg. 22:218, 1964.
2. Giansanti, J. S., Someren, A., and Waldron, C. A.: Odontogenic adenomatoid tumor (adenoameloblastoma). Oral Surg. 30:69, 1970.
3. Courtney, R. M. and Kerr, D. A.: The odontogenic adenomatoid tumor. A comprehensive study of twenty new cases. Oral Surg. 39:424, 1975.
4. Bedrick, A. E., Solomon, M. P., and Ferber, I.: The adenomatoid odontogenic tumor: An unusual clinical presentation. Oral Surg. 48:143, 1979.
5. Schlosnagle, D. C. and Someren, A.: The ultrastructure of the adenomatoid odontogenic tumor. Oral Surg. 52:154, 1981.

Odontoma

Age: Teenagers, young adults
Sex: Slight male predilection

Clinical and Radiographic Features: A mixed odontogenic tumor emulating all the hard tissue products of a mature tooth germ, the odontoma is probably the most common type of odontogenic tumor or hamartoma. While usually located pericoronal to an impacted tooth, the odontoma may also arise from odontogenic progenitor cells within the periodontal ligament and become located between tooth roots. There is no pain, and cortical expansion is either not discernible or present only to a limited degree. Radiographically, the lesion may present one of two patterns. When a target pattern with a lucent halo prevails, the central opacities assume tooth form configurations. This variety has been called *compound composite odontoma* and is frequently interposed between anterior teeth. The *compound complex odontoma* is more common in the posterior region, is less commonly inter-radicular, and manifests a well-localized opacity with frayed margins, a "sunburst" pattern.

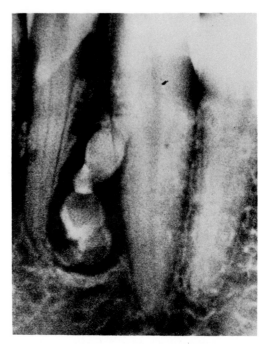

FIG. 10–9. Multiple tooth-form radiopacities situated between the tooth roots, typical features encountered in odontomas.

Microscopic Features: Enamel matrix, dentin, cementum, and bone are arranged in tooth-germ-like configurations or admixed in haphazard fashion. Odontogenic epithelium, odontoblasts, and pulp mesenchyme are also present. The soft tissue components show no proliferative activity. Some odontomas exhibit a central radiolucent zone, being cystic (dilated odontome). Oftentimes, the features of a Gorlin cyst are present in addition to the odontoma.

Differential Diagnosis: The compound composite variety with tooth forms is easily recognized radiographically. The compound complex type may present radiologic features in common with the other odontogenic tumors included here, as well as residual osteitis and cementoma, ossifying or cementifying fibroma, and Gorlin cyst. Both types may develop a dentigerous cyst from the follicular wall.

Treatment: Odontomas are generally encapsulated by a fibrous lining and can be enucleated. Since dentigerous cysts and even other odontogenic neoplasms can arise from the odontogenic epithelial component of odontomas, they should be removed.

References

1. Gorlin, R. J., et al.: Odontogenic tumors. Cancer *14*:73, 1961.
2. Cobos, L., et al.: Compound and complex odontomas. Odontol Chile *15*:33, 1966.
3. Budnick, S. D.: Compound and complex odontomas. Oral Surg. *42*:501, 1976.
4. Slootweg, P. G.: An analysis of the interrelationship of the mixed odontogenic tumors—ameloblastic fibroma, ameloblastic fibro-odontoma, and the odontomas. Oral Surg. *51*:266, 1981.
5. Goldberg, H., et al.: Cystic complex composite odontoma. Report of two cases. Oral Surg. *51*:16, 1981.

Central Ossifying or Cementifying Fibroma

Age: Teenagers, young adults
Sex: No predilection

Clinical and Radiographic Features: The ossifying and cementifying fibromas are mesenchymal neoplasms of the jaws; they may differentiate along osseous, cemental, or both osseous and cemental lines. The neoplasm is usually located in the body or anterior region of the mandible or maxilla and classically produces expansion, usually in a buccal plane. Pain is not a feature; the overlying alveolar mucosa is generally intact, devoid of ulceration. Radiographically, expansion is usually demonstrable along the inferior border of the mandible; on occlusal films the buccal plate is bulged. The tumor displays sharply delineated margins and is usually unilocular, although multilocular patterns are not uncommon. The central zone contains opaque calcific flecks or a dense radiopaque conglomerate mass. Divergence of adjacent tooth roots is a common finding. Whereas the majority of ossifying and cementifying fibromas are slow-growing lesions, occasionally these tumors are extremely aggressive with rapid growth, a marked tendency for expansion, and a potential for reaching massive proportions. This type of lesion has been referred to as *aggressive juvenile ossifying fibroma*.

Microscopic Features: A fibro-osseous microscopic pattern with a hypercellular fibroblastic stroma prevails. Ossifying fibroma contains irregular osteoid spicules or retiform trabeculae often rimmed by osteoblasts. Ovoid and curvilinear tra-

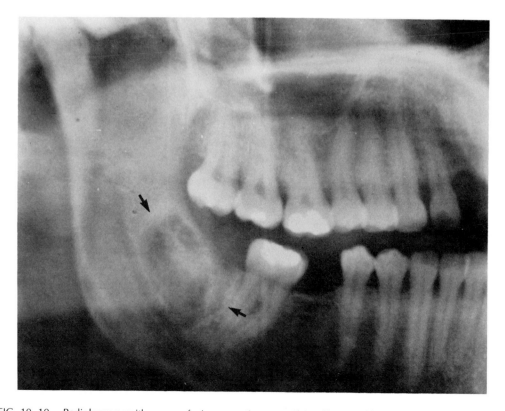

FIG. 10–10.   Radiolucency with opaque foci representing an ossifying fibroma of bone.

beculae that polarize with a microlamellar or quilted pattern are typical of cementifying fibromas. Alternatively, some lesions show both types of trabeculae. The active juvenile variant may not be readily segregated on the basis of histopathologic features, although pronounced hypercellularity is an indication of rapid proliferative capability.

Differential Diagnosis: The expansile target pattern typical of ossifying and cementifying fibromas may be seen with the calcifying epithelial odontogenic cyst, odontogenic adenomatoid tumor, and some of the mixed odontogenic tumors. Lesions at an early stage may not show dense opacities; rather, faint calcified flecks float within an expanding radiolucency. In these cases, the differential diagnosis should include Pindborg tumor as well as the aforementioned entities. Biopsy will disclose the characteristic histomorphology.

Treatment: Surgical enucleation is rarely followed by recurrence for relatively small lesions. Large expansile tumors with root divergence or resorption and thin cortical boundaries may require en bloc resection to prevent recurrence. The juvenile aggressive ossifying fibroma, as determined histologically and radiographically with clinical observation of rapid growth, should be resected.

References

1. Hamner, J. E., et al.: Cemento-ossifying fibroma of the maxilla. Oral Surg. 26:579, 1968.
2. Eversole, L. R., Sabes, W. R., and Rovin, S.: Fibrous dysplasia; a nosologic problem in the diagnosis of fibro-osseous lesions of the jaws. J. Oral Pathol. 1:189, 1972.
3. Martis, C. and Karakasis, D.: Cemento-ossifying fibroma of the mandible. J. Oral Surg. 33:364, 1975.
4. Taylor, N. D., Watkins, J. P., and Bear, S. E.: Recurrent cementifying fibroma of the maxilla: report of case. J. Oral Surg. 35:204, 1977.
5. Walter, J. M., et al.: Aggressive ossifying fibroma of the maxilla: review of the literature and report of case. J. Oral Surg. 37:276, 1979.

Benign Osteoblastoma

Age: Children and teenagers
Sex: Male predilection

Clinical and Radiographic Features: A tumor that generally arises in the long bones and vertebrae, the osteoblastoma may occasionally arise in the maxillofacial complex. It is a benign neoplasm of osteoblastic origin with a rapid growth rate capable of expansion and facial deformity. Radiographically, it is relatively well circumscribed,

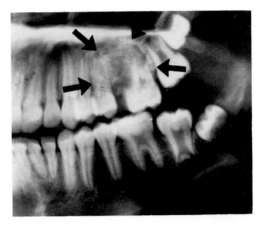

FIG. 10–11. Powdered radiopaque foci located between maxillary teeth in an osteoblastoma. (From Kent, J. N., et al.: Benign osteoblastoma of the maxilla. Oral Surg. 27:208, 1969.)

although the tumor margins may be scalloped. Centrally, radiopaque foci are encountered. Adjacent teeth are displaced and root resorption is usually encountered. While the disease is rare, there may be a predilection for the maxilla.

Microscopic Features: Dispersed throughout an areolar fibrous marrow are irregular or retiform arrangements of thin osteoid trabeculae rimmed to the point of stratification by plump basophilic osteoblasts. Osteoclasts are present as well, and the marrow is generally well vascularized.

Differential Diagnosis: Expansile inter-radicular radiopacities as seen in benign osteoblastoma may be encountered in central ossifying or cementifying fibromas and certain mixed odontogenic tumors. Biopsy is required to achieve a definitive diagnosis.

Treatment: Benign osteoblastoma is an aggressive neoplasm; while enucleation may be attempted, recurrence is a distinct possiblility. If the lesion recurs, en bloc resection is recommended to eradicate the disease.

References

1. Borello, E. D. and Sedano, H. O.: Giant osteoid osteoma of the maxilla. Oral Surg. 23:563, 1967.
2. Kent, J. N., et al.: Benign osteoblastoma of the maxilla. Oral Surg. 27:209, 1969.
3. Brady, C. L. and Browne, R. M.: Benign osteoblastoma of the mandible. Cancer 30:329, 1972.
4. Miller, A. S., et al.: Benign osteoblastoma of the jaws: report of three cases. J. Oral Surg. 38:694, 1980.
5. Smith, R. A., et al.: Comparison of the osteoblastoma in gnathic and extragnathic sites. Oral Surg. 54:285, 1982.

PERICORONAL RADIOPACITIES

Odontogenic Adenomatoid Tumor

Age: Teenagers
Sex: Female predilection

Clinical and Radiographic Features: More than three-quarters of all odontogenic adenomatoid tumors arise from reduced enamel epithelium surrounding the crown of an impacted anterior tooth. Some cases have been extraosseous. The maxillary cuspid is the most commonly affected tooth. Clinically, expansion of the buccal and palatal or lingual plates is seen in the absence of pain. Radiographically, the lesion is usually a well-delineated corticated radiolucency containing calcific flecks. The pericoronal lesion, as opposed to a simple dentigerous cyst, tends to originate low on the root rather than from the dentinoenamel junction. Occasionally, a classic target pattern is seen, whereby a circumferential halo envelops a dense, central, round radiodense mass.

Microscopic Features: The tumor is composed of swirled spindle-shaped epithelial cell conglomerates with focal duct-like configurations lined by columnar cells. Dystrophic calcifications are distributed throughout. A dense fibrous wall confines the neoplastic element.

Differential Diagnosis: A pericoronal radiolucency with an opaque center occurring in the anterior segment of the jaws in teenage females invariably represents odontogenic adenomatoid tumor. Nevertheless, the differential diagnosis must include other odontogenic tumors included in this section, since they may assume similar radiologic characteristics. Biopsy is necessary for a definitive diagnosis.

Treatment: Simple surgical excision is curative. Recurrence is almost nonexistent.

References

1. Abrams, A. M., Melrose, R. J., and Howell, F. W.: Adenomeloblastoma. A clinical pathologic study of ten new cases. Cancer 22:175, 1968.
2. Giansanti, J. S., Someren, A., and Waldron, C. A.: Odontogenic adenomatoid tumor (adenoameloblastoma). Oral Surg. 30:69, 1970.
3. Courtney, R. M. and Kerr, D. A.: The odontogenic adenomatoid tumor. A comprehensive study of twenty new cases. Oral Surg. 39:424, 1975.
4. Tsaknis, P. J., Carpenter, W. M., and Shade, N. L.: Odontogenic adenomatoid tumor: report of case and review of the literature. J. Oral Surg. 35:146, 1977.
5. Schlosnagle, D. C. and Someren, A.: The ultrastructure of the adenomatoid odontogenic tumor. Oral Surg. 52:154, 1981.

Calcifying Epithelial Odontogenic Tumor

Age: Middle-aged adults
Sex: No predilection

Clinical and Radiographic Features: The calcifying epithelial odontogenic (Pindborg) tumor is an aggressive odontogenic neoplasm of epithelial derivation. Most cases are associated with an impacted tooth, and the mandibular body or ramus is by far the most common site of origin. Pain is usually not a complaint. The chief sign is cortical expansion. Radiographically, expanded cortices

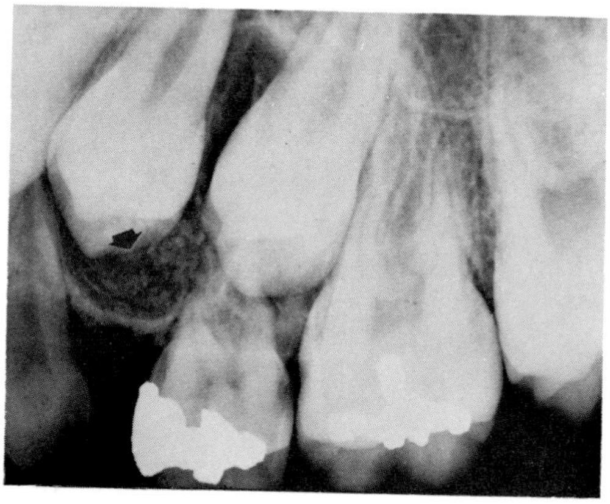

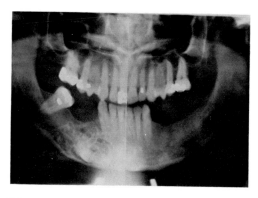

FIG. 10–12. Pericoronal radiopaque flecks associated with an impacted premolar representing odontogenic adenomatoid tumor. (From Abrams, A. M., Melrose, R. J., and Howell, F. W.: Adenoameloblastoma: Pathologic study of ten cases. Cancer 22:175, 1968.)

FIG. 10–13. Pericoronal radiolucency with opaque conglomerates associated with an impacted bicuspid represents calcifying epithelial odontogenic tumor. (From Gargiulo, E. A., Ziter, W. D., and Mastrocola, R.: Calcifying epithelial odontogenic tumor: report of case and review of literature. J. Oral Surg. 29:862, 1971. Copyright American Dental Association, reprinted by permission.)

can be visualized in buccal, lingual, and vertical dimensions. The lesion is usually radiolucent with poorly defined or, at the least, noncorticated borders. It may appear unilocular, multilocular, or moth-eaten. Multiple radiopaque foci can be detected within the radiolucent zone in the form of flecks, conglomerates, or diffuse opacities yielding a "driven-snow" appearance. Root divergence and resorption are common findings. The impacted tooth usually shows arrested root development and is often significantly displaced by the tumor.

Microscopic Features: Sheets, nests and cords of eosinophilic epithelial cells prevail, bearing no resemblance to tooth germ primordia. Nuclear pleomorphism may be marked despite the benignity of the tumor. Neoplastic cells are oriented about amyloid droplets or conglomerates. Concentrically laminated Leisegang calcifications similar to psammoma bodies are a classic finding. A variety of so-called *atypical* variants are encountered; the primary variant is a clear cell lesion that is composed of sheets and islands of cells with vacuolated cytoplasm and associated amyloid deposits with calcification.

Differential Diagnosis: The radiography of Pindborg tumor may simulate a variety of both benign and malignant lesions of the jaws. The more well-delineated tumors must be microscopically differentiated from the other benign odontogenic neoplasms included in this section. Lesions with expansile mixed radiolucent/radiopaque patterns lacking margination must be differentiated from osteogenic and chondrogenic sarcomas; however, these malignancies are rarely associated with an impacted tooth.

Treatment: Calcifying epithelial odontogenic tumors are aggressive and may reach large proportions. Their behavior is not unlike that of ameloblastoma. En bloc resection, hemimandibulectomy, or partial maxillectomy, depending on tumor size, are the treatment methods required to eradicate the disease.

References

1. Pindborg, J. J.: The calcifying epithelial odontogenic tumor; review of the literature and report of an extraosseous case. Acta Odontol. Scand. 24:419, 1966.
2. Chaudhry, A. P., et al.: Calcifying epithelial odontogenic tumor. Cancer 30:519, 1972.
3. Krolls, S. E. and Pindborg, J. J.: Calcifying epithelial odontogenic tumor. A survey of 23 cases and discussion of histomorphologic variations. Arch. Pathol. 98:206, 1974.
4. Franklin, C. D. and Pindborg, J. J.: The calcifying epithelial odontogenic tumor. A review and analysis of 113 cases. Oral Surg. 42:753, 1976.
5. Sadeghi, E. M., and Hopper, T. L.: Calcifying epithelial odontogenic tumor. J. Oral & Maxillofacial Surg. 40:225, 1982.

Ameloblastic Fibrodentinoma

Age: Teenagers, young adults
Sex: No predilection

Clinical and Radiographic Features: This rare mixed odontogenic tumor represents an ameloblastic fibroma that has differentiated to the extent that dentin is elaborated. Expansion is often present, but pain is not a feature. The lesion invariably arises in association with an impacted tooth; depending upon the degree of dentinal calcification, it may appear radiolucent with central opaque flecks or may assume a target configuration. It may be unilocular or multilocular with well-defined margins. A variant form occurs in children and is located peripherally as a gingival swelling.

Microscopic Features: Dispersed throughout an embryonic hypercellular hypocollagenous mesenchymal element are linear cords of cuboidal epithelium that tend to open, creating tooth germ configurations with a central stellate reticulum element. In juxtaposition to these epithelial nests are sheets of eosinophilic hyalinized material representing dentinoid. Occasionally, tubules are demonstrable. Cell nuclei may be entrapped within this product.

Differential Diagnosis: Pericoronal lucencies with central opacities as seen in ameloblastic fibrodentinoma are also typical of other odontogenic neoplasms included in the section. Biopsy is required to secure a definitive diagnosis.

Treatment: Simple surgical nucleation is the treatment of choice. Recurrence is uncommon.

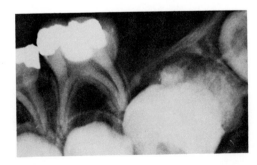

FIG. 10–14. Ameloblastic fibrodentinoma arising in association with an impacted first molar showing a pericoronal radiopacity.

References

1. Pindborg, J. J. and Clausen, F.: Classification of odontogenic tumors; suggestion. Acta Odontol. Scand. *16*:293, 1958.
2. Gorlin, R. J., et al.: Odontogenic tumors. Cancer *15*:73, 1961.
3. Azaz, B., Ulmansky, M., and Lewin-Epstein, J.: Dentinoma. Report of a case. Oral Surg. *24*:659, 1967.
4. Eversole, L. R., Tomich, C. A., and Cherrick, H. M.: Histogenesis of odontogenic tumors. Oral Surg. *32*:569, 1971.
5. McKelvy, B. D. and Cherrick, H. M.: Peripheral ameloblastic fibrodentinoma. J. Oral Surg. *34*:826, 1976.

Ameloblastic Fibro-odontoma

Age: Teenagers
Sex: No predilection

Clinical and Radiographic Features: The ameloblastic fibro-odontoma, referred to in the past simply as ameloblastic odontoma, is an aggressive mixed odontogenic neoplasm that is analogous to an ameloblastic fibroma capable of elaborating all of the hard tissues found in a mature tooth. Clinically, the mandibular body and ramus regions are the most frequent sites of origin, and expansion is the chief sign. Radiographically, most are associated with the crown of an impacted tooth. The lesion may reach large proportions yet is well demarcated. It may be unilocular or multilocular and contains multiple radiopaque foci with irregular configurations.

Microscopic Features: Calcified and uncalcified matrices of dentin, enamel, and cementum prevail in haphazard arrangement. A significant portion of the tumor is composed of proliferating epithelial and mesenchymal soft tissue with features identical to those of ameloblastic fibroma. Inductive changes with dentinoid and a mantle of enamel matrix are interposed between the epithelial and mesenchymal tissues in focal regions.

Differential Diagnosis: Large well-defined radiolucencies with multifocal central opacities in association with an impacted tooth, usually a molar, are typically seen with ameloblastic fibrodentinoma and odontoameloblastoma as well as with ameloblastic fibro-odontoma. Microscopic examination is therefore required.

Treatment: Surgical enucleation is the treatment of choice. Recurrence may develop, but is uncommon.

References

1. Hooker, S. P.: Ameloblastic odontoma: an analysis of twenty-six cases. Oral Surg. *24*:375, 1967 (abstract).
2. Worley, R. D. and McKee, P. E.: Ameloblastic odontoma: report case. J. Oral Surg. *30*:764, 1972.
3. Hanna, P. J., Regezi, J. A., and Hayward, J. R.: Ameloblastic fibro-odontoma: Report of case with light and electron microscopic observations. J. Oral Surg. *34*:820, 1976.

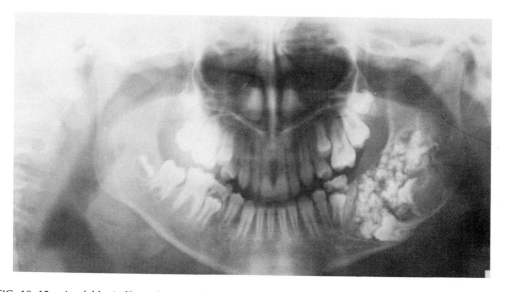

FIG. 10–15. Ameloblastic fibro-odontoma showing an expansile well-circumscribed radiolucency with multiple opaque foci in association with an impacted molar. (From Woorley, R. D. and McKee, P. E.: Ameloblastic odontoma: report of case. J. Oral Surg. *30*:764, 1972. Copyright American Dental Association, reprinted by permission.)

4. Miller, A., et al.: Ameloblastic fibro-odontoma. Report of seven cases. Oral Surg. *41*:354, 1976.

5. Hutt, P. H.: Ameloblastic fibro-odontoma: report of a case with documented four year follow-up. J. Oral & Maxillofacial Surg. *40*:45, 1982.

Odontoma

Age: Teenagers, young adults
Sex: No predilection

Clinical and Radiographic Features: The odontoma, a mixed odontogenic tumor with the capability of elaborating all dental tissues found in a mature tooth, is self-limiting in its growth potential. It is the most common pericoronal radiopacity. Expansion, if present at all, is limited. Lesions located high in the alveolus may tend to erupt, with ulceration, fistulization, and inflammation. Radiographically, a pericoronal radiolucency with well-defined or corticated borders is seen. The center contains tooth-like calcified masses (composite type) or round, oval, or sunburst masses (complex type). When odontoma are associated with impacted teeth, they are usually mandibular molars.

Microscopic Features: Enamel matrix, tubular dentin, and cementum are associated with their complementary soft tissue elements, odontogenic epithelium, odontoblasts, and cementoblasts respectively. The calcified components may or may not assume tooth-form configurations.

Differential Diagnosis: When tooth-like opacities are present within a unilocular radiolucency, a radiographic diagnosis can often be rendered. The complex varieties or larger pericoronal lesions must be microscopically differentiated from other odontogenic neoplasms such as Pindborg tumor, ameloblastic fibrodentinoma, ameloblastic fibro-odontoma, and odontoameloblastoma.

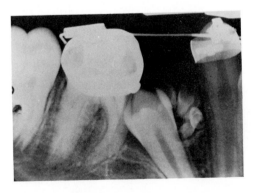

FIG. 10–16. Tooth-like forms of an odontoma located around the crown of an impacted premolar.

Treatment: Surgical enucleation is easily achieved because of encapsulation by follicular fibrous tissue. The lesion should be removed, since odontomas may prevent eruption, displace adjacent teeth, or develop dentigerous cysts.

References

1. Gorlin, R. J., et al.: Odontogenic tumors. Cancer *14*:73, 1961.
2. Cobos, L., et al.: Compound and complex odontomas. Odontol. Chile *15*:33, 1966.
3. Regezi, J. A., Kerr, D. A., and Courtney, R. M.: Odontogenic tumors; analysis of 706 cases. J. Oral Surg. *36*:771, 1978.
4. Minderjahn, A.: Incidence and clinical differentiation of odontogenic tumors. J. Maxillofacial Surg. *7*:142, 1979.
5. Gardner, D. G. and Dort, L. C.: Dysplastic enamel in odontomas. Oral Surg. *47*:238, 1979.

Odontoameloblastoma

Age: Teenagers and young adults
Sex: No predilection

Clinical and Radiographic Features: An extremely rare mixed odontogenic tumor, the odontoameloblastoma is an aggressive neoplasm capable of producing significant expansion and facial asymmetry. The tumor is composed of all tissue components of a normal tooth and can be considered an aggressive variant of the odontoma. Radiographically, an impacted tooth with a well-circumscribed expansile radiolucency containing multifocal radiopaque foci is demonstrated. The central opacities often resemble malformed teeth. They may arise in either jaw with a tendency to locate in the body area in association with an impacted molar, which is usually markedly displaced by the lesion. Root divergence or resorption may be discernible.

Microscopic Features: Decalcified specimens show a diverse array of calcified tissue matrices: enamel, dentin, and cementum. These are often arranged in morphologic structures that resemble developing anomalous teeth. The hard tissues are admixed and associated with odontogenic epithelium, which in many regions is proliferative, displaying an ameloblastoma-like histomorphology. These ameloblastomatous islands are embedded in mature collagenous stroma.

Differential Diagnosis: Odontoma and odontogenic adenomatoid tumor are rarely as aggressive as odontoameloblastoma; nevertheless, they should be included in the differential radiographic diagnosis. Ameloblastic fibro-odontoma, ameloblastic fibrodentinoma, and calcifying epithelial odontogenic tumor may all appear radio-

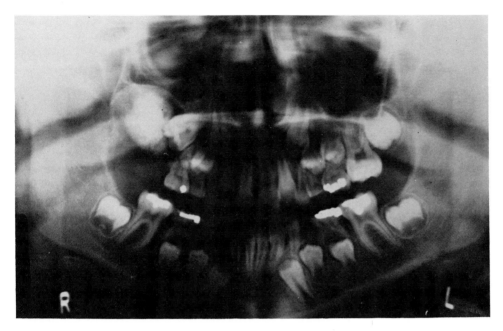

FIG. 10–17.   Odontoameloblastoma associated with an impacted molar.

graphically indistinguishable from odontoameloblastoma.

Treatment: Since few cases of this tumor have been reported, a reliable prognostic index cannot be based upon previous experiences. Reported cases often recur. Thorough enucleation is recommended and, if a recurrence develops, resection may be required.

References

1. Clausen, F.: Les odontomes ameloblastiques. Rev. Stomatol. Chir. Maxillofac. 60:590, 1959.
2. Frissell, G. T. and Shafer, W. G.: Ameloblastic odontoma; report of a case. Oral Surg. 6:1129, 1953.
3. Pindborg, J. J., Kramer, I. R., and Torloni, H.: International histological classification of tumors, no. 5. Histological typing of odontogenic tumors, jaw cysts, and allied lesions. Geneva World Health Organization, 1970.
4. La Briola, J. D., et al.: Odontoameloblastoma. J. Oral Surg. 38:139, 1980.

GROUND-GLASS RADIOPACITIES

Fibrous Dysplasia

Age: Teenagers and young adults
Sex: No predilection

Clinical and Radiographic Features: Fibrous dysplasia is the most common disease of the jaws to manifest a ground-glass radiographic pattern. It may exist as a solitary lesion (the monostotic form), as multiple lesions involving many bones of the jaws and cranium (the craniofacial form), or throughout the skeleton (the polyostotic variety). The latter may be complicated by endocrine defects, including precocious puberty, goiter, and café-au-lait macular pigmentations of the skin. This form of polyostotic fibrous dysplasia is known as Albright's syndrome. When long bones are affected, deformed limbs and pathologic fractures are frequent findings. The monostotic variant is by far the most common type seen when the jaw is affected. The disease is a painless expansile dysplastic process of osteoprogenitor connective tissue. Slow growth is seen with progressive facial deformity. Pain and paresthesia are generally lacking. The maxilla is most often the site of involvement. When the mandible is affected, the radiographic pattern is more apt to be multicystic or mottled. The maxillary lesion is monotonously ground-glass or "orange-peel" in configuration, shows expansion, and characteristically lacks margination. Rather, the dysplastic process appears to blend subtly into the adjacent trabecular bone. The lesion does not cross the midline and shows a tendency to limit itself to one bone, crossing sutures only occasionally. The antrum is often obliterated, and involvement of the orbital floor may displace the globe.

Microscopic Features: Dispersed throughout a

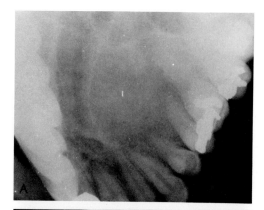

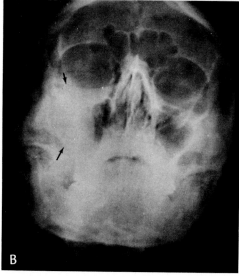

FIG. 10–18. *A:* Ground-glass lesion in maxilla and *B:* similar-appearing ground-glass opacity of antrum and maxilla in fibrous dysplasia.

hypercellular fibrous stroma are irregular haphazardly arranged osseous trabeculae with no structural arrangement; however, a retiform pattern may be discerned in some cases. With polarized light, most of the trabeculae show a woven bone pattern, but the presence of lamellar trabeculae does not militate against a diagnosis of fibrous dysplasia.

Differential Diagnosis: The ground-glass pattern of fibrous dysplasia may be encountered in the early stages of osteitis deformans and in hyperparathyroidism. Osteitis deformans characteristically crosses the midline, is a disease of the elderly, and produces significantly elevated serum alkaline phosphatase levels. During early or active growth stages of fibrous dysplasia, serum alkaline

phosphatase may be elevated as well. Hyperparathyroidism is more apt to manifest brown tumors of the jaws than ground-glass lesions. A skeletal survey should be taken to rule out polyostotic lesions.

Treatment: Treatment should be deferred, if possible, until skeletal maturity is reached. Attempts to intervene surgically during the lesional growth phase may actually activate the process. Fibrous dysplasia tends to become arrested and static at the same time that the epiphyseal growth centers close. A rare aggressive form of the disease known as *active juvenile fibrous dysplasia* shows rapid aggressive growth, particularly in the maxilla, and may invade the cranial base. Extremely aggressive clinical behavior in the face of cellularly active disease requires partial maxillectomy to achieve control. Taking the aforementioned features into consideration, it is recommended that children with a diagnosis of fibrous dysplasia be followed quarterly with clinical, radiographic, and periodic study-model evaluation to determine whether accelerated or diminished growth is taking place.

References

1. Zimmerman, D. C., Dahlin, D. C., and Stafne, E. C.: Fibrous dysplasia of the maxilla and mandible. Oral Surg. *11*:55, 1958.
2. Eversole, L. R., Sabes, W. R., and Rovin, S.: Fibrous dysplasia; a nosologic problem in the diagnosis of fibro-osseous lesions of the jaws. J. Oral Pathol. *1*:189, 1972.
3. Waldron, C. A. and Giansanti, J. S.: Benign fibro-osseous lesions of the jaws: a clinical-radiologic-histologic review of sixty-five cases. I. Fibrous dysplasia of the jaws. Oral Surg. *35*:190, 1973.
4. Obisesan, A. A., et al.: The radiologic features of fibrous dysplasia of the craniofacial bones. Oral Surg. *44*:949, 1977.
5. Nance, F. L., Fonseca, R. J., and Burkes, E. J., Jr.: Technetium bone imaging as an adjunct in the management of fibrous dysplasia. Oral Surg. *50*:199, 1980.

Osteitis Deformans (Paget's Disease of Bone)

Age: Elderly adults
Sex: Male predilection

Clinical and Radiographic Features: Osteitis deformans is a dysplastic bone disease that classically occurs in the elderly and involves replacement of normal bone by an irregular osseous growth, with an increase in osteoblastic activity. The long bones, pelvis, and cranium are predilected sites that show expansion and deformity. As skull lesions develop, foramina become con-

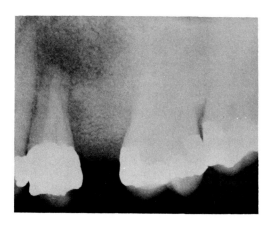

FIG. 10–19. Ground-glass radiopacity of maxilla with periapical clearing around premolar in early osteitis deformans.

stricted, leading to such cranial nerve neuropathies as blindness, deafness, and facial palsy. Skull lesions begin in early stages as focal radiolucencies, so-called osteitis circumscripta. Later, the cranium enlarges with fuzzy radiopaque conglomerates, producing the classic cotton-wool pattern. In the jaws, the maxilla is more often involved than the mandible, and the early stages show a uniform ground-glass appearance with faint poorly demarcated periapical clearing (ill-defined radiolucencies). The teeth remain vital. The cotton-wool pattern eventually replaces the ground-glass appearance, and teeth may develop hypercementosis. The maxillary lesions cross the midline to involve both quadrants and clinically manifest progressive expansion, which in turn leads to diastema formation in dentulous patients. Giant cell tumors similar to giant cell granuloma are occasionally encountered in patients with Paget's disease, appearing as expansile multilocular radiolucencies. Osteomyelitis and an increased risk for development of osteogenic sarcoma are complications.

Microscopic Features: A fibro-osseous microscopic pattern is seen in the early stages of osteitis deformans; a hypercellular fibrous stroma supports irregular osteoid trabeculae rimmed by osteoblasts on one side with resorbing osteoclasts on the opposite side. Vascularity is prominent, and osteoclastic giant cells are often encountered in fibrous areas removed from any osseous trabeculae. Mosaic bone is usually encountered even in the early stages, yet is far more prevalent in lesions of long standing.

Differential Diagnosis: A uniform bilateral maxillary ground-glass pattern with expansion and periapical clearing in an elderly patient is nearly diagnostic for Paget's disease. Alkaline phosphatase, calcium, and phosphorus levels should be obtained; bone biopsy is recommended. Alkaline phosphate is characteristically elevated, while calcium and phosphorus levels are within normal limits. Whereas fibrous dysplasia and hyperparathyroidism may show similar radiographic features, the former is seen in young persons and is restricted to one quadrant, and the latter fails to expand bone and is characterized by an elevated serum calcium.

Treatment: No effective treatment is available. Calcitonin is effective only temporarily. Patients developing periapical inflammation or requiring tooth extraction should be given antibiotics because widespread osteomyelitis, which is difficult to control, is a complication.

References

1. Cooke, B. E. D.: Paget's disease of the jaws; fifteen cases. Ann. R. Coll. Surg. Engl. *19*:223, 1956.
2. Tillman, H. H.: Paget's disease of bone; a clinical, radiological, and histomorphological study of twenty-four cases involving the jaws. Oral Surg. *15*:1225, 1962.
3. Morgan, G. A. and Morgan, P. R.: Oral and skull manifestations of Paget's disease. J. Can. Dent. Assoc. *35*:208, 1969.
4. Brady, F. A., Roser, S. M., and Sapp, J. P.: Osteomyelitis of the mandible as a complicating factor in Paget's disease of bone. Br. J. Oral Surg. *17*:33, 1979.
5. Guyer, P. B.: The clinical relevance of radiologically revealed Paget's disease of bone (osteitis deformans). Br. J. Surg. *66*:438, 1979.

Hyperparathyroidism

Age: Middle-aged adults
Sex: Female predilection

Clinical and Radiographic Features: The jaw manifestations of hyperparathyroidism are rare and, when present, are encountered only late in the course of the disease. The result of an adenoma of the parathyroid gland with increased output of parathormone, the characteristic laboratory finding is an elevation in serum calcium with a decreased level of phosphorus. Elevated calcium leads to precipitation of mineral in tissues (metastatic calcification), particularly in the bladder; this leads to nephrocalcinosis and urolithiasis. Elevated calcium levels also cause muscular weakness and lethargy. Mobilization of calcium from bone results in osteitis fibrosa cystica, a general-

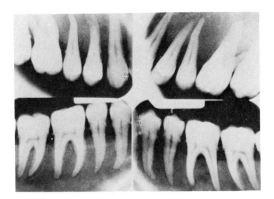

FIG. 10–20. Ground-glass appearance of bone in hyperparathyroidism.

ized demineralization; subperiosteal resorption in the middle phalanges is a characteristic finding. When the jaw is involved, multilocular radiolucencies representing giant cell brown tumors may be seen, or a diffuse ground-glass nonexpansile pattern may be encountered. The lamina dura is missing, and the teeth become mobile. The same changes can be seen in secondary hyperparathyroidism, which evolves subsequent to renal insufficiency and in which excessive urinary loss of calcium evokes a compensatory parathyroid hyperplasia.

Microscopic Features: A fibro-osseous pattern prevails in the ground-glass lesion whereby fibrous stroma replaces normal bone and is stippled with irregular osseous trabeculae showing excessive osteoclastic activity.

Differential Diagnosis: Whereas the ground-glass pattern of hyperparathyroidism may be similar to that seen in fibrous dysplasia and osteitis deformans, expansion is lacking. The loss of lamina dura in conjunction with the ground-glass appearance in an isolated jaw quadrant may occasionally be seen in metastatic carcinoma or even primary sarcomas of the jaws. A bone chemistry profile, including calcium, phosphorus, and alkaline phosphatase, should be obtained even when clinical symptomatology (urolithiasis, muscular weakness) points to a diagnosis of hyperparathyroidism.

Treatment: Once it has been determined that the cause for the ground-glass lesion is hyperparathyroidism (usually by an elevated serum calcium level), the patient should be referred to an internist to determine whether a primary neoplasm or renal disease is causative. Parathyroid adenomas are treated surgically. Even after elimination of the dis-

ease, the ground-glass pattern in the jaws may persist.

References

1. Silverman, S., Jr., et al.: The dental structures in primary hyperparathyroidism. Oral Surg. *15*:425, 1962.
2. Silverman, S. Jr., Ware, W. H., and Gillooly, C.: Dental aspects of hyperparathyroidism. Oral Surg. *26*:184, 1968.
3. Walsh, R. F. and Karmiol, M.: Oral roentgenographic findings in osteitis fibrosa generalisata associated with chronic renal disease. Oral Surg. *28*:273, 1969.
4. Fletcher, P. D., Scopp, I.W., and Hersh, R. A.: Oral manifestations of secondary hyperparathyroidism related to long-term hemodialysis therapy. Oral Surg. *43*:218, 1977.

Osteopetrosis

Age: Childhood onset

Sex: No predilection

Clinical and Radiographic Features: Osteopetrosis, also known as marble bone disease or Albers-Schönberg disease, is inherited as an autosomal dominant trait (benign form) or as an autosomal recessive trait (malignant form). The

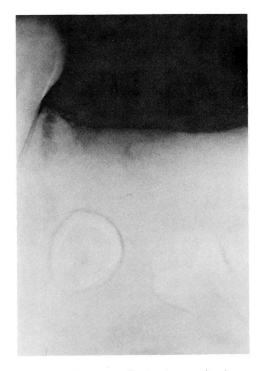

FIG. 10–21. Dense opacification in generalized osteopetrosis (marble bone disease). (Courtesy of Dr. J. Campbell.)

former may develop later in life; the severe recessive form is present from birth, and life expectancy rarely exceeds 20 years. The disease is apparently the result of defective osteoclastic activity; unchecked osteoblastic activity leads to excessive osteogenesis. Radiographically, trabeculation is obscured by an extremely dense opacification of medullary bone. The bone may appear so dense that dental root morphology is obscured. Excessive endosteal bone formation results in a myelophthisic anemia and pancytopenia. Neural compression accounts for neurologic sensory and motor function deficits, and the long bones become brittle and are subject to fracture. Hepatosplenomegaly with extramedullary hematopoiesis, hydrocephalus, and mental retardation may be encountered.

Microscopic Features: Medullary bone resembles cortex with thick anastomosing lamellar trabeculae obliterating soft tissue marrow.

Differential Diagnosis: The other entities included as ground-glass opacities are finely granular and should not be confused radiographically with osteopetrosis, which is strikingly radiodense. Familial historic genetic mapping may uncover affected relatives of the propositus.

Treatment: There is no effective treatment. Periapical infections may progress to severe osteomyelitis. Dental sepsis and extraction of teeth in affected individuals should be treated in conjunction with antibiotic therapy.

References

1. Gomez, L. S. A., et al.: The jaws in osteopetrosis (Albers-Schönberg disease): Report of case. J. Oral Surg. 24:67, 1966.
2. Smith, N. H.: Albers-Schönberg disease (osteopetrosis): report of case and review of the literature. Oral Surg. 22:699, 1966.
3. Thompson, R. D., et al.: Manifestations of osteopetrosis. J. Oral Surg. 27:63, 1969.
4. Cangiano, R., Meoney, J., and Stratigos, G. T.: Osteopetrosis: report of case. J. Oral Surg. 30:217, 1972.
5. Nitzan, D. W. and Marmary, Y.: Osteomyelitis of the mandible in a patient with osteopetrosis. J. Oral & Maxillofacial Surg. 40:377, 1982.

MULTIFOCAL CONFLUENT (COTTON-WOOL) RADIOPACITIES

Osteitis Deformans (Paget's Disease of Bone)

Age: Elderly adults

Sex: Male predilection

Clinical and Radiographic Features: Osteitis deformans is a dysplastic bone disease of the aged that is more severe in females than males yet affects males more frequently than females. It is polyostotic in distribution; when the long bones and spine are severely involved, deformity and crippling results. The skull and maxilla are rarely spared, with expansile overgrowth that is uniformly symmetrical. Osteoblastic hyperactivity prevails, with resultant excess secretion of osteoblastic alkaline phosphatase. The enzyme may be detected in elevated serum levels often approaching tenfold elevations over normal amounts. As the craniofacial bones expand, the skull and upper face enlarge, with resulting increase in hat size, inability to wear dentures, or if the patient is dentulous, diastema formation. Bone enlargement in the area of neural foramina results in bizarre nerve deficits such as hearing loss, blindness, and facial palsy. While the early stages appear as ground-glass radiopacities, as the disease progresses osteoblastic activity prevails, with the appearance of multifocal radiopacities in the maxilla, yielding a cotton-wool pattern. The process is generalized throughout the maxilla and calvarium, and is bilateral. Hypercementosis is a common finding. The jaws are susceptible to infection of odontogenic origin; therefore, widespread osteomyelitis may develop. Patients with Paget's disease are at risk for malignant transformation to osteogenic sarcoma or fibrosarcoma central in bone.

Microscopic Features: A fibro-osseous pattern predominates with irregular osseous trabeculae implanted in a hypercellular vascular marrow. Concomitant osteoblastic and osteoclastic rimming trabeculae is a dominant feature. Large dense and compact trabeculae are riddled with basophilic resting and reversal lines, producing a jigsaw-puzzle arrangement. Occasionally, giant cell lesions accompany Paget's disease.

Differential Diagnosis: The cotton-wool, multifocal radiodense conglomerates seen in osteitis deformans may also be encountered in florid cemento-osseous dysplasia and Gardner's syndrome. The osseous lesions are restricted to the maxillofacial complex in these disorders, whereas in Paget's disease of bone, the skull, long bones, and vertebrae are usually involved as well. The jaw lesions of Paget's are usually maxillary with only occasional involvement of the mandible, as opposed to florid cemento-osseous dysplasia, which is more common in the mandible. The presence of supernumerary teeth and other features of Gardner's syndrome are unique, allowing for differentiation on a clinicoradiologic basis. Alkaline

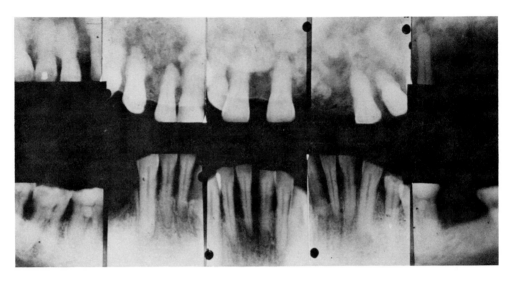

FIG. 10–22. Multiple confluent radiopacities of the maxilla in osteitis deformans. (Courtesy of Dr. H. Cherrick.)

phosphatase elevations are a feature of Paget's disease and are not significantly elevated in other diseases considered in the differential diagnosis. In addition, the mosaic bone pattern observed microscopically is not featured in other diseases.

Treatment: There is no effective treatment for osteitis deformans. When dental abscess occurs, necessitating extraction, antibiotic coverage should be provided to circumvent the complication of osteomyelitis. Follow-up both clinically and radiographically for sarcomatous change is indicated.

References

1. Stafne, E. C. and Austin, L. R.: A study of dental roentgenograms in cases of Paget's disease (osteitis deformans), osteitis fibrosa cystica and osteoma. J. Am. Dent. Assoc. 25:1210, 1938.
2. Gardner, A. R., et al.: Study of 24 cases of Paget's disease involving the maxilla and mandible with reference to dentistry. J. Calif. Dent. Assoc. 39:105, 1963.
3. Rosenmertz, S. K. and Schare, H. J.: Osteogenic sarcoma arising in Paget's disease of the mandible. Oral Surg. 28:304, 1968,
4. Feig, H. I., et al.: Chronic osteomyelitis of the maxilla secondary to Paget's disease. Oral Surg. 28:320, 1969.
5. Guyer, P. B.: The clinical relevance of radiologically revealed Paget's disease of bone (osteitis deformans). Br. J. Surg. 66:438, 1979.

Florid Cemento-osseous Dysplasia (Diffuse Sclerosing Osteomyelitis)

Age: Middle-aged adults
Sex: Female predilection

Clinical and Radiographic Features: Florid cemento-osseous dysplasia occurs predominantly in middle-aged Negro females and has been postulated to represent a low-grade inflammatory lesion of the jaws resulting from pulpal or periapical infection, hence the term *diffuse sclerosing osteomyelitis.* Alternatively, an infectious source is usually not identifiable. For this reason, the condition has been suggested to represent a dysplastic process of periodontal ligament (cementoblastic) origin unique to the Negro race. Nevertheless, it is occasionally seen in members of other races. Radiographically, one or all four jaw quadrants can be affected, although there is a tendency to be limited to or more extensive in the mandible. The jaws possess multiple confluent radiopacities yielding a cotton-wool pattern. More often than not, the jaws are edentulous. Sequestrum formation with a surface nodularity may be demonstrable, but expansion of the cortices is lacking or present to a limited degree. The alkaline phosphatase is usually within normal limits. The pathologic osseous tissue is susceptible to infection, with development of acute osteomyelitis with bony sequestration and fistula formation.

Microscopic Features: A fibro-osseous histologic pattern prevails in areas devoid of acute inflammation. A hypercellular fibrous stroma supports curvilinear trabeculae that show the polarization microscopic features of cementum; however, some examples are composed predominantly of bone. Mononuclear inflammatory cells, if present at all, are sparse.

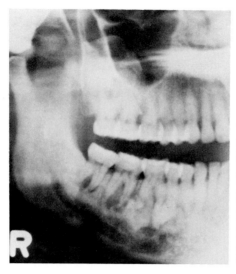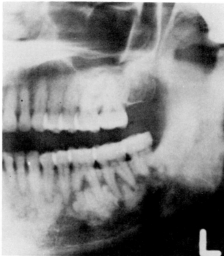

FIG. 10–23. Cotton-wool appearing opacities in mandible representing florid cemento-osseous dysplasia.

Differential Diagnosis: The cotton-wool radiography of diffuse sclerosing osteomyelitis or diffuse cemental dysplasia is easily confused with that of osteitis deformans. The former is primarily mandibular, extragnathic osseous lesions are absent, and the alkaline phosphatase is normal; in Paget's disease the dysplastic osseous process is polyostotic, alkaline phosphatase is elevated, and the maxillary quadrants are affected exclusively or more extensively than those of the mandible. Gardner's syndrome must also be included in the differential diagnosis. The cotton-wool osteomas of this syndrome are rarely limited to the jaws, the sinuses being a common site of localization. In addition, the other manifestations of Gardner's syndrome are diagnostic.

Treatment: No treatment is required. Should osteomyelitis of an acute nature evolve, antibiotic therapy with surgical removal of sequestra and debridement is recommended.

References

1 Bhaskar, S. N. and Cutright, D. E.: Multiple enostosis: report of cases. J. Oral Surg. 26:321, 1968.

2. Waldron, C. A., Giansanti, J. S., and Browand, B. C.: Sclerotic cemental masses of the jaws (so-called chronic sclerosing osteomyelitis, sclerosing osteitis, multiple enostosis, and gigantiform cementoma). Oral Surg. 39:590, 1975.

3. Melrose, R. J., Abrams, A. M., and Mills, B. G.: Florid osseous dysplasia. A clinical-pathologic study of thirty-four cases. Oral Surg. 41:62, 1976.

4. Jacobsson, S. and Heyden, G.: Chronic sclerosing osteomyelitis of the mandible: histologic and histochemical findings. Oral Surg. 43:357, 1977.

5. Sedano, H. O., Kuba, R., and Gorlin, R. J.: Autosomal dominant cemental dysplasia. Oral Surg. 54:643, 1982.

Gardner's Syndrome

Age: Young adults
Sex: No predilection

Clinical and Radiographic Features: Inherited as an autosomal dominant trait, Gardner's syndrome is characterized by multiple osteomas of the jaws and sinuses, supernumerary teeth, desmoid (fibrous) tumors of skin, epidermal inclusion cysts and intestinal polyps with a predilection for malignant transformation into adenocarcinomas. The intestinal polyps are limited to colorectal mucosa and can be detected on gastrointestinal radiologic analysis and proctoscopic examination. The skin lesions are multiple and appear as nodular smooth-surfaced lesions located primarily on the trunk and back. The manifestations include multiple supernumerary teeth and odontomas, most of which are impacted. The osteomas are demonstrable on jaw, panographic, and Water's sinus radiographs, as multiple diffuse and confluent radiopacities, which may involve all four jaw quadrants. The antra and frontal sinuses often contain similar irregular radiodensities. Since the osteomas may reside both centrally and in parosteal locations, clinically detectable indurated protuberances can be identified on palpation.

Microscopic Features: The osteomas are composed of dense lamellar Haversian bone with scant fibrous stroma.

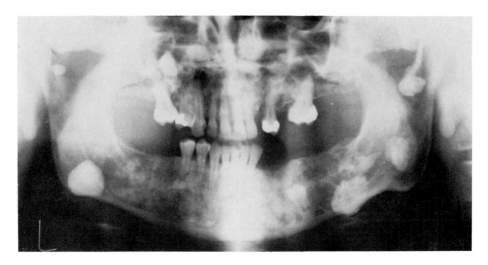

FIG. 10–24.   Multiple radiodense masses of the jaws in the Gardner syndrome. (Courtesy of Dr. S. Levin.)

Differential Diagnosis: The multifocal cotton-wool radiodensities of Gardner's syndrome are similar radiologically to the lesions encountered in Paget's disease and diffuse sclerosing osteomyelitis. A tendency for localization of osteomas in the sinuses, the presence of supernumerary teeth, and the other features of the syndrome are sufficient to rule out these other entities.

Treatment: The osteomas may be removed if they interfere with function or present a cosmetic problem. Supernumerary teeth and odontomas should be removed. Patients should be referred to a gastroenterologist since intestinal adenocarcinoma is the most serious aspect of this syndrome.

References

1. Gorlin, R. J. and Chaudhry, A. P.: Multiple osteomatosis, fibromas and fibrosarcomas of the skin and mesentery, epidermoid inclusion cysts of the skin, leiomyomas and multiple intestinal polyposis. N. Engl. J. Med. 236:1151, 1969.
2. Gardner, E. J.: Follow-up study of a family group exhibiting dominant inheritance for a syndrome including intestinal polyposis, osteomas, fibromas, and epidermal cysts. Am. J. Hum. Genet. 14:376, 1962.
3. Neal, C. J.: Multiple osteomas of the mandible associated with polyposis of the colon (Gardner's syndrome). Oral Surg. 28:628, 1969.
4. Redding, S. W., Carr, R. F., and Foti, C. E.: Gardner's syndrome: report of case. J. Oral Surg. 39:50, 1981.
5. Ida, M., Nakamura, T., and Utsunomiya, J.: Osteomatous changes and tooth abnormalities found in the jaws of patients with adenomatosis coli. Oral Surg. 52:2, 1981.

Mandibular Tori and Exostoses

Age;   Middle-aged adults
Sex: Female predilection

Clinical and Radiographic Features: Mandibular tori are bony excrescences located in the premolar region on the lingual alveolus; exostoses are similar developmental osseous nodules found at the mucobuccal fold on the maxillary buccal alveolar ridge. Both, if large enough, are visible radiographically as multiple, usually bilateral, ovoid radiodensities superimposed over the premolar and molar roots. These lesions are quite common, occurring in nearly 8 percent of the population, and have a familial tendency. They may continue to grow slowly with advancing years.

Microscopic Features: The osseous nodules are composed of a thickened outer cortical plate of Haversian bone. Medullary trabeculae extend internally and are admixed with an intervening fibroadipose marrow.

Differential Diagnosis: Exostoses and mandibular tori may radiographically simulate the jaw lesions of osteitis deformans, osteomyelitis and Gardner's syndrome. Tori and exostoses, as opposed to these other diseases, manifest radiopacities located near the crest of the alveolus without extension below root apices. When the radiographic findings are compared with the clinical features a definitive diagnosis is easily rendered.

Treatment: No treatment is required unless the bony nodules interfere with function or placement of a prosthetic appliance. In these instances, they may be removed surgically.

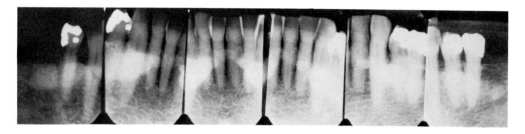

FIG. 10–25. Diffuse indiscrete opacities at the alveolar crest in the mandible representing mandibular tori.

References

1. Kolas, S., et al.: The occurrence of torus palatinus and torus mandibularis in 2,478 dental patients. Oral Surg. 6:1134, 1953.
2. Suzuki, M., and Sakai, T.: A familial study of torus palatinus and torus mandibularis. Am. J. Phys. Anthropol. *18*:263, 1960.
3. Summers, C. J.: Prevalance of tori. J. Oral Surg. 26:718, 1968.
4. Blakemore, J. R., Eller, D. J., and Tomaro, A. J.: Maxillary exostoses. Oral Surg. *40*:200, 1975.

CORTICAL REDUNDANCIES (ONION-SKIN PATTERNS)

Garre's Periostitis

Age: Children and teenagers

Sex: No predilection

Clinical and Radiographic Features: Garre's periostitis represents a reactive periosteal proliferative inflammatory response to infection or trauma. In the jaws, the most common source is inflammation of odontogenic origin. A soft tissue or parotid abscess overlying periosteum may also stimulate periosteal osteogenesis. A new bone is formed, expansion becomes evident; radiograph-

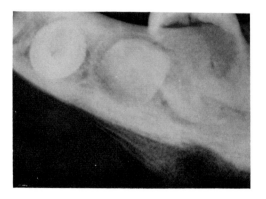

FIG. 10–26. Redundant cortical layering located adjacent to a carious molar in this occlusal x-ray, typical for Garre's periostitis.

ically, a redundant cortical layering phenomenon is usually but not invariably encountered. A constant radiographic feature is preservation of the normal boundary of the cortex subjacent to the expanded region. The disease is essentially confined to the mandibular body when the jaws are affected. Toothache or dull bone pain may cause the patient to seek dental consultation.

Microscopic Features: A fibro-osseous histologic pattern prevails, with a cellular fibroblastic stroma interposed between irregular or parallel trabeculae of woven or lamellar bone. Scattered mononuclear inflammatory cells are often observed.

Differential Diagnosis: The cortical layering with expansion seen in Garre's periostitis is also encountered in Caffey's disease and Ewing's sarcoma. Since Garre's periostitis is an inflammatory disorder, an infectious source, usually a carious molar tooth with a periapical radiolucency, can be identified. Caffey's disease is seen in infants, is bilateral, and involves numerous bones of the appendicular skeleton. A biopsy is recommended to rule out Ewing's sarcoma.

Treatment: The periosteal proliferative response becomes arrested and will remodel to normal contour once the infectious process responsible for its genesis has been eliminated.

References

1. Pell, G. J., et al.: Garre's osteomyelitis of the mandible. J. Oral Surg. *13*:248, 1955.
2. Suydam, M. J. and Mikity, V. G.: Cellulitis with underlying inflammatory periostitis of the mandible. Am. J. Roentgenol. Radium Ther. Nucl. Med. *106*:133, 1969.
3. Ellis, D. J., Winslow, J. R., and Indovina, A. A.: Garre's osteomyelitis of the mandible. Oral Surg. 44:183, 1977.
4. Eversole, L. R., et al.: Proliferative periostitis of Garre; its differentiation from other neoperiostoses. J. Oral Surg. *37*:725, 1979.
5. Eisenbud, L., Miller, J., and Roberts, I. L.: Garre's proliferative periostitis occurring simultaneously in

four quadrants of the jaws. Oral Surg. *51*:172, 1981.

Infantile Cortical Hyperostosis

Age: Infants

Sex: No predilection

Clinical and Radiographic Features: Inherited as an autosomal dominant trait, infantile cortical hyperostosis or Caffey-Silverman disease begins before 6 months of age as a polyostotic cortical hyperostosis. The thickened cortices reflect exaggerated periosteal osteogenesis, which has been suggested to evolve subsequent to tissue hypoxia resulting from genetically defective periosteal vessels. Recently it has been proposed that all infants exhibit an accelerated appositional bone growth spurt, and periosteal redundancy is merely an exaggerated form of this growth phase, which is radiographically demonstrable in some infants. Clinically, the overlying soft tissues are tender, warm, and swollen. The swellings are bilateral and are particularly obvious about the mandible. Fever and leukocytosis are generally apparent. Radiographically, the body and ramus manifest expansion with onion-skin cortical redundancy. Within a few months, the generalized condition resolves spontaneously .

Microscopic Features: The microscopic features of the osseous lesions have not been well delineated.

Differential Diagnosis: The polyostotic symmetrical distribution of cortical redundancies of infancy permit differentiation from other diseases manifesting similar radiographic features. Familial fibrous dysplasia or cherubism shows bilateral mandibular expansion. However, cortical redundancy is not a feature; the jaw lesions of cherubism are multilocular and expansile.

Treatment: No treatment is necessary as the disease spontaneously regresses. Despite this fact, some residual jaw deformity may predispose to malocclusion.

References

1. Burbank, P. M., Lovestedt, S. A., and Kennedy, R. L. J.: The dental aspects of infantile cortical hyperostosis. Oral Surg. *11*:1126, 1958.,
2. Holman, G. H.: Infantile cortical hyperostosis; a review. Q. Rev. Pediatr. *17*:24, 1962.
3. Shopfer, C. E.: Periosteal bone growth in normal infants; preliminary report. Am. J. Roentgenol. *97*:154, 1966.
4. Ditkowsky, S. P., et al.: Normal periosteal reactions and associated soft tissue findings. Relationship to infantile colic and to the Caffey syndrome. Clin. Pediatr. *9*:515, 1970.

Generalized Cortical Hyperostosis

Age: Childhood onset

Sex: No predilection

Clinical and Radiographic Features: Generalized cortical hyperostosis or Van Buchem's disease is inherited as an autosomal recessive trait. The disease is characterized by generalized thickening of the cortical table throughout the skeleton, primarily the tubular bones, the calvaria and the mandible. The hyperostotic changes become evident during the second decade of life. The jaw is squared and enlarged. Thickening of the cranial base may eventually lead to foramina narrowing with attending neurologic deficits including facial paralysis, optic atrophy, and hearing loss. Alkaline phosphatase becomes elevated in the serum. Radiographically, the cortices show a two- or three-fold thickening. *Sclerostosis* is a variant form that favors the calvaria, mandible, and clavicles along with syndactyly. Typical facies are observed in infancy and include a long face with high forehead, hypertelorism, enlarged head, and mandibular prognathism.

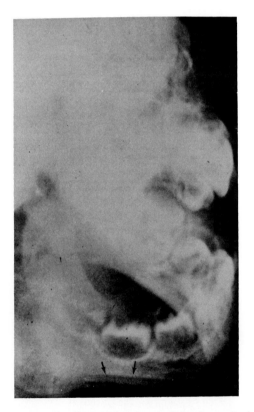

FIG. 10–27. Cortical layering in infantile cortical hyperostosis. (Courtesy of Dr. S. Rovin.)

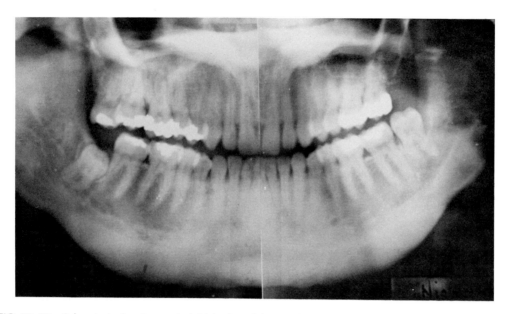

FIG. 10–28.   Sclerostosis showing marked thickening of the mandibular cortex. (Courtesy of Dr. J. Ditmer.)

Microscopic Features: Grossly, the cortices are markedly thickened with irregular grooving and osteophyte formation. The cortical haversian bone is markedly thickened yet histologically unremarkable.

Differential Diagnosis: Sclerostosis and Van Buchem's disease are similar, but they can be differentiated on the basis of the digital anomalies observed in sclerostosis. Osteopetrosis may manifest similar changes, yet the entire medullary bone is hyperostotic and yields a diffuse, rather than strictly cortical, opacification.

Treatment: There is no effective treatment.

References

1. Van Buchem, F. S. P., et al.: An uncommon familial systemic disease of the skeleton: hyperostosis corticalis generalisata familaris. Acta Radiol. 44:109, 1955.
2. Fosmoe, R. J., et al.: Van Buchem's Disease. Radiology 90:771, 1968.
3. Truswell, A. S.: Osteopetrosis with syndactyly: a morphologic variant of Albers-Schönberg's disease. J. Bone Joint Surg. 40-B:208, 1958.
4. Van Buchem, F. S., et al.: Hyperostosis corticalis generalisata. Amer. J. Med. 33:387, 1962.

Juxtacortical Osteogenic Sarcoma

Age: Adults

Sex: Male predilection

Clinical and Radiographic Features: Also termed parosteal osteogenic sarcoma, the juxtacortical neoplasm apparently arises from perios-

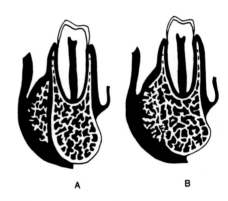

FIG. 10–29.   Juxtacortical osteogenic sarcoma. A: Periosteal pattern. B: Confluent pattern.

teal osteoblasts, and elaboration of tumor bone is peripheral. The mandible is affected more often than the maxilla, and the prognosis of this type of osteogenic sarcoma is much more favorable than that of its endosteal counterpart. Pain may be featured; however, the most common complaint is alveolar swelling with a history of rapid growth. Radiographically, a mottled appearance of opacification is observed on periapical films. Occlusal radiographs reveal the characteristic features. An onion-skin appearance is usually not apparent; instead an irregular opacification is observed, and radially protruding osteophytic spicules can be identified. Cortical invasion with erosion may be featured. Occasionally, the periosteal new growth is clearly demarcated from cortex by an interposed radiolucent band. Such lesions are referred to as periosteal osteogenic sarcoma.

Microscopic Features: Most of these neoplasms are well differentiated; others are anaplastic. Pleomorphic osteoblasts and a hypercellular stroma are observed with formation of irregular trabeculae, which are also hypercellular. Chondroid foci are present in half the cases.

Differential Diagnosis: Both proliferative periostitis and infantile cortical hyperostosis show onion-skin patterns as opposed to irregular osteophytic changes. Myositis ossificans and fasciitis ossificans should be considered in the radiographic diagnosis.

Treatment: Despite the peripheral orientation of the tumor, an en bloc resection of the underlying mandible or maxilla should be performed. Adjunctive chemotherapy should be considered for those lesions with invasion of the endosteum. Anaplastic invasive tumors behave poorly, similar to those lesions arising centrally. Patients with well-differentiated peripheral tumors have shown a 75 percent 5-year survival.

References

1. Solomon, M. P., et al.: Parosteal osteogenic sarcoma of the mandible: existence masked by diffuse periodontal inflammation. Arch. Otolaryngol. *101*:754, 1975.
2. Unni, K. K., et al.: Parosteal osteogenic sarcoma. Cancer *37*:2466, 1976.
3. Ahuja, S. C., et al.: Juxtacortical (parosteal) osteogenic sarcoma: Histologic grading and prognosis. J. Bone Joint Surg. *59-A*:632, 1977.
4. Newland, J. R. and Ayala, A. G.: Parosteal osteosarcomas of the maxilla. Oral Surg. *43*:727, 1977.
5. Bras, J. M., et al.: Juxtacortical osteogenic sarcoma of the jaws. Review of the literature and report of a case. Oral Surg. *50*:535, 1980.

IRREGULAR, ILL-DEFINED EXPANSILE RADIOPACITIES

Calcifying Epithelial Odontogenic Tumor

Age: Middle-aged adults
Sex: No predilection

Clinical and Radiographic Features: The Pindborg or calcifying epithelial odontogenic tumor is a neoplasm of epithelial origin. Clinically, depending upon the size and duration, cortical expansion or facial asymmetry heralds its presence. Radiographically, the tumor may manifest many patterns, one of the predominant ones being a mixed radiolucent-radiopaque expansile lesion

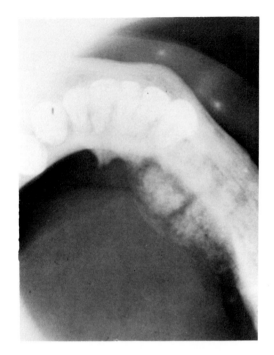

FIG. 10–30. Diffuse expansile radiodensity of a mandibular calcifying epithelial odontogenic tumor. (Courtesy of Dr. R. Middleton.)

with irregular configuration. The margins are poorly defined, and osteophytic spicules may project outward, yielding a sunray pattern. Most cases are associated with an impacted tooth, and the body or ramus regions of the mandible are favored sites.

Microscopic Features: The neoplastic epithelial element exists in sheets or islands of eosinophilic or clear polygonal cells with vesicular nuclei. Often bizarre and pleomorphic nuclear elements are encountered, but this feature has no bearing on the prognosis. Within the stroma and often in intimate association with the epithelial islands are amorphous globules of amyloid material. Circular and ovoid laminated calcifications or Leisegang rings are seen in most tumors.

Differential Diagnosis: When the Pindborg tumor appears radiographically as an expansile illdefined lesion with irregular radiodense conglomerates and spicules, malignant neoplasms of bone should be considered in the differential diagnosis. If an impacted tooth is encompassed by a lesion with the aforementioned features, Pindborg tumor should be the foremost consideration. Biopsy is required in any case.

Treatment: Pindborg tumor is aggressive and

will recur if adequate therapy is not instituted. Large lesions require resection, hemimandibulectomy or partial maxillectomy, while smaller tumors may be cured by en bloc or marginal resection.

References

1. Pindborg, J. J.: A calcifying epithelial odontogenic tumor. Cancer 11:838, 1958.

2. Vap, D. R., Dahlin, D. C., and Turlington, E. G.: Pindborg tumor: The so-called calcifying epithelial odontogenic tumor. Cancer 25:629, 1970.

3. Chaudhry, A. P. et al.,: Calcifying epithelial odontogenic tumor. A histochemical and ultrastructural study. Cancer 30:519, 1972.

4. Krolls, S. O. and Pindborg, J. J.: Calcifying epithelial odontogenic tumor. A survey of 23 cases and discussion of histomorphologic variations. Arch. Pathol. 98:206, 1974.

5. Leipzig, B. and Yau, P. C.: Pindborg tumor of the mandible. Otolaryngol. Head Neck Surg. 90:69, 1982.

Osteogenic and Chondrogenic Sarcoma

Age: Teenagers and young adults

Sex: Male predilection

Clinical and Radiographic Features: Both osteogenic and chondrogenic sarcomas of the jaws are rare. They show similar radiographic features, although sarcomas of chondroblastic origin tend to be more radiolucent. When the tumor cartilage or osteoid calcifies, both chondrosarcoma and osteosarcoma can manifest irregular, poorly marginated radiopaque foci. Osteogenic sarcomas show a sunray or sunburst pattern of osteophytic radiodense spicules in 25 percent of the cases. Expansion of the alveolar cortices is demonstrable both clinically and radiographically. The mandible is more often affected than the maxilla. Pain, paresthesia, and loosening of teeth in the region of tumor are common complaints. Both sarcomas tend to metastasize via hematogenous routes.

Microscopic Features: Osteogenic sarcomas are histologically divided into three groups: osteoblastic, chondroblastic, and fibroblastic. This classification has no bearing on prognosis. The tumor may differentiate along all three cell lines; yet, regardless of the preponderance of fibrous and cartilaginous elements, the sine qua non of osteogenic sarcoma is the elaboration of neoplastic osteoid matrix. Tumor osteoid is found in all osteogenic sarcomas, including the chondroblastic variant. Chondrosarcomas fail to elaborate tumor osteoid. The cellular element is composed in both instances of pleomorphic angulated, polygonal or spindle-shaped cells.

Differential Diagnosis: Irregular, poorly marginated radiopacities should always suggest a tentative diagnosis of osteogenic or chondrogenic sarcoma. Pindborg tumor, particularly if an impacted tooth is associated with the lesion, and metastatic carcinoma must be considered in the differential radiographic diagnosis. Biopsy is required to arrive at a definitive diagnosis.

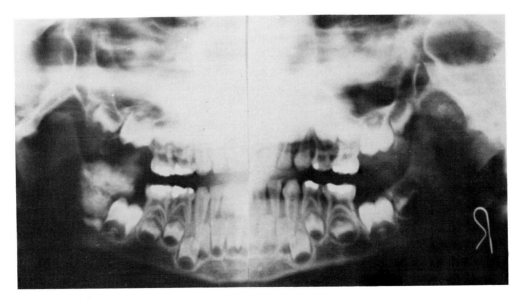

FIG. 10–31.   Irregular expansile radiopacity of the posterior mandible overlying and displacing developing teeth, representing an osteogenic sarcoma.

Treatment: The prognosis for osteogenic sarcoma is better for mandibular (70 percent 5-year survival) than for maxillary tumor (50 percent 5-year survival). Information of this nature does not exist for chondrosarcoma of the jaws. The treatment consists of maxillectomy with preservation of the orbit if extent of disease allows. Mandibular tumors are treated with intraosseous radium needles with external radiation when soft tissues are involved (10,000 rads total dosage). Following radiation, en bloc resection or hemimandibulectomy is performed.

References

1. Chaudhry, A. P., et al.: Chondrogenic tumors of the jaws. Am. J. Surg. *102:*403, 1961.
2. Garrington, G. E., et al.: Osteosarcoma of the jaws: analysis of 56 cases. Cancer 20:377, 1967.
3. Finklestein, J. B.: Osteosarcoma of the jaw bones. Radiol. Clin. North Amer. *8:*425, 1970.
4. Caron, A. S., Hajdu, S. I., and Strong, E. W.: Osteogenic sarcoma of the facial and cranial bones. A review of forty three cases. Am. J. Surg. *122:*719, 1971.
5. Russ, J. E. and Jesse, R. H.: Management of osteosarcoma of the maxilla and mandible. Am. J. Surg. *140:*572, 1980.

Metastatic Carcinoma

Age: Middle-aged and elderly adults

Sex: Depends upon primary site

Clinical and Radiographic Features: Carcinoma arising in the lung, breast, thyroid, prostate, and colon tends to metastasize to bone. When the jaws become a metastatic depot these malignancies may become deposited in marrow spaces and actually simulate osteoblastic acitivity. The body and ramus areas of the mandible are most frequently involved. The chief clinical finding is

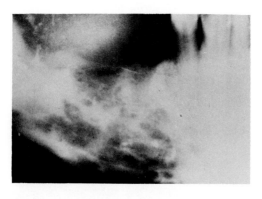

FIG. 10–32. Osteoblastic metastasis from carcinoma of the breast showing a moth-eaten radiolucent pattern admixed with multiple irregular opaque foci.

paresthesia of the lower lip. Radiographically, expansion is usually obvious, as are focal radiolucent zones admixed with irregular radiopaque foci. The margins of the metastatic lesion are poorly defined. Metastatic carcinoma is the most common malignant tumor of the jaws.

Microscopic Features: The microscopic features are variable depending upon the tissue site of origin. In general, nests, cords, or sheets of neoplastic epithelial cells show pleomorphism, anaplasia, and numerous mitotic figures. The tumor cells are dispersed within a fibrous stroma and lie in juxtaposition to dense and irregular osseous trabeculae.

Differential Diagnosis: The irregular, poorly marginated radiopacities as seen in osteoblastic metastatic carcinomas are also seen in Pindborg tumor, osteogenic sarcoma, and chondrosarcoma. A history of cancer elsewhere in the body helps to limit the differential diagnosis; however, microscopic confirmation is necessary. On the other hand, the jaw metastasis may be the first indication of a primary tumor of internal organs.

Treatment: The primary tumor must be identified, as well as other sites of metastasis; and a skeletal survey is indicated to detect other osseous foci of disease. The prognosis is extremely poor. The patient should be managed by an oncologist.

References

1. Castigliano, S. G. and Rominger, C. J.: Metastatic malignancy of the jaws. Am. J. Surg. 87:496, 1954.
2. Clausen, F. and Poulsen, H.: Metastatic carcinoma to the jaws. Acta Pathol. Microbiol. Scand. *57:*361, 1963.
3. Mesa, M. C.: Metastatic prostatic carcinoma to the mandible: report of case. J. Oral Surg. *35:*133, 1977.

SUPERIMPOSED SOFT TISSUE RADIOPACITIES

Sialolithiasis

Age: Middle-aged adults

Sex: Male predilection

Clinical and Radiographic Features: Salivary stones are calcium phosphate salts that crystallize about a central nidus of gelled mucin, desquamated epithelial cells, or bacterial colonies. They are most frequently formed within the submandibular ducts, but may arise within the parotid gland or minor salivary gland ducts of the lips or buccal mucosa. When a major duct becomes occluded, swelling with sialadenitis ensues and pain while eating is a common complaint. Many patients may be asymptomatic. Milking the involved

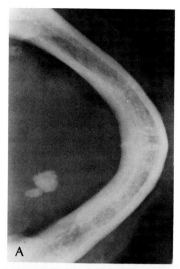

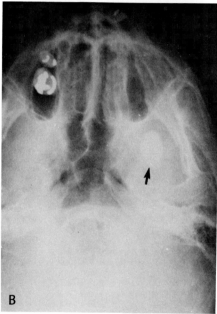

FIG. 10–33. *A:* Occlusal radiograph of a sialolith. *B:* Submental vertex showing a calcified submandibular gland.

gland fails to elicit flow. When submandibular sialoliths become large they produce a radiopacity that may become superimposed over the mandible on dental films. They are well circumscribed, oval or elongated, or if the entire gland becomes filled with intraductal stones, they may show a cauliflower pattern radiographically. An occlusal radiograph will locate the stone in the soft tissue of the oral floor. There is no relationship between

hyperparathyroidism and a tendency to form salivary calculi.

Microscopic Features: The decalcified stone shows concentric laminations without viable cellular elements. The ducts show sialodochitis with squamous, mucous, or respiratory epithelial metaplasia. The gland displays acinar degeneration with fibrous and mononuclear leukocytic infiltration representing a chronic sclerosing sialadenitis.

Differential Diagnosis: When a stone is superimposed over the body of the mandible, a central lesion manifesting a radiopaque appearance must be included in the differential diagnosis. Occlusal and soft tissue films will rule out the possibility of a central lesion. Other soft tissue lesions, which may manifest a superimposed radiopacity, must also be considered.

Treatment: Small stones may be manipulated manually through the duct orifice. Larger ones may require surgical extirpation. If recurrent sialadenitis with a purulent discharge develops after removal, sialadenectomy is usually indicated.

References

1. Tholen, E. F.: Sialolithiasis. J. Oral Surg. *7:*63, 1949.
2. Levy, B. M., ReMine, W. H., and DeVine, K. D.: Salivary gland calculi: Pain, swelling associated with eating. J. Am. Med. Assoc. *181:*1115, 1962.
3. Elmostehy, M. R.: Parotid salivary calculus. Oral Surg. *26:*18, 1968.
4. Rust, T. A. and Messerly, C. D.: Oddities of salivary calculi. Oral Surg. *28:*862, 1969.
5. El Deeb, M., Holte, N., and Gorlin, R. J.: Submandibular salivary gland sialoliths perforated through the oral floor. Oral Surg. *51:*134, 1981.

Phlebolithiasis

Age: No predilection
Sex: No predilection

Clinical and Radiographic Features: Phleboliths are calcified thrombi that form within the lumina of dilated vascular channels. They are most frequently encountered in hemangiomas and varices. The vascular lesions can be visualized clinically and are generally palpable, particularly when phleboliths are present. When these lesions arise in tissues such as the cheek, lips, and tongue, the calcifications, which may be multiple, will be demonstrable on dental radiographs. The stones appear as circular or oval well-demarcated focal radiopaque foci.

Microscopic Features: Vascular channels are dilated and intraluminal thrombi are present. Within these thrombosed regions, dystrophic and laminated calcific foci are observed.

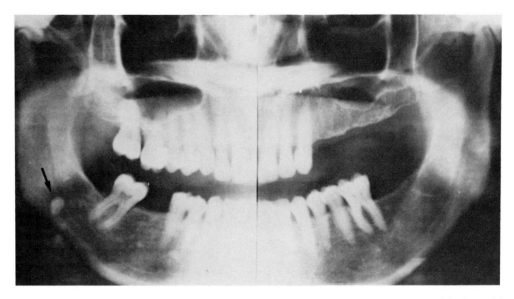

FIG. 10–34. Multiple superimposed radiopaque foci representing phleboliths in a hemangioma of the base of the tongue.

Differential Diagnosis: Phleboliths with radiographically demonstrable calcifications must be differentiated from central osseous lesions. Occlusal and soft tissue radiographs will rule out this possibility. Other soft tissue disorders manifesting radiopacities must be included in the differential radiographic diagnosis. Clinical examination will disclose the presence of a vascular lesion unless it is deep seated; in these instances biopsy is indicated.

Treatment: Since most hemangiomas show a cessation in growth potential, no treatment is required provided the diagnosis has been confirmed. Surgical removal may be indicated if function is compromised by the tumor or if cosmesis is a concern.

References
1. Parker, L. A. and Frommer, H. H.: Phleboliths; report of case. Oral Surg. *18*:476, 1964.
2. O'Riordan, B.: Phleboliths and salivary calculi. Br. J. Oral Surg. *12*:119, 1974.

Foreign Bodies

Age: No predilection
Sex: No predilection

Clinical and Radiographic Features: Foreign objects are introduced into the oral soft tissues as a result of traumatic or iatrogenic injuries. Dental amalgam and metal fragments from automobile accidents or assault are the more frequently encountered foreign bodies that are demonstrable

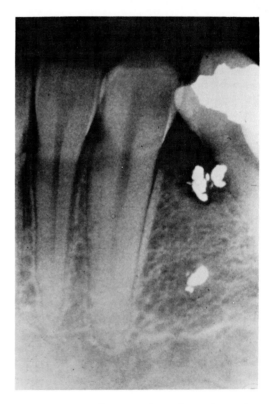

FIG. 10–35. Amalgam particles in the gingiva producing superimposed irregular dense radiopacities.

radiographically. When these metallic objects become lodged within the buccal mucosa, lips, tongue, alveolar ridges, or gingiva they appear as irregular ragged radiopacities superimposed over the maxilla or mandible. Many foreign bodies are easily visualized clinically as discolorations or swellings, or they may be palpable.

Microscopic Features: Metallic foreign bodies cannot be processed for routine microscopy. The surrounding tissue may be fibrous, granulomatous with giant cells, or acutely inflamed, depending on the chemical and physical properties of the foreign object.

Differential Diagnosis: Foreign-body radiopacities superimposed over bone are usually readily identifiable because of irregular outline or configuration of the metal deposit. In addition, the opacity is generally more dense and homogeneous than that of calcific lesions. Soft tissue films and biopsy will provide a definitive diagnosis.

Treatment: The foreign body should be excised, particularly if a fistula or swelling is present. Amalgam pigmentation seen clinically in conjunction with a radiopacity does not require treatment.

References

1. Blum, T.: Foreign bodies in and about the jaws. Dent. Cosmos 63:12227, 1921.
2. Stafne, E. C. and Gibilisco, J. A.: *Oral Roentgenographic Diagnosis,* 4th Ed. Philadelphia, W. B. Saunders Co., 1975, Chapter 22.
3. Eliasson, S. T. and Holte, N. O.: Rubber base impression material as a foreign body: report of case. Oral Surg. 48:379, 1979.
4. Alexander, J. M.: An unusual case of trismus. Oral Surg. 47:419, 1979.
5. Beasley, W. R.: Foreign body in the right condyle area. Report of a case. Oral Surg. 52:241, 1981.

Calcified Lymph Nodes

Age: Adults

Sex: No predilection

Clinical and Radiographic Features: In the head and neck area, submandibular, cervical, and digastric nodes are most often enlarged during infectious processes. Occasionally, a node or group of nodes with long-standing lymphadenopathy will undergo fibrosis and subsequently devlop foci of dystrophic calcification. Scrofula, or tuberculous lymphadenitis, is probably the most prevalent disease process to eventuate in nodal calcification. Actinomycosis, cat-scratch fever, and other chronic infectious diseases may also eventually become quiescent with dystrophic calcification of sclerotic nodes. Radiographically, a single ovoid calcification or clustered calcifications may be en-

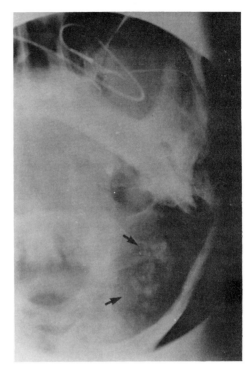

FIG. 10–36. Calcified tuberculous nodes. Sialogram shows parotid gland above nodal calcifications.

countered in regions where groups of lymph nodes are typically found.

Microscopic Features: The normal architecture of the lymph node is usually obliterated; however, the periphery may occasionally be represented by aggregates of lymphocytes and atrophic germinal centers. The cental zone is occupied by dense collagenous connective tissue with confluent deposits of calcification.

Differential Diagnosis: Calcified lymph nodes will radiographically resemble sialoliths, phleboliths, or foreign bodies. Sialography is often helpful in that the calcified node is not asociated with the duct tree. A history of scrofula or other diseases associated with chronic lymphadenitis aids in arriving at a definitive diagnosis, particularly when the radiopacities are located in an area known to be populated by lymph nodes.

Treatment: No treatment is required.

Reference

1. Wood, N. K. and Goaz, P. W.: Periapical radiopacities. In *Differential Diagnosis of Oral Lesions.* St. Louis, C. V. Mosby Co., 1980, p. 559.

Myositis Ossificans

Age: Adults
Sex: Male predilection

Clinical and Radiographic Features: Ossification of muscle occurs in a generalized form that begins in childhood and becomes progressively more extensive with ensuing age. In this form intestinal smooth muscle, skeletal muscle, and fascia undergo calcification. The facial muscles may be involved. Etiology is unknown. The second form, seen in a single muscle, is more often encountered in the perioral musculature and is secondary to trauma (traumatic myositis ossificans). The traumatic episode is thought to produce an intramuscular hematoma, which organizes and susequently calcifies. The masseter, temporal, pterygoid, and geniohyoid muscles have been reported to be involved by this process. The affected muscle shows rapid enlargement subsequent to trauma and then becomes indurated. Motion may be limited. Radiographically, the muscle involved shows a radiopaque zone that may be discrete or show frayed margins. Myositis ossificans in the masseter, pterygoids, or muscles in the floor of the mouth will manifest a radiopacity superimposed over the mandible.

Microscopic Features: Osteoid trabeculae are rimmed by osteoblasts, and the intervening fibrous tissue is hypercellular. The overall picture is one of extremely active osteoplasia that has been mistaken for sarcoma. The ossified zone is surrounded by muscle fibers. Mononuclear inflammatory cells are occasionally present in limited number.

Differential Diagnosis: The history and clinical features usually indicate the radiopaque mass is external to bone. Radiographic views from various angles will usually locate the lesion in the soft tissues in the vicinity of muscle. Sialoliths can be eliminated from consideration on the basis of location and symptoms, particularly with the aid of occlusal x-rays. In addition, most sialoliths and phleboliths are focal, small calcific structures, while the opacity seen in myositis ossificans is generally large and diffuse.

Treatment: Once a tentative diagnosis is established the muscle can be entered surgically and the calcified mass excised; a portion of the adjacent normal-appearing muscle must also be obtained. A biopsy is needed to confirm the clinical diagnosis. Recurrence is uncommon.

References

1. Goodsell, J. O.: Traumatic myositis ossificans of the masseter muscle: review of the literature and report of a case. J. Oral Surg. 20:116, 1962.
2. Vernale, C. A.: Traumatic myositis ossificans of the masseter muscle. Oral Surg. 26:8, 1968.
3. Narang, R. and Dixon, R. A., Jr.: Myositis ossificans: Medial pterygoid muscle—a case report. Br. J. Oral Surg. 12:229, 1974.
4. Plezia, R. A., Mintz, S. M., and Calligaro, P.: Myositis ossificans traumatica of the masseter muscle. Report of a case. Oral Surg. 44:351, 1977.
5. Mulherin, D. and Schow, C. E., Jr.: Traumatic myositis ossificans after genioplasty. J. Oral Surg. 38:786, 1980.

ANTRAL OPACITIES

Maxillary Sinusitis

Age: Adults
Sex: No predilection

Clinical and Radiographic Features: Sinusitis is a common disease and is usually allergic. Many cases of acute sinusitis and some cases of chronic sinusitis are associated with or caused by infectious organisms; chief among these are *Haemophilus influenzae*, *Streptococcus pneumoniae*, and rhinovirus. Allergic sinusitis is generally secondary to rhinitis, in which the lateral nasal mucous membranes become edematous leading to blockage of the ostium. The affected sinus fills with mucous secretion and if also infected, a purulent aspirate can be obtained. Repeated bouts of inflammation with periodic blockage and drainage

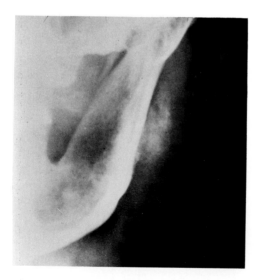

FIG. 10–37. Soft tissue opacity in masseteric region representing myositis ossificans. (From Plezia, R. A., Mintz, S. M., and Calligaro, P.: Myositis ossificans traumatica of the masseter muscle. Oral Surg. 44:351, 1977.)

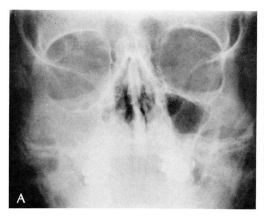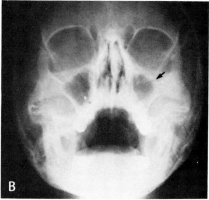

FIG. 10–38. *A:* Unilateral diffuse antral opacification in chronic sinusitis. *B:* Hyperplastic sinus membrane in chronic sinusitis.

can lead to a thickening of the sinus membrane. Fluid-filled sinuses appear as a diffuse opacification; transillumination of the sinuses reveals a dull or opaque appearance when a fiberoptic light source is placed against the palate in a darkened room. When the upper sinus is pneumatized while fluid occupies the lower region, a discrete fluid level can be identified on Water's projections. Chronic recurrent sinusitis often discloses patency with a thickened membrane. In general, a membrane thickening greater than 8 mm is associated with symptoms. Many asymptomatic patients exhibit a mild to moderate thickening radiographically. The chief symptom of active chronic sinusitis is dull pain that is referred to all posterior maxillary teeth, which are sensitive to percussion. When the head is lowered, the pain intensifies. Acute infectious sinusitis is associated with moderate to severe maxillary pain and pressure, both of which occur spontaneously and on palpation.

Microscopic Features: An aspirate in cases of acute infectious sinusitis will show neutrophils, whereas subacute or chronic infectious lesions will contain a preponderance of mononuclear cells. The mucous membranes in chronic sinusitis are edematous with a leukocytic infiltrate containing many eosinophils. Polypoid excrescences are common and show similar histologic changes to hyperplastic mucosal thickening.

Differential Diagnosis: Osseous destruction is not usually a feature of chronic sinusitis. Nevertheless, neoplastic processes may cause diffuse homogeneous opacification; however, pain is not usually featured. Failure of the opacification to resolve following conventional therapy for sinusitis warrants exploration, sinoscopy, and biopsy. Dental sources of infection should be ruled out.

Treatment: A therapeutic trial employing nasal decongestants and antihistamine should be initiated. Should the symptoms and radiographic opacification fail to resolve within four or five days, an aspirate should be obtained in order to evaluate the presence of leukocytes. Furthermore, a culture and sensitivity test should be performed to explore an infectious etiology; appropriate antibiotic therapy, usually ampicillin or amoxicillin, should follow.

References

1. Fascenelli, F. W.: Maxillary sinus abnormalities: radiographic evidence in an asymptomatic population. Arch Otolaryngol. *90:*190, 1969.
2. Waite, D. E.: Maxillary sinus. Dent. Clin. North Amer. *15:*349, 1971.
3. Axelsson, A. and Brorson, J. E.: The correlation between bacterological findings in the nose and maxillary sinus in acute maxillary sinusitis. Laryngoscope *83:*2003, 1973.
4. Axelsson, A., and Jensen, C.: The roentgenologic demonstration of sinusitis. Am. J. Roentgenol. *122:*621, 1974.
5. Evans, F. O., Jr., et al.: Sinusitis of the maxillary antrum. N. Engl. J. Med. *293:*735, 1975.

Antral Mucosal Cyst (Polyp)

Age: Middle-aged adults
Sex: No predilection

Clinical and Radiographic Features: The mucosal cyst of the antrum represents an inflammatory polyp without an epithelial lining and is therefore not a true cyst. Furthermore, this lesion should

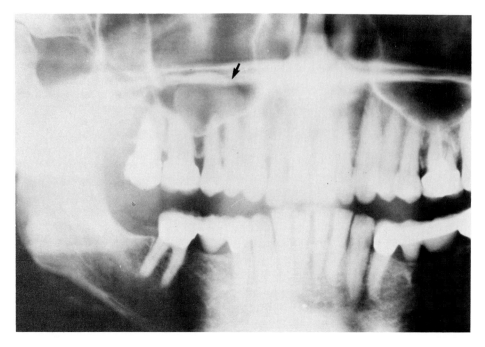

FIG. 10–39.   Antral mucosal cyst.

not be confused with a true mucocele of the sinuses, which, unlike the mucosal cyst, exhibits aggressive behavior. The antral mucosal cyst should be referred to as an inflammatory mucosal polyp. Usually no symptoms are present; however, there may be a history of nasal discharge, congestion, or other symptoms of chronic sinusitis. Radiographically, panoramic, Caldwell and Water's views reveal a smooth-surfaced, dome-shaped homogenous opacity that emanates from the antral floor. On anterior-posterior views, an air space usually separates the polyp from the lateral sinus bony wall. Bone erosion or expansion is not featured. The maxillary teeth underlying the sinus lesion are vital.

Microscopic Features: The antral retention polyp lacks an epithelial lining. The sinus respiratory epithelium occupies the surface and is distended by an underlying mass of areolar and myxomatous fibrous or granulation tissue. Mucoid lakes are often observed and are compartmentalized by intervening delicate fibrovascular septa. Ductal ectasia of the tubuloacinar glands is common, and a mild inflammatory cell infiltrate composed of lymphocytes, plasma cells, neutrophils, and eosinophils prevails throughout.

Differential Diagnosis: Antral mucosal polyps appear identical to antral polyps associated with spread of odontogenic infection. Periapical cysts or granulomas with sinus extension can be ruled out by vitalometer testing. Most neoplasms fail to show a discrete dome-shaped opacity emanating from the sinus floor. Osteomas, antroliths, and odontomas are more discrete and are generally more opacified than antral mucosal polyps.

Treatment: Symptoms rarely exist; thus no treatment is necessary. Periodic follow-up radiographs should be obtained; most lesions spontaneously resolve within 1 year.

References

1. Wright, R. W.: Round shadows in the maxillary sinuses. Laryngoscope 56:455, 1946.
2. Kwapis, B. W. and Whitten, J. B.: Mucosal cysts of the maxillary sinus. J. Oral Surg. 29:561, 1971.
3. Halstead, C. L.: Mucosal cysts of the maxillary sinus: report of 75 cases. J. Am. Dent. Assoc. 87:1435, 1973.
4. Myall, R. W. T., Eastep, P. B., and Silver, J. B.: Mucous retention cysts of the maxillary antrum. J. Am. Dent. Assoc. 89:1338, 1974.
5. Gothberg, T. K. A., et al.: A clinical study of cysts arising from mucosa of the maxillary sinus. Oral Surg. 41:52, 1976.

Sinus Mucocele

Age: Middle-aged adults
Sex: No predilection

Clinical and Radiographic Features: The sinus

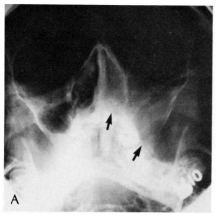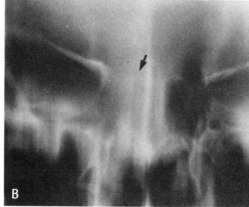

FIG. 10–40. Sinus mucocele showing A: antral and nasal opacification and B: sphenoethmoidal opacification with erosion of the bony walls.

mucocele is usually located in the frontal or anterior ethmoidal sinus, yet occasionally involves the antrum. Rare cases of pansinus involvement have been reported. While the etiology is unknown, the most plausible cause is blockage of the sinus openings with mucous retention. There is usually a history of surgery, trauma, or recurrent sinusitis. Frontoethmoidal lesions expand and displace the eye laterally and inferiorly. A crepitant bulge can usually be detected in the frontal region. Radiographically, diffuse opacification is seen along with effacement of the septate configuration. Erosion of the sinus walls may be preceded or accompanied by reactive osteosclerosis. Rarely, a proliferative osteomyelitis is observed with dense opacification and obliteration of the sinus air spaces. An acute infection may also evolve (mucopyocele). When the antrum is involved, diffuse opacification is seen along with osseous destruction. Clinically, the teeth may loosen and the ipsilateral eye may exhibit proptosis. Computerized tomography is extremely useful for determining extent of disease.

Microscopic Features: Although the sinus lining usually maintains a pseudostratified columnar ciliated appearance, foci of squamous metaplasia may be present. An inflammatory cell infiltrate is frequently encountered in the submucosa.

Differential Diagnosis: When a mucocele arises in the antrum, the diffuse opacification with erosion of the sinus walls cannot be reliably differentiated from tumor. Aspiration that reveals a mucoid secretion suggests mucocele. A Caldwell-Luc procedure with sinus exploration and biopsy should be performed.

Treatment: Frontal sinus and ethmoidal mucoceles may extend intracranially. A modified Lynch-Howarth surgical procedure is recommended along with establishment of a wide and patent nasofrontal duct. Antral lesions should be treated in similar fashion, employing a Caldwell-Luc approach and maintaining a large and patent antronasal opening.

References

1. Schuknecht, H. F. and Lindsay, J. R.: Benign cyst of the paranasal sinuses. Arch. Otolaryngol. 49:609, 1949.
2. Zizmor, J. and Noyek, A. M.: Cysts, benign tumors and malignant tumors of the paranasal sinuses. Otolaryngol. Clin. North Am. 6:487, 1973.
3. Natrig, K. and Larsen, T. E.: Mucocele of the paranasal sinuses: a retrospective clinical and histological study. J. Laryngol Otol. 92:1075, 1978.
4. Hesselink, J. R., et al.: Evaluation of mucoceles of the paranasal sinuses with computed tomography. Radiology 133:397, 1979.
5. Jacobson, A. L., Lawson, W., and Biller, H. F.: Bilateral pansinus mucocele with bilateral orbital and intracranial extension. Otolaryngol. Head Neck Surg. 90:507, 1982.

Periapical Infection with Antral Polyps

Age: Adults

Sex: No predilection

Clinical and Radiographic Features: Because of the close proximity of the maxillary molar root apices to the antrum, periapical spread of infection often results in perforation. Acute pulpal infections may drain, causing an acute sinusitis. Radiographically, the entire antrum becomes opacified with intact bony margins. Apical granulomas and cysts

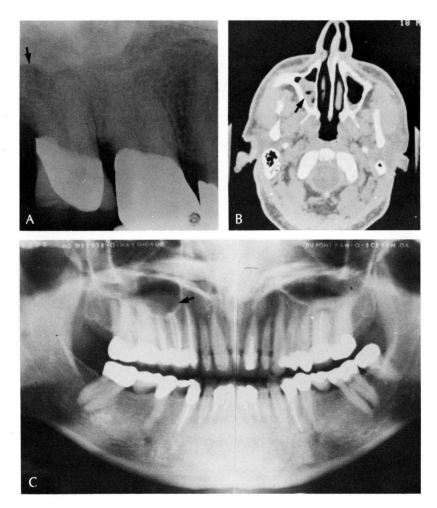

FIG. 10–41. Periapical infection with sinus involvement. *A:* periapical radiolucency involving second molar. *B:* CT scan from same patient shown in A with antral soft tissue opacification. *C:* Sinus polyp secondary to odontogenic infection.

may expand the antral floor cortex or erode and become confluent with the mucosal lining, thus creating an elevated dome-shaped soft tissue opacity. Radiographically, when cortices are expanded, a halo effect about the root apex is observed (apical radiolucency with an egg-shell-like cap). When the inflammatory tissue perforates the cortex, a smooth-surfaced dome-shaped homogenous opacity emanates from the antral floor.

Microscopic Features: Antral polyps secondary to odontogenic infection are composed of extremely loose mucoid areolar granulation tissue exhibiting a leukocytic infiltrate. The surface is covered by respiratory epithelium. Apical periodontal cysts protruding into the antrum may fuse with sinus lining so that both stratified squamous

and respiratory epithelial tissues comprise the cyst lining.

Differential Diagnosis: Antral polyps associated with necrotic teeth appear identical radiographically to antral mucosal cysts. Pulp vitality testing is essential to uncover the etiology. The apical periodontal ligament space is often, yet not invariably, widened in instances involving infected teeth. Because both of these lesions appear as smooth-surfaced dome-shaped opacities arising from the antral floor, confusion with the more generalized opacifications represented by other antral lesions should not be problemmatic.

Treatment: Once the incriminating tooth has been treated endodontically or extracted, the antral lesion will resolve. Occasionally, however, an osseous protuberance will evolve during healing.

References

1. Matilla, K.: Roentgenological investigations into the relation between periapical lesions and conditions of the mucous membrane of the maxillary sinus. Acta Odontol. 23:5, 1965.
2. Ericson, S. and Welander, N.: Local hyperplasia of maxillary sinus mucosa after elimination of adjacent periapical osteitis. Odont. Rev. 17:153, 1966.
3. Worth, H. M. and Stoneman, D. W.: Radiographic interpretations of antral mucosal changes due to localized dental infection. J. Can. Dent. Assoc. 38:111, 1972.
4. Halstead, C. L.: Mucosal cysts of the maxillary sinus: report of 75 cases. J. Am. Dent. Assoc. 87:1435, 1973.
5. Fireman, S. M. and Noyek, A. M.: Dental anatomy and radiology of the maxillary sinus: symposium on the maxillary sinus. Otolaryngol. Clin. North Am. 9:83, 1976.

Antral Mycoses

Age: Adults
Sex: No predilection

Clinical and Radiographic Features: Fungal sinusitis generally affects only debilitated patients such as juvenile brittle diabetics and immunosuppressed individuals. The Phycomycetes and Aspergillus organisms may become opportunistic pathogens in the milieu of the immunologically compromised patient, particularly in mucormycosis. Maxillary enlargement with ocular displacement, loosening of maxillary teeth, and palatal perforation are later manifestations. Radiographically, the antral walls and orbital floor may exhibit bony erosion, and the entire antrum will be faintly opacified.

Microscopic Features: The sinus membrane is infiltrated by mononuclear inflammatory cells, and the antral contents are represented by necrotic debris that is laced with hyphae. The organisms are readily identifiable with periodic acid-Schiff staining. Spores are prominent in aspergillosis.

Differential Diagnosis: The opacification and osseous destruction observed in mucormycosis and aspergillosis are reminiscent of carcinoma. A history of advanced overt diabetes or systemic cancer in a patient receiving chemotherapy should arouse suspicion of antral mycosis. Biopsy is the most rapid method of diagnosis; however, culture of the sinus contents is recommended to specifically identify and differentiate the two organisms.

Treatment: Aggressive therapy is indicated since widespread mycotic osteomyelitis can result in massive sequestration of bone. The underlying systemic problem should be controlled if at all feasible, and systemic antifungal therapy with amphotericin B or ketokonazole should be administered. Both Aspergillus and Phycomycete infections should also be treated by surgical curettage.

References

1. Iwamoto, H., Katsura, M., and Fujimaki, T.: Mycosis of the maxillary sinuses. Laryngoscope 82:903, 1972.
2. Zinneman, H. H.: Sino-orbital Aspergillosis: Report of a case and review of the literature. Minn. Med. 55:661, 1972.
3. Gonty, A. A. and Page, L. R.: Aspergillosis of the maxillary sinus. Oral Surg. 43:350, 1977.
4. Blitzer, A., et al.: Patient survival factors in paranasal sinus mucormycosis. Laryngoscope 90:635, 1980.
5. Breiman, A., Sadowsky, D., and Friedman, J.: Mucormycosis. Discussion and report of a case involving the maxillary sinus. Oral Surg. 52:375, 1981.

Displaced Teeth, Roots, and Foreign Bodies

Age: Adults
Sex: No predilection

Clinical and Radiographic Features: Teeth or root fragments within the sinus are usually readily identifiable by their morphology and radiologic identification of a pulp chamber or root canal shadow. They may radiographically appear in this location as a consequence of (1) traumatic dis-

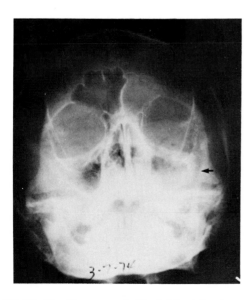

FIG. 10–42. Mucormycosis. The left frontal and maxillary sinuses are opacified, and osseous destruction is evident in the lateral and superior antral walls (arrows).

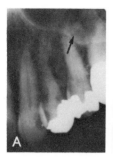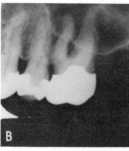

FIG. 10–43. A: Root tip in sinus. B: Same patient depicted in A showing superimposition of root tip over mesial molar root.

placement, (2) displacement of fractured root tips following exodontia, (3) developmental displacement, or (4) superior displacement by an enlarging dentigerous cyst. Water's views are not as efficacious as periapical, Caldwell, and lateral sinus views. When teeth or roots lie within the sinus cavity, they may change positions with head movement. More often, the tooth fragment is trapped between the antral bony floor and the lining membrane; in these instances, a change in head position will not alter the localization radiographically. Unerupted teeth appearing to lie within the sinus often are not, in actuality, within the sinus itself. Rather they are encased in bone and will show a periodontal ligament space with an eggshell-thin cortex interposed between tooth and sinus cavity. Last, it should be stressed that during surgery a tooth may be displaced into the infratemporal space, or a root tip may become lodged between the periosteum and outer cortical table. A variety of radiographic projections and tomography will help to pinpoint the precise location. Root tips lying free within the sinus may serve as an infectious source with resultant sinusitis and diffuse opacification. Rarely, other foreign bodies may reside within the sinus. Impression material forced through an oral-antral fistula and traumatically placed metals are more common.

Microscopic Features: Not applicable.

Differential Diagnosis: Focal opacities representing teeth or roots may be confused radiographically with osteoma, exostosis, or antrolith. Usually the opacity is recognizable by virtue of its morphology as tooth structure.

Treatment: Using a Caldwell-Luc approach, intrasinus teeth and/or root tips should be removed surgically. A longstanding asymptomatic displaced root fragment may be left in place and followed on a regular basis.

References

1. Jones, E. H. and Steel, J. S.: Roots in the maxillary sinus. Aust. Dent. J. 14:8, 1969.
2. Lee, F. M. S.: The displaced root in the maxillary sinus. Oral Surg. 29:491, 1970.
3. Van Wowern, N.: Oroantral communications and displacements of roots into the maxillary sinus. J. Oral Surg. 29:622, 1971.
4. Herd, J. R.: The tooth root within the maxillary sinus. Aust. Dent. J. 19:77, 1974.

Antrolith/Rinolith

Age: Adults
Sex: No predilection

Clinical and Radiographic Features: Stones arising in the antral cavities are uncommon. They may develop around a nidus, which usually represents a foreign body such as a tooth root; on the other hand, no particular material may be identified as serving as the nidus for mineralization. Microbial colonies in bacterial and mycotic antral infections may serve as a matrix for calcification as well. The antrolith may be associated with dull pain or ache, mimicking sinusitis. Radiographically, a dense, irregular yet well-defined mass can be identified in the antrum, usually resting on the antral floor. Stones may develop within the nasal cavity; they will be obvious on panoramic films, Water's radiographs, and tomograms.

Microscopic Features: Decalcified specimens are composed of dystrophic calcified amorphous matrices. The adjacent antral membrane may be polypoid with a submucosal inflammatory cell infiltrate.

Differential Diagnosis: A radiopacity with well-defined margins located in the antrum can

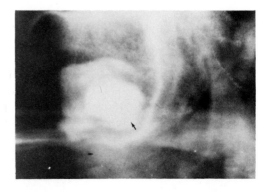

FIG. 10–44. Focal opacity in the antrum representing a calcareous deposit. (From Karges K. A., et al.: Antrolith; report of case and review of literature. J. Oral Surg. 29:813, 1971. Copyright American Dental Association, reprinted by permission.)

be differentiated from an antral retention cyst. A root fragment located in the antrum is perhaps more common. The osteomas in Gardner's syndrome often localize within the sinuses as well.

Treatment: Antroliths should be removed because they irritate the sinus lining and predispose to sinusitis.

References

1. Lord, O. C.: Antral rhinoliths. J. Laryngol. *59:*218, 1944.
2. Karges, M. A., Eversole, L. R., and Poindexter, B. J., Jr.: Antrolith; report of case and review of literature. J. Oral Surg. *29:*813, 1971.
3. Crist, R. D. and Johnson, R. L.: Antrolith: report of case. J. Oral Surg. *30:*694, 1972.
4. Allen, G. A. and Liston, S. L.: Rhinolith: unusual appearance on panoramic radiograph. J. Oral Surg. *37:*54, 1979.
5. Blaschke, D. D. and Brady, F. A.: The maxillary antrolith. Oral Surg. *48:*187, 1979.

Odontoma

Age: Teenagers and adults

Sex: No predilection

Clinical and Radiographic Features: Occasionally, a maxillary odontoma will develop in the maxillary bones of the sinus wall. Alternatively, some odontomas actually lie free within the sinus cavity without an enveloping osseous encasement. Free odontomas within the sinus often manifest symptoms of dull aching pain and nasal discharge by predisposing to a chronic sinusitis. Radiographically, the opacity may be focal; more often, multifocal confluent opacities are clustered, and a fully formed unerupted tooth lies in juxtaposition to the hamartomatous element. Free odontomas change position when the head is moved during procurement of various maxillary films. If the odontoma is encased in bone or entrapped under the sinus membrane, no positional change will occur.

Microscopic Features: Haphazardly arranged dental hard tissues including enamel matrix, dentin, and cementum are present and often histologically mimic miniature tooth buds. Dental pulp with an odontoblastic layer is usually identifiable, and odontogenic epithelium lies adjacent to enamel matrix. A fibrous follicle is also present.

Differential Diagnosis: Composite odontomas with multiple tooth-like configurations are easily

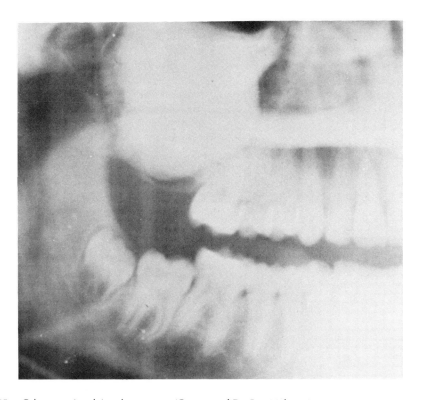

FIG. 10–45.   Odontoma involving the antrum. (Courtesy of Dr. Ray Melrose.)

recognized radiographically. Complex varieties may be confused radiographically with osteoma or antrolith, thus a definitive diagnosis necessitates biopsy.

Treatment: A Caldwell-Luc approach with surgical removal is the treatment of choice. Any associated tooth should be removed in continuity. In addition, any polypoid lesions resulting from irritation by the tumor should be excised.

References

1. Caton, R. B., Marble, H. B., Jr., and Topazian, R. G.: Complex odontoma in the maxillary sinus. J. Oral Surg. *36:658,* 1973.
2. Osborne, T. P., et al.: Odontoma containing ghost cells in the maxillary sinus. Oral Surg. *38:819,* 1974.
3. Currori, R. C., Messer, J. E., and Abramson, A. L.: Complex odontoma of the maxillary sinus: report of case. J. Oral Surg. *33:45,* 1975.
4. Sander, B., Halliday, R., and McKelvey, B.: Odontoma of the antrum presenting as a maxillary sinusitis. J. Oral Med. *31:60,* 1976.
5. Griffith, C. R. and Imperato, A. A.: Large antral odontoma as the cause of acute maxillary sinusitis: report of case. J. Am. Dent. Assoc. *94:107,* 1977.

Osteomas and Exostoses

Age: Adults
Sex: No predilection

Clinical and Radiographic Features: Ossified bodies (osteomas) and bony excrescences (exostoses) may be found within the antrum, although they are more common in the frontal and ethmoidal sinuses. Antral cases are quite rare, and the etiology is obscure. Identification of an osteoma in the antrum should alert the clinician to the possibility of Gardner's syndrome, characterized by supernumerary teeth, osteomas of the jaws and sinuses, desmoid tumors of the skin, and premalignant adenomatous polyposis coli. Antral osteomas may predispose to sinusitis with symptoms of maxillary pain and nasal discharge. Radiographically, osteomas may be seen as single or multiple round or oval radiopacities. A concomitant sinusitis may show a fluid level or diffuse opacification of the affected sinus. Exostoses are firmly adherent and confluent with the sinus wall, usually the lateral wall.

Microscopic Features: Osteomas and exostoses are both composed of mature lamellar bone. They are usually ovoid bodies with an outer cortical margin that encases a medullary trabecular zone. The marrow spaces are represented by areolar fibrous or adipose tissue. When multiple osteomas occur, the ossified bodies are usually dis-

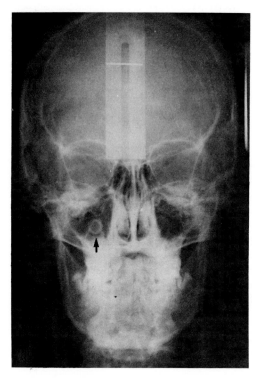

FIG. 10–46.   Osteoma.

crete, being separated from one another by mature fibrous tissue.

Differential Diagnosis: Osteomas may be radiographically indistinguishable from antroliths or complex odontomas. Once biopsy has confirmed a diagnosis of osteoma, paranasal sinus radiographic series and jaw films should be obtained to uncover osteomatous lesions. Should they be discovered, a workup for Gardner's syndrome should be undertaken.

Treatment: The Caldwell-Luc approach should be used to remove the lesion along with hyperplastic sinus membrane or polyps. As mentioned previously, Gardner's syndrome should be ruled out by referral to an internist or gastroenterologist.

References

1. Karmody, C. S.: Osteoma of maxillary sinus. Laryngoscope *79:427,* 1969.
2. Leopard, J. P.: Osteoma of the maxillary antrum. Br. J. Oral Surg. *10:73,* 1972.
3. Herd, J. R.: Exostoses of the sinus wall: a diagnostic problem. Aust. Dent. J. *19:269,* 1974.
4. Liston, L. S., Barker, B. F., and Cocayne, D. R.: Multiple osteomas of the maxillary sinus. J. Oral Surg. *37:113,* 1979.
5. Fu, Y. S. and Perzin, K. H.: Non-epithelial tumors

of the nasal cavity, paranasal sinuses, and naso-pharynx: A clinicopathologic study. Osseous and fibro-osseous lesions, including osteoma, fibrous dysplasia, ossifying fibroma, osteoblastoma, giant cell tumor and osteosarcoma. Cancer *33*:1289, 1974.

Benign Mesenchymal Neoplasms

Age: Adults

Sex: No predilection

Clinical and Radiographic Features: Benign neoplasms of connective tissue origin arising in the antrum are rare. Vascular and nerve sheath neoplasms are more frequently encountered; these lesions arise primarily within the submucosa of the sinus membrane. Intraosseous neoplasms of the maxilla may expand and displace the lateral sinus wall medially; ossifying and cementifying fibromas as well as maxillary odontogenic tumors may behave in this fashion. Ameloblastomas of the maxilla can perforate into the antral space.

Primary benign neoplasms will grow to fill the sinus air space with symptoms of swelling and nasal congestion. Radiographically, diffuse opacification is observed; in larger neoplasms, the sinus walls may exhibit expansion with bowing in all dimensions, particularly obvious along the medial wall on sinus films. Osseous erosion and perforation can also occur with benign neoplasms.

Microscopic Features: The histologic features vary depending upon the cell of origin. The reader is referred to the chapter on oral soft tissue swellings for microscopic descriptions of vascular and neural sheath neoplasms.

Differential Diagnosis: The diffuse opacifications seen in benign mesenchymal neoplasms along with symptoms of congestion may be confused with sinusitis. When expansion and erosion are present, mycotic infections and malignant tumors must be considered, and immediate exploration with biopsy is recommended.

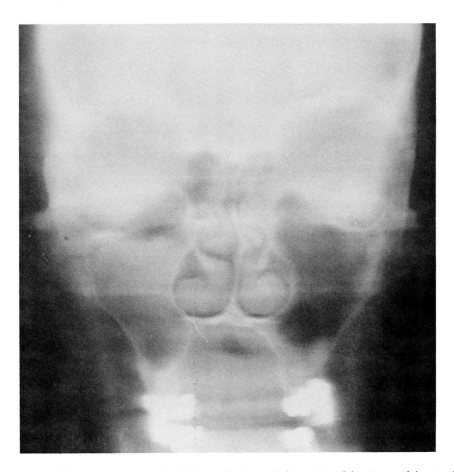

FIG. 10–47.   Maxillary sinus tomogram showing opacification and destruction of the sinus roof due to a benign neoplasm.

Treatment: Most benign neoplasms of connective tissue origin can be treated by curettage or excision. Osseous invasion or large destructive lesions may require hemimaxillectomy.

References

1. Fu, Y. S. and Perzin, K. H.: Non-epithelial tumors of the nasal cavity, paranasal sinuses, and nasopharynx: A clinicopathologic study. I. General features and vascular tumors. Cancer 33:1275, 1974.
2. Agarwal, M. K., et al.: Neurilemmoma of the maxillary sinus. J. Oral Surg. 38:698, 1980.
3. Shugar, J. M., et al.: Peripheral nerve sheath tumors of the paranasal sinuses. Head Neck Surg. 4:72, 1981.
4. Dolan, K. D. and Smoker, W. R. K.: Paranasal sinus radiology, part 4B: Maxillary sinuses. Head Neck Surg. 5:428, 1983.

Inverted Papilloma

Age: Middle-aged adults
Sex: Male predilection

Clinical and Radiographic Features: Unlike the common inflammatory nasal and antral polyp, the inverted or Schneiderian papilloma represents a true neoplastic process arising from the ectodermally derived epithelium. It arises from the lateral nasal wall, either in the region of the middle turbinate or ethmoidal recess. The lesion invades the submucosa and frequently, either via the ostium or by bony erosion, extends into the antral or ethmoidal sinus. Clinically, the most common symptom is nasal obstruction. Radiographically, the affected sinus is opacified; maxillary tomograms often disclose destruction of the medial antral wall with opacification of the nasal cavity. Importantly, carcinoma is associated with inverted papilloma in 10 to 15 percent of the cases. The common fungiform papilloma is limited to the nasal septum and does not invade the maxillary sinus.

Microscopic Features: Inverted papillomas, as the term implies, grow in inverted fashion into the subjacent sinus and nasal submucosa. Budding folds of stratified squamous epithelium are frequently covered by a single row of ciliated columnar cells. Microcysts with mucin are located throughout the spinous cell layer. A rare variant termed cylindrical papilloma may also invade the antrum. The inverted architecture prevails; however, the tumor element is represented by eosinophilic columnar cells, which may show surface cilia.

Differential Diagnosis: Complete antral opacification with inverted papilloma may be encountered in many other benign and malignant lesions of the maxillary sinus. A concurrent opaque mass in the ipsilateral nasal cavity suggests inverted papilloma; however, biopsy is required for a definitive diagnosis.

Treatment: Inverted papillomas are aggressive, and over 60 percent recur following simple excision (polypectomy). CT scans or paranasal sinus tomograms are recommended in order to determine the extent of disease. Lateral rhinotomy offers the greatest chance for cure. Interestingly, this lesion tends to recur more often in females.

References

1. Hyams, V. J.: Papillomas of the nasal cavity and paranasal sinuses. A clinicopathological study of 315 cases. Ann. Otol. Rhinol. and Laryngol. 80:192, 1971.
2. Snyder, R.N. and Perzin, K. H.: Papillomatosis of

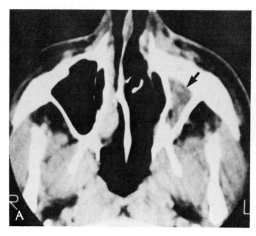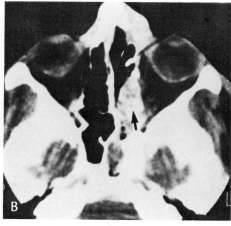

FIG. 10–48.   Inverted papilloma. CT scans showing *A:* antral involvement and *B:* ethmoid sinus involvement.

nasal cavity and paranasal sinuses (Inverted papilloma, squamous papilloma). A clinicopathologic study. Cancer 30:668, 1972

3. Vrabec, D. P.: The inverted Schneiderian papilloma: A clinical and pathological study. Laryngoscope 85:186, 1975.

4. Suh, K. W., et al.: Inverting papilloma of the nose and paranasal sinuses. Laryngoscope 87:35, 1977.

Antral Carcinoma

Age: Elderly adults

Sex: Male predilection

Clinical and Radiographic Features: Maxillary sinus carcinoma rarely manifests worrisome signs or symptoms in the early stages. Patients may complain of unilateral dull sinus pain along with nasal discharge, which masquerade as sinusitis. The majority of cases represent squamous cell carcinoma; transitional cell or anaplastic carcinoma and adenocarcinoma of lining cell origin are less common. Occasionally, adenocarcinomas of tubuloacinus origin occur in the antrum and show histopathologic features similar or identical to salivary tumors. As these malignant tumors proliferate, they fill the sinus cavity and in later stages induce osseous destructive changes. Medial growth will perforate into the nasal cavity, supe-

rior growth may displace the eye with diplopia, posterior extension into the pterygopalatine and pterygomandibular spaces may cause trismus, and inferior extension will cause loosening of maxillary teeth with palatal enlargement or perforation. Infraorbital paresthesia may be featured, and facial expansion can occur. Radiographically, opacification is observed; with conventional sinus radiographs, sinus tomograms, and CT scans, osseous destructive changes can be identified in advanced cases. Extension into other sinuses and cranial base involvement may be extant at the time of admission. Despite the advanced stage and diffuse extent of disease, palpable nodes in the submandibular and upper neck regions are encountered in less than 20 percent of these patients.

Microscopic Features: Squamous cell carcinoma, which is most common, shows proliferating islands and cords of epidermal cells with keratin formation that is generally not abundant. Occasionally, adjacent tissue represents inverted papilloma that has undergone carcinomatous transformation. Adenocarcinomas show tubular and ductal differentiation. Both adenoid cystic and mucoepidermoid carcinoma may be encountered.

Differential Diagnosis: Early tumors may exhibit opacification without destruction of the bony walls and may therefore simulate sinusitis. When osseous destruction is witnessed, sarcomas and mycotic infections must be included in the radiographic diagnosis. Persistent opacification following conventional therapy for sinusitis should be explored and biopsied.

Treatment: Most antral cancers are advanced (T3, T4) by the time they are discovered. Maxillectomy with exploration and surgical excision of tumor in contiguous sinus cavities followed by postoperative external radiation (7500 rads) offers the best chance for cure. Five-year survival for T3 and T4 lesions is about 75 percent and 35 percent respectively.

References

1. Larsson, L. G. and Mårtensson, G.: Maxillary antral cancers. J. Am. Med. Assoc. 219:342, 1972.

2. Sakai, S., Shigematzu, Y., and Fuchihata, H.: Diagnosis and TNM classification of maxillary sinus carcinoma. Acta Otolaryng. 74:123, 1972.

3. Jackson, R. T., Fitz-hugh, G. S., and Constable, W. C.: Malignant neoplasms of the nasal cavities and paranasal sinuses (retrospective study). Laryngoscope 87:726, 1977.

4. Ahmad, K., Cordoba, R. B., and Fayes, J. W.: Squamous cell carcinoma of the maxillary sinus. Arch. Otolaryngol. 107:48, 1981.

5. Hartenian, K. M. and Stenger, T. G.: Carcinoma of

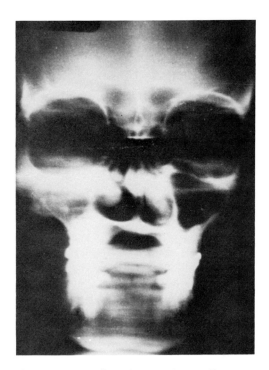

FIG. 10–49. Maxillary sinus carcinoma. Tomogram showing opacification.

the maxillary sinus: report of case. J. Oral Surg. 36:898, 1978.

Antral Sarcoma

Age: Adults
Sex: Male predilection

Clinical and Radiographic Features: Malignant lymphomas and extramedullary plasmacytomas are the most common malignant mesenchymal tumors found to arise in the maxillary sinus. Malignant fibrous histiocytoma, rhabdomyosarcoma, and fibrosarcoma may also occur; occasionally, metastatic neoplasms are located in the antrum. These malignant mesenchymal neoplasms share common clinical and radiographic findings that are similar to those observed in antral carcinoma. As the neoplasm proliferates with the sinus, expansion with facial swelling may be encountered along with extension of a mass into the nasal fossa, superior displacement of the eye, and palatal swelling with loosening of the maxillary teeth. Infraorbital paresthesia and epistaxis are common signs and symptoms, particularly with lymphoma

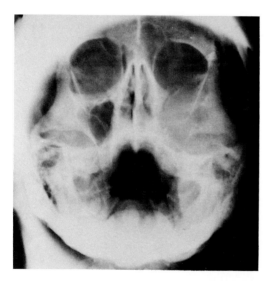

FIG. 10–50. Malignant fibrous histiocytoma of the maxillary sinus showing opacification, expansion, and osseous destruction of the sinus walls.

and plasmacytoma. Radiographically, diffuse opacification is seen with expansion and sinus wall osseous destruction. Water's views and tomograms will often show opacification of the ipsilateral nasal cavity, and CT scans will aid in determining extent of disease.

Microscopic Features: Lymphomas are characterized by sheets of neoplastic lymphoblasts and may be diffuse or nodular. Malignant reticulosis, which represents a specific form of lymphoma that affects the upper air passages, may also be encountered. Extramedullary plasmacytomas are composed of diffuse sheets of plasma cells with a scant vascular stroma. Many lesions of this nature are associated with or progress to multiple myeloma. Malignant spindle cells with bizarre nuclei are seen in fibrosarcoma, malignant fibrous histiocytoma, and rhabdomyosarcoma.

Differential Diagnosis: Clinical evidence of epistaxis in conjunction with antral disease represents an ominous finding. Radiographically, expansile and osseous destructive changes occurring in malignant mesenchymal sinus tumors cannot be differentiated from carcinoma. Biopsy is required for a definitive diagnosis.

Treatment: Lymphoma and plasmacytoma respond to 6000 rads of external beam radiation therapy. Spindle cell malignancies require radical maxillectomy. A thorough workup for involvement of other organ systems and bones should be undertaken.

References

1. Prasanna, N. M. and Mendelsohn, M.: Maxillary sinus sarcomas. Can. J. Otolaryngol. 4:704, 1975.
2. Shabel, S. I., et al.: Extramedullary plasmacytoma. Radiology 128:625, 1978.
3. Fu, Y. S. and Perzin, K. H.: Non-epithelial tumors of the nasal cavity, paranasal sinuses and nasopharynx. A clinicopathologic study. X. Malignant lymphoma. Cancer 43:611, 1979.
4. Merrick, R. E., Rhone, D. P., and Chilis, T. J.: Malignant fibrous histiocytoma of the maxillary sinus. Case report and literature review. Arch. Otolaryngol. 106:365, 1980.
5. Dolan, K. D. and Smoker, W. R. K.: Paranasal sinus radiology, part 4B: Maxillary sinuses. Head Neck Surg. 5:428, 1983.

11
Dental Defects

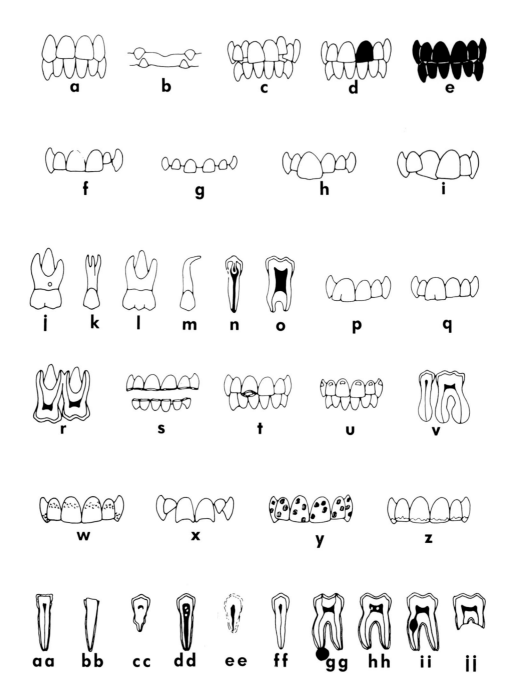

Dental Defects

a, Limited hypodontia; b, Severe hypodontia; c, Hyperdontia; d, Focal pigmentation; e, Generalized pigmentation; f, Localized microdontia; g, Generalized microdontia; h, Localized macrodontia; i, Generalized macrodontia; j, Enamel pearl; k, Accessory roots; l, Accessory cusps; m, Dilaceration; n, Dens-in-dente; o, Taurodontia; p, Fusion; q, Gemination; r, Concrescence; s, Attrition; t, Abrasion; u, Erosion; v, Hypercementosis; w, Enamel hypoplasia; x, Congenital syphilis; y, Fluorosis; z, Snow-capped teeth; aa, Amelogenesis imperfecta; bb, Dentinogenesis imperfecta; cc, Dentin dysplasia I; dd, Dentin dysplasia II; ee, Odontodysplasia; ff, Cemental agenesis (hypophosphatasia); gg, Vitamin D refractory rickets; hh, Pulp stones; ii, Internal resorption; jj, External resorption

11
Dental Defects

ALTERATIONS IN NUMBER: MISSING TEETH

Hypodontia
Incontinentia Pigmenti
Hyalinosis Cutis et Mucosae
Mandibulo-oculo-facial Dyscephaly
Hereditary Ectodermal Dysplasia
Chondroectodermal Dysplasia

ALTERATIONS IN NUMBER: SUPERNUMERARY TEETH

Hyperdontia
Cleidocranial Dysplasia
Gardner's Syndrome

ALTERATIONS IN MORPHOLOGY

Microdontia and Macrodontia
Accessory Cusps and Roots
Dental Transposition
Enamel Pearl
Dilaceration
Dens Invaginatus
Taurodontism
Gemination
Fusion
Concrescence
Attrition
Abrasion
Erosion
Hypercementosis

ALTERATIONS IN STRUCTURE

Dental Caries
Enamel Hypoplasia
Congenital Syphilis
Dental Fluorosis
Snow-capped Teeth
Amelogenesis Imperfecta, Hypoplastic Types
Amelogenesis Imperfecta, Hypomaturation/
   Hypocalcification Types
Syndrome-Associated Enamel Defects

Dentinogenesis Imperfecta
Dentin Dysplasia Type I
Dentin Dysplasia Type II
Regional Odontodysplasia
Hypophosphatasia
Vitamin D Refractory Rickets
Denticles and Pulp Calcification
Internal Resorption
Idiopathic External Resorption

ENLARGED PULP CHAMBERS/ROOT CANALS*

Vitamin D Refractory Rickets
Dentin Dysplasia Type II
Dentinogenesis Imperfecta, Brandywine Type
Pseudohypoparathyroidism
Regional Odontodysplasia

OBLITERATED PULP CHAMBERS/ROOT CANALS*

Dentinogenesis Imperfecta
Dentin Dysplasia Type I

ALTERATIONS IN ERUPTION/EXFOLIATION TIMES

Premature Eruption
Delayed Eruption
Impaction
Premature Exfoliation

PIGMENTATIONS

Erythroblastosis Fetalis
Biliary Atresia
Porphyria
Dental Fluorosis
Tetracycline Staining
Extrinsic Staining
Focal Pigmentation
Dental Caries*
Dentinogenesis Imperfecta*
Dentin Dysplasia Type II*
Amelogenesis Imperfecta*

---

*Refer to "Alterations in Structure" for detailed description.

The anomalies of teeth have been categorized conventionally to include defects in number, morphology, and hard tissue structure. Most dental defects are strictly local, while others are inheritable disorders associated with other anomalies of the jaws and/ or other organ systems. Most of the dental defects outlined here are familial or follow definite Mendelian patterns of inheritance. Some are associated with life-threatening diseases.

It should be noted that age predilection has

been omitted for many of the entities included in this chapter. This omission is intentional as it can be inferred that the defect makes its appearance at the time the dentition has completed development or the teeth have erupted, thereby being initially observable in children.

The most common disorders showing missing teeth are simple uncomplicated cases of hypodontia. Missing teeth are seen in incontinentia pigmenti, a potentially fatal disease of females.

Supernumerary teeth are common. Gardner's syndrome is a potentially lethal disease associated with supernumerary and impacted teeth.

Common defects in size and morphology of teeth include accessory cusps, enamel pearl, dilaceration, and dens invaginatus.

The most common anomalies in dental structure are enamel hypoplasia, snow-capped teeth and dental fluorosis. Hypophosphatasia, associated with premature exfoliation and cemental agenesis, is a potentially lethal metabolic bone disease.

Alterations in eruption and exfoliation processes are included in this chapter, as are diseases that cause the deposition of pigments either in or on dental hard tissues.

ALTERATIONS IN NUMBER: MISSING TEETH

Hypodontia

Sex: No predilection

Clinical Features: Hypodontia may involve both deciduous and permanent teeth but is far more often encountered in the latter. The third molars, any or all of them, are the most frequently observed congenitally missing teeth. The maxillary lateral incisors and second mandibular bicuspids are also frequently missing. Rarely does partial anodontia affect the mandibular lateral incisors and first molars. When deciduous teeth are involved, the maxillary lateral incisors are most often affected. When this occurs, the corresponding permanent succedaneous teeth are usually missing as well. Hypodontia shows a definite familial tendency. Occasionally, numerous congenitally missing teeth are encountered in children who received radiation to the jaws as infants for therapeutic reasons. Tooth germs are quite sensitive to radiation and low doses may arrest or cause abortion of odontogenesis.

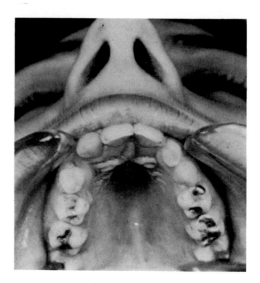

FIG. 11–1.   Partial anodontia with retention of deciduous molars.

Two specific syndromes, both of which are rare, are associated with localized hypodontia. Böök's syndrome is characterized by premature whitening of the hair, hyperhidrosis of the palms and soles, and aplasia of the premolars and third molars. It is inherited as an autosomal dominant trait. Rieger's syndrome, also an autosomal dominant hereditary disorder, shows oligodontia and microdontia associated with iridial hypoplasia and anterior synechiae; occasionally, glaucoma is a complication. Missing teeth also occur in a variety of other rare syndromes.

Treatment: When teeth are congenitally missing, the occlusion is usually defective. Orthodontic therapy may be indicated.

References

1. Dolder, E.: Deficient dentition. Dent. Res. 56:142, 1937.
2. Böök, J. A.: Clinical and genetic studies of hypodontia. I. Premolar aplasia, hyperhidrosis, and canities prematura. A new hereditary syndrome in man. Am. J. Hum. Genet. 2:240, 1950.
3. Grahnen, H. and Granath, L. E.: Numerical variations in primary dentition. Odontol. Revy 12:342, 1961.
4. Feingold, M., et al.: Rieger's syndrome. Pediatrics 44:564, 1969.
5. Chosach, A., Eidelman, E., and Cohen, T.: Hypodontia: a polygenic trait—a family study among Israeli Jews. J. Dent. Res. 54:16, 1975.

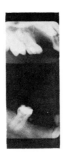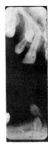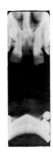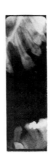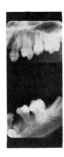

FIG. 11–2. Hypodontia with coronal defects in incontinentia pigmenti. (Courtesy of Dr. R. Gorlin.)

Incontinentia Pigmenti

Sex: Exclusively in females

Clinical Features: Incontinentia pigmenti is transmitted as an X-linked dominant trait and is lethal for males; only females with the disease survive infancy. Vesicular and erythematous skin lesions appear shortly after parturition, becoming keratotic. The characteristic lesions are diffuse reticulated slate-gray macules that cover broad areas of the skin. Skeletal, ocular, and neurologic disorders accompany the disease. White lesions may be seen on the oral mucosa. Delayed eruption, conical crown forms, and oligodontia are the chief dental anomalies seen.

Treatment: The disease cannot be treated. The dental defects may be corrected with orthodontic and prosthetic therapy.

References
1. Gorlin, R. J. and Anderson, J. A.: The characteristic dentition of incontinentia pigmenti. J. Pediatr. *57*:78, 1960.
2. Russell, D. L. and Finn, S. B.: Incontinentia pigmenti (Bloch-Sulzberger syndrome): A case report with emphasis on dental manifestations. J. Dent. Child. *34*:494, 1967.
3. Baddour, H. M., Steed, D. L., and Tilson, H. B.: Incontinentia pigmenti: report of case. J. Oral Surg. *39*:57, 1981.

Hyalinosis Cutis et Mucosae

Sex: No predilection

Clinical Features: Hyalinosis cutis et mucosae, also known as lipoid proteinosis and the Urbach-Wiethe syndrome, is inherited as an autosomal recessive disorder characterized by pathologic accumulation of glycoproteins in most bodily tissues. Hoarseness or a weak cry from infancy develops due to vocal cord infiltration. The skin develops vesicles that, after healing, appear as acneform scars with altered pigmentation; later, pale yellow nodules evolve. Multiple papules or nodules de-

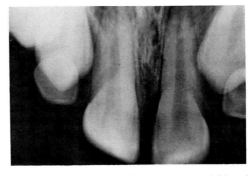

FIG. 11–3. Missing lateral incisors in a child with hyalinosis cutis et mucosae.

velop in the oral cavity, particularly on the tongue, buccal mucosa, and soft palate. Intracranial calcifications, particularly of the dorsum sellae, and seizures occur, as does decreased sensitivity to pain. Reported dental defects include hypodontia, primarily involving the maxillary lateral incisors and premolars.

Treatment: There is no known treatment for the systemic manifestations. Missing teeth may be replaced prosthetically.

References
1. Hofer, P. A.: Urbach-Wiethe disease. A review. Acta Derm. Venereol. *53* (Suppl. *71)*:5, 1971.
2. Jensen, A. D., Khodadoust, A., and Emery, J. M.: Lipoid proteinosis: report of a case with electron microscopic findings. Arch. Ophthalmol. *88*:273, 1972.
3. Finkelstein, M. W., Hammond, H. L., and Jones, R. B.: Hyalinosis cutis et mucosae. Oral Surg. *54*:49, 1982.

Mandibulo-oculo-facial Dyscephaly

Sex: No predilection

Clinical Features: The mandibulo-oculo-facial dyscephaly syndrome, also known by the eponym Hallermann-Streiff syndrome, is characterized by

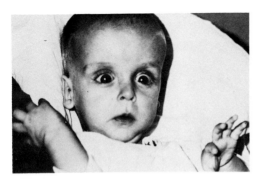

FIG. 11–4. Mandibulo-oculo-facial dyscephaly. (Courtesy of Dr. Ray Stewart.)

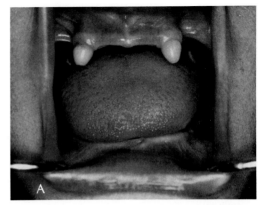

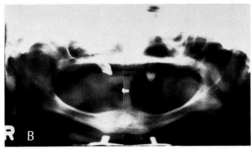

FIG. 11–5. Ectodermal dysplasia. A: Clinical photograph showing the presence of maxillary cuspids only. B: Panorex radiograph. (From Bartlett, R. C., Eversole, L. R., and Adkins, R. S.: Autosomal recessive hypohidrotic ectodermal dysplasia: Dental manifestations. Oral Surg. 33:736, 1972.)

brachycephaly with frontal bossing, small face, beak-like nose, mandibular retrognathia, temporomandibular joint anomalies, open sutures, and microphthalmia with blue sclera. Hypotrichosis with absent brows, cutaneous atrophy, spinal deformities, and mild retardation are also featured. Hypodontia is seen with retention of deciduous teeth, although supernumerary teeth can also be present. Dental malformations are also commonly encountered. The syndrome is usually sporadic.

Treatment: As long as the deciduous dentition remains sound, it can be retained. Severe caries and malocclusion, which are common in this syndrome, should be treated accordingly. The craniofacial anomalies can be treated by orthognathic and plastic surgery.

References
1. Hoefnagel, D. and Benirschke, K.: Dyscephalia mandibulo-oculo-facialis (Hallermann-Streiff syndrome). Arch. Dis. Child. 40:57, 1965.
2. Hutchinson, M. et al.: Oral manifestations of oculomandibulodyscephaly with hypotrichosis (Hallermann-Streiff syndrome). Oral Surg. 31:234, 1971.
3. Judge, C. and Chakanouskis, J. E.: The Hallermann-Streiff syndrome. J. Ment. Defic. Res. 15:115, 1971.

Hereditary Ectodermal Dysplasia

Sex: Male predilection

Clinical Features: Usually inherited as an X-linked recessive trait, ectodermal dysplasia is seen in males. One of the few inherited structural defects to show genetic heterogenicity, ectodermal dysplasia may also show an autosomal dominant form of transmission whereby females manifest the trait. Ectodermal appendages including hair, teeth, and sweat glands either fail to develop or are rudimentary. Children may be completely bald or possess lanugo hair. Heat intolerance is a common finding because of the sweat gland agenesis.

Complete anodontia is sometimes seen; however, in most cases, the cuspids are present, albeit malformed, with conical crown structure. Salivary hypoplasia with xerostomia is sometimes seen.

Treatment: In most affected children, prosthetic appliances are well tolerated; if xerostomia is severe, dentures with a soft liner may be employed. However, in some cases prostheses cannot be tolerated. Because affected children cannot stand hot humid climates, relocation to cool climates and/or air-conditioned living quarters are recommended.

References
1. Upshaw, B. Y. and Montgomery, H.: Hereditary anhidrotic ectodermal dysplasia: A clinical and pathologic study. Arch. Dermatol. Syph. 60:1170, 1949.
2. Reed, W. B., et al.: Clinical spectrum of anhidrotic ectodermal dysplasia. Arch. Dermatol. 102:134, 1970.
3. Bartlett, R. C., Eversole, L. R., and Adkins, R. S.: Autosomal recessive hypohidrotic ectodermal dysplasia: Dental manifestations. Oral Surg. 33:736, 1972.

4. Nakata, M., et al.: A genetic study of anodontia in x-linked hypohidrotic ectodermal dysplasia. Am. J. Hum. Genet. *32*:908, 1980.
5. Goepferd, S. J. and Carroll, C. E.: Hypohidrotic ectodermal dysplasia: a unique approach to esthetic and prosthetic management. J. Am. Dent. Assoc. *102*:867, 1981.

Chondroectodermal Dysplasia

Sex: No predilection

Clinical Features: Inherited as an autosomal recessive trait, the Ellis-van Creveld syndrome or chondroectodermal dysplasia represents a developmental disorder involving both epidermal and mesodermal tissues. The skin anomalies include dysplasia of the nails and hair. Sweat glands may be normal. Congenital absence of some or numerous teeth and fusion of the upper lip to the anterior maxillary alveolar ridge are noted. Eruption is often retarded. As with ectodermal dysplasia, the teeth that do form often evince conical crown forms. The mesodermal defects are most prominent in endochondral bones. The limbs are short, and polydactyly is observed on both hands and feet. These same features are typical of chondroplastic dwarfism. Congenital heart defects are present in half of the individuals affected with the syndrome. The dental anomalies are similar to those encountered in ectodermal dysplasia. Chondroplastic dwarfism in conjunction with ectodermal defects and hypodontia are the diagnostic features of chondroectodermal dysplasia.

Treatment: If their root length is adequate, the existing teeth may be utilized as abutments for either removable or fixed dental prostheses. When congenital heart disease is present and oral surgical procedures are required, prophylactic antibiotic coverage should be instituted to prevent subacute bacterial endocarditis.

References
1. McKusick, V. A., et al.: Dwarfism in the Amish. I. The Ellis-van Creveld syndrome. Bull. Hopkins Hosp. *115*:306, 1964.
2. Winter, G. B. and Geddes, M.: Oral manifestations of chondroectodermal dysplasia (Ellis-van Creveld syndrome). Report of a case. Br. Dent. J. *122*:103, 1967.
3. Biggerstaff, R. H. and Mazaheri, M.: Oral manifestations of the Ellis-van Creveld syndrome. J. Am. Dent. Assoc. *77*:1090, 1968.
4. Lynch, J. I., et al.: Congenital heart disease and chondroectodermal dysplasia. Am. J. Dis. Child. *115*:80, 1968.
5. Blackburn, M. G. and Belliveau, R. E.: Ellis-van Creveld syndrome: a report of previously undescribed anomalies in two siblings. Am. J. Dis. Child. *122*:267, 1971.

ALTERATIONS IN NUMBER: SUPERNUMERARY TEETH

Hyperdontia

Sex: No predilection

Clinical Features: Simple hyperdontia is not uncommon. The supernumerary teeth may be eumorphic but are usually heteromorphic. The most common supernumerary tooth is the mesiodens, which is formed in the midline of the maxilla, either erupted or impacted, and may occur singly or in pairs. It is heteromorphic with conical crown form. Maxillary fourth molars, also generally heteromorphic, may be located behind the third molars (distomolars), or they may erupt laterally on the buccal aspect of the normal maxillary molar dentition (paramolars). Maxillary lateral incisors, mandibular incisors, and bicuspids occasionally are supernumerary; extra cuspids are rarely encountered. Extra deciduous teeth are rare.

Treatment: Supernumerary teeth that have erupted usually are afunctional and should be extracted. Impacted supernumerary teeth may interfere with normal tooth position and can develop dentigerous cysts. For this reason, they too should be surgically extracted as soon as they are identified.

References
1. Webster, R. L.: Two cases of hereditary supernumeraries in same family. Int. J. Orthod. *13*:620, 1927.
2. Stafne, E. C.: Supernumerary teeth. Dent. Cosmos *74*:653, 1932.
3. Järvinen, S. and Lehtinen, L.: Supernumerary and congenital missing primary teeth in Finnish chil-

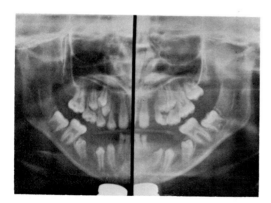

FIG. 11–6. Hypodontia in chondroectodermal dysplasia. (Courtesy of Dr. Stefan Levin.)

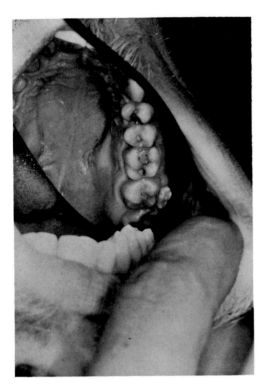

FIG. 11–7. Supernumerary fourth molar (paramolar) in the maxilla.

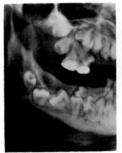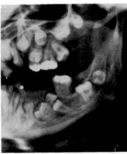

FIG. 11–8. Multiple impactions and supernumerary teeth in cleidocranial dysplasia. (Courtesy of Dr. Stefan Levin.)

dren. An epidemiologic study. Acta Odontol. Scand. *39*:83, 1981.
4. Bodin, I., Julin, P., and Thomsson,M.: Hyperodontia III. Supernumerary anterior teeth. Dentomaxillofac. Radiol. *10*:35, 1981.
5. Bodin, I., Julin, P., and Thomsson, M.: Hyperodontia IV. Supernumerary premolars. Dentomaxillofac. Radiol. *10*:99, 1981.

Cleidocranial Dysplasia

Sex: No predilection

Clinical Features: Cleidocranial dysplasia may occur sporadically or as an autosomal dominant trait. The disease affects the bones of the shoulder and craniofacial complex. The cranial fontanels remain open into adult life, the frontal eminence is prominent with bossing, and the maxillary sinuses are rudimentary. The clavicles may be absent or hypoplastic so that the patient may be able to adduct the shoulders almost to the point of touching. Other bones may show anomalous development as well. The oral manifestations are striking, particularly on dental radiographs. The deciduous teeth may show delayed exfoliation, and both dental arches are virtually filled with

unerupted permanent and supernumerary teeth. It has been suggested that the defect in eruption is linked to the absence or paucity of cementum on the permanent tooth roots.

Treatment: Deciduous tooth retention and numerous impactions provide for a monumental orthodontic problem. Removal of the deciduous teeth does not usually allow for eruption of the secondary dentition. Attempts to surgically uncover, wire, and orthodontically erupt the impacted teeth may be successful.

References
1. Miles, P. W.: Cleidocranial dysostosis: A survey of six new cases and 126 from the literature. J. Kans. Med. Soc. *41*:462, 1940.
2. Kalliala, E. and Taskinen, P. J.: Cleidocranial dysostosis; report of six typical cases and one atypical case. Oral Surg. *15*:808, 1962.
3. Douglas, B. C., and Greene, H. L.: Cleidocranial dysostosis. J. Oral Surg. *27*:41, 1969.
4. Järvinen, S.: Dental findings in three cases of cleidocranial dysostosis. Proc. Finn. Dent. Soc. *76*:56, 1980.
5. Trimble, L. D., West, R. A., and McNeill, R. W.: Cleidocranial dysplasia: comprehensive treatment of the dentofacial abnormalities. J. Am. Dent. Assoc. *105*:661, 1982.

Gardner's Syndrome

Sex: No predilection

Clinical Features: Gardner's syndrome is a complex disorder with anomalies involving a variety of tissues, the most significant of which are multiple intestinal polyps of the colon; these are premalignant and eventually evolve into adenocarcinoma. Other defects include osteomas of the facial bones, soft tissues, and sinuses; multiple epidermoid cysts of skin; fibrous (desmoid) tumors of skin; and multiple impacted permanent and supernumerary teeth. The disease is inherited as an

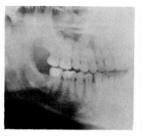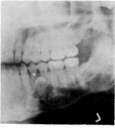

FIG. 11–9. Supernumerary teeth in Gardner's syndrome. (Courtesy of Dr. H. M. Cherrick.)

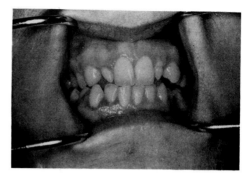

FIG. 11–10. Microdontia of the maxillary lateral incisors.

autosomal dominant trait. The osteomas are obvious on radiographs and often produce clinically demonstrable indurated swellings. The skin lesions are multiple and consist of smooth-surfaced movable nodules.

Treatment: The primary concern in Gardner's syndrome is detection of the entity so that the patient can be referred to a gastroenterologist for management of the potentially malignant intestinal polyps. The maxillofacial osteomas may require surgical removal, and orthodontic therapy may be instituted to restore the occlusion.

References

1. Duncan, B. R., Dohner, V. A., and Priest, J. H.: The Gardner syndrome: Need for early diagnosis. J. Pediatr. 72:497, 1968.
2. Rayne, J.: Gardner's syndrome. Br. J. Oral Surg. 6:11, 1968.
3. Coli, R. D., et al.: Gardner's syndrome. Am. J. Dig. Dis. 15:551, 1970.
4. Sitzmann, F. and Bruning, H.: Multiple odontome bei Garner-Syndrom. Dtsch. Zahnaerztl. Z 32:781, 1977.
5. Ida, M., Nakamura, T., and Utsanomiya, J.: Osteomatous changes and tooth abnormalities in the jaw of patients with adenomatosis coli. Oral Surg. 52:2, 1981.

ALTERATIONS IN MORPHOLOGY

Microdontia and Macrodontia

Sex: No predilection

Clinical Features: Variations in the size of teeth may be generalized, involving the entire dentition, or localized to one or a few teeth; the latter is more common. Generalized microdontia, extremely rare, is encountered among pituitary dwarfs, whereas macrodontia may be a feature of pituitary gigantism. Macrodontia restricted to half the teeth in unilateral distribution is a feature of facial hemihypertrophy. Localized microdontia most often affects the maxillary lateral incisors,

with formation of conical crown forms. The disorder is usually familial. Third molars are commonly small and malformed as well. Localized macrodontia is less often observed than microdontia. The incisors are most commonly affected, but geminated or fused teeth may show features that could be confused with true macrodontia.

Treatment: Microdontia and macrodontia of a localized nature are usually of no consequence. Orthodontics may be required if an arch length problem develops. Crown and bridge prosthodontic reconstruction may be employed to achieve an esthetic appearance.

References

1. Bowden, D. E. and Goose, D. H.: Inheritance of tooth size in Liverpool families. J. Med. Genet. 6:55, 1969.
2. Baum, B. J. and Cohen, M. M.: Patterns of size reduction in hypodontia. J. Dent. Res. 50:779, 1971.
3. Shafer, W. G., Hine, M. L., and Levy, B. M.: A Textbook of Oral Pathology, 4th ed. Philadelphia, W. B. Saunders Co., 1983, pp. 37–38.
4. Burke, R. S.: Megadontism and partial gemination. Oral Surg. 42:703, 1976.
5. Ruprecht, A. and Singer, D. L.: Macrodontia of the mandibular left first premolar. Oral. Surg. 48:573, 1979.
6. Hayward, J. R.: Cuspid gigantism. Oral Surg. 49:500, 1980.

Accessory Cusps and Roots

Sex: No predilection

Clinical Features: Accessory cusps are commonly encountered on the lingual surface of maxillary first molars as the so-called cusps of Carabelli. Indeed, rudimentary forms may affect as many as 90 percent of all such teeth in Caucasians, although they are extremely rare among Eskimos and Asians. Buccal accessory cusps are occasion-

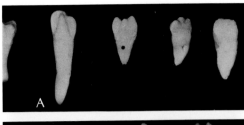

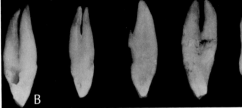

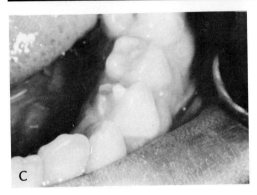

FIG. 11–11. *A:* Accessory cusps on cuspid and premolar teeth. *B:* Accessory roots. *C:* Dens evaginatus.

ally encountered on both molars and premolars. Dens evaginatus represents an accessory cusp emanating occlusally from the central groove of premolars and molars. This anomaly is rare and is most often encountered among Eskimos. A pulp horn may extend into this central occlusal cusp. Excluding the cusp of Carabelli, the most common accessory cusp represents an anomalously enlarged lingual tubercle on an incisor. Accessory roots are most frequently seen on maxillary molar teeth, secondly on mandibular molars. Premolars and maxillary cuspids and incisors may have accessory or appendicial roots; however, mandibular cuspid or incisor accessory roots are extremely rare.

Treatment: Accessory cusps are rarely in occlusion so that no treatment is required unless, in the case of buccal accessory cusps, periodontal pocket formation is encountered. In this case, tooth reduction and placement of a restoration to avoid exposure of dentin are recommended. Dens evaginatus may pose a problem, as the cusps are in occlusion. It must be remembered that pulp horns extend into these areas. A knowledge of the existence of accessory roots is significant when endodontic therapy is required.

References

1. Kraus, B. X.: Carabelli's anomaly of the maxillary molar teeth. Am. J. Hum. Genet. *3:*348, 1951.
2. Lau, I. C.: Odontomes of the axial core type. Br. Dent. J. *99:*219, 1955.
3. Dehlers, F. A. C., Lee, K. W., and Lee, E. C.: Dens evaginatus (evaginated odontome). Dent. Pract. *17:*239, 1967.
4. Krolls, S. O. and Donalhue, A. H.: Double-rooted maxillary primary canines. Oral Surg. *49:*379, 1980.
5. Speiser, A. M. and Bikofsky, V. M.: Premolars with double occlusal surfaces. J. Am. Dent. Assoc. *103:*600, 1981.

Dental Transposition

Sex: No predilection

Clinical Features: Teeth may erupt into inappropriate positions. A second premolar may be interposed between a first and second molar, or a cuspid may erupt into position between the premolars. Although rare, a tooth may erupt into the opposite quadrant. Many examples of so-called "transposition" are instances of supernumerary teeth, particularly in the molar region. These supernumerary molars are small and malformed and often show occlusal anatomy analogous to premolars. Data regarding any genetic tendency for true transposition are insufficient.

Treatment: If crowding and malocclusion are not significant, no treatment is required. Otherwise, extraction and/or orthodontic therapy may be indicated.

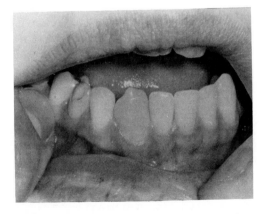

FIG. 11–12.   Transposition of lateral incisor and canine.

References

1. Raphael, D. M.: Transposed supernumerary premolars. Oral Surg. 46:598, 1978.
2. Patel, J. R.: Transposed and submerged teeth. Oral Surg. 46:599, 1978.
3. Abbott, D. M., Svirsky, J. A., and Yarborough, B. H.: Transposition of the permanent mandibular canine. Oral Surg. 49:97, 1980.
4. Winter, A. A.: Pseudotranspositioning. Oral Surg. 49:188, 1980.

Enamel Pearl

Sex: No predilection

Clinical Features: Enamel pearls or droplets are white dome-shaped calcific concretions of enamel, usually located at the furcation areas of molar teeth. Maxillary molars are most often affected. Encountered fairly frequently, enamel pearls probably represent a histologic abnormality occurring in Hertwig's sheath: The sheath epithelium retains ameloblastic potential in a focal area so that a nodule of enamel forms in place of cementum. Occasionally, a dentin core extends into the enamel-surfaced excresence.

Treatment: Treatment is necessary only when periodontal disease involves a furcation area with an enamel pearl. Since the region is difficult to maintain in a hygienic state, the pearl should be removed with dental burrs or stones.

References

1. Turner, J. G.: A note on enamel nodules. Br. Dent. J. 78:39, 1945.
2. Cavanha, A. O.: Enamel pearls. Oral Surg. 19:373, 1965.

Dilaceration

Sex: No predilection

Clinical Features: Dilaceration refers to a defect in root development whereby a bend or curve develops. This flaw, which is not the result of a true laceration of Hertwig's sheath, probably evolves subsequent to trauma or some defect in development that alters the angulation of the tooth germ during root formation. The angulation may occur at any location along the root. Any tooth,

deciduous or permanent, may show this anomaly. Dilaceration of the coronal portion of the tooth has also been reported.

Treatment: No treatment is required. When extraction or endodontic therapy is necessary, a knowledge of this defect and its identification on dental radiographs will aid in circumventing complications that could occur when these procedures are performed on such anomalous teeth.

References

1. Schulze, C.: In *Thoma's Oral Pathology,* 6th Ed., edited by R. J. Gorlin and H. M. Goldman. St. Louis, C. V. Mosby Co., 1970, Vol. I, pp.105–106.
2. Shafer, W. G., Hine, M. K., and Levy, B. M.: *A Textbook of Oral Pathology,* 4th Ed. Philadelphia, W. B. Saunders Co., 1975.
3. Rengaswamy, V.: Bilateral dilaceration of maxillary central incisors. Oral Surg. 47:200, 1979.
4. Ligh, R. A.: Coronal dilaceration. Oral Surg. 51:567, 1981.

Dens Invaginatus (Dens in Dente)

Sex: No predilection

Clinical Features: Dens invaginatus represents a defect in morphologic development whereby the coronal enamel and dentin become inverted into the pulp chamber. The defect, which is generally localized to a single tooth, occasionally involves multiple teeth and frequently involves the same tooth bilaterally. The coronal invagination may be limited to the crown region, or it may extend deeply into the radicular pulp. The defect is most often encountered in the maxillary lateral incisor and in mesiodens. Clinically, the incisor may manifest only an enlarged lingual pit. The defect is easily demonstrated radiographically as an invaginated radiopaque ribbon-like enamel structure, giving the impression of a small tooth within the coronal pulp cavity. The invaginated core is patent; food debris with accompanying microorganisms enter this canal, predisposing the affected tooth to caries, pulp infection, and periapical disease.

Treatment: When dens invaginatus is encountered shortly after eruption, prophylactic restoration of the invaginated channel is recommended to prevent pulpal necrosis.

References

1. Shafer, W. G.: Dens in dente. NY Dent. J. 19:220, 1953.
2. Poyton, H. G. and Morgan, G. A.: Dens in dente. Dent. Radiogr. Photogr. 39:27, 1966.
3. Conklin, W. W.: Bilateral dens invaginatus in the mandibular incisor region. Oral Surg. 45:905, 1978.

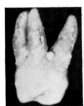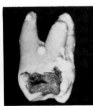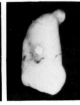

FIG. 11–13. Molar teeth with enamel pearls.

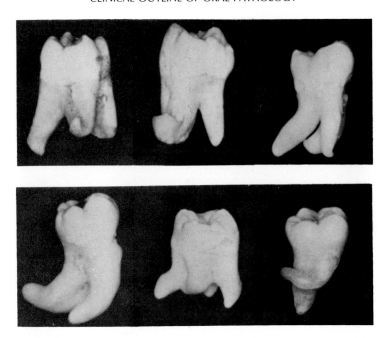

FIG. 11–14.   Dilaceration of roots.

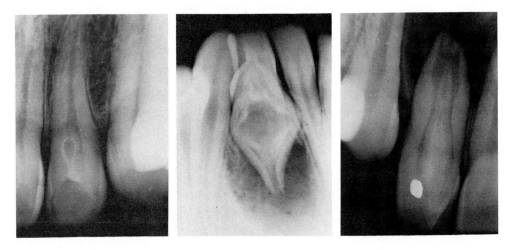

FIG. 11–15.   Dens invaginatus.

4. Burton, D. J., Saffos, R. O., and Scheffer, R. B.: Multiple bilateral dens in dente as a factor in the etiology of multiple periapical lesions. Oral Surg. 49:496, 1980.

Taurodontism

Sex: No predilection

Clinical Features: Taurodontism means *bull teeth;* the term is appropriate because this human dental defect involves a markedly elongated pulp chamber with rudimentary root formation mim- icking, to some extent, the normal morphology of the ungulate dentition. The defect is observable only in dental radiographs, there being no clini- cally obvious malformation. Molars are affected and give the appearance of having been "stretched," with the root furcation occurring at the apical third. One or more molars may show this change. Taurodonts may be encountered in patients suffering from various developmental craniofacial deformities. Specifically, in the tri- chodento-osseous syndrome, hypoplastic-hypo-

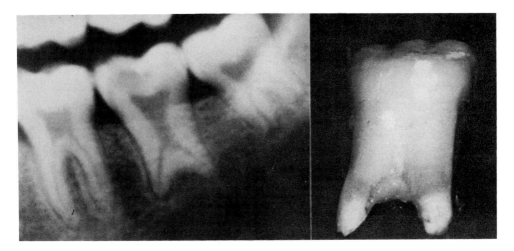

FIG. 11–16. Taurodontism.

calcified amelogenesis imperfecta, kinky hair, and cortical osteosclerosis are seen along with taurodontism. Interestingly, similar dental morphology has been encountered among fossil hominoids, particularly the Neanderthals.

Treatment: No treatment is required. The enlarged pulp chamber is of significance when endodontic therapy is required.

References

1. Mangion, J. J.: Two cases of taurodontism in modern human jaws. Br. Dent. J. *113*:309, 1962.
2. Hamner, J. E., III, Witkop, C. J., and Metro, P. S.: Taurodontism. Report of a case. Oral Surg. *18*:409, 1964.
3. Crawford, J. L.: Concomitant taurodontism and amelogenesis imperfecta in the American Caucasian. J. Dent. Child. *37*:83, 1970.
4. Holt, R. D. and Brook, A. H.: Taurodontism: a criterion for diagnosis and its prevalence in mandibular first permanent molars in a sample of 1,115 British school children. J. Int. Assoc. Dent. Child. *10*:41, 1979.
5. Milazzo, A. and Alexander, S. A.: Fusion, gemination, oligodontia and taurodontism. J. Pedod. 6:194, 1982.

Gemination

Sex: No predilection

Clinical Features: Gemination is the result of either schizodontism, the splitting of a tooth germ during development, or synodontism, the fusion of a normal tooth bud with one from a developing supernumerary tooth. Both forms represent abortive attempts at forming supernumerary buds. The deciduous mandibular incisors and permanent maxillary incisors are most often affected. Gemi-

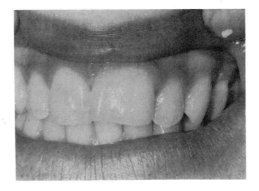

FIG. 11–17. Gemination.

nation may be distinguished from fusion by the fact that the full complement of teeth is present in the former whereas a tooth is missing in the latter. Geminate teeth usually show doubling of both the crown and root. The crown may be excessively widened or may actually show an indentation or groove delineating the two crown forms. A hereditary pattern is sometimes evident.

Treatment: Gemination of anterior teeth represents a prosthetic challenge. Depending upon the morphologic character of the defect, a fixed anterior bridge may be constructed, utilizing the anomalous tooth as an abutment. Alternatively, to ensure an adequate esthetic result, the affected teeth may have to be extracted and the cuspids utilized as abutments.

References

1. Clayton, J. M.: Congenital dental anomalies occurring in 3,557 children. J. Dent. Child. *23*:206, 1956.

2. Tannenbaum, K. A. and Alling, E. E.: Anomalous tooth development. Oral Surg. *16*:883, 1963.
3. Levitas, T. C.: Gemination, fusion, twinning and concrescence. J. Dent. Child. *32*:93, 1965.
4. Hitchin, A. D. and Morris, L.: Geminated odontome. J. Dent. Res. *45*:575, 1966.
5. Svirsky, J. A.: Bilateral gemination. Oral Surg. *47*:300, 1979.

Fusion

Sex: No predilection

Clinical Features: Fusion represents a junction at the level of dentin between juxtaposed normal tooth germs, so that one enlarged anomalous crown form exists in place of two normal teeth. A single enlarged root or two roots are observed. A hereditary pattern is often encountered. Either deciduous or permanent teeth can be affected; however, the anomaly has been reported to be more common in deciduous teeth. In both dentitions, the incisors are most often affected.

Treatment: Depending upon the morphologic features of the fused teeth, a fixed prosthetic appliance may include the anomalous tooth as an abutment, or the tooth may be extracted with subsequent bridge fabrication to achieve optimal esthetics.

References
1. Moody, E. and Montgomery, L. B.: Hereditary tendencies in tooth formation. J. Am. Dent. Assoc. *21*:1774, 1934.
2. Clayton, J. M.: Congenital dental anomalies occurring in 3,557 children. J. Dent. Child. *23*:206, 1956.
3. Saito, T.: A genetic study on the degenerative anomalies of deciduous teeth. Jpn. J. Hum. Genet. *4*:27, 1959.
4. Eidelman, E.: Fusion of maxillary primary central and lateral incisors bilaterally. Pediatr. Dent. *3*:346, 1981.
5. Delany, G. M. and Goldblatt, L. I.: Fused teeth: a

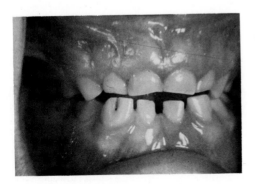

FIG. 11–18.   Fusion of deciduous lateral incisor and canine. (Courtesy of Dr. R. Adams.)

multidisciplinary approach to treatment. J. Am. Dent. Assoc. *103*:732, 1981.

Concrescence

Sex: No predilection

Clinical Features: Concrescence represents union between juxtaposed teeth at the level of the cementum; there is no interdental combination. The maxillary molars are usually affected by this developmental abnormality. Confluency of cementum between adjacent teeth may occur with two normal molars, yet is perhaps more often en-

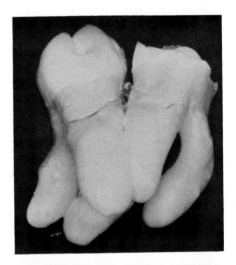

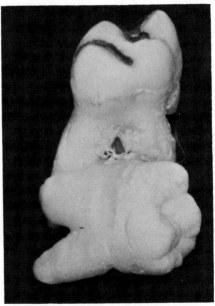

FIG. 11–19.   Concrescence in molar teeth.

countered between a normal molar and a supernumerary molar (i.e., paramolar, distomolar). Concrescence may occur in both impacted and erupted teeth.

Treatment: Concrescent teeth are either in malocclusion or impacted, usually necessitating extraction. If such a condition is suspected from radiographic features, care during extraction is necessary, particularly to avoid fracturing excessive amounts of alveolar bone.

References

1. Schulze, C.: In *Thoma's Oral Pathology*, 6th Ed., edited by R. J. Gorlin and H. M. Goldman. St. Louis, C. V. Mosby Co., 1970, Vol. 1, p. 121.
2. Levitas, T. C.: Gemination, fusion, twinning and concrescence. J. Dent. Child. *32*:93, 1965.

Attrition

Age: Adults, particularly the elderly
Sex: No predilection

Clinical Features: Attrition represents the physiologic loss of tooth structure. The pattern of loss is characteristic in that the enamel and dentin become abraded on their occlusal and incisal surfaces in a generalized fashion. The process is related to diet, and is seen in individuals who partake of a food such as maize or use their teeth in the preparation of hides. It is therefore common among older American Indians and Eskimos. Tooth wear has been correlated with erosive degenerative changes in the temporomandibular joint among aboriginals. It may be difficult to differentiate between attrition and bruxism with abrasion by noting only the pattern of tooth wear.

Treatment: No treatment is required as secondary dentin proceeds at a rate commensurate with the attritional wear. When the crowns are worn down to the gingival margin, an overdenture may be constructed to improve function.

References

1. Sicher, H.: The biology of attrition. Oral Surg. 6:406, 1953.
2. Davies, G. N.: Social customs and their effect on oral diseases. J. Dent. Res. 42:209, 1963.
3. Richards, L. C. and Brown, T.: Dental attrition and degenerative arthritis of the temporomandibular joint. J. Oral Rehabil. 8:293, 1981.
4. Goldman, H. M.: An atlas of acquired dental defects. Compend. Cont. Educ. Dent. 3:275, 1982.

Abrasion

Age: Adults
Sex: No predilection

Clinical Features: Abrasion represents the pathologic wear of tooth structure. The location of tooth structure loss is in keeping with the nature of the etiology or habit responsible for excessive abrasion. Notching of incisors is seen in hairdressers who hold bobby pins between their teeth; grooving of both maxillary and mandibular incisors is observed in pipe smokers; cervical abrasion occurs in individuals who brush excessively in a horizontal plane. In the last instance, pulp exposure may ensue. Isolated foci of abrasion are observed in patients with occlusal prematurities appearing as cuspal wear facets. A common occlusal anomaly leading to widespread abrasion occurs in patients who show incisal guided protrusive movement. The incisal portion of the mandibular incisors shows abrasion, as do the incisal and lingual surfaces of the maxillary incisors and cuspids. It is important to recognize that abrasion

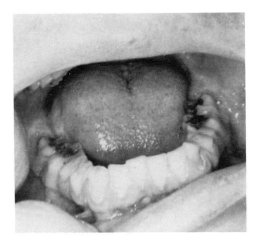

FIG. 11–20. Physiologic tooth wear or attrition.

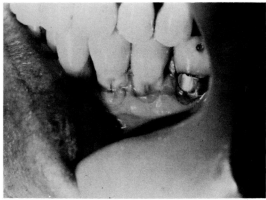

FIG. 11–21. Pathologic tooth wear or abrasion resulting from overzealous brushing.

related to occlusal disharmony may be associated with advancing periodontal disease about the affected teeth. Patients with bruxism display generalized abrasion that mimics physiologic attrition in its distribution.

Treatment: Limited forms of abrasion require elimination of the incriminating habit and restoration of normal tooth contour if function or esthetics is a problem. Abrasion related to malocclusion may require occlusal rehabilitation and a complete periodontal evaluation. Nightguard appliances may limit abrasion in patients with bruxism.

References

1. Ervin, J. C. and Bucher, E. M.: Prevalence of tooth root exposure and abrasion among dental patients. Dent. Items Interest 66:760, 1944.
2. Smith, J. F.: Pathological wear of the teeth. SC Dent. J. 20:9, 1962.
3. Harrington, J. H. and Terry, I. A.: Automatic and hard tooth brushing abrasion studies. J. Am. Dent. Assoc. 68:343, 1964.
4. Goldman, H. M.: An atlas of acquired dental defects. Compend. Cont. Educ. Dent. 3:275, 1982.

Erosion

Age: Adult predilection

Sex: No predilection

Clinical Features: Erosion represents the demineralization of tooth structure as a result of chemical action, usually that of acidic compounds. While a definite history of oral contact with acids can be elicited in most instances, occasionally a cause is not readily apparent. The more common agents associated with erosion are chronic vomiting, habitual carbonic acid intake from cola or soft drinks, or habitual contact with citric acid as in lemon sucking. When vomiting is the cause, a smooth homogeneous loss of enamel with exposure of dentin is observed on the lingual surfaces. Both facial and lingual loss of surface tooth structure can be seen in persons who imbibe acidic fruits or beverages. Idiopathic erosion occurs on the cervical and middle thirds of the incisors, cuspids, and bicuspids as a smooth cupped-out depression.

Treatment: Areas of erosion may be sensitive and should be restored with conventional operative procedures.

References

1. Shulman, E. and Robinson, G. B. G.: Salivary citrate content and erosion of teeth. J. Dent. Res. 27:541, 1948.
2. Allan, D. N.: Enamel erosion with lemon juice. Br. Dent. J. 122:300, 1967.

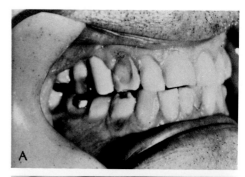

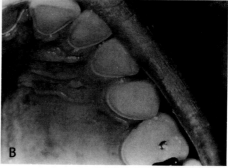

FIG. 11–22   A: Idiopathic erosion of facial enamel. B: Lingual erosion in anorexia nervosa with chronic vomiting.

3. House, R. C., et al.: Perimolysis: unveiling the surreptitious vomiter. Oral Surg. 51:152, 1981.
4. Andrews, F. F.: Dental erosion due to anorexia nervosa with bulimia. Br. Dent. J. 152:89, 1982.
5. Stege, P., Visco-Dangler, L., and Rye, L.: Anorexia nervosa: review including oral and dental manifestations. J. Am. Dent. Assoc. 104:648, 1982.

Hypercementosis

Age: Middle-aged and elderly adults

Sex: No predilection

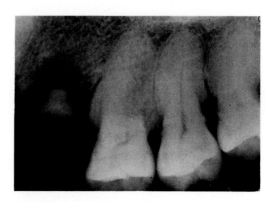

FIG. 11–23. Hypercementosis.

Clinical Features: Excessive deposition of secondary cementum may develop on one tooth or may be generalized. Generally no cause can be found; occasionally, contributing factors can be detected (periapical inflammation and hypofunction as seen when an opposing tooth is missing). Pain is not a feature. The roots show laminated layers of secondary cementum, usually of the lamellar type, which is most extensive in the apical third of the root. The radiographic features are characteristic, showing bulbous enlarged roots. Generalized hypercementosis is seen in conjunction with a ground-glass- or cotton-wool-appearing alveolar bone in osteitis deformans. A serum alkaline phosphatase assay is helpful.

Treatment: No treatment is required. Extraction of teeth with hypercementosis may require sectioning to facilitate removal.

References

1. Gardner, B. S. and Goldstein, H.: The significance of hypercementosis. Dent. Cosmos *73*:1065, 1931.
2. Weinberger, A.: The clinical significance of hypercementosis. Oral Surg. *7*:79, 1954.
3. Malkin, M.: Hypercementosis: report of an unusual case. NY State Dent. J. *27*:32, 1961.
4. Humerfelt, A. and Reitan, K.: Effects of hypercementosis on the movability of teeth during orthodontic treatment. Angle Orthodont. 6:179, 1966.
5. Lumerman, H. and Tamagna, J. A.: Hypercementosis. Oral Surg. *24*:208, 1967.

ALTERATIONS IN STRUCTURE

Dental Caries

Sex: No predilection

Clinical Features: Dental caries represents the most common disease to affect the teeth. Most evidence supports a bacterial etiology whereby teeth accumulate material known as plaque which provides a carbohydrate substrate for acid-producing bacteria, primarily Streptococcus mutans. Acid generation induces a chemical demineralization of hydroxyapatite crystals in the enamel. When the enamel has been penetrated other microorganisms gain access to the protoplasm of the dentinal tubules, and the carious process proceeds pulpally. Once the pulp has been invaded by bacteria, inflammation ensues; ultimately, necrosis with spread of infection occurs through the apical foramen or accessory root canals. In children, pits and fissures are the most common sites along with interproximal areas. Clinically, pit and fissure caries is characterized by either a chalky appearance or a brown discoloration. A sharp dental explorer can be forced into a carious fissure or pit and will

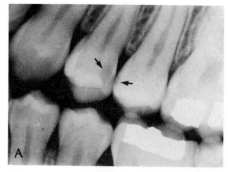
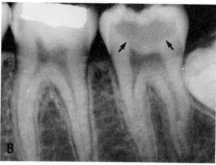

FIG. 11–24.   Radiographs depicting dental caries. *A*: Proximal caries on premolars. *B*: Occlusal caries on second molar.

be retained, requiring somewhat forceful removal. Interproximal caries can often be detected as pits or irregularities upon instrument exploration; however, bite-wing radiographs are the major diagnostic aid. Immediately below the point of tooth-to-tooth contact, a funnel-shaped radiolucency can be detected with its apex directed toward the dentin. Dentinal caries also appears triangular and undermines the overlying intact enamel. Cervical caries on the facial or buccal gingival one-third of the crown is more frequently encountered among adults. It may involve cementum and extend below the marginal gingiva. Cervical caries begins as white opaque areas that become discolored brown or yellow-brown. Severe or rampant caries occurs in children who eat excessive amounts of candy and other sweets. In adults, severe caries occurs in xerostomia secondary to the Sjögren syndrome or following radiation therapy for head and neck cancer.

Treatment: All carious enamel and dentin must be removed prior to restoration with amalgam, cast gold, or resin materials. Pit and fissure sealants effectively prevent dental decay among children. Patients with xerostomia due to immunopathic sialadenitis or radiation should be treated with daily fluoride gel.

References

1. Losee, F. L.: Dental caries in abutting or bilaterally corresponding tooth surfaces. J. Am. Dent. Assoc. 35:323, 1947.
2. Savara, B. S. and Suher, T.: Study of dental caries in children 1 to 6 years of age as related to socio-economic level and food habits. J. Dent. Res. 32:680, 1953.
3. Darling, A. I.: The pathology and prevention of caries. Brit. Dent. J. 107:287, 1959.
4. Backer-Dirks, O.: Longitudinal dental caries in children 9–15 years of age. Arch. Oral Biol. 6:94, 1961.
5. Frank, R. M., et al.: Acquired dental defects and salivary gland lesions after irradiation for carcinoma. J. Am. Dent. Assoc. 70:868, 1965.

Enamel Hypoplasia

Sex: No predilection

Clinical Features: Damage to ameloblasts during odontogenesis, if severe, will result in defective enamel formation. A variety of infectious, nutritional, chemical, and traumatic factors play a role. (Because of their unique characters, congenital syphilis and dental fluorosis are considered separately.) Perhaps the most common form of enamel hypoplasia is seen in isolated permanent teeth, whereby caries with periapical spread of infection or trauma to a deciduous tooth results in damage to ameloblasts forming the crown of the subjacent developing permanent tooth. The affected tooth, so-called Turner's tooth, is yellow or brown, and the enamel surface is pitted or chalky. Occasionally, many teeth show pitting or rough, poorly calcified enamel matrices. In these instances, one of the childhood infectious diseases

associated with prolonged elevated temperature may have resulted in ameloblastic injury, in which case only that portion of the teeth under development at the time of infection manifests hypoplastic changes. Enamel hypoplasia with a similar distribution as that seen with febrile childhood infections may occur in rickets, congenital hypoparathyroidism, and birth injuries.

Treatment: When the pulp chambers have receded to an appropriate level, permanent restorations may be fabricated. In the interim, resin restorative materials may be periodically placed to achieve a desirable esthetic appearance.

References

1. Shelling, D. H. and Anderson, G. M.: Relation of rickets and Vitamin D to the incidence of dental caries, enamel hypoplasia and malocclusion in children. J. Am. Dent. Assoc. 23:840, 1936.
2. Via, W. F., Jr.: Enamel defects induced by trauma during tooth formation. J. Oral Surg. 25:49, 1968.
3. Morningstar, C. H.: Effect of infection of deciduous molar on the permanent tooth germ. J. Am. Dent. Assoc. 24:786, 1937.
4. Porteous, J. R.: Appearance of chronologic hypoplasia. Oral Surg. 48:282, 1979.

Congenital Syphilis

Sex: No predilection

Clinical Features: Congenital syphilis is contracted in utero from a mother who has active treponemal infection. The clinical manifestations are protean, as the infection may involve virtually any tissue or organ, particularly bone, tooth, and nerve. Saber shins, rhagedes, frontal bossing, and saddle nose are common structural anomalies. Hutchinson's triad consists of blindness, deafness, and dental anomalies. The classic dental changes involve the maxillary incisors and first permanent molars. The central incisors are notched, the laterals are peg shaped, and the molars manifest a crumpled, discolored occlusal surface (so-called mulberry molars). Not all patients manifest all components of Hutchinson's triad, nor do they all

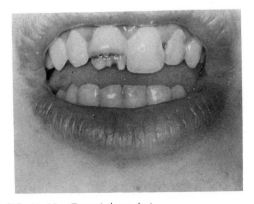

FIG. 11–25.   Turner's hypoplasia.

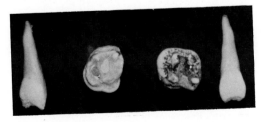

FIG. 11–26.   "Screwdriver" centrals and "mulberry" molars in congenital syphilis.

show the three dental anomalies together. The fact that children with congenital syphilis may continue to carry spirochetes, may be infectious, and may show any of the signs of acquired syphilis is extremely important .

Treatment: Children should be referred to a pediatrician to determine whether or not active disease persists. The anomalous teeth may be restored by the usual operative procedures.

References

1. Brauer, J. C. and Blackstone, C. H.: Dental aspects of congenital syphilis. J. Am. Dent. Assoc. *28*:1633, 1941.
2. Sarnat, B. G. and Shaw, N. G.: Dental development in congenital syphilis. Am. J. Orthodont. (Oral Surg. Sect.) *29*:270, 1943.
3. Putkonen, T.: Dental changes in congenital syphilis. Acta Derm. Venerol. *42*:44, 1962.
4. Fiumara, N. J. and Lessell, S.: Manifestations of late congenital syphilis. Arch. Dermatol. *102*:78, 1970.

Dental Fluorosis

Sex: No predilection

Clinical Features: When fluoride levels in the drinking water exceed one part per million, mottling of enamel may occur. Certain regions of the world have natural drinking water supplies in which the fluoride content is extremely high. Fluoride in concentrated levels is toxic to ameloblasts; during amelogenesis cell damage will lead to defective enamel formation. The affected teeth, deciduous or permanent, will vary considerably regarding the extent of hypoplasia. The surface may be chalky, opaque, and flecked or the enamel may show extensive flaking, fracturing, and brown or black pigmentation. The condition is generalized, affecting all teeth exposed to excess fluoride during development.

Treatment: No treatment can remineralize the defective surface. Temporary resin restorations should be employed during childhood, and full-coverage fixed prostheses can be fabricated after the pulp chamber has sufficiently receded. Treatment is elective because the teeth are not any more susceptible to decay than the normal dentition.

References

1. Black, G. V. and McKay, F. A.: Mottled teeth: An endemic developmental imperfection of the enamel of teeth heretofore unknown in the literature of dentistry. Dent. Cosmos *58*:129, 1916.
2. Dean, H. T.: Chronic endemic fluorosis. J. Am. Med. Assoc. *107*:1269, 1936.
3. Dean, H. T. and Arnold, F. A.: Endemic dental fluorosis or mottled teeth. J. Am. Dent. Assoc. *30*:1278, 1943.
4. McClure, F. S. and Lipkins, R. C.: Fluorine in human teeth studied in relation to fluorine in the drinking water. J. Dent. Res. *30*:172, 1951.

Snow-capped Teeth

Sex: No predilection

Clinical Features: This autosomal dominantly inherited disorder is relatively common. The incisors, cuspids, and occasionally even posterior teeth manifest a white chalky-appearing opaque discoloration of the incisal and occlusal third of the crown. This opacified region of the enamel reflects an anomaly of mineralization; however, the involved hard tissue is neither structurally weakened nor more susceptible than normal tooth structure to caries. Recently, a rare X-linked form of snow-capped teeth has been described and has been classified as a form of amelogenesis imperfecta, hypomaturation type. This form resembles the common variety in that the incisal one-third

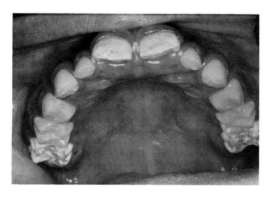

FIG. 11–27. Fluorosis prior to age one with hypoplastic enamel of incisors and molars. (Courtesy of Drs. R. Abrams and R. Sobel.)

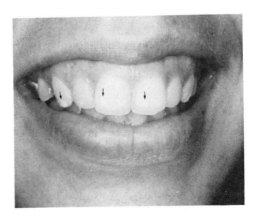

FIG. 11–28. Opaque regions on incisal one-third of maxillary central incisors and cuspids representing snow-capped teeth.

of the teeth exhibit an opaque appearance; it differs in that a brownish discoloration also is observed. Scanning electron microscopic studies indicate a structural defect in the outer prismless enamel layer.

Treatment: No treatment is required.

References

1. Witkop, C. J., Jr.: Snow-capped teeth (marker). In *Birth Defects Atlas and Compendium*, The National Foundation, edited by D. Bergsma. Baltimore, Williams and Wilkins, 1973, p. 812, entry 743.
2. Witkop, C. J., Jr.: Heterogeneity in inherited dental tracts, gingival fibromatosis and amelogenesis imperfecta. South. Med. J. *64*(Suppl. 1):16, 1971.
3. Winter, G. B. and Brook, A. H.: Enamel hypoplasia and anomalies of the enamel. Dent. Clin. North Am. *19*:3–24, 1975.
4. Witkop, C. J., Jr. and Sauk, J. J., Jr.: Heritable defects of enamel. In *Oral Facial Genetics*, edited by R. E. Stewart and G. H. Prescott. St. Louis., C. V. Mosby Co., 1976, pp. 187–188.
5. Escobar, V. H., Goldblatt, L. I., and Bixler, D.: A clinical, genetic and ultrastructural study of snow-capped teeth: Amelogenesis imperfecta, hypomaturation type. Oral Surg. *52*:607, 1981.

Amelogenesis Imperfecta, Hypoplastic Types

Sex: Predilection varies according to mode of inheritance.

Clinical Features: Two major forms of amelogenesis imperfecta (AI) exist; the hypoplastic types exhibit a deficient amount of surface enamel while the hypomaturation forms show adequate enamel thickness with defective mineralization. This subdivision is often confusing because both hypoplastic and hypomineralized enamel may coexist. The hypoplastic forms have been subcategorized according to clinical, microscopic, and genetic features. This group has the following general features: The enamel is thin, teeth fail to evince mesiodistal contacts, and pitting or fissuring, either horizontal or vertical, occurs. The *autosomal dominant pitted hypoplastic variety* affects both primary and secondary dentitions that manifest multiple pinpoint pits randomly distributed over the crowns. *Autosomal dominant local hypoplastic AI* is characterized by horizontal rows of pits located on the middle one-third of the crown; the immediately adjacent enamel is hypocalcified, and the occlusal third is usually unaffected. The *autosomal dominant smooth hypoplastic form* is devoid of pits, being smooth and approximately one-fourth normal thickness; clinically, newly erupted teeth are yellow and later appear opaque white or slightly brown. Radiographically, the

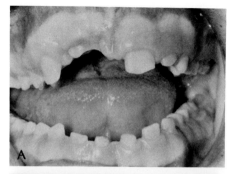
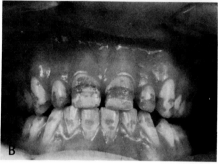

FIG. 11–29. *A*: Amelogenesis imperfecta, smooth hypoplastic type. *B*: Amelogenesis imperfecta, local hypoplastic type showing midcoronal pitting.

teeth may appear to be devoid of enamel. The *autosomal dominant rough hypoplastic form* is represented by hard granular white or yellow-white enamel, one-fourth normal thickness, that chips away from the underlying dentin. There is some degree of incisal flare. Radiographically, the enamel layer is readily identified yet extremely thin. In contrast, the *autosomal recessive rough hypoplastic type* is nearly devoid of enamel and is also termed enamel agenesis. The surface exhibits a granular, ground-glass appearance and a yellow discoloration. Impaction with resorption is frequently witnessed. Last, *X-linked dominant smooth hypoplastic AI* varies according to sex. Hemizygous males show smooth yellowish-brown thin enamel with marked abrasion; a thin opaque enamel capping is observed radiographically. Female heterozygotes show vertically banded fissures, alternating with enamel striations of normal thickness (Lyonization effect). These vertical stria are radiographically evident. In all forms of amelogenesis imperfecta, there is a tendency for development of anterior open bite.

Treatment: Full crown prostheses are recommended for esthetic reasons and to eliminate sensitivity. Dentitions affected by amelogenesis imperfecta are not inherently caries prone.

References

1. Weinman, J. P., Svoboda, J. R., and Woods, R. W.: Disturbances of enamel formation and calcification. J. Am. Dent. Assoc. *32*:397, 1945.
2. Darling, A. I.: Some observations on amelogenesis imperfecta and calcification of the dental enamel. Proc. R. Soc. Med. *49*:759, 1956.
3. Witkop, C. J., Jr. and Rao, S.: Inherited defects of tooth structure. D. Bergsma, ed.: Orofacial Structures., Birth Defects *11*:153, 1971.
4. Witkop, C. J., Jr., and Sauk, J. J., Jr.: Heritable defects of enamel. In *Oral Facial Genetics*, edited by R. E. Stewart and G. H. Prescott. St. Louis. C. V. Mosby Co., 1976, pp.151–226.
5. Winter, G. B. and Brooks, A. H.: Enamel hypoplasia and anomalies of the enamel. A. E. Poole, ed.: Symposium on Genetics. Dent. Clin. North Am. *19*:3, 1975.

Amelogenesis Imperfecta, Hypomaturation/Hypocalcification Types

Sex: Predilection varies according to mode of inheritance.

Clinical Features: Hypomaturation and hypocalcification forms of amelogenesis imperfecta (AI)

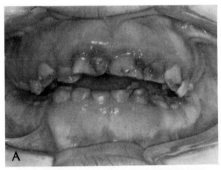

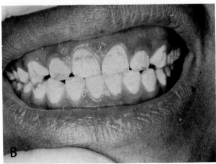

FIG. 11–30. *A*: Amelogenesis imperfecta, pigmented hypomaturation type. *B*: Amelogenesis imperfecta, hypocalcified type.

exhibit normal enamel thickness with mesiodistal contacts, yet are poorly mineralized, mottled, discolored, and tend to show chipping of enamel away from the dentin. The hypocalcified enamel is no more radiodense than dentin. *Autosomal dominant hypocalcified AI* is the most common form, occurring once in every 20,000 births. The enamel is normal in thickness yet is soft, cheesy, and crumbly, being penetrable with a dental explorer. Newly erupted teeth are without luster and are opaque white or orange. The enamel wears away rapidly, and calculus deposition is often a striking feature. Radiographically, multiple moth-eaten foci are observed over the crowns. An *autosomal dominant hypomaturation-hypoplastic form* of AI occurs in conjunction with taurodontism, which may represent a variation of expressivity of the trichodento-osseous syndrome (see Syndrome-Associated Enamel Defects). *X-linked recessive hypomaturation AI* affects both primary and adult dentitions. Males show more severe changes. The permanent teeth are nearly normal in thickness and are in contact, yet are yellowish-brown and mottled. The cervical collar is minimally involved. In females, wavy vertical banding is seen and has the appearance of dripping wax. These stria are not seen radiographically. *Autosomal recessive pigmented hypomaturation AI* affects both primary and adult dentitions. Although thickness approaches normalcy, the enamel chips, particularly around restorations, and is brown. The incisal and occlusal surfaces are usually eroded. These teeth tend to accumulate calculus that fluoresces red-violet. Radiographically, the enamel layer is poorly defined.

Treatment: Full coverage prostheses are indicated for esthetic reasons. In addition, full crowns minimize calculus deposition, which predisposes to gingival and periodontal inflammation.

References

1. Sauk, J. J., Jr., Lyon, H. W., and Witkop, C. J., Jr.: Electron optic microanalysis of two gene products in enamel of females heterozygous for X-linked hypomaturation amelogenesis imperfecta. Am. J. Hum. Genet. *24*:267, 1972.
2. Witkop, C. J., Jr, Kuhlmann, W., and Sauk, J. J., Jr.: Autosomal recessive pigmented hypomaturation amelogenesis imperfecta. Oral Surg. *36*:367, 1973.
3. Giansanti, J. S.: A kindred showing hypocalcified amelogenesis imperfecta: report of case. J. Am. Dent. Assoc. *86*:675,1973.
4. Witkop, C. J., Jr., and Sauk, J. J., Jr.: Heritable defects of enamel. In *Oral Facial Genetics*, edited by R. E. Stewart and G. H. Prescott. St. Louis. C. V. Mosby Co., 1976, pp. 151–226.

5. Winter, G. B. and Brooks, A. H.: Enamel hypoplasia and anomalies of the enamel. A. E. Poole, ed.: Symposium on Genetics. Dent. Clin. North Am. 19:3, 1975.

Syndrome-Associated Enamel Defects

Sex: Predilection varies according to mode of inheritance.

Clinical Features: A vast number of rare syndromes have been described in which dental anomalies have been observed. Some of these syndromes show enamel defects as the sole dental anomaly; others affect enamel as well as other dental tissues. *Epidermolysis bullosa* occurs in at least four genetic forms and is a bullous disease of skin and mucous membranes. Dental defects are observed in some of these forms and consist of thin hypoplastic enamel with random pitting, yielding a honeycomb pattern. The *mucopolysaccharidoses (MPS)* are heritable diseases of defective mucopolysaccharide metabolism. In type IV, Morquio's syndrome, the enamel is defective, being hypoplastic with pointed peak-like cusp tips. The teeth are grey and pitted, and the pits tend to be vertically oriented. The teeth in type III, Sanfilippo's syndrome, exhibit loss of enamel with excessive and defective dentinogenesis, yielding radiographic evidence of pulp obliteration. In *tuberous sclerosis,* linear enamel pits may pock the facial enamel surfaces; these pits are usually apparent as punctate radiolucencies. *Oculodento-osseous dysplasia* is characterized by microphthalmus, iridal anomalies, bony anomalies of the digits and syndactyly, thickened mandibular bone, and enamel hypoplasia. The teeth show large multifocal hypoplastic defects and pitting, yielding a moth-eaten pattern radiographically. In the *amelo-onychohypohidrotic syndrome,* defective nails with subungual hyperkeratosis are seen in conjunction with sweat gland hypofunction, seborrheic dermatitis, and severe hypoplastic-hypocalcified enamel. Many resorbing unerupted teeth are observed in this syndrome.

The *trichodento-osseous syndrome* also shows enamel defects in conjunction with morphologic dental anomalies. These patients have tightly curled, kinky hair, with osteosclerosis of bone cortices. The enamel is hypoplastic and hypocalcified, lacking mesiodistal contact with pitting. Taurodontism is a feature, and many of the teeth remain unerupted. In *vitamin D refractory rickets,* the incisal or occlusal one-third is hypoplastic with granular enamel. The pulp chambers are large and pulp horns extend to the dentinoenamel junction. *Pseudohypoparathyroidism* exists in two forms. In both forms parathyroid hormone levels are intact; however, there is an inability to eliminate phosphate through the kidneys. Males are more severely affected in this X-linked disease. Features include round facies, short neck, short fourth metacarpals, falx cerebri and basal ganglia calcifications, and hypocalcemia with tetany. In addition, isolated secondary teeth, usually molars and premolars, show pitted enamel defects, are wedge shaped, and have short roots with wide root canals and open apices. There are numerous other syndromes not mentioned here that show dental anomalies.

Treatment: The dental defects included here

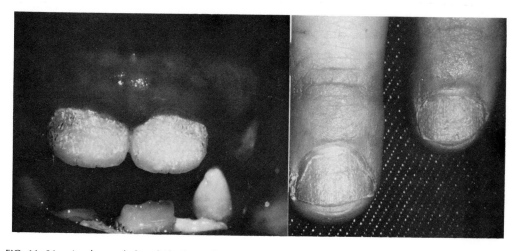

FIG. 11–31.   Amelo-onychohypohidrotic syndrome. (Courtesy of Dr. R. Sobel.)

are all characterized by enamel hypoplasia with pitting and can be restored with full crowns.

References

1. Arwill, T., Bergenholtz, A., and Olsson, O.: Epidermolysis bullosa hereditaria. III. A histologic study of the teeth in the polydysplastic, dystrophic, and lethal forms. Oral Surg. *19*:723, 1965.
2. Levin, L. S., Jorgenson, R. J., and Salinas, C. F.: Oral findings in the Morquio syndrome (mucopolysaccharidosis IV). Oral Surg. *39*:390, 1975.
3. Hoff, M., et al.: Enamel defects associated with tuberous sclerosis: a clinical and scanning-electronmicroscope study. Oral Surg. *40*:261, 1975.
4. Gorlin, R. J., Meskin, L. H., and Geme, J. W.: Oculo-dento-digital dysplasia. J. Pediatr. *63*:69, 1963.
5. Witkop, C. J., Jr., Brearley, L. J., and Gentry, W. C., Jr.: Hypoplastic enamel, onycholysis, and anhidrosis inherited as an autosomal dominant trait: a review of ectodermal dysplasia syndromes. Oral Surg. *39*:71, 1975.
6. Crawford, J. L.: Concomitant taurodontism and amelogenesis imperfecta in the American Caucasian. J. Dent. Child. *37*:83, 1970.
7. Croft, L. K., Witkop, C. J., Jr., and Glas, J. E.: Pseudohypoparathyroidism. Oral Surg. *20*:758, 1965.
8. Wright, J. T.: Epidermolysis bullosa: Dental and anesthetic management of two cases. Oral Surg. *57*:155, 1984.

Dentinogenesis Imperfecta

Sex: No predilection

Clinical Features: Dentinogenesis imperfecta is inherited as an autosomal dominant trait and is occasionally associated with osteogenesis imperfecta with blue sclera. Not all osteogenesis imperfecta (OI) syndromes are associated with dentinal defects. Furthermore, there is no correlation between dentinogenesis imperfecta and severity of the osseous diseases in OI; rather, it appears that OI pedigrees either consistently exhibit dentinogenesis imperfecta or show no evidence of heritable dental disease. Dentinogenesis imperfecta without associated osseous disease is encountered more frequently than OI-associated disease. Both deciduous and permanent dentitions are affected. The teeth show a yellowish to blue-gray opalescent, polished appearance. The defective dentin pervades both the coronal and radicular regions. A severe form of dentinogenesis imperfecta was first described in a triracial isolate group in Maryland. Opalescent bell-shaped crowns are seen; radiographically, dentin is rudimentary with large pulp chambers (shell teeth, Brandywine type, Shields type III). Originally it was thought that a defective dentinoenamel junc-

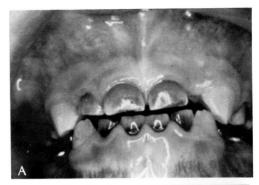
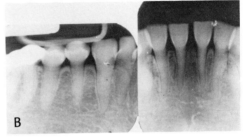

FIG. 11–32. *A:* Dentinogenesis imperfecta with opalescent teeth, which are subject to enamel fragmentation and advanced abrasion. (Courtesy of Dr. R. Sobel.) *B:* Radiographs showing obliteration of root canals.

tion was extant; scanning electronmicroscope studies have disclosed a normal junction. There is a propensity for enamel loss, and the cleavage of enamel likely occurs within defective dentin underlying the dentinoenamel junction. The exposed dentin rapidly abrades in many instances so that the coronal surface may fail to extend beyond the gingival crest. Radiographically, the cervix region is constricted, the roots are spiked, and the pulp chambers and root canals manifest calcific obliteration. Since dentinal tubules are haphazardly arranged and often devoid of odontoblastic processes, the teeth are not particularly sensitive even when most of the enamel surface has been lost. Microscopically, the pulp chamber is nearly obliterated yet does exist. The dentinal tubules are poorly formed and fail to radiate in parallel fashion; rather, they are serpentine and haphazardly arranged.

Treatment: Affected teeth are not more prone than normal teeth to dental caries. Full crowns can be fabricated, even at an early age, because of the small, obliterated pulp chambers. It should be noted that root fractures are not uncommon. When severe abrasion exists, an overdenture may be considered.

References

1. Heys, F. M., Blattner, R. J., and Robinson, H. B. G.: Osteogenesis imperfecta and odontogenesis imperfecta: Clinical and genetic aspects in eighteen families. J. Pediatr. *56*:234, 1960.
2. Bixler, D., Conneally, P. M., and Christen, A. G.: Dentinogenesis imperfecta; genetic variations in a six-generation family. J. Dent. Res. *48*:1196, 1969.
3. Witkop, C. J., Jr., and Rao, S.: Inherited defects in tooth structure. Birth Def. *7*:170, 1971.
4. Bixler, D.: Heritable disorders affecting dentin. In *Oral Facial Genetics,* edited by R. E. Stewart and G. H. Prescott. St. Louis. C. V. Mosby Co., 1976, pp. 230–37.
5. Levin, L. S.: The dentition in the osteogenesis imperfecta syndromes. Clin. Orthop. *159*:65, 1981.

Dentin Dysplasia Type I

Sex: No predilection

Clinical Features: Dentin dysplasia type I is inherited as an autosomal dominant trait that affects both the deciduous and permanent dentitions. It represents a peculiar disturbance in the development of radicular dentinogenesis in that the coronal morphology and histology are normal. Unlike dentinogenesis imperfecta, enamel fragmentation is not encountered. Clinically, the crowns usually appear normal, yet in some individuals there is a subtle opalescent gray discoloration. Radiographically, the roots are rudimentary with tapering and blunting. The root canals are obliterated and the pulp chambers are malformed, appearing as horizontal crescents. Periapical radiolucencies of unknown origin underlie many of the teeth. The microscopic appearance of extracted teeth is pathognomonic. The coronal dentin shows normal tubular orientation while the radicular dentin is whorled, giving the appearance of cascading waterfalls. The pulp chamber and

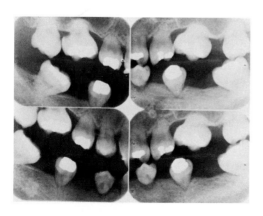

FIG. 11–33.   Dentin dysplasia type I.

root canal cannot be identified. The short roots are functionally unstable, so that loosening of teeth is a feature. Dentin dysplasia type I has been reported to occur in conjunction with diffuse generalized osteosclerosis in some patients.

Treatment: No specific treatment is recommended. When teeth are lost as a result of shortened roots, adjacent teeth should not be used as prosthetic abutments.

References

1. Rushton, M. A.: A case of dentinal dysplasia. Guys Hosp. Rep. *89*:369, 1939.
2. Sauk, J. J., Jr., et al.: An electron optic analysis and explanation for the etiology of dentinal dysplasia. Oral Surg. *33*:763, 1972.
3. Wesley, R. K., et al.: Dentin dysplasia type I. Clinical, morphologic, and genetic studies of a case. Oral Surg. *41*:516, 1976.
4. Morris, E. and Augsburger, R. H.: Dentine dysplasia with sclerotic bone and skeletal anomalies inherited as an autosomal dominant trait. A new syndrome. Oral Surg. *43*:267, 1977.
5. Petrone, J. A. and Noble, E. R.: Dentine dysplasia type I: a clinical report. J. Am. Dent. Assoc. *103*:891, 1981.

Dentin Dysplasia Type II

Sex: No predilection

Clinical Features: Dentin dysplasia type II, coronal type, is inherited as an autosomal dominant disorder. The deciduous teeth are amber-gray and translucent in appearance with radiographic evidence of pulp chamber and root canal obliteration, thereby resembling dentinogenesis imperfecta. The permanent dentition is clinically normal; radiographically pronounced cervical constriction is not featured. Large, flame-shaped pulp chambers contain many denticles; root canals may be partially obliterated.

Treatment: No special treatment is required, as enamel fracturing is not a problem and root length is essentially normal.

References

1. Shields, E. D., Bixler, D., and El-Kafrawy, A. M.: A proposed classification for heritable human dentine defects with a description of a new entity. Arch. Oral Biol. *18*:543, 1973.
2. Giansanti, J. S. and Allen, J. D.: Dentin dysplasia type II, or dentin dysplasia, coronal type. Oral Surg. *38*:911, 1974.
3. Wald, C. and Diner, H.: Dysplasia of the dental pulp: report of a case. J. Dent. Child. *41*:212, 1974.
4. Witkop, C. J., Jr.: Hereditary defects of dentin. Dent. Clin. North Am. *19*:25, 1975.
5. Burkes, E. J., Aquilino, S. A., and Bost, M. E.: Dentin dysplasia II. J. Endodontics *5*:277, 1979.

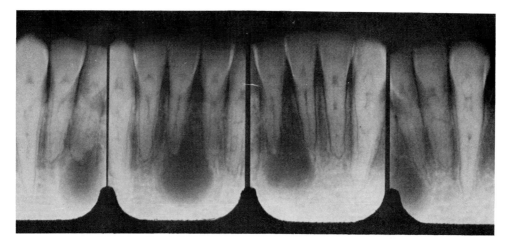

FIG. 11–34. Dentin dysplasia type II showing denticles. (Courtesy of Dr. J. Campbell.)

Regional Odontodysplasia

Sex: No predilection

Clinical Features: Occurring as a sporadic anomaly, regional odontodysplasia is a localized developmental dental defect restricted to a single tooth or group of contiguous teeth in one quadrant. The involved teeth are usually the central and lateral incisors and cuspid in the maxilla. They fail to erupt completely. On radiographs both enamel and dentin formation are deficient, yielding a subdued appearance with patent dilated pulp chambers. The appearance accounts for the term *ghost teeth.* The cause is unknown; however, the distribution in the maxilla often corresponds to the neurovascular supply, suggesting that an ischemic phenomenon may be responsible. In fact, many cases have been reported in which vascular nevi

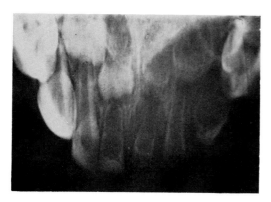

FIG. 11–35. Ghost teeth of odontodysplasia. (From Gardner, D. G. and Sapp, J. P.: Regional odontodysplasia. Oral Surg. *35:*351, 1973.)

involve the area of the face that harbors the hypoplastic teeth. Both permanent and deciduous predecessors may be affected. Microscopically, large pulp chambers are noted and the dentin is thin and globular. The enamel layer is attenuated and disrupted. The reduced enamel epithelium persists, and the follicular connective tissue contains many enameloid droplet calcifications.

Treatment: The teeth are nonfunctional; because eruption is not evident or is only partial, extraction with fabrication of a prosthetic appliance is recommended.

References

1. Rushton, M. A.: Odontodysplasia. "Ghost teeth." Br. Dent. J. *119:*109, 1965.
2. Alexander, W. N., Lilly, G. E., and Irby, W. B.: Odontodysplasia. Oral Surg. *22:*814, 1966.
3. Gardner, D. G. and Sapp, J. P.: Regional odontodysplasia. Oral Surg. *35:*351, 1973.
4. Lustmann, J., Klein, H., and Ulmansky, M.: Odontodysplasia. Report of two cases and review of the literature. Oral Surg. *39:*781, 1975.
5. Walton, J. L., Witkop, C. J., Jr., and Walker, P. O.: Odontodysplasia. Report of three cases with vascular nevi overlying the adjacent skin of the face. Oral Surg. *46:*676, 1978.

Hypophosphatasia

Sex: No predilection

Clinical Features: Inherited as an autosomal recessive trait, hypophosphatasia represents an enzyme-deficiency metabolic bone disease characterized by absence or diminution of alkaline phosphatase in osteoblasts, intestines, and kidneys, among other tissues. It occurs in infantile, juvenile, and adult forms; the infantile form has

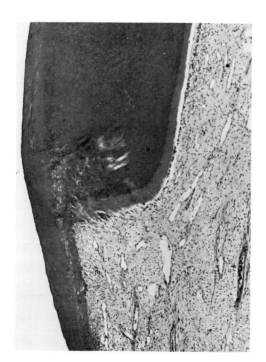

FIG. 11–36. Histologic section of exfoliated tooth showing cemental agenesis and apical defect in dentin formation in hypophosphatasia. (Courtesy of Dr. C. Witkop.)

the worst prognosis. Those individuals capable of survival show osteomalacia with hypomineralization similar to that seen in acquired rickets. The chief dental manifestation is premature tooth loss from cemental agenesis with lack of secure periodontal fiber attachment to the teeth. In addition, the teeth are often hypocalcified with large pulp chambers resembling shell teeth or odontodysplasia. Both primary and secondary teeth are affected. Histologically, a thin layer of dentin is observed with cemental agenesis. Serum alkaline phosphatase is lowered; in many cases, hypercalcemia and urinary phosphoethanolamine are demonstrable.

Treatment: No successful treatment is available. High-dose vitamin D therapy has been employed with limited success.

References
1. Sobel, E. H., et al.: Rickets, deficiency of "alkaline" phosphatase activity and premature loss of teeth in childhood. Pediatrics *11*:309, 1953.
2. Houpt, M. I., Kenny, F. M., and Listgarten, M.: Hypophosphatasia: Case reports. J. Dent. Child. *34*:126, 1970.
3. Poland, E., III, et al.: Histochemical observations in hypophosphatasia. J. Dent. Res. *51*:333, 1972.
4. Beumer, J., et al.: Childhood hypophosphatasia and

the premature loss of teeth. Oral Surg. *35*:631, 1973.
5. Kjellman, M., et al.: Five cases of hypophosphatasia with dental findings. Int. J. Oral Surg. *2*:152, 1973.

Vitamin D Refractory Rickets

Sex: Males are affected more severely.

Clinical Features: Vitamin D refractory or hypophosphatemic rickets is a heritable disorder with X-linked dominant transmission. The clinical features, osteomalacia causing osseous deformi-

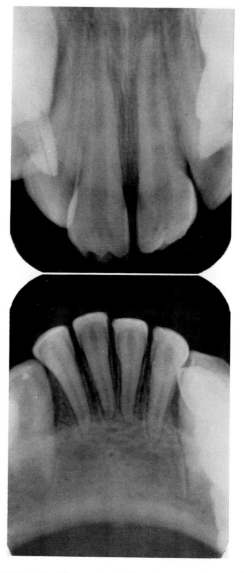

FIG. 11–37. Elongated pulp horns in region of coronal fissures in vitamin D refractory rickets. (Courtesy of Drs. R. Wesley and J. Delaney.)

ties similar to those seen in ordinary rickets, do not show resolution with administration of vitamin D. Serum phosphorus levels are depressed. Patients lack an enzyme necessary for conversion of intestinally absorbed vitamin D_3 into the active $1\alpha-25$ dihydroxyvitamin D_3. The resultant deficit in active vitamin leads to poor phosphate absorption and deficient mineralization of osteoid. There is also some evidence to support a defect in renal tubular handling of phosphate. Affected children have difficulty walking. Globular dentin is prominent; fissures develop and extend from the pulp horns, which are elongated, to the cusp tips. These fissures are patent, allowing oral microorganisms to gain access to the pulp chamber in the absence of caries. This, in turn, leads to periapical disease, demonstrated radiographically, with clinical evidence of widespread fistulae. The supportive alveolar bone often shows an osteoporotic pattern of trabeculation. The long-bone epiphyseal plates show pericartilaginous deposition with failure to mineralize.

Ordinary rickets fails to show the dental defects encountered in hypophosphatemic rickets, and the former disease responds rapidly to vitamin D therapy.

Differential Diagnosis: Widespread dental abscess formation may be seen in diabetes of juvenile onset, yet diabetes rarely becomes severe enough to produce these changes in young children. Serum phosphorus levels and a skeletal radiographic survey should be done with children showing widespread periapical disease in the absence of dental caries. The presence of a familial pattern also helps to limit the differential diagnosis.

Treatment: Administration of $1\alpha-25$ dihydroxyvitamin D_3 will result in marked improvement. The patient should be referred to an internist or endocrinologist. Occlusal sealants will not prevent pulpal and periapical infection. Complete pulpectomy of affected teeth is recommended with placement of zinc oxide and engenol.

References

1. Archard, H. O. and Witkop, C. J., Jr.: Hereditary hypophosphatemia (vitamin D-resistant rickets) presenting primary dental manifestations. Oral Surg. 22:184, 1966.
2. Tracy, W. E., et al.: Analysis of dentin pathogenesis in vitamin D-resistant rickets. Oral Surg. 32:38, 1971.
3. Sauk, J. J. and Witkop, C. J., Jr.: Electron optic analysis of human dentin on hypophosphatemic vitamin D-resistant rickets. Oral Surg. 32:38, 1971.
4. Vasilakis, G. J., Nygaard, V. K., and DiPalma, D. M.: Vitamin D resistant rickets. A review and case report of an adolescent boy with a history of dental problems. J. Oral Med. 35:19, 1980.
5. Rakocz, M., Keating, J., III, and Johnson, R.: Management of the primary dentition in vitamin D-resistant rickets. Oral Surg. 54:166, 1982.

Denticles and Pulp Calcification

Age: Adults
Sex: No predilection

Clinical Features: Pulpal calcifications are identified on dental roentgenograms and may be located either within the pulp chamber, appearing as focal intrapulpal radiopacities, or within the root canals, as diffuse radiopacities giving the appearance of calcific obliteration. The calcifications in the coronal pulp chamber are referred to as *denticles* or *pulp stones*, while root canal calcification has been referred to as *calcific metamorphosis of pulp.* In either case, no cause can be identified either locally or systemically. The teeth are vital, even when canals appear to be obliterated, and there is no relationship between pulp calcification and facial pain. Denticles are classified as "true" if composed of dentin or

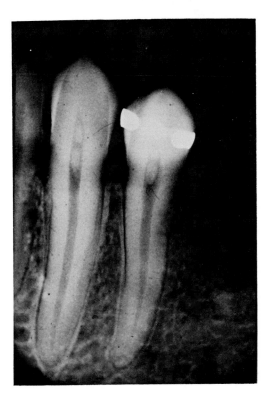

FIG. 11–38. Pulp stones.

"false" if composed of laminated dystrophic calcific concretions. Furthermore, either type may be attached or free, depending on whether the calcified mass is confluent with the normal tooth dentin. Type II dentin dysplasia is characterized by large pulp chambers with denticle formation. Microscopically, calcific metamorphosis of the root canal is characterized by multifocal dystrophic calcifications that tend to align themselves in a vertical plane throughout the radicular pulp.

Treatment: No treatment is required.

References

1. Stafne, E. C. and Szabo, S. E.: The significance of pulp nodules. Dent. Cosmos 75:160, 1933.
2. Hill, T. J.: Pathology of dental pulp. J. Am. Dent. Assoc. 21:820, 1934.
3. Johnson, P. L. and Bevelander, G.: Histogenesis and histochemistry of pulpal calcifications. J. Dent. Res. 35:714, 1956.
4. Stafne, E. C. and Gibilisco, J. A.: Oral Roentgenographic Diagnosis, 4th Ed. Philadelphia, W. B. Saunders Co., 1975, ch. 5.

Internal Resorption

Age: Young adults
Sex: No predilection

Clinical Features: As opposed to most of the diseases showing structural deformities, internal resoprtion is acquired later in life and fails to follow any hereditary pattern. The cause is unknown, although trauma has been suggested. Caries with pulpitis may be present, but this is not a prerequisite. Pain is not a feature when caries is absent. When internal resorption develops in the coronal pulp, the tooth may resorb to the point where the vascularity of the pulp tissue is observed through a thin dental hard tissue layer with a pink appearance (pink tooth of Mummery). Radiographs show a circular or ovoid radiolucency within the region of the pulp chamber either in the coronal or, more commonly, in the radicular region. The maxillary central incisors are most often afflicted. Internal resorption may accompany external resorption, particularly with impacted teeth. Microscopically, the pulp chamber contains viable fibrous connective tissue, which in unexposed pulps is devoid of inflammation. The dentin shows scalloping with osteoclastic resorption. Attempts at repair may exist, with deposition of osteodentin over zones of resorption.

Treatment: No treatment is required. Endodontic therapy is not feasible because of the inaccessibility of the resorbed recesses to instrumentation. As the disease progresses root fracture may occur, thus necessitating extraction. Often the resorption becomes static.

References

1. Selley, W. G.: Idiopathic internal resorption of upper central incisor. Br. Dent. J. 100:357, 1956.
2. Sweet, A. P. S.: Internal resorption, a chronology. Dent. Radiogr. Photogr. 38:75, 1965.
3. Toplis, J. W.: Idiopathic internal resorption of deciduous teeth. Br. Dent. J. 149:111, 1980.
4. Horn, A. B.: Tooth resorption and root canal therapy. Oral Surg. 52:325, 1981.
5. Frank, A. L.: External-internal progressive resorption and its nonsurgical correction. J. Endod. 7:473, 1981.

Idiopathic External Resorption

Age: Adults
Sex: No predilection

Clinical Features: The cementum and underlying dentin may show resorption as a consequence of pressure or trauma generated by tumors and cysts, orthodontic forces, reimplantation or periapical inflammation. Impacted teeth of long standing may also show internal and external resorption of both coronal and radicular hard tissues. Resorption of roots on erupted teeth where no cause can be determined is termed idiopathic resorption. Some degree of root resorption probably occurs in nearly all adults; however, it is minimal. Occasionally, for no apparent reason,

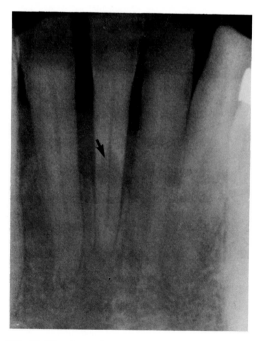

FIG. 11–39.   Internal resorption manifesting an intradental radiolucency.

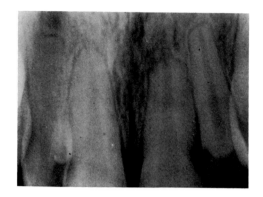

FIG. 11–40.   Idiopathic external resorption.

many teeth will show advanced resorption with blunting of the roots. The maxillary premolars, incisors, and molars are most often affected. Neither periodontal disease nor periapical inflammation bears any relationship to idiopathic generalized resorption. The apices show osteoclast-mediated resorption of cementum and dentin, with no alteration in the periodontal ligament or underlying periodontal bone that replaces the zone previously occupied by dental root structure.

Treatment: No form of treatment has been shown to arrest the process. Resorption may proceed progressively until the involved teeth become loose. Extraction may then become necessary.

References

1. Massler, M. and Perreault, J. G.: Root resorption in the permanent teeth of young adults. J. Dent. Child. *21*:158, 1954.
2. Kerr, D. A., Courtney, R. M., and Burkes, E. J.: Multiple idiopathic root resorption. Oral Surg. *29*:552, 1970.
3. Yaacob, H. B.: Idiopathic external resorption of teeth. Can. Dent. Assoc. J. *46*:578, 1980.
4. Newman, G. W.: Possible aetiologic factors in external root resorption. Am. J. Orthodont. *67*:522, 1975.
5. Goldman, H. M.: An atlas of acquired dental defects. Compend. Cont. Educ. Dent. *3*:275, 1982.

ALTERATIONS IN ERUPTION/EXFOLIATION TIMES

Premature Eruption

Sex: No predilection

Clinical Features: Early eruption of teeth may occur with both deciduous and permanent dentitions in the absence of any underlying systemic disorder. Indeed, 10 percent of the population may manifest precocious eruption as early as 3 months for deciduous and 4 years for permanent denti-

tions. Natal or neonatal teeth are deciduous teeth, usually mandibular incisors, that are present at birth or erupt soon thereafter. This condition seems to be genetically determined and is most frequently encountered among isolated tribes and ethnic groups. Often, prematurely erupted deciduous teeth fail to complete root development and are prematurely exfoliated. A variety of craniofacial syndromes are associated with premature eruption of teeth: clefts, oculomandibulodyscephaly, chondroectodermal dysplasia, and hemifacial hypertrophy. Hyperthyroidism of congenital or childhood onset may also be associated with early eruption.

References

1. Bodenhoff, J. and Gorlin, R. J.: Natal and neonatal teeth; folklore and fact. Pediatrics *32*:1087, 1963.
2. Spouge, J. D. and Feasby, W. H.: Erupted teeth in the newborn. Oral Surg. *22*:198, 1966.
3. Dixon, G. H. and Stewart, R. E.: In *Oral Facial Genetics,* edited by R. E. Stewart and G. H. Prescott. St. Louis, C. V. Mosby Co., 1976, pp. 142–45.

Delayed Eruption

Sex: No predilection

Clinical Features: Great variation exists with regard to eruption dates; thus, delayed eruption may not herald the presence of any underlying disorder but may merely represent a variation in normal physiology. Certain systemic illnesses and syndromes may be associated with generalized delayed eruption, and these conditions must be considered when a patient exhibits alteration in eruption dates. In particular, patients with *cleidocranial dysostosis* show hypoplastic or aplastic clavicles, cranial anomalies, and multiple unerupted and supernumerary teeth. In *cryptodontic brachymetacarpia,* the metacarpals and metatarsals are shortened and teeth fail to erupt. Many of the syndromes described in conjunction with enamel defects show retarded eruption or unerupted teeth. Hypothyroidism and hypopituitarism (pituitary dwarfism) are often associated with delayed eruption. Multiple impacted teeth are encountered in cleidocranial dysplasia and Gardner's syndrome. Generalized delayed eruption may also be encountered in mongolism, rickets, vitamin D refractory rickets, lead poisoning, and osteopetrosis. Isolated or individual teeth showing retarded eruption often indicate the presence of an intrabony odontogenic neoplasm or cyst, requiring radiographs to determine whether or not a radiolucent or radiopaque lesion is associated with the impacted tooth. In addition to impaction, congenitally missing teeth will of course give the impression that eruption is retarded. This may be generalized in hereditary ectodermal dysplasia and chondroectodermal dysplasia.

References

1. Pindborg, J. J.: *Pathology of the dental hard tissues.* Philadelphia, W. B. Saunders Co., 1970.
2. Shokeir, M. H.: Complete failure of eruption of all permanent teeth: an autosomal dominant disorder. Clin. Genet. 5:322, 1974.
3. Dixon, G. H. and Stewart, R. E.: In *Oral Facial Genetics,* edited by R. E. Stewart and G. H. Prescott. St. Louis, C. V. Mosby Co., 1976, pp. 142–45.
4. Pearl, M. and Roland, N. M.: Delayed primary dentition in a case of congenital lead poisoning. ASDC J. Dent. Child. 47:269, 1980.

Impaction

Sex: No predilection

Clinical Features: Impaction or retention of teeth is one of the most common developmental dental defects encountered in man. Failure of teeth to erupt may be the result of a physical barrier, unexplained loss of eruption force, or a tumor or cyst of the jaws arising from odontogenic or nonodontogenic tissues. The mandibular third molars and maxillary canines are most frequently involved, followed by the maxillary third molars. Maxillary central incisors, mandibular canines, and premolars in both arches are also retained with some degree of frequency. Supernumerary teeth such as mesiodens and premolars often fail to erupt. Multiple impactions and supernumerary teeth are encountered in cleidocranial dysostosis, which is characterized by the aforementioned dental defect in conjunction with agenesis or hypoplasia of the clavicles and craniofacial anomalies including Wormian bones, open fontanels, hypoplastic sinuses, and other defects of both membranous and endochondral bones. Gardner's syndrome is also associated with multiple dental impactions. Impacted teeth are also seen in various forms of amelogenesis imperfecta and in syndromes associated with enamel defects. The significance of impacted teeth rests with the latent potential of the follicular tissues to undergo cystic or neoplastic transformation.

References

1. Blum, T.: Malposed teeth; their classification, pathology and treatment. Int. J. Orthod. 9:122,1923.
2. Dachi, S. F. and Howell, F. V.: A survey of 3,874 routine full-mouth radiographs. II. A study of impacted teeth. Oral Surg. 14:1165, 1961.
3. Fielding, A. F., Douglass, A. F., and Whitley, R. D.: Reasons for early removal of impacted third molars. Clin. Prevent. Dent. 3:19, 1981.
4. Brockbank, J.: Change in position of unerupted mandibular third molars. Oral Surg. 51:461, 1981.
5. Shaw, B. M., Schneider, S. S., and Zeger, J.: Surgical management of ankylosed impacted maxillary canines. J. Am. Dent. Assoc. 102:497, 1981.

Premature Exfoliation

Sex: No predilection

Clinical Features: Premature loss of deciduous teeth in conjunction with precocious eruption is usually of no clinical significance since the succedaneous dentition also commonly erupts early. Premature exfoliation limited to a localized region may be an ominous sign. Loosening of either deciduous or permanent teeth in children, teenagers, or young adults may be indicative of an underlying destructive process of the alveolar bone: leukemia, sarcoma, histiocytosis X, or a benign neoplasm. Generalized premature loss of the incisors and molars is a feature of periodontosis; when seen in conjunction with palmar-plantar hyperkeratosis, the Papillon-Lefevre syndrome should be considered. Generalized early tooth loss is also encountered in hypophosphatasia, juvenile onset diabetes, cyclic neutropenia, agranulocytosis, acrodynia, scurvy, and dentin dysplasia. Full-mouth dental radiographs or a panorex film should be obtained when teeth become loose prior to their normal exfoliation times.

References

1. Cohen, D. W. and Morris, A. L.: Periodontal manifestations of cyclic neutropenia. J. Periodontol. 32:159, 1961.
2. Gorlin, R. J., Sedano, H., and Anderson, V. E.: The syndrome of palmar-plantar hyperkeratosis and premature periodontal destruction of the teeth. J. Pediatr. 65:895. 1964.
3. Ritchie, B. M.: Hypophosphatasia. A metabolic dis-

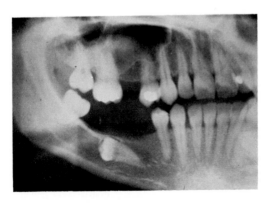

FIG. 11–41.   Impacted mandibular tooth.

ease with important dental manifestations. Arch. Dis. Child. *39*:584, 1964.

4. Kjellman, M., et al.: Five cases of hypophosphatasia with dental findings. Int. J. Oral Surg. *2*:151, 1973.

PIGMENTATIONS

Erythroblastosis Fetalis

Sex: No predilection

Clinical Features: Hemolytic anemia develops in infants when an Rh-positive fetus is nurtured in the womb of an Rh-negative mother who has developed anti-Rh antibodies from a previous pregnancy. When antibodies pass the placental membrane and enter the fetal circulation they agglutinate fetal erythrocytes, bind complement, and cause hemolysis. This same immunologic lesion may evolve as a consequence of ABO isoantigen incompatibility, in which the fetus is A, B, or AB and the mother lacks A or B isoantigens. If the anemia is prolonged, hemolyzed erythrocytes liberate hemosiderin pigment, which may become deposited in developing dentin matrices. Teeth at a comparable stage of development (usually only deciduous) will then show pigmentation; they are brown, black, green, or blue in appearance. The pigment is transmitted from the deeper layers of dentin. When icterus develops, hypoplasia of enamel may be seen.

Differential Diagnosis: The pigment of erythroblastosis is not associated with a chalky enamel surface as is often encountered in fluorosis. Staining from tetracycline occurs more often in permanent teeth, is yellow, and fluoresces with ultraviolet light. Red fluorescence is seen in porphyria. Bilirubin-stained teeth are also green, so that various other forms of neonatal jaundice

must be considered. Extrinsic stains can be removed with scalers.

Treatment: No treatment is required. Upon exfoliation, the permanent teeth are usually of normal color.

References

1. Thursfield, H.: Green teeth subsequent to a prolonged jaundice in the first weeks of life. Proc. R. Soc. Med. *5*:147, 1912.
2. Kesson, C. W.: Green teeth following icterus gravis neonatorum. Proc. Roy. Soc. Med. *42*:561, 1949.
3. Tank, G.: Two cases of green pigmentation of deciduous teeth associated with hemolytic disease of the newborn. J. Am. Dent. Assoc. *42*:302, 1951.
4. Marsland, E. A. and Gerrard, J. W.: Intrinsic staining of teeth following icterus gravis. Brit. Dent. J. *94*:305, 1953.
5. Grahnén, H. and Granath, L. E.: Effect of hyperbilirubinemia on primary teeth; a clinical study. Odont. Rev. *13*:337, 1962.

Biliary Atresia

Sex: No predilection

Clinical Features: Atresia of the biliary ducts, or other liver disorders such as neonatal hepatitis, may cause retention of either conjugated or unconjugated bilirubin. The bile pigments become elevated in serum and may then become incorporated into the organic matrices of developing teeth. In the icterus state the deposited bilirubin imparts a green color to the deciduous teeth. If the child is able to thrive and if the jaundice can be corrected, he or she will have a normal secondary dentition. The prognosis with biliary atresia is poor. Other forms of neonatal jaundice such as erythroblastosis and hepatitis are reversible in most cases.

Differential Diagnosis: The diagnosis of biliary

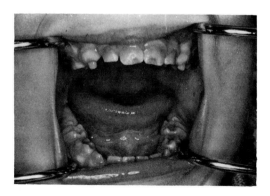

FIG. 11–42. Teeth in erythroblastosis fetalis darkened as a result of hemosiderin pigment deposition in dentin. (Courtesy of Drs. R. Abrams, R. Adams, and R. Sobel.)

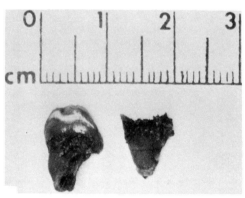

FIG. 11–43. Exfoliated teeth stained green by bilirubin pigment in biliary atresia.

atresia is made on the basis of biochemical and radiologic studies for liver function. A conjugated hyperbilirubinemia prevails, and cholangiograms disclose a rudimentary biliary tree. Liver biopsy may also be required to make the diagnosis. Fever with jaundice in newborns may indicate neonatal hepatitis. Needle biopsies may aid in obtaining a definitive diagnosis. By the time the patient is seen by the dentist, a diagnosis has usually been rendered.

Treatment: Provided that jaundice has been corrected, the secondary dentition will be normal.

References

1. Baden, E.: In *Thoma's Oral Pathology*, 6th Ed. edited by R. J. Gorlin and H. M. Goldman. St. Louis, C. V. Mosby Co., 1970, Vol. 1, pp. 191–192.
2. Shapiro, B. M., Gallagher, R. E., and Needleman, H. L.: Dental management of the patient with biliary atresia. Report of two cases. Oral Surg. *40*:742, 1975.

Porphyria

Sex: No predilection

Clinical Features: Accumulations of porphyrin compounds in tissues may result from certain infections or from an inborn error in metabolism. The most important form associated with dental pigmentation is congenital erythropoietic porphyria, which is inherited as an autosomal recessive trait. The first sign is red coloration of the urine by uroporphyrin. Photosensitivity becomes progressively worse as the child ages and a vesiculobullous dermatitis develops. Both deciduous and permanent dentitions show pigmentation, usually brown. Under ultraviolet light the teeth show a striking red fluorescence. Ground sections disclose porphyrin pigments deposited in enamel, dentin, and cementum.

Differential Diagnosis: The stain in porphyria

often has a reddish tinge. Under fluorescent light the red fluorescence is pathognomonic. The cutaneous manifestations of porphyria, in conjunction with other clinical features of the disease, allow for differentiation from other disorders that show dental pigmentation.

Treatment: No treatment is available. The discolored teeth may be cosmetically restored with porcelain-veneered crowns.

References

1. Schmid, R., Schwartz, S., and Sundberg, R. D.: Erythropoietic (congenital) porphyria: a rare abnormality of the normoblasts. Blood *10*:416, 1955.
2. Waldenstrom, J. and Haeger-Aronsen, B.: Different patterns of human porphyria. Br. Med. J. *2*:272, 1963.
3. Hearing, R. G., et al.: Congenital erythropoietic porphyria. Am. J. Med. *45*:624, 1968.
4. Trodahl, J. N., Schwartz, S., and Gorlin, R. J.: The pigmentation of dental tissues in erythropoietic (congenital) porphyria. J. Oral Pathol. *1*:159, 1972.

Dental Fluorosis

Sex: No predilection

Clinical Features: Fluorosis, a common cause of dental pigmentation, is discussed with structural dental defects. In addition to the hypoplastic changes, a mottled or blotchy brown pigmentation is present in the enamel layers. Both deciduous and permanent teeth are affected if excess fluoride is consumed in drinking water during the period of tooth development. Concentrations in excess of one part per million are required to produce dental mottling. Severe pigmentation is usually not seen unless the fluoride concentration exceeds five parts per million.

Differential Diagnosis: Dental fluorosis is usu-

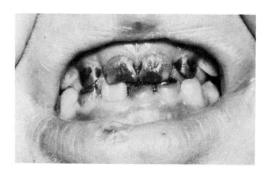

FIG. 11–44.   Porphyrin deposits in porphyria. (Courtesy of Dr. R. Gorlin.)

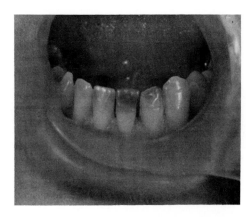

FIG. 11–45.   Teeth with fluorosis showing brown pigmentation.

ally associated with chalky enamel surfaces, and the pigmentation is generally irregular and blotchy, as opposed to that of other dental pigmentations. The pigment shows no fluorescent properties. A history of residence in a geographic region known to contain high levels of fluoride in the water is significant in limiting the differential diagnosis.

Treatment: Teeth with fluorosis pigmentation can be restored with esthetic porcelain crowns.

References

1. Black, G. V. and McKay, F. S.: Mottled teeth: An endemic developmental imperfection of the enamel of teeth heretofore unknown in the literature of dentistry. Dent. Cosmos *58*:129, 1916.
2. Dean, H. T.: Chronic endemic dental fluorosis. J. Am. Med. Assoc. *107*:1269, 1936.
3. Dean, H. T. and Arnold, F. A.: Endemic dental fluorosis or mottled teeth. J. Am. Dent. Assoc. *30*:1278, 1943.
4. McClure, F. S. and Lipkins, R. C.: Fluorine in human teeth studied in relation to fluorine in the drinking water. J. Dent. Res. *30*:172, 1951.

Tetracycline Staining

Sex: No predilection

Clinical Features: Tetracycline antibiotics act as a vital dye, being incorporated into bone and dentin during osteogenesis and dentinogenesis respectively. The antibiotic becomes highly concentrated in dentin and renders the teeth yellow or yellowish-brown. Under ultraviolet light, a bright yellow or yellowish-green fluorescence is observed. Discoloration as seen clinically is dependent upon dose and duration of drug administration. The drug is deposited only during dentinogenesis. Most examples of severe discolorations are seen in children requiring long-term antibiotic therapy; relatively short courses of drug use usually fail to produce any significant clinical

manifestations. Ground sections of teeth examined under fluorescent microscopy show linear deposits in dentin corresponding temporally to drug intake.

Differential Diagnosis: When staining is seen as a result of tetracycline administration, it is generally diffuse and uniform as opposed to that of fluorosis, which is brown and mottled. Tetracycline fluoresces yellow whereas porphyria is red. A history of drug use is, of course, the key in making the diagnosis.

Treatment: Severely discolored anterior teeth may be cosmetically corrected by porcelain-veneered crowns.

References

1. Baden, E.: In *Thoma's Oral Pathology*, 6th Ed., edited by R. J. Gorlin and H. M. Goldman. St. Louis, C. V. Mosby Co., 1970, Vol. 1, pp. 189–191.
2. Shafer, W. G., Hine, M. K., and Levy, B. M.: *A Textbook of Oral Pathology*, 4th Ed. Philadelphia, W. B. Saunders Co., 1983, p. 581.
3. Witkop, C. J., Jr., and Wolf, R. O.: Hypoplasia and intrinsic staining of enamel following tetracycline therapy. J. Am. Med. Assoc. *185*:1009, 1963.
4. Bridges, J. B., et al.: Tetracyclines and teeth. Br. Dent. J. *126*:306, 1969.
5. Primosch, R. E.: Tetracycline discoloration, enamel defects, and dental caries in patients with cystic fibrosis. Oral Surg. *50*:301, 1980.

Extrinsic Staining

Sex: No predilection

Clinical Features: Extrinsic staining is generally confined to the cervical enamel whereby extrinsic pigments become incorporated into dental plaque or calculus deposits. The color of the deposit varies according to the agent responsible. In children, green stain is most frequent. It is common and most prominent on maxillary anterior teeth. The

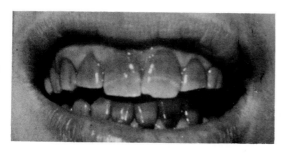

FIG. 11–46. Brownish-yellow pigmentation in teeth of a patient receiving tetracycline over a long period of time. (Courtesy of Drs. R. Abrams, R. Adams, and R. Sobel.)

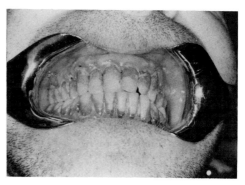

FIG. 11–47. Extrinsic orange stain limited to the cervical third of the teeth.

cause has not clearly been identified but may represent chlorophyll or deposits of chromogenic bacteria. Orange stain, also seen in children, is believed to evolve as a result of colonization by chromogenic bacteria. Neither green nor orange stains have any pathogenic consequences. Rarely, black or brown stains are encountered on deciduous teeth and, as with green or orange stains, chromogenic bacteria are probably responsible. In adults, brown or black stains are usually attributable to tobacco or caffeine.

Differential Diagnosis: Extrinsic stains can be differentiated from the other forms of dental pigmentation included here on the basis of location, being confined to the cervical third of the tooth crown, and the fact that they can be scaled from the tooth surface.

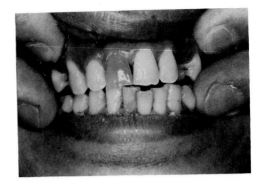

FIG. 11–48.   Focal dental pigmentation in pulp necrosis of central incisor.

References

1. Ayers, P.: Green stain. J. Am. Dent. Assoc. *26*:2, 1939.
2. Boyle, P. E. and Dinnerman, M.: Natural vital staining of the teeth of infants and children. Am. J. Orthodont. Oral Surg. *27*:377, 1941.
3. Leung, S. W.: Naturally occurring stains on the teeth of children. J. Am. Dent. Assoc. *41*:191, 1950.
4. Van Reenen, J. F.: Tobacco; the effects of its use with special reference to the mouth and dental elements; a survey of the literature. J. Dent. Assoc. S. Afr. *9*:334, 1954.
5. Sutcliffe, P.: Extrinsic tooth staining in children. Dent. Pract. *17*:175, 1967.

Focal Pigmentation

Sex: No predilection

Clinical Features: Pigmentation of a single tooth is seen in pulp necrosis and internal coronal resorption. In pulp necrosis, the affected tooth shows a brown or gray discoloration, which results from deposition of hemosiderin pigment and necrotic tissue products. Radiographs will usually disclose the presence of a periapical radiolucency. Coronal internal resorption has no known etiology, yet may be the result of trauma. The affected tooth appears pink ("pink tooth" of Mummery) due to pulpal enlargement subsequent to internal resorption of dentin. A radiograph will disclose focal pulp chamber enlargement.

Differential Diagnosis: The other pigmentations listed here are generalized or involve more than one tooth. Internal coronal resorption can be easily differentiated from the pigmentation associated with pulp necrosis on the basis of color differences, radiographs, and response to pulp testing.

Treatment: Because pink teeth with coronal internal resorption fracture easily, pulp extirpation with endodontic therapy and a prosthetic crown are indicated. Pigmented nonvital teeth should be treated similarly, and the discoloration can be managed by peroxide bleaching.

References

1. Sweet, A. P. S.: Internal resorption, a chronology. Dent. Radiogr. Photogr. *38*:75, 1965.
2. Nuttling, E. B. and Poe, G. S.: Chemical bleaching of discolored endodontically treated teeth. Dent. Clin. N. Amer., p. 655, Nov. 1967.

12
Facial Pain and
Neuromuscular Disorders

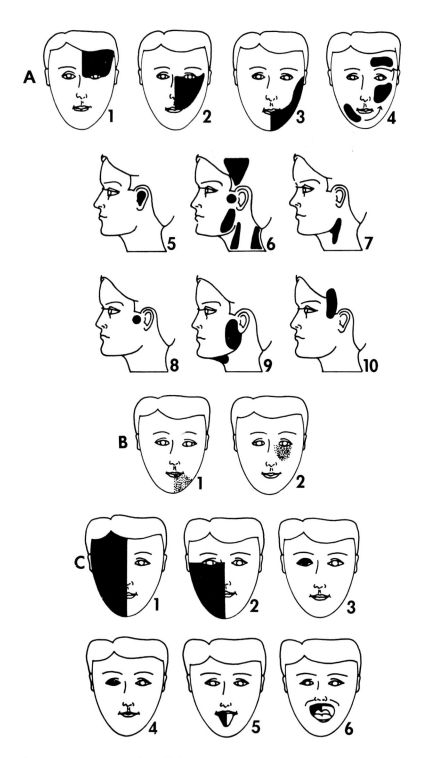

Pain and Neuromuscular Disorders

A-1, Ophthalmic division pain; A-2, Maxillary division pain; A-3, Mandibular division pain; A-4, Wandering pain; A-5, Otologic pain; A-6, Myofacial pain; A-7, Upper cervical pain; A-8, TMJ internal derangement; A-9, Sialogenic pain; A-10, Temporal pain; B-1, Mental nerve paresthesia/hypoesthesia; B-2, Infraorbital paresthesia/hypoesthesia; C-1, Peripheral nerve VII paralysis; C-2, CNS nerve VII paralysis; C-3, Horner's syndrome; C-4 ,Ophthalmoplegia; C-5, Nerve XII paralysis; C-6, V Motor paralysis, X paralysis

12
Facial Pain and Neuromuscular Disorders

OPHTHALMIC DIVISION PAIN

Odontogenic Infection
Frontal Sinusitis
Myogenic Pain‡
Postherpetic Neuralgia*
Trigeminal Neuralgia*
Cranial Base and CNS Neoplasms*
Vascular Occlusive Disease and Aneurysms

MAXILLARY DIVISION PAIN

Odontogenic Infection
Maxillary Sinusitis
Pathologic Jawbone Cavities
Traumatic Neuroma†
Antral and Maxillary Neoplasms
Cluster Headache
Trigeminal Neuralgia
Postherpetic Neuralgia
Causalgia
Cranial Base and CNS Neoplasms
Atypical Facial Pain

MANDIBULAR DIVISION PAIN

Odontogenic Infection
Trigeminal Neuralgia*
Postherpetic Neuralgia*
Causalgia*
Pathologic Jawbone Cavities*
Traumatic Neuroma
Subacute Thyroiditis
Cranial Base and CNS Neoplasms*
Stomatodynia/Glossopyrosis
Atypical Facial Pain*
Cardiogenic Facial Pain

WANDERING FACIAL PAIN

Atypical and Psychogenic Pain*
Myogenic Pain‡

OTOGENIC PAIN

Acute Otitis Media
Chronic Otitis Media
Herpes Zoster Oticus
Middle Ear Neoplasms
Odontogenic Infection†

NECK AND THROAT PAIN

Stylohyoid Syndrome
Hyoid Syndrome
Subacute Thyroiditis†
Glossopharyngeal Neuralgia
Carotidynia
Superior Laryngeal Neuralgia
Laryngeal Neoplasms

TMJ REGION PAIN

Myogenic Pain
Type I Internal Derangement
Type II Internal Derangement
Type III Internal Derangement
Meniscus Perforation
Osteoarthritis
Rheumatoid Arthritis
Acute Infectious Arthritides
Miscellaneous Arthritides
Condylar Fracture
Synovial Chondromatosis
Pigmented Villonodular Synovitis
Odontogenic Infection†
Otitis Media§

SIALOGENIC PAIN

Sialolithiasis
Endemic Parotitis
Acute Suppurative Sialadenitis

TEMPORAL PAIN

Migraine
Myogenic Pain
Giant Cell Arteritis

PARESTHESIA

Mental Paresthesia
Infraorbital Paresthesia

LOCALIZED MOTOR DEFICITS

Facial Paralysis
Horner's Syndrome
Ophthalmoplegia
Hypoglossal Paralysis

---

*Refer to Maxillary Division Pain.
†Refer to Mandibular Division Pain.
‡Refer to TMJ Region Pain.
§Refer to Otogenic Pain.

Soft Palate Paralysis

LIMITED AND DEVIANT MANDIBULAR OPENING

Muscle Splinting
Myogenic Pain‡
Internal TMJ Derangement‡
Post-Injection/Post-Infection Trismus
Conversion Trismus
Subcondylar Fracture‡
Ankylosis
Hecht-Beals-Wilson Syndrome
Coronoid Hyperplasia
Condylar Hyperplasia

TMJ Region Neoplasms
Scleroderma
Tetanus

GENERALIZED MOTOR FUNCTION DISORDERS

Auriculotemporal Syndrome
Jaw-winking Syndrome
Motor System Disease
Multiple Sclerosis
Muscular Dystrophies
Myotonias
Congenital Facial Diplegia
Hemifacial Atrophy
Myasthenia Gravis

Pain in the maxillofacial region is usually and significantly a symptom heralding the presence of an infectious or inflammatory disease process. The more prevalent sources of facial pain include odontogenic infections, trauma, periodontal infections (abscess), sinusitis, otitis, salivary destruction, internal derangements of the temporomandibular joint (TMJ), and myofascial psychofunctional disorders. Most organic diseases manifest acute pain, whereas rare pain syndromes and psychogenic pain disorders are chronic. Patients who have organic disorders usually present obvious clinical signs uncovered by a thorough dental, oral, and facial physical examination. After appropriate tests have been performed (including sensitivity testing of teeth to hot and cold stimuli, percussion of teeth, occlusal stressing and fiberoptic evaluation for cracked teeth, vitalometric testing, and periodontal probing), a diagnosis can usually be rendered.

Many of the diseases included in this chapter show no identifiable organic lesions. They represent defects in sensory perception, vasodilatory phenomena, or symptoms associated with psychological disorders such as endogenous depression, conversion reactions, stress-associated myospasm, or delusionary phenomena. As mentioned previously, most of these disorders have not been found to be associated with any histopathologic alteration in the tissues and are usually characterized by chronic pain. Furthermore, paroxysmal chronic pain is more often seen as a symptom of trigeminal neuralgia or vasoactive pain (cluster or migrainous facial pain).

In order to aid the clinician in developing a differential diagnosis, the pain symptoms are classified according to location. The more common entities such as organic pain of odontogenic, periodontal, sinus, and salivary origin are described first, followed by the more esoteric entities representing vasoactive, neuralgic, and psychogenic disorders.

When no organic source for facial pain can be detected, the clinician is always concerned that a brain tumor or abscess is potentially causative. Lethal nervous system malignancies rarely cause facial pain; yet, when they do there is usually a persistent paresthesia with a concomitant deficit in motor function of ocular, facial, or masticatory muscles.

Many pain disorders share common symptoms. The specific disorders can often be differentiated from one another on the basis of the character, location, and duration of sensory alterations considered in conjunction with the physical and radiographic findings. A definitive diagnosis of some diseases requires an extensive workup, cranial nerve function tests, therapeutic trials, laboratory data, and expert psychiatric analysis. The characteristics allowing for a definitive diagnosis along with recommendations for the workup protocol are outlined for each entity.

The diagnosis of chronic facial pain can be problematic and evasive. In addition, those patients with psychiatric disorders are frequently demanding, abrasive, and otherwise difficult to manage; a team approach is recommended in such cases. Furthermore, the clinician should be advised that more than one process may be involved, and therefore more than one diagnosis may be made. For example, a given patient may suffer from concurrent myogenic pain, an internal derangement of the TMJ, and migraine headaches.

This chapter also includes motor function disorders that involve the muscles of facial expression and mastication. The gnathologic apparatus may be affected by diseases causing pain in the temporomandibular joint (TMJ) area. Some of these TMJ pain problems exhibit an attending motor defect such as limitation in opening or deviant function. Alternatively, jaw functional movements may exist in the absence of pain. TMJ diseases are included here under both categories. In addition, rare neurologic and muscular disease processes of a systemic nature can affect the facial musculature. Differentiation among the specific disorders requires evaluation of the muscle groups involved in paralysis or deviant function.

OPHTHALMIC DIVISION PAIN

Odontogenic Infection

Age: No predilection

Sex: No predilection

Clinical Features: Frontal pain of odontogenic origin is rare. It represents referred pain from an acute pulpitis or acute apical periodontitis associated with the maxillary incisors or canines. Pain is usually experienced in the infected tooth as well, yet occasionally may be referred solely to the medial supraorbital area. The frontal pain is a constant moderate ache with or without throbbing. Patients complaining of medial frontal pain should be examined for an incriminating anterior maxillary tooth; thus evaluation for dental caries, tooth percussion sensitivity, pulp test response, and periapical radiographic changes is required.

Differential Diagnosis: Odontogenic infection is easily differentiated from the other entities included here if the clinician is aware that dental infections can refer pain to this region.

Treatment: The infected tooth should be treated endodontically and subsequently restored with a crown of porcelain fused to metal. When evidence of suppuration is observed it is advisable to obtain a culture with sensitivity. When facial

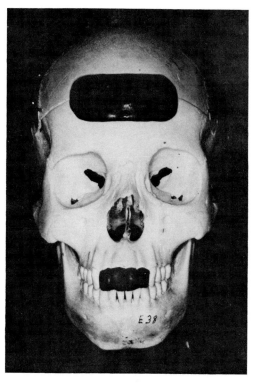

FIG. 12–1. Frontal pain referral from anterior maxillary odontogenic infection.

swelling and fever are present antibiotic therapy is indicated: a one-week course of penicillin or erythromycin for patients with penicillin allergy. In the absence of response, the possibility of staphylococcal or anaerobic infection must be considered with selection of appropriate antibiotics (e.g., cloxacillin or clindamycin, respectively).

References

1. Robertson, S., Goodell, H., and Wolff, H. G.: The teeth as a source of headache and other pain. Arch. Neurol. Psychiatr. 57:277, 1947.
2. Sicher, H.: Problems of pain in dentistry. Oral Surg. 7:149, 1954.
3. Glick, D. H.: Locating referred pulpal pains. Oral Surg. 15:613, 1962.
4. Olsen, R. E., Morello, J. A., and Keiff, E. D.: Antibiotic treatment of oral anaerobic infections. J. Oral Surg. 33:619, 1976.

Frontal Sinusitis

Age: Primarily adults

Sex: No predilection

Clinical Features: The frontal sinuses may be chronically inflamed due to allergy; patients will generally be asymptomatic, although some will

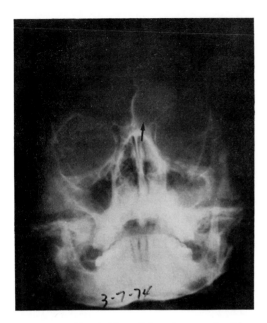

FIG. 12–2. Clouded frontal sinus in acute sinusitis.

complain of pressure or a mild dull ache. Allergic frontal sinusitis is rarely localized; the other sinus cavities are also inflamed, and chronic rhinitis is usually observed. Acute frontal sinusitis is usually infectious; it frequently occurs after water is forced into the nose, thus affecting swimmers. A deviated septum or presence of nasal polyps also may predispose to frontal sinusitis. The patient will complain of severe throbbing pain in the medial supraobital region. Water's sinus radiographs will generally exhibit opacification as a result of accumulation of a purulent exudate within the sinus cavity. Lowering the head will often exacerbate or intensify the pain. *Hemophilus influenzae* and anaerobic organisms are the more prevalent microbial agents. If left untreated, swelling and redness of the upper eyelid may be seen and brain abscess can occur.

Differential Diagnosis: Acute frontal sinusitis may be confused with referred pain of odontogenic origin. Dental examination and evaluation of sinus films will aid in arriving at a diagnosis. Myogenic pain involving the frontalis muscle is usually bilateral, dull, and diffuse; elevated electromyographic readings from the frontalis muscle will be encountered. The other disorders listed here manifest specific symptoms, allowing for exclusion from the differential diagnosis of acute ophthalmic division pain.

Treatment: Because the nasofrontal communication is usually blocked due to edema, a nasal decongestant spray should be used in conjunction with antibiotics. Penicillin or one of the cephalosporins is the antibiotic of choice. When the patient's response is poor, the sinus may require irrigation or surgical intervention.

References

1. Wilson, W. R. and Montgomery, W. M.: Infections and granulomas of the nasal airways and paranasal sinuses. In *Otolaryngology*, 2nd Ed., edited by M. M. Paparella and D. A. Shumrick. Philadelphia, W. B. Saunders Co., 1980, p. 1972.
2. Lehman, R. H.: Frontal sinus surgery. Acta Otolaryngol. (Suppl.) *270*, 1970.
3. Frederick, J. and Brande, A. I.: Anaerobic infection of the paranasal sinuses. N. Engl. J. Med. *290*:135, 1974.

Vascular Occlusive Disease and Aneurysms

Age: Adults
Sex: No predilection

Clinical Features: Thrombosis of the internal or common carotid may cause unilateral cranial edema with headache occurring on the affected side. Transient ischemia may also be associated with pain. Aneurysms and arteriovenous malformations have been associated with headache often mimicking migraine with contralateral visual disturbances; intracranial bruit is usually detectable. Ruptured aneurysms will lead to subarachnoid hemorrhage and often follow sexual intercourse or physical exertion. Other neurologic deficits are often encountered, including hemiparesis, third nerve palsy or palsy involving other cranial motor nerves. While some of these CNS vascular lesions cause parietal or occipital headache, many patients will complain of unilateral frontal and retro-orbital pain, which is frequently throbbing in nature.

Differential Diagnosis: When the classic signs and symptoms of both cluster and tension headache are lacking and frontal sinus and odontogenic pain sources have been excluded, a CNS lesion, either vascular or neoplastic, should be suspected. This is particularly true when other neurologic deficits can be detected.

Treatment: When other pain syndromes have been eliminated and a vascular occlusive or aneurysmal source is suspected, referral to a neurologist is recommended. A spinal tap, CT scans, and carotid angiograms are of great importance diagnostically for localizing the lesion.

References

1. Grindal, A. B. and Toole, J. F.: Headache and transient ischaemic attacks. Stroke 5:603, 1974.

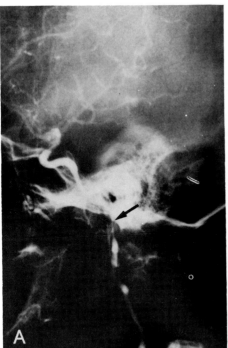 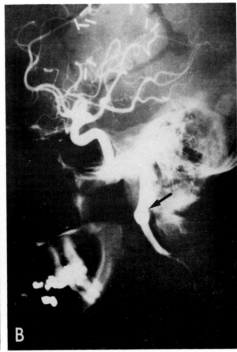

FIG. 12–3. Frontal area pain is occasionally associated with *A:* vascular occlusive disease or *B:* aneurysms (angiograms of carotid).

2. Mathew, N. T.: Headache of neurologic origin. In *Headache and Head Pain,* edited by R. E. Ryan, Sr. and R. E. Ryan, Jr. St. Louis, C. V. Mosby Co., 1978, Chap. 13.
3. Lance, J. W.: *Mechanisms and Management of Headache.* 3rd Ed., London, Butterworths, 1978, chap. 7.

MAXILLARY DIVISION PAIN

Odontogenic Infection

Age: No predilection

Sex: No predilection

Clinical Features: Maxillary teeth with pulpitis or pulp necrosis with acute apical periodontitis will exhibit pain in the maxilla. The pain will be localized to the infected tooth or may be diffusely distributed over the malar region. It is a dull aching pain or may progress to severe throbbing. The tooth will be sensitive to heat, cold, and/or percussion. Periapical radiographs should be obtained to evaluate for apical widening of the periodontal ligament space or a gross periapical radiolucency. When radiographs are negative and no carious lesions are encountered, fiberoptic examination for cracks should be performed. Local infiltration anesthesia may be used diagnostically.

Differential Diagnosis: A variety of pain syndromes affect the second division region of the trigeminal nerve. These disorders generally manifest characteristic symptoms, yet many of them mimic toothache. Identification of an acutely infected or necrotic tooth, relief of pain by infiltration anesthesia, and favorable response to analgesic drugs allow for a definitive diagnosis.

Treatment: Root canal therapy or extraction, when the affected tooth is nonrestorable, is the treatment of choice. When patients are febrile or show facial swelling, 10-day treatment with penicillin or erythromycin, in the presence of penicillin allergy, is advisable. Patients who do not respond should be reevaluated for staphylococcal penicillinase-positive organsims or anaerobes, especially bacteroides. In these instances, penicillinase-resistant antibiotics or clindamycin should be prescribed respectively.

References

1. Robertson, S., Goodell, H., and Wolff, H. G.: The teeth as a source of headache and other pain. Arch. Neurol. Psychiatr. 57:277, 1947.
2. Sicher, H.: Problems of pain in dentistry. Oral Surg. 7:149, 1954.
3. Glick, D. H.: Locating referred pulpal pains. Oral Surg. 15:613, 1962.

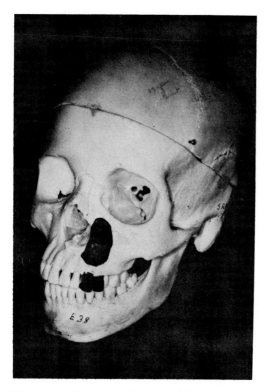

FIG. 12–4. Paranasal pain referred from maxillary odontogenic infection.

4. Chow, A. W., et al.: Oralfacial odontogenic infections. Ann. Intern. Med. 88:392, 1978.
5. Kannangara, D. W., Thadepelli, H., and McQuiter, J. L.: Bacteriology and treatment of dental infections. Oral Surg. 50:103, 1980.

Maxillary Sinusitis

Age: Adults

Sex: No predilection

Clinical Features: Chronic maxillary sinusitis is usually allergic in origin and develops secondary to chronic rhinitis. As the nasal mucous membranes become congested and edematous secondary to allergen:IgE mediated inflammation, the ostium of the maxillary sinus becomes occluded. The sinus membranes may become inflamed and thickened, or the antral cavity may partially or entirely fill with secretions. The pain is dull, aching, and constant. All posterior maxillary teeth on the affected side will ache and be sensitive to percussion; malar tenderness to percussion also may be witnessed. Pain increases when the head is lowered between the knees. Nasal examination discloses edematous and erythematous mucous membranes over the lateral wall and turbinates.

Water's sinus radiographs or maxillary sinus tomograms fail to show osseous destruction or expansion. The sinus membrane is thickened, a fluid level may be detected, or the entire antral cavity may be diffusely opacified. Acute sinusitis, which is usually infectious in origin, manifests similar radiographic changes; the patient experiences intense acute throbbing pain. In addition, a periodic purulent nasal discharge may be experienced and should be cultured. *Hemophilus influenzae, Streptococcus pneumoniae,* and *Staphylococcus aureus* are the bacteria most frequently cultured. Occasionally, acute sinusitis is caused by odontogenic infection, thus necessitating a thorough dental examination.

Differential Diagnosis: Chronic maxillary sinusitis may have features suggesting odontogenic infection. Cluster headaches and trigeminal neualgia are severe and paroxysmal. Neoplasms of sinus or cranial base origin generally manifest a sensory and/or motor deficit. Dull aching pain with rhinitis, congestion, and pandental percussion sensitivity in the affected maxilla along with radiographic evidence of nondestructive antral disease are usually adequate signs and symptoms for diagnosis. If osseous destruction or expansion is noted radiographically, an antral biopsy should be performed.

Treatment: Chronic sinusitis should be treated with nasal decongestant sprays such as neosynephrine and antihistamines. Occasionally, sinus irrigation and lavage will be necessary. Acute sinusitis should be treated promptly with penicillin or erythromycin, in the presence of penicillin allergy; if a purulent exudate is present, culture and sensitivity tests are required.

References

1. Evans, F. O., Jr., et al.: Sinusitis of the maxillary antrum. N. Engl. J. Med. 293:735, 1975.
2. Eichel, B. S.: The medical and surgical approach in management of the unilateral opacified antrum. Laryngoscope 87:737, 1977.
3. Ryan, R. E., Jr. and Kern, E. B.: Rhinologic causes of facial pain and headache. Headache 18:44, 1978.

Pathologic Jawbone Cavities

Age: Middle-aged and elderly adults

Sex: No predilection

Clinical Features: The existence of radiologically nondemonstrable bone cavities in extraction site foci within the jaws has been reported to be etiologically related to both atypical facial pain and trigeminal neuralgia. The maxilla is more

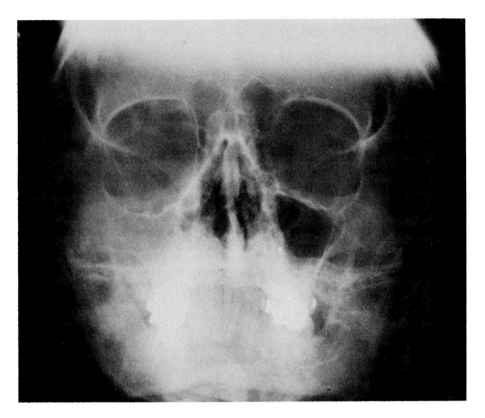

FIG. 12–5. Clouded sinus in chronic maxillary sinusitis.

commonly affected than the mandible; however, many patients experience both maxillary and mandibular pain. The focus is usually located within one jaw with upper-to-lower or lower-to-upper pain referral patterns. Patients may complain of classic trigeminal neuralgia symptoms with an identifiable trigger zone, or they may present with constant, dull, aching, or burning pain with unilateral distribution. The pain develops after tooth extraction either immediately or many years later. In the absence of odontogenic or antrogenic infection, radiographs are used to identify edentulous zones on the ipsilateral side for diagnostic infiltration anesthesia. Three percent mepivicaine, .25 ml, is injected subperiosteally over the suspected site. Abolition of pain then warrants surgical exploration of the edentulous region. Failure to achieve pain relief by local infiltration anesthesia requires readministration to a closely adjacent site until pain ablation is achieved, thereby precisely pinpointing the location of the suspected bone cavity. Surgery will reveal cavitation of the medullary region with soft tissue contents. His-

tologically, these bone cavities are represented by vascular connective tissue and occasionally exhibit a mononuclear inflammatory cell infiltrate. Microbiological studies have disclosed the presence of a mixed aerobic anaerobic flora.

Differential Diagnosis: Odontogenic and antrogenic sources of pain should be ruled out initially. Reported pain referral patterns associated with pathologic bone cavities are often diffuse and may extend beyond the alveolus to involve the maxillary, temporal or TMJ regions; therefore, myogenic facial pain, internal derangements of the TMJ, and temporal arteritis should be considered in the differential diagnosis. Elimination of pain with local infiltration anesthesia over an extraction site supports a diagnosis of bone cavity–related neuralgia.

Treatment: One week prior to surgery the patient is given 1,600,000 units of penicillin daily, and this treatment must continue for 1 month following disappearance of pain. The edentulous site is approached surgically after a flap reflection. The contents are curetted and the space is packed with gauze impregnated with 500 mg tetracycline/ml sterile water. This packing is replaced until healthy granulation tissue appears, after which the packing is removed. Chloromycetin also has been used in the packing. It should be noted that most studies reporting this form of treatment for facial pain have not included follow-up evaluation over 18 months for the majority of patients; however, a small number of cases have been pain free for 2 to 5 years.

References

1. Ratner, E. J., et al.: Jawbone cavities and trigeminal and atypical facial neuralgias. Oral Surg. *48*:3, 1979.
2. Roberts, A. M. and Person, P.: Etiology and treatment of idiopathic trigeminal and atypical facial neuralgias. Oral Surg. *48*:298, 1979.
3. Shaber, E. P. and Krol, A. J.: Trigeminal neuralgia— A new treatment concept. Oral Surg. *49*:286, 1980.

Antral and Maxillary Neoplasms

Age: Predilection dependent on nature of disease
Sex: Male predilection

Clinical Features: Maxillary and antral neoplasms are often asymptomatic in the early stages of proliferation. Pain may develop later in the course of the disease and is usually accompanied by paresthesia. Infraorbital paresthesia and pain occur when the neoplasm, usually a malignant tumor, grows superiorly to involve the sinus roof. Antral carcinomas often undergo foci of necrosis with secondary infection, which can result in release of endogenous pain mediators. The pain is usually deep seated and may be maxillary, retro-orbital or dental in distribution. Water's radiographs, maxillary sinus tomograms, and CT scans

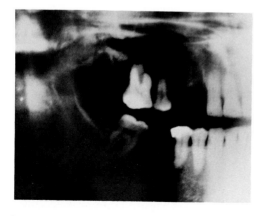

FIG. 12–6. Antral carcinoma with alveolar bone resorption around maxillary teeth.

will disclose diffuse antral opacification with sinus wall erosion.

Differential Diagnosis: Pain associated with sinus cancer is usually coexistent with paresthesia. Occasionally, no sensory deficit will be encountered. In these instances, the pain symptoms will mimic odontogenic pain or acute sinusitis. Radiographic opacification along with sinus wall erosion or expansion warrants a Caldwell-Luc access with biopsy.

Treatment: Most sinus tumors with pain and paresthesia are malignant. Squamous cell carcinoma and adenocarcinoma are managed by hemimaxillectomy. Because the tumor may perforate into the nasal cavity, other paranasal sinuses, or the cranium, a thorough clinical and radiographic evaluation is needed to determine the extent of disease and the form of treatment.

References

1. Boles, R.: Paransal Sinuses and Facial Pain. In *Facial Pain,* 2nd Ed., edited by E. C. Alling III and P. E. Mahan. Philadelphia, Lea & Febiger, 1977, pp. 120–122.
2. Frazell, E. L. and Lewis, J. S.: Cancer of the nasal cavity and accessory sinuses; a report of the management of 416 patients. Cancer *16*:1293, 1963.

Cluster Headache

Age: Middle-aged adults
Sex: Male predilection

Clinical Features: A variety of eponymic designations, which relate to the precise location of pain, have been applied to a group of midface' vasoactive headaches (Vail's syndrome, Horton's headache, Sluder's neuralgia, Charlin's syndrome). Sphenopalatine neuralgia, vidian neuralgia, petrosal neuralgia, and ciliary neuralgia are all forms of midface cluster or vasoactive headaches. Two clinical presentations are observed. The *chronic* form persists throughout the year, whereas the *episodic* form is seasonal with pain attacks being more frequent in the spring. In both forms the nature of the pain attacks is similar. The pain is severe and sharp, lasting 15 to 20 minutes, being unilaterally located in the maxilla, retro-orbital, or supraorbital region. There is no trigger zone. The attacks occur once or twice daily, and nocturnal episodes following REM sleep are common. There are no visual scotomata or other "aura" prodromal changes as seen in classic migraines. The concurrent observation of ipsilateral conjunctival erythema, palpebral edema, lacrimation, and nasal stuffiness is significant diagnostically. Patients with cluster headache often ex-

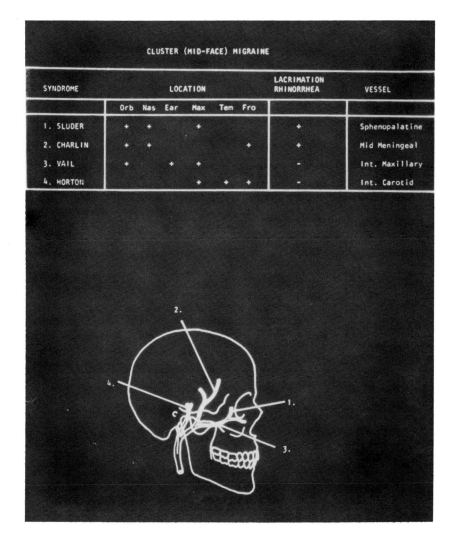

SYNDROME	LOCATION						LACRIMATION RHINORRHEA	VESSEL
	Orb	Nas	Ear	Max	Tem	Fro		
1. SLUDER	+	+		+			+	Sphenopalatine
2. CHARLIN	+	+			+		+	Mid Meningeal
3. VAIL	+		+	+			-	Int. Maxillary
4. HORTON			+	+	+		-	Int. Carotid

CLUSTER (MID-FACE) MIGRAINE

FIG. 12–7. Vessels involved in vasodilation cluster headache.

hibit a ruddy facial complexion. Alcoholism, peptic ulcer, and hypertension are also common concomitants. While the cause is unknown, vasodilation of the cranial or internal maxillary artery branches is thought to be pathogenetically related to the condition. Platelet-rich plasma serotonin and histamine are elevated while the platelet count is decreased during attacks. Electroencephalograms, CT scans, and radionucleotide brain scans are usually normal.

Differential Diagnosis: Cluster headaches, being paroxysmal, may be confused with trigeminal neuralgia involving the maxillary division. Absence of a trigger zone, presence of autonomic signs and symptoms (lacrimation, nasal stuffiness, conjunctival erythema) and other aforementioned features are characteristic for cluster headache. The other lesions causing maxillary pain fail to manifest the episodic paroxysmal symptoms of cluster headache.

Treatment: In the past, the treatment of choice has been sublingual ergotamine tartrate or cafergot rectal suppositories, which are used during a pain attack. Methysergide and prednisone are effective in the prevention of cluster headache, and calcium channel blockers have been shown to be efficacious. Administration of 100 percent oxygen at 7 liters per minute flow is more effective for aborting pain if given at the onset of the attack. Importantly, ergot alkaloids are contraindicated in patients with hypertension, cardiac, or cerebral vascular occlusive disease.

References

1. Friedman, A. and Mikropoulos, H. E.: Cluster headaches. Neurology 8:63, 1958.
2. Kudrow, L.: Prevalence of migraine, peptic ulcer, coronary heart disease and hypertension in cluster headache. Headache 16:66, 1976.
3. Kudrow, L.: Cluster headache: diagnosis and management. Headache 19:142, 1979.
4. Medina, J. L., Diamond, S., and Fareed, J.: The nature of cluster headache. Headache 19:309, 1979.
5. Kudrow, L.: Response of cluster headache attacks to oxygen inhalation. Headache 21:1, 1981.

Trigeminal Neuralgia

Age: Middle-aged and elderly adults
Sex: Slight female predilection

Clinical Features: Trigeminal neuralgia or tic douloureux is a pain syndrome involving the trigeminal nerve divisions and is of unknown etiology. It has been speculated that this neuralgia is the result of ganglionic compression over the petrous ridge or by an artery or vein. Electron microscopic evidence of myelin degeneration of nerves is observed; these findings support a peripheral etiology and suggest a herpetic ganglioneuritis. The clinical symptoms are unique and diagnostic. The pain is sudden, paroxysmal, severe, and stabbing; it follows one or more divisions of the trigeminal nerve. The right side of the face is most frequently affected, and the pain is precipitated by touching a specific area of the skin or mucous membrane referred to as a "trigger zone." A patient's trigger zone is localized consistently in the same region, usually at the lip commissure or the nasal ala. Local anesthetic infiltration of the trigger zone will temporarily cause the pain to abate. During the early onset of pain paroxysms, a discrete trigger zone may not be apparent. In addition to pain, many patients experience paresthesia along the involved nerve division. Most cases are unilateral with 5 percent of patients developing bilateral involvement. It should be noted that the symptoms of trigeminal neuralgia are occasionally encountered in association with a CNS neoplasm. Also, trigeminal neuralgia is known to occur in a minority of patients with multiple sclerosis and progressive systemic sclerosis (scleroderma).

Differential Diagnosis: Sharp stabbing paroxysmal pain with identification of a discrete trigger zone allows for a straight-forward clinical diagnosis. Atypical trigeminal neuralgias, which have no discrete trigger zone, may be confused with other facial pain syndromes such as midface cluster headache and psychogenic atypical facial pain. Eventually, a trigger zone will become evident in most instances. Since neoplasia may, albeit rarely, underlie the condition, both brain and CT scans are recommended.

Treatment: The treatment of choice is carbamazepine or carbamazepine with Dilantin. High doses of carbamazepine induce bone marrow suppression, thus necessitating regular blood count monitoring. Some patients cannot tolerate the drugs and are candidates for thermal nucleolysis, peripheral neurectomy, or vascular decompression neurosurgical intervention. Surgical treatment is temporary when peripheral neurectomies are performed, offering, on the average, 1½ to 2 years of pain relief. Radiofrequency thermal nucleolysis to specific tracts within the trigeminal ganglion is effective, yet pain often recurs within 1 or 2 years. Because the procedure is not particularly invasive, it can be readministered. Vascular decompression of the ganglion is also effective, yet not universally.

References

1. Peet, M. M. and Schneider, R. C.: Trigeminal neuralgia: a review of six hundred and eighty-nine cases with a follow-up study on sixty-five percent of the group. J. Neurosurg. 9:367, 1952.
2. Kerr, F. W. L.: Pathology of trigeminal neuralgia: light and electron microscopic observations. J. Neurosurg. 26:151, 1967.
3. Jannetta, P. J.: Trigeminal neuralgia and hemifacial spasm—etiology and definitive treatment. Trans. Am. Neurol. Assoc. 100:89, 1975.
4. Quinn, J. H. and Weil,. T.: Trigeminal neuralgia: treatment by repetitive peripheral neurectomy. Supplemental report. J. Oral Surg. 33:591, 1975.
5. Sweet, W. H.: Treatment of facial pain by percutaneous differential thermal trigeminal rhizotomy. Prog. Neurol. Surg. 7:153, 1976.
6. Taarhj, P.: Decompression of the posterior trigeminal root in trigeminal neuralgia. A 30-year follow-up review. J. Neurosurg. 57:14, 1982.

Postherpetic Neuralgia

Age: Middle-aged and elderly adults
Sex: No predilection

Clinical Features: Varicella-zoster infection, causing herpes zoster or shingles, results in a painful vesicular eruption along sensory nerve pathways. The virus initially infects sensory ganglia and subsequently disseminates along the sensory nerve terminals in skin or mucosa. The lesions persist for 2 to 3 weeks and are accompanied by a stinging pain. When the trigeminal ganglion is infected the lesions generally localize in the region

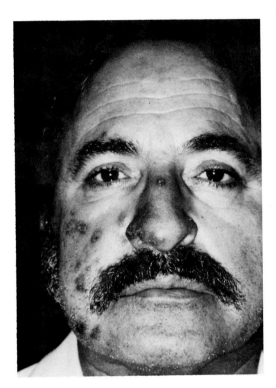

FIG. 12–8. Herpes zoster vesicular lesions precede the onset of postherpetic neuralgia.

of the ophthalmic division; however, both maxillary and mandibular divisions may be involved. In older patients, the pain may persist after the lesions have resolved; if this symptom prevails after 6 to 8 weeks, the condition represents postherpetic neuralgia. The character of the pain changes somewhat in that stinging is replaced by burning, aching, and paresthesia. This pain is usually chronic and persistent. Scarified zones in areas of old vesicular lesions are hypesthetic when pinched with a needle. The pain may persist for months or even years following infection and, needless to say, results in tremendous emotional upset. Occasionally, paroxysmal stabbing pains mimic trigeminal neuralgia, although trigger zones are lacking.

Differential Diagnosis: The pain of postherpetic neuralgia is limited to a single division of the trigeminal nerve in most instances, and is restricted to the superficial skin or mucosal surfaces. Nevertheless, it may be confused with trigeminal neuralgia or even cluster headache. A history of vesicular eruption (shingles) is diagnostic.

Treatment: Postherpetic neuralgia is difficult to

control. Cutaneous stimulation with an electric physiologic stimulator offers some degree of palliation. Chlorprothixene, one of the thioxanthenes, administered in 25-mg doses 3 to 4 times daily is often effective.

References

1. Sugar, O. and Bucy, P. C.: Postherpetic trigeminal neuralgia. Arch. Neurol. Psychiatr. 65:131, 1951.
2. Russell, W. R., et al.: Treatment of post-herpetic neuralgia. Lancet 1:242, 1957.
3. Woodforde, J. M., et al.: Treatment of post-herpetic neuralgia. Med. J. Aust. 2:869, 1965.
4. Farber, G. A. and Burks, J. W.: Chlorprothixene therapy for herpes zoster neuralgia. S. Med. J. 67:808, 1974.
5. Kramer, P. W.: The management of postherpetic neuralgia with chlorprothixene. Surg. Neurol. 15:102, 1981.

Causalgia

Age: Adults

Sex:; No predilection

Clinical Features: This rare facial pain syndrome is usually localized to the extremities following an episode of severe trauma. Facial causalgia is characterized by hyperesthesia of the affected skin; often, a trophic response is observed with erythema and dermatitis. The pain is burning and may be deep, yet there is invariably a superficial component. A light touch or even a blast of air will provoke a hyperesthetic response. The pain may be constant or episodic, and in some cases cutaneous erythema is observed during intensity peaks; this vasodilation phenomenon subsequently wanes. Facial trauma or surgery usually precedes onset of the syndrome. The mechanism is not clearly understood; however, mediation by the sympathetic nervous system appears to be an important factor. Afferent nociceptor pathways are apparently stimulated by locally released catecholamines. A stellate ganglion block with bupivacaine will cause relief of symptoms and is therefore the most important diagnostic tool when causalgia is suspected.

Differential Diagnosis: A variety of facial pain syndromes should be included in the differential diagnosis. Many cases of causalgia have probably gone undiagnosed, being labeled as atypical facial pain. Hyperesthesia, burning pain, vasodilatory cutaneous signs, and a history of facial surgery or trauma should alert the clinician to the probability of causalgia. Abolition of pain subsequent to a stellate ganglion block will confirm the diagnosis.

Treatment: Biweekly stellate ganglion blocks, confirmed by initiation of Horner's syndrome, will

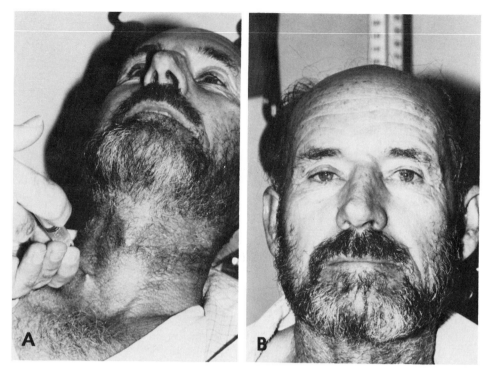

FIG. 12–9.   Causalgia. *A:* Stellate ganglion block. *B:* Resultant Horner's syndrome and pain relief.

often be curative after six to ten injections. If relief is not achieved, surgical stellate ganglion sympathectomy may be required. This will, of course, result in a permanent hemifacial sympathetic blockade with ptosis, miosis, and anhidrosis.

References

1. Elfenbaum, A.: Causalgia in dentistry: an abandoned pain syndrome. Oral Surg. *7:*594, 1954.
2. Hanowell, S. T. and Kennedy, S. F.: Phantom tongue pain in causalgia: a case presentation and treatment. Anesth. Analg. *58:*436, 1979.
3. Khoury, R., Kennedy, S. F., and Macnamara, T. E.: Facial causalgia: report of case. J. Oral Surg. *38:*782, 1980.

Cranial Base and CNS Neoplasms

Age: Adults
Sex: No predilection

Clinical Features: Neurologic deficits are encountered in neoplastic processes that encroach on cranial nerves above or below the exit through the cranial base foramina. Metastatic tumors to the cranial base or middle fossa, cerebellopontine angle tumors, and nasopharyngeal tumors will often compress or invade one or two, or all three divisions of the trigeminal nerve, thus resulting in paresthesia, hypesthesia, and/or pain. The fact that a sensory deficit or pain symptom is rarely encountered in the absence of a motor deficit is significant. While a variety of eponymic syndromes have been described depending upon the localization of signs and symptoms, the commonality is tumor compression of nerves. Many of these eponymic syndromes exhibit overlapping features that are confusing to the clinician; therefore, a topographical nosology is more practical. Malignant disease of the orbit, the *orbital syndrome,* causes supraorbital pain and hypesthesia, blurred vision or diplopia, ptosis, and/or ophthalmoplegia. Tumors encroaching on the cavernous sinus, the *parasellar syndrome,* compress the first division of the fifth nerve as well as nerves three, four, and six; the result is frontal pain and ophthalmoplegia. The *middle fossa syndrome* occurs in patients with neoplastic disease in the region of the gasserian ganglion. While hypesthesia, paresthesia, and pain of the second and third divisions are common, numbness without pain also is encountered. Ocular muscle paralysis is common, and paresis of the masticatory muscles may be detected (i.e., deviated mandibular opening, mas-

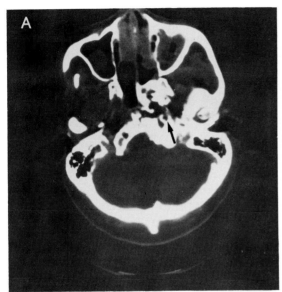
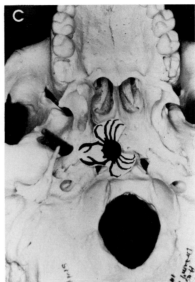
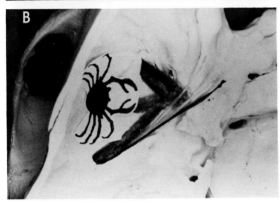

FIG. 12–10. *A:* CT scan illustrating a cranial base chondrosarcoma with sphenoid sinus extension. *B:* Site of tumor in parasellar syndrome in relation to trigeminal and ocular motor nerves. *C:* Site of nasopharyngeal/cranial base tumor in relation to V-3 and motor root of the trigeminal nerve.

seteric weakness, unilateral soft palate paralysis, etc.). Foramina or intracranial extension by a nasopharyngeal carcinoma may cause similar signs and symptoms including a unilateral hearing deficit due to eustachian tube extension. The *jugular foramen syndrome* is characterized by dysphagia, hoarseness, glossopharyngeal neuralgia-like pain, palate weakness, and vocal cord paralysis. Hypoglossal weakness is also common, but it occurs more frequently in the *occipital condyle syndrome,* which is heralded by occipital pain that is exacerbated by neck flexion.

Differential Diagnosis: Malignant neoplasia that is primary within the central nervous system, secondary to nasopharyngeal extension, or metastatic may cause facial pain and be confused with a variety of local pain syndromes. The triad of sensory deficit (numbness or paresthesia), pain, and motor deficit (ocular, masticatory, facial, or glossal) constitutes an ominous finding. Although routine radiographs often fail to uncover a lesion, CT scans will reveal a pathologic process. A history of cancer may indicate the probability of cranial base metastasis.

Treatment: Any patient with pain, numbness, and cranial nerve motor weakness should be evaluated by a neurologist; a CT scan of the cranium should be performed. Treatment will be determined when the process has been definitively diagnosed.

References

1. Thomas, J. E. and Yoss, R. E.: The parasellar syndrome: problems determining etiology. Mayo Clin. Proc. 45:617, 1970.
2. Horowitz, S.: Isolated facial numbness. Ann. Intern. Med. 80:49, 1974.
3. Svien, H. J., Baker, H. L., and River, M. H.: Jugular foramen syndrome and allied syndromes. Neurology 13:797, 1963.
4. Greenberg, H. S.: Metastasis to the base of the skull: clinical findings in 43 patients. Neurology 31:530, 1981.

Atypical Facial Pain

Age: Middle-aged adults
Sex: Female predilection

Clinical Features: Atypical facial pain occurs in the maxilla or the mandible, but current evaluative and diagnostic methods do not reveal an organic cause. The diagnosis requires exclusion of other known pain syndromes including the true neuralgias, vasoactive headaches, and myogenic pain disorders. Then one is left with a pain patient whose signs, symptoms, or chemical and laboratory findings do not allow for a definitive diagnosis. By exclusion, one attaches the appellation "atypical facial pain," which probably includes a heterogeneous constellation of disorders. *Pathologic jawbone cavities* have been identified in some of these patients and are discussed separately. The symptoms of atypical pain are inconsistent from one patient to the next. Some patients complain of localized dull aches; others say the pain is dull and wanders from one site to another; yet others complain of paroxysms of acute pain without a trigger zone. Many instances of atypical facial pain probably represent symptoms of a psychiatric disorder, usually depression or histrionic personality. *Post-herpetic ganglioneuritis* associated with herpes simplex may be responsible for some instances of atypical pain, particularly when mild paresthesia is present or motor weakness of facial muscles is observed. There is no hard data to support a viral etiology; however, demyelinating peripheral lesions can follow herpes hominis infections and could eventuate in pain, paresthesia, and seventh or fifth nerve motor weakness. *Atypical odontalgia* can be included as a form of atypical facial pain. Patients complain of aching pain in a tooth or group of teeth in which objective pulp testing and radiographs fail to show evidence of pulpal disease. These patients are insistent and demand endodontic therapy or extraction. Typically, endodontic therapy is given, but pain persists; then apicoectomy is performed, but pain

continues. Ultimately, the tooth is removed; subsequently, the patient complains of pain in an adjacent tooth. In these instances, psychogenic causes should be suspected. The clinician should consider depression and conversion symptoms with secondary gain or guilt complex.

Differential Diagnosis: The symptoms encountered in atypical facial pain can mimic organic, neuralgic, vasoactive, or myogenic pain syndromes. The clinician is obliged to rule out odontogenic, antrogenic, and sialogenic sources first. Secondly, muscle palpation and muscle trigger point tenderness should be assessed with subcutaneous or intramuscular local anesthesia to evaluate elimination of myogenic referred pain to teeth or the jaws. When edentulous regions are observed, a pathologic bone cavity should be considered; selective infiltration anesthesia is useful diagnostically. While central neural or cranial base neoplasms may cause facial pain, they rarely do so in the absence of paresthesia or motor deficit.

Treatment: Unfortunately, and by definition, the causal process is unknown. When a psychogenic origin is suspected, patients rarely accept this diagnosis and refuse psychiatric care. A 6-week trial of tricyclic antidepressant therapy is recommended. This treatment has been beneficial for some patients with atypical facial pain.

References

1. Marbach, J. J., et al.: Incidence of phantom tooth pain: An atypical facial neuralgia. Oral Surg. 53:190, 1982.
2. Kreisberg, M. K.: Atypical odontalgia: differential diagnosis and treatment. J. Am. Dent. Assoc. 104:852, 1982.
3. Brooke, R. I.: Atypical odontalgia. Oral Surg. 49:196, 1980.
4. Denaley, J. F.: Atypical facial pain as a defense against psychosis. Am. J. Psychol. 133:1151, 1976.
5. Adour, K. K., Hilsinger, R. L., Jr., and Byl, F. M.: Herpes simplex polyganglionitis. Otolaryngol. Head Neck Surg. 88:270, 1980.

MANDIBULAR DIVISION PAIN

Odontogenic Infection

Age: No predilection
Sex: No predilection

Clinical Features: The most common cause of mandibular pain is odontogenic infection. The pain is usually sharp and severe in acute pulpitis. Sensitivity to heat, cold, and percussion is characteristic. The pain often awakens the patient or prevents sleep. In most instances, clinical and radiographic examination will disclose a large car-

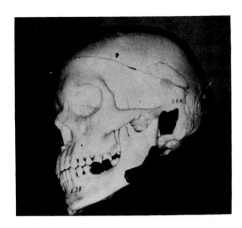

FIG. 12–11. Pain referral routes to TMJ, ear, and mandibular angle from mandibular odontogenic infection.

ious lesion encroaching on the pulp or pulp horns. Acute pain during mastication or when firm lateral pressure is applied to cusps and the presence of cold sensitivity are indicative of tooth fracture. Fiberoptic light examination will often uncover a fracture line; however, some fractures underlie restorations, thus necessitating removal of the material prior to fiberoptic examination. Dull chronic aching pain is more often associated with periapical disease related to a necrotic tooth. Alternatively, many patients with pulp necrosis and periapical granulomas or cysts are pain free or have a history of pain that eventually resolved. Radiographs will uncover a periapical radiolucency, and the tooth will fail to respond to electrical pulp test stimulation. Most teeth with pulp necrosis are grossly carious. A maxillary tooth seldom refers pain to the mandible. Furthermore, the pain, particularly in molar teeth, may be referred to the TMJ and ear.

Differential Diagnosis: Most mandibular pains are of odontogenic origin; therefore, a dental source should be sought before other pain syndromes involving the third division of the trigeminal nerve are considered. The suspected tooth (teeth) should be tested with heat, cold, percussion, electrical stimulation, and fiberoptics; radiographs should be obtained. When no dental source can be uncovererd in the mandible, the maxillary dentition should be evaluated. Periodontal probing should be undertaken, after all dental sources are ruled out, if a periodontal abscess cannot be found easily. Failure to uncover either a dental or periodontal source of the pain

will direct attention to other pain syndromes included in this section.

Treatment: Restorable teeth should be treated endodontically. In some cases, cracked teeth can be managed by full crown coverage; however, large cracks may require extraction. When fever or a facial swelling is present, penicillin or erythromycin (when patients are allergic to penicillin) should be prescribed for 10 days. Response failure may indicate penicillinase-producing organisms or anaerobes. In these instances, penicillinase resistant antibiotics or clindamycin should be used respectively.

References:
1. Glick, D. H.: Locating referred pulpal pains. Oral Surg. *15*:613, 1962.
2. Chow, A. W., et al.: Oralfacial odontogenic infections. Ann. Intern. Med. *88*:392, 1978.
3. Kannangara, D. W., Thadepelli, H., and McQuiter, J. L.: Bacteriology and treatment of dental infections. Oral Surg. *50*:103, 1980.

Traumatic Neuroma

Age: Middle-aged and elderly adults
Sex: Male predilection

Clinical Features: Severance of a nerve trunk will result in axonal degeneration of the distal segment with regeneration by the proximal axonal segment, which canalizes the distal nerve sheath tract. When the severed nerve ends are not readily approximated, the regenerating axon may, in the process of searching for the distal sheath, become hyperplastic and tortuous, creating a painful nodule. Traumatic neuromas of soft tissue are usually

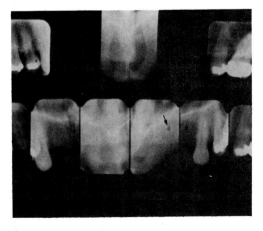

FIG. 12–12. Small radiolucency in anterior maxilla representing a traumatic neuroma causing severe pain. These lesions are actually more common in the mandible.

detected visually as swelling, or they are palpable. Compression will initiate pain. Occasionally, traumatic neuromas arise central in bone subsequent to tooth extraction or alveolar bone trauma. The pain is deep, intraosseous,and can be moderate or severe. The canine and mental foramen areas are the most common sites; the pain can be triggered by denture pressure or digital compression over the involved area, simulating a trigger zone in trigeminal neuralgia. Local anesthesia will eliminate the symptoms. Occasionally, a radiolucency can be seen on periapical films.

Differential Diagnosis: When compression of a palpable nodule overlying the mental foramen or alveolus causes a pain paroxysm, traumatic neuroma should be suspected. Alternatively, centrally located neuromas are not palpable, and the pain episodes may mimic trigeminal neuralgia or be classified as atypical facial pain. Any radiolucency in the vicinity of the pain should be tested for abolition of pain by local infiltration anesthesia; pending a positive result, the area should be explored surgically.

Treatment: Painful nodules or radiolucent foci suspected of representing traumatic neuroma should be excised. A definitive diagnosis requires microscopic confirmation. Step serial sections may be needed to identify the neuromatous tissue in marrow curettings.

References

1. Robinson, M. and Slavkin, H. C.: Dental amputation neuromas. J. Am. Dent. Assoc. 70:662, 1965.
2. Trodahl, J. M. and Carroll, G. W.: Traumatic neuroma of the mandibular ridge. Oral Surg. 24:563, 1967.
3. Rasmussen, O. C.: Painful traumatic neuromas in the oral cavity. Oral Surg. 49:191, 1980.

Subacute Thyroiditis

Age: Middle-aged adults
Sex: Female predilection

Clinical Features: Subacute thyroiditis usually evolves subsequent to an upper respiratory infection; the prevailing evidence supports a viral etiology, probably coxsackievirus. The pain, which is located in the thyroid region, is aggravated by swallowing or turning the head. Pain radiation to the mandible, ear, and/or occipital region is a common finding; indeed, the patient's chief complaint may be jaw pain. Other symptoms include nervousness, palpitations, and lassitude. Fever may be severe. Palpation of the thyroid will disclose diffuse swelling and acute tenderness. The overlying skin is often erythematous. Occasion-

ally, the disease is asymptomatic. Most patients are euthyroid with normal thyroid function tests. The condition usually resolves of its own accord within 4 to 6 weeks.

Differential Diagnosis: Acute thyroiditis with mandibular pain being the primary complaint may be mistaken for a variety of organic and functional diseases involving the mandibular nerve distribution. In addition, the styloid and hyoid syndromes, carotidynia, and cardiogenic pain may be suspected. Elevated temperature and exquisite pain on palpation of the thyroid gland will usually suffice for the clinical diagnosis. Tenderness and pain on palpation are rarely featured in goiter, Graves' disease, Hashimoto's thyroiditis, or thyroid neoplasia.

Treatment: Palliative care includes the use of analgesics and antipyretics. The disease is self-limited and while thyrotoxicosis has been reported to occur, most patients fail to suffer from any residual thyrometabolic complications.

References

1. Papapetrou, P. D. and Jackson, I.: Thyrotoxicosis due to "silent" thyroiditis. Lancet 1:361, 1975.
2. Volpe, R.: Acute and subacute thyroiditis. Pharmac. Ther. 1:171, 1976.
3. Ingbar, S. H. and Woeber, K. A.: The Thyroid Gland. In Textbook of Endocrinology, 6th Ed., edited by R. H. Williams. Philadelphia, W. B. Saunders, 1981, pp. 241–243.
4. Smith, M. J. A. and Myall, R. W. T.: Subacute thyroiditis as a cause of facial pain. Oral Surg. 43:59, 1977.

Stomatodynia/Glossopyrosis

Age: Middle-aged and elderly adults
Sex: Female predilection

Clinical Features: Burning mouth or tongue (glossopyrosis) is a common symptom and in younger patients is usually associated with one of the vesiculo-bullous-ulcerative diseases. Older patients may also present with this symptom in the absence of oral lesions. Rarely, burning tongue is a symptom in patients with organic diseases including pernicious anemia and diabetes mellitus. In the former, the tongue is often beefy red and denuded of papillae. Most elderly patients with stomatodynia suffer from psychiatric illness with chronic depression being the most prevalent diagnosis. Loss of enthusiasm, sleep disturbances, loss of libido and concurrent anxiety are often present. Patients with long-standing endogenous depression will usually manifest an elevated blood cortisol after challenge with oral steroids (dexamethasone suppression test). Guilt, conversion reactions, and overt schizophrenia may be encountered; many of these patients are cancerophobic as well.

Differential Diagnosis: A fasting blood sugar or, preferably, a two-hour postprandial glucose should be obtained along with a hemogram in order to rule out diabetes and megaloblastic anemia, respectively. Negative laboratory findings and normal-appearing oral soft tissues lead to a diagnosis of psychogenic stomatodynia. A psychiatric workup augmented with psychometric testing (e.g., MMPI) and a dexamethasone suppression test will aid in establishing a diagnosis of depressive illness.

Treatment: Once a diagnosis of depression has been confirmed, treatment with one of the tricyclic antidepressants should be instituted. Doxepin, 100 mg 2 hours before retiring, can be prescribed for one week; a final dosage of 200 to 250 mg per day will affect an elevation in mood with resolution of pain symptoms for most patients. Beneficial results usually require 3 or 4 weeks of therapy. When medical treatment has proven efficacious, psychotherapy should be considered.

References

1. Ziskin, D. E. and Moulton, R.: Glossodynia: a study of idiopathic orolingual pain. J. Am. Dent. Assoc. 33:1422, 1946.
2. Schoenberg, B.: Psychogenic aspects of the burning mouth. New York Dent. J. 33:467, 1967.
3. Schoenberg, B., et al.: Chronic idiopathic orolingual pain. Psychogenesis of burning mouth. New York State. J. Med. 71:1832, 1971.
4. Brooke, R. I. and Seganski, D. P.: Aetiology and investigation of the sore mouth. J. Canad. Dent. Assn. 43:504, 1977.

Cardiogenic Facial Pain

Age: Middle-aged and elderly adults
Sex: Male predilection

Clinical Features: While myocardial ischemia classically produces angina pectoris with referred pain over the left shoulder and down the arm, the pain is occasionally referred to the left mandible. Indeed, some patients may complain of jaw pain without a substernal component. Pain referred to the mandible has been explained on the basis of converging nociceptor pathways from cardiac pain fibers that ascend the cord subsequent to synapsing in the thoracic dorsal horn and communicate with neurons located in the subnucleus caudalis of the trigeminal nerve. Typically, the pain is precipitated by exertion or stress and is usually described as an ache. Administration of a nitroglycerin tablet sublingually will usually, yet not invariably, relieve the symptoms. An electrocardiogram will often display S-T or T wave anomalies indicative of myocardial ischemia. It should be emphasized that a normal resting ECG does not rule out coronary vascular disease.

Differential Diagnosis: Since many common local processes can cause mandibular pain, a cardiogenic etiology is often overlooked. Pain on exertion or left mandibular pain with concurrent chest pain should arouse suspicion of coronary ischemia.

Treatment: Referral to a physician is recommended when cardiac origin is suspected. Resting and stress ECG readings will then aid in establishing the diagnosis, and appropriate medical management will serve to control the jaw symptoms.

References

1. Paine, R.: Vascular facial pain. In Facial Pain, 2nd Ed., edited by Charles C. Alling III and Parker E. Mahan. Philadelphia, Lea & Febiger, 1977, ch. 4.
2. Matson, M. S.: Pain in orofacial region associated with coronary insufficiency. Oral Surg. 16:284, 1963.
3. Norman, J. E.: Facial pain and vascular disease. Some clinical observations. Brit. J. Oral Surg. 8:138, 1970.
4. Natkin, E., Harrington, G. W., and Mandel, M. A.: Anginal pain referred to the teeth. Oral Surg. 40:678, 1975.

OTOGENIC PAIN

Acute Otitis Media

Age: Children and young adults
Sex: No predilection

Clinical Features: Acute inflammation of the middle ear is usually bacterial in origin with beta hemolytic streptococci, *Streptococcus pneumoniae*, and *Hemophilus influenzae* being the pre-

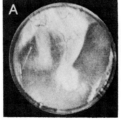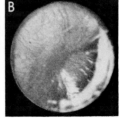

FIG. 12–13. Tympanic membrane in *A:* Normal ear. *B:* Acute otitis media with bulging drum and loss of landmarks. (Reprinted by permission from Dr. R. A. Buckingham, *Some Pathological Conditions of the Eye, Ear and Throat,* Abbott Laboratories, 1955.)

dominant infectious organisms. Viral agents are rarely responsible, yet may predispose to bacterial infection by inducing eustachian tube edema and obstruction. Pain is severe and persistent; otoscopic examination reveals a bulging hyperemic tympanic membrane. Conductive hearing loss is a feature; the eustachian tube mucosa in the nasopharynx is usually hyperemic. Eventually, the patient becomes febrile and may manifest an exudate with perforation of the drum. Coalescent mastoiditis develops, and opacification of the middle ear chamber and mastoid air cells can be detected radiographically. Subsequent to perforation and drainage, the lesion may resolve, or complications such as subperiosteal abscess, dural abscess, or brain abscess may evolve.

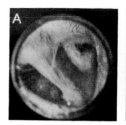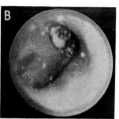

FIG. 12–14. Tympanic membrane in *A:* Normal ear. *B:* Cholesteatoma with chronic otitis media showing sloughing of pars flaccida, attic erosion, and inflamed pars tensa. (Reprinted by permission from Dr. R. A. Buckingham, *Some Pathological Conditions of the Eye, Ear and Throat,* Abbott Laboratories, 1955.)

Differential Diagnosis: Acute otitis media is usually not confused with other otalgic disorders because of the classic clinical changes that involve the tympanic membrane along with acute severe persistent pain.

Treatment: Penicillin or erythromycin therapy is indicated; myringotomy may help to relieve pain when exudation has not yet occurred. Referral to an otolaryngologist is recommended.

References

1. Coffey, J. D.: Otitis media in the practice of pediatrics; bacteriologic and clinical observations. Pediatrics *38:*25, 1966.
2. Yules, R. B.: Differential diagnosis of referred otalgia. Eye Ear Nose Throat Mon. *46:*587, 1967.
3. Klein, J. O. and Teele, D. W.: Isolation of viruses and mycoplasmas from middle ear effusions. A review. Ann. Otol. Rhinol. Laryngol. *85*(Suppl *25):* 140, 1976.
4. Giebink, G. S. and Quie, P. G.: Otitis media: the spectrum of middle ear inflammation. Ann. Rev. Med. *29:*285, 1978.

Chronic Otitis Media

Age: Adults
Sex: No predilection

Clinical Features: Chronic otitis media is far more complex than acute infectious otitis. The onset may be insidious, and pain is not common. *Staphylococcus aureus* and *Bacillus proteus* are most frequently cultured. Many factors are believed to predispose to chronic otitis, including progression of acute otitis, eustachian tube obstruction, and allergy. Ear pain, if present, is dull and usually mild to moderate. Occasionally, acute exacerbations with sharp pain will surface. Persistent otitis media of long standing is accompanied by destructive changes within the middle ear and mastoid air cells. Otoscopic examination

may disclose a perforation of the pars tensa, and a discharge may or may not be seen. Small perforations may not interfere with normal hearing; however, hearing loss will occur with larger perforations. In chronic tubotympanic otitis, the perforation may be filled with edematous polypoid mucosa. Otitis represented by excessive middle ear keratinization (keratoma, cholesteatoma) is probably the result of drum perforation with epidermal migration from the meatus. Retraction and pitting with loss of ossicle definition are indicative of disease. Chronic otitis can become severely destructive.

Differential Diagnosis: Chronic otalgia can be seen in referred pain of odontogenic origin or in diseases of the temporomandibular joint. Changes in the tympanic membrane warrant a thorough otologic evaluation. In the absence of drum changes, pain with hearing loss suggests middle ear disease. Significantly, otitis media can result from tubal obstruction secondary to nasopharyngeal carcinoma. In histiocytosis X, histiocytic infiltrates involve the middle ear; however, pain is usually not a complaint.

Treatment: When clinical signs and symptoms indicate chronic otitis media, referral to an otolaryngologist is indicated. Surgery is often necessary, particularly when keratoma is present.

References

1. Freidman, I.: Epidermoid cholesteatoma and cholesterol granuloma. Ann. Otol. *68:*57, 1959.
2. McGuckin, F.: Nonmalignant destructive ear disease. Arch. Otolaryngol. *78:*358, 1963.
3. Thomas, R.: The chronic ear. Renewed argument. J. Laryngol. *81:*1071, 1967.
4. Schuknecht, H. F.: *Pathology of the Ear.* Cambridge, Harvard University Press, 1974.
5. Howie, V. W., Ploussard, J. H., and Sloyer, J.: The

"otitis prone" condition. Am. J. Dis. Child. *129*:676, 1975.

Herpes Zoster Oticus

Age: Middle-aged and elderly adults

Sex: Male predilection

Clinical Features: Also known as geniculate ganglion neuralgia or the Ramsay-Hunt syndrome, herpes zoster oticus causes aural and postauricular pain. Pain is acute and burning and often represents a prodromal symptom preceding the onset of a vesicular eruption involving the postauricular cleft. The external ear canal receives sensory innervation from geniculate ganglion fibers of the seventh nerve that innervate the aural skin and travel with branches of the tenth nerve. Branches from the auriculotemporal also innervate the auditory canal anteriorly. Regardless of which nerves are affected by the varicella-zoster virus, the signs and symptoms are the same. A coexistent ipsilateral facial paralysis frequently follows the vesicular eruption. Vesicles are occasionally seen in the ipsilateral pharynx.

Differential Diagnosis: Prior to onset of the aural vesicular eruption, the diagnosis may be enigmatic, simulating other diseases causing otalgia. Within a few days the vesicles appear; a cytologic smear will disclose viral epithelial cell changes. Elevated serum varicella-zoster antibody titers can be detected following appearance of vesicles.

Treatment: The disease is self-limited and will resolve of its own accord. Facial paralysis may require 4 to 6 weeks to resolve. Intramuscular ACTH for 5 days has been reported to facilitate resolution.

References

1. Blackley, B., Friedman, I., and Wright, I.: Herpes zoster auris associated with facial palsy and auditory nerve symptoms: A case report with histopathological findings. Acta Otolaryngol. *63*:533, 1967.
2. Harner, S. G., Heiny, B. A., and Newell, R. C.: Herpes zoster oticus. Arch. Otol. *92*:632, 1970.
3. Jurgens, E. H. and Jurgens, P. E.: Syndromes Involving Facial Pain. In *Facial Pain*, 2nd Ed., edited by C. C. Alling III and P. E. Mahan. Philadelphia, Lea & Febiger, 1977, p. 231.

Middle Ear Neoplasms

Age: Adults

Sex: Male predilection

Clinical Features: Neoplastic and neoplasm-like proliferations of the middle ear, temporal bone, and mastoid air cells are usually painless; however, otalgia can be a major complaint, particularly when secondary infection occurs. Histiocytosis X and granulomatous inflammatory diseases are the more frequently encountered reactive lesions. Pain with erosion of the mastoid region and acute mastoiditis is more often encountered in histiocytosis X. Glomus jugulare tumors, meningiomas, facial nerve neuromas, squamous cell carcinomas, and adenocarcinomas are the common primary tumors in this region; acute ear pain, particularly nocturnal, is often reported by patients with squamous cancer. Metastatic lesions and invasion by tumors arising from contiguous tissues of the brain, meninges, external ear, nasopharynx, and parotid gland can also cause bone destruction, otitis media, and otalgia. Visual inspection of the tympanic membrane often discloses drum perforation, a retrotympanic mass, or suppurative otitis. Invasion of the temporal bone, inner ear, and facial canal will cause a variety of signs and symptoms including unilateral pulsatile tinnitus, neurosensory hearing loss, and paresis of cranial nerves VII, IX, X, XI, and XII.

Differential Diagnosis: Differentiation of tumor from other lesions causing otalgia is not always straightforward on clinical grounds alone. Cranial nerve deficits, hearing loss, and tinnitus should arouse suspicion of tumor. Angiography and tomography will then be employed, and if significant bony destruction is observed, biopsy is indicated.

Treatment: Most middle ear complex tumors are treated by surgical resection. Referral to an otolaryngologist or head and neck surgeon is recommended; the extent of disease along with the specific microscopic diagnosis will help to determine the treatment.

References

1. House, H. P.: Early detection of middle ear malignancy. Ann. Otol. *58*:789, 1949.
2. Hudson, W. R. and Kenan, P. D.: Otologic manifestations of histiocytosis X. Laryngoscope *59*:678, 1969.
3. Spector, G. J., Maisel, R. H., and Ogura, J. H.: Glomus tumors in the middle ear. I. An analysis of 46 patients. Laryngoscope *83*:1652, 1973.
4. Neely, J. G.: Neoplastic involvement of the facial nerve. Otolaryngol. Clin. North Am. *7*:385, 1974.
5. Conley, J. J. and Schuller, D. E.: Malignancies of the ear. Laryngoscope *86*:1147, 1976.

NECK AND THROAT PAIN

Stylohyoid Syndrome (Eagle's Syndrome)

Age: Middle-aged adults

Sex: No predilection

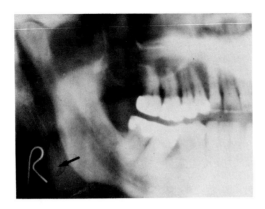

FIG. 12–15. Calcified stylohyoid ligament associated with upper lateral neck pain.

Clinical Features: Eagle's syndrome is characterized by pain during mandibular movement or twisting of the head and neck; it is stabbing, originates in the tonsillar region and radiates to the region of the TMJ and base of the tongue. When the jaws are closed, the pain subsides. The pain is caused by dystrophic calcification of the stylohyoid ligament. Lateral jaw or panographic radiographs will demonstrate a slender radiopaque spicule emanating from the region of the styloid process. Other elongated protuberances, such as the hamular process and cervical transverse process, may impinge upon nerves in their vicinity, thus causing pain and discomfort. It should be noted that calcified stylohyoid ligaments are frequent and are usually asymptomatic.

Differential Diagnosis: Pain associated with a calcified stylohyoid ligament may simulate the pain associated with other causes of TMJ and upper cervical pain. When the pain originates in the throat or tonsillar region, glossopharyngeal neuralgia must be considered in the differential diagnosis; however, a trigger zone is not present in Eagle's syndrome and pain is elicited upon mandibular opening. Radiographs will disclose the presence of a calcified stylohyoid ligament.

Treatment: Symptomatic elongated styloid processes can be surgically removed, using an intraoral approach.

References

1. Odenheimer, K.: Symptomatic calcified stylohyoid ligaments. In *Oral and Maxillofacial Surgery,* 5th Ed., edited by W. H. Archer. Philadelphia, W. B. Saunders Co., 1975, pp. 1728–1729.
2. Gossman, J. R., Jr., and Tarsitano, J. J.: The styloid and stylohyoid syndrome. J. Oral Surg. *35:*555, 1977.
3. Correll, R. W., et al.: Mineralization of the stylo-hyoid-stylomandibular ligament complex. A radiographic incidence study. Oral Surg. *48:*286, 1979.
4. Solfanelli, S. X., Braun, T. W., and Sotereanos, T. C.: Surgical management of a symptomatic fractured, ossified stylohyoid ligament. Oral Surg. *52:*569, 1981.

Hyoid Syndrome

Age: Middle-aged and elderly adults
Sex: Female predilection

Clinical Features: The hyoid syndrome results from elongation of the greater cornu with impingement upon adjacent laryngeal tissues. Pain is experienced in the lateral neck/carotid area at the tip of the greater hyoid cornu. Pain may be acute, particularly when the neck is turned or the patient swallows. Ipsilateral referred pain to the ear is common, and syncope may be a feature. Many patients experience a chronic persistent dull ache and the sensation that a foreign body is lodged in the throat. Lateral movement of the hyoid bone elicits pain. Significantly, radiographs may disclose an elongated cornu, and a calcified stylohyoid ligament is usually not evident.

Differential Diagnosis: Carotidynia, styloid syndrome, and superior laryngeal neuralgia will mimic hyoid syndrome because they manifest pain in virtually the same location. The clinical features and tenderness on palpation or lateral displacement of the hyoid bone allow for a definitive diagnosis.

Treatment: Surgical excision of the affected greater cornu is the treatment of choice. This is usually performed through a cutaneous incision, which follows local anesthetization.

References

1. Brown, L. A.: Hyoid bone syndrome. South Med. J. *47:*1088, 1954.
2. Steinmann, E. P.: Styloid syndrome in absence of an elongated process. Acta Otolaryngol. *66:*347, 1968.
3. Kopstein, E.: Hyoid syndrome. Arch. Otolaryngol. *101:*484, 1975.
4. Lim, R. Y.: The hyoid bone syndrome. Otolaryngol. Head Neck Surg. *90:*198, 1982.

Glossopharyngeal Neuralgia

Age: Middle-aged adults
Sex: No predilection

Clinical Features: Affecting the left side of the face more often than the right, glossopharyngeal neuralgia appears to represent a disorder similar to tic douloureux but involving cranial nerve IX. Excruciating, stabbing. and paroxysmal pain develops after stimulation of a trigger zone located in the tonsil region or throat. Swallowing may stimulate an attack. Pain evolves at the base of the tongue or in the pharynx, radiating to the ear. Other signs, such as coughing and even syncope, may appear during an attack. A minority of affected patients also suffer from trigeminal neuralgia.

Differential Diagnosis: Paroxysmal pain in the throat and base of the tongue differentiates glossopharyngeal neuralgia from trigeminal neuralgia. Few organic lesions will cause paroxysms of pain; however, a thorough physical examination of the pharynx and hypopharynx should be undertaken to rule out infection or neoplasm. The cocaine test is useful in making the diagnosis. Application of 10 percent cocaine to the site of pain almost invariably eliminates the symptoms in glossopharyngeal neuralgia.

Treatment: Phenytoin and carbamazepine are the drugs of choice; however, they are usually less effective in glossopharyngeal neuralgia than in trigeminal neuralgia. When medical treatment fails, surgical sectioning of the rootlets of nerve IX may be required. Some neurosurgeons also recommend sectioning of laryngeal fibers from nerve X, which may also contribute to the pain paroxysms.

References

1. Laskiewicz, A.: Anatomical and clinical considerations on some rare forms of glossopharyngeal neuralgias. Acta Otolaryngol. 43:545, 1953.
2. Bohn, E. and Strang, R. R.: Glossopharyngeal neuralgia. Brain 85:371, 1962.
3. Brzustowicz, R. J.: Combined trigeminal and glossopharyngeal neuralgia. Neurology 5:1, 1955.
4. Orton, C. I.: Glossopharyngeal neuralgia: Its diagnosis and treatment. Br. J. Oral Surg. 9:228, 1972.
5. Rushton, J. G., Stevens, J. C., and Miller, R. H.: Glossopharyngeal (vagoglossopharyngeal) neuralgia. A study of 217 cases. Arch. Neurol. 38:201, 1981.

Carotidynia

Age: Middle-aged adults
Sex: Female predilection

Clinical Features: Carotidynia is believed to represent a vasodilation-mediated pain response located in the vicinity of the common carotid artery directly below the bifurcation area. In this respect, it is probably closely related to the other atypical facial pain syndromes described as midface cluster headaches. The pain may be unilateral or bilateral, lasting for a few days or a week, with localization in the lateral neck, ear, and angle of the mandible. It is intense and can be accentuated when the carotids are manually pressed posterolaterally against the cervical transverse processes. Inhalation of 100 percent oxygen may cause pain relief, such as that encountered with midface cluster headaches. In most instances, the disorder is self-limiting with spontaneous remission of symptoms.

Differential Diagnosis: The localization of pain in the region of the carotid artery is considered to represent carotidynia only when all organic disease has been eliminated from consideration. Neoplasms, aneurysms, and inflammatory conditions of the lateral pharynx must be ruled out, as must odontogenic inflammation arising from infected mandibular teeth. Parotitis, sialadenitis, arteritis, and otitis may all exhibit pain centered around the carotid bifurcation and angle of the mandible.

Treatment: Ergotamine tartrate administered as an anal suppository will induce transient vasoconstriction and relief of pain. This drug should not be given to patients who are pregnant or hypertensive. Most cases eventually resolve of their own accord.

References

1. Fay, T.: Atypical facial neuralgia, a syndrome of vascular pain. Ann. Otol. Rhinol. Laryngol. 41:1030, 1932.
2. Campbell, J. and Evans, J. P.: Carotidynia. Neurology 3:391, 1953.
3. Roseman, D. M.: Carotidynia. A distinct syndrome. Arch. Otolaryngol. 85:81, 1967.
4. Raskin, N. H. and Prusiner, S.: Carotidynia. Neurology 27:43, 1977.
5. Scheitler, L. E. and Balciunas, B. A.: Carotidynia. J. Oral & Maxillofac. Surg. 40:121, 1983.

Superior Laryngeal Neuralgia

Age: Adults
Sex: No predilection

Clinical Features: Superior laryngeal neuralgia, like trigeminal and glossopharyngeal neuralgias, is a pain syndrome of unknown etiology characterized by acute lancinating paroxysmal pain, which is localized above the thyroid cartilage in the region of the hyoid bone. The disorder is usually unilateral; however, bilateral cases have been reported. A trigger mechanism prevails; an acute pain attack, which lasts a few seconds, can be precipitated by yawning, swallowing, sneezing, or touching the skin over the hyoid bone. During a pain attack the patient may exhibit uncontrolled swallowing and belching. Local anesthesia in the region of the hypothyroid membrane or in the pyriform sinus will ablate the pain when trigger zones are stimulated; this represents an important diagnostic finding.

Differential Diagnosis: Superior laryngeal neuralgia may be confused with glossopharyngeal neuralgia. The former is localized to the thyrohyoid region, whereas the latter affects the base of the tongue and supraglottic region of the pharynx. Local disease of the larynx should be ruled out by palpation of the neck and thyroid area, and laryngoscopy should be performed. The absence of organic pathosis along with a history of acute lancinating pain with a trigger mechanism is usually sufficient for a definitive diagnosis. Nevertheless, the hyoid syndrome may evince similar if not identical features. The hyoid should be palpated and shifted laterally; if this maneuver does not elicit pain, a true neuralgia of the superior laryngeal nerve is the likely diagnosis.

Treatment: Carbamazepine (Tegretol), 200 to 1200 mg daily, is usually adequate for control; the drug can be withdrawn slowly. Periodic blood counts should be obtained. Surgical intervention with nerve resection should be reserved for those who cannot be managed medically.

References

1. Echols, D. H. and Maxwell, J. H.: Superior laryngeal neuralgia relieved by operation. J. Am. Med. Assoc. *103*:2027, 1934.
2. Smith, L. A., Moersh, H. J., and Love, J. G.: Superior laryngeal neuralgia. Mayo Clinic Proc. *16*:164, 1941.
3. Brownstone, P. K., Ballenger, J. J., and Vick, N. A.: Bilateral superior laryngeal neuralgia. Its successful treatment with carbamazepine. Arch. Neurol. *37*:525, 1980.

Laryngeal Neoplasms

Age: Middle-aged and elderly adults

Sex: Male predilection

Clinical Features: Most neoplastic processes that arise in the larynx originate on the true or false cords and pyriform recess. Benign neoplasms rarely are painful. Malignant laryngeal tumors usually result in hoarseness without pain. Nevertheless, pain can be a sign of larynx cancer, particularly in large necrotic squamous carcinomas and in smaller tumors of the aryepiglottic fold, vallecula, and epiglottis. The pain is often referred to the ear. Invasion of cartilage or contiguous laryngeal soft tissues may produce induration with loss of the normal laryngeal cartilage crepitus on palpation. Direct or indirect laryngoscopy should be performed in patients with hoarseness, with or without upper cervical or larynx pain. White ker-

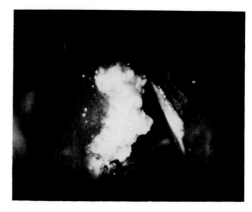

FIG. 12–16.   Keratotic squamous cell carcinoma of the true cord associated with hoarseness and throat pain.

atotic, red, ulcerated, and tumefactive lesions should arouse suspicion of carcinoma and warrant biopsy.

Differential Diagnosis: Pain associated with larynx cancer is usually a mild to moderate dull ache, yet may manifest occasional sharp twinges. When throat pain is present, laryngitis or one of the other pain syndromes listed here is more likely than cancer. Regardless, cancer should be considered as a potential cause of laryngeal pain, particularly among smokers.

Treatment: Laryngeal carcinoma is treated according to clinical staging and should be managed by a head and neck surgeon in conjunction with a radiotherapist.

References

1. Ogura, J. H. and Thawley, S. E.: Cysts and Tumors of the Larynx. In *Otolaryngology*, 2nd Ed., edited by M. M. Paparella and D. A. Shumrick. Philadelphia, W. B. Saunders, Co., 1980, p. 2518.
2. Micheau, C., et al.: Modes of invasion of cancer of the larynx. A statistical, histological and radioclinical analysis of 120 cases. Cancer *38*:346, 1976.
3. English, G. M.: Malignant Neoplasms of the Larynx. In *Otolaryngology, A Textbook*, edited by G. M. English. Hagerstown, Harper and Row Publishers, 1976, chap. 48.

TMJ REGION PAIN

Myogenic Pain

Age: Young and middle-aged adults

Sex: Female predilection

Clinical Features: Myogenic pain represents one of the most common disorders causing facial pain. It is included with TMJ pain because myospasm can refer pain to the joint region with or without diffuse distribution over the facial mus-

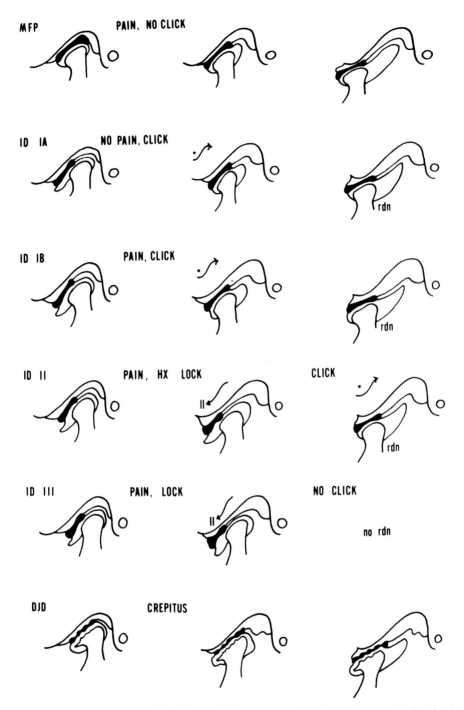

FIG. 12–17 Classification of functional and internal derangements of TMJ. (MFP—myogenic facial pain, ID—internal derangement, DJD—degenerative joint disease, RDN—reduction of meniscus). See text for explanation.

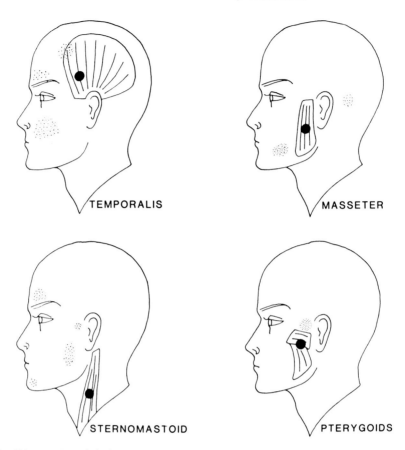

FIG. 12–18.   Trigger points (dark dot) and pain referral patterns (stippled areas) in myogenic pain of masticatory and strap muscles.

culature. Nevertheless, localized pain due to myospasm without a more diffuse distribution over the masseteric and temporal regions is not common in the absence of joint sounds. When it does occur, the patient complains of a dull ache in the TMJ area; it is chronic and usually persistent. Often the pain is worse in the morning, in nocturnal bruxism, or in the late afternoon if parafunctional clenching or bruxing habits are correlated with work stress. The mandible may or may not deviate to the affected side; a full range of opening is observed, although maximal opening may be painful. The patient should be evaluated for myogenic TMJ pain by palpating the muscles for trigger point tenderness. The lateral pterygoid is most often involved, followed by the masseter and temporalis. Persistent digital pressure on the muscle trigger point will usually intensify the joint pain, and local anesthetic infiltration of the muscle will eliminate the pain. In uncomplicated my-

ogenic facial pain, clicking or popping cannot be palpated or auscultated.

Differential Diagnosis: Internal derangements can be excluded from the differential when no joint sounds are detectable and a full range of opening is observed. Organic lesions such as arthritis can be ruled out when joint swelling is absent or when tomograms fail to show pathologic changes indicative of arthritis. Muscle splinting secondary to a high restoration or odontogenic infection should be ruled out by conducting a thorough dental examination.

Treatment: Myogenic TMJ pain can be managed in a variety of ways. All modalities are directed toward minimizing myospasm and parafunctional activities. Electromyographic biofeedback with stress management behavioral medicine is highly effective. Occlusal splints may be employed, especially for nocturnal bruxism and clenching. Ultrasound applied over affected muscles may also relieve myogenic pain. Last, trigger point injections of a local anesthetic without a vasoconstrictor into affected muscle may be useful as an adjunctive management technique.

References

1. Travell, J. G.: Temporomandibular joint pain referred from muscles of the head and neck. J. Prosthet. Dent. *10*:745, 1960.
2. Travell, J. G.: Mechanical headache. Headache *7*:23, 1967.
3. Laskin, D. M.: Etiology of pain dysfunction syndrome. J. Am. Dent. Assoc. *79*:153, 1969.
4. Kraus, H.: *Clinical Treatment of Back and Neck Pain.* New York, McGraw-Hill, 1970.
5. Murphy, G. J.: Electrical physical therapy in treating TMJ patients. J. Craniomand. Prac. *1*:68, 1983.

Type I Internal Derangement

Age: Young and middle-aged adults

Sex: Female predilection

Clinical Features: Type I derangements may be subdivided into two variants. Type IA is characterized by clicking or popping of the affected joint without pain, whereas type 1B is characterized by clicking or popping with pain. Both opening and closing clicks occur, and the fact that they are detected at different condylar positions is important. The pain may be a constant dull ache in the joint area, or it may be periodic and sharp, particularly when the patient eats hard or tough foods. Notably, the patient has no history of locking. The problem is usually unilateral, yet can be bilateral. On opening, the mandible often deviates to the affected side, the click occurs, and the mandible then shifts to the midline, reaching a full open position. The pathogenesis of this disorder is re-

lated to anterior displacement of the TMJ meniscus. The etiology has not been clarified and is probably multifactorial. Bruxing, clenching, occlusal disharmony, yawning, mandibular trauma, and overextension of the joint due to intubation or prolonged opening have been implicated. It should be stressed that many patients with a type 1B internal derangement may manifest concurrent myospasm with trigger point tenderness of masticatory and/or strap muscles of the neck. Tomograms fail to show pathologic osseous changes; however, the condyle(s) on the affected side(s) may appear to be retroposed, a finding that is not always consistent. Arthrograms and/or CAT scans may be used to confirm anterior displacement of the disc.

Differential Diagnosis: Uncomplicated myogenic pain can be ruled out when no joint sounds are apparent. A history of locking or a persistent closed lock places the derangement into type II and III respectively. Tomograms should be obtained to rule out degenerative joint disease.

Treatment: Evidence indicates that this type of derangement may be reversible. Alternatively, some patients become progressively worse, and progress to type II or III derangements, and ultimately develop degenerative joint disease. Because muscle spasm may occur in conjunction with clicking or pain and clicking, the muscles should be palpated for trigger point tenderness, and electromyographic scanning is advisable. Splint therapy, along with muscle relaxation and stress management strategies, is the treatment of choice. Occlusal equilibration may be performed, particularly if the occlusion tends to retropose the mandible. Alternatively, recent studies tend to minimize the role of occlusion in the etiology of this disorder.

References

1. Laskin, D. M.: Etiology of pain dysfunction syndrome. J. Am. Dent. Assoc. *79*:153, 1969.
2. Wilkes, C. H.: Structural and functional alterations of the temporomandibular joint. Northwest Dent. *57*:287, 1978.
3. Farrar, W. B.: Characteristics of the condylar path in internal derangement of the TMJ. J. Prosthet. Dent. *39*:319, 1978.
4. Farrar, W. B. and McCarty, W. L., Jr.: Inferior joint space arthrography and characteristics of condylar paths in internal derangement of the TMJ. J. Prosthet. Dent. *41*:548, 1979.
5. Brownstein, S. L., Tomasetti, B. J., and Ryan, D. E.: Internal derangements of the temporomandibular joint: correlation of arthrogra-

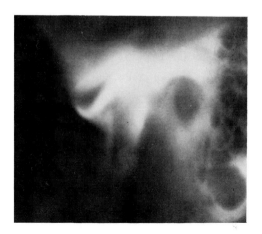

FIG. 12–19. Arthrogram illustrating anterior displacement of the meniscus in a type 1B internal derangement.

phy with surgical findings. J. Oral Surg. *39:*572, 1981.

Type II Internal Derangement

Age: Young and middle-aged adults
Sex: Female predilection

Clinical Features: Anterior displacement of the meniscus with clicking or popping and pain in the affected joint(s) along with a history of locking characterize the type II internal derangement. The displaced disc in patients with a history of locking may not be a reversible phenomenon. The retrodiscal tissues (bilaminar zone) have been overdistended, and the meniscus cannot be firmly positioned over the condylar head. At surgery, the entire meniscus may be found to be loose ("floppy disc"). Patients may complain of transient closed lock whereby they are unable to open more than 15 to 25 mm, yet with automanipulation of the mandible they are able to open full range. In these instances, the displaced disc precludes translation of the condyle, yet reduction of the disc is ultimately achieved. Alternatively, transient open locks may occur, presumably due to entrapment of a reduced disc. An open lock should not be confused with true subluxation of the condyles, which lock anterior to a steep eminence. The mandible may deviate laterally on opening, and in some patients the deviation corrects at the fully open position. Pain is usually dull and aching, but sharp episodes can occur during transient locking or when hard foods are eaten. In addition, muscle trigger points and elevated electromyographic readings may be noted, as patients with type II derangements sometimes manifest coexistent myogenic pain.

Differential Diagnosis: The other TMJ pain syndromes listed here usually can be eliminated with the confirmation that locking occurs, yet is transitory.

Treatment: The reversibility of type II derangements is usually unpredictable. Splint therapy with muscle relaxation and stress therapy should be attempted. If no progress is achieved after 6 months or if the patient proceeds to a type III derangement with persistent, nonreducing closed lock, surgical intervention with meniscus repositioning is recommended.

References

1. Farrar, W. B. and McCarty, W. L., Jr.: Inferior joint space arthrography and characteristics of condylar paths in internal derangement of the TMJ. J. Prosthet. Dent. *41:*548, 1979.
2. Katzberg, R. W., et al.: Arthrotomography of the temporomandibular joint. AJR *134:*995, 1980.
3. Westesson, P. L.: Double-contrast arthrotomography of the temporomandibular joint. J. Oral Maxillofac. Surg. *41:*163, 1983.

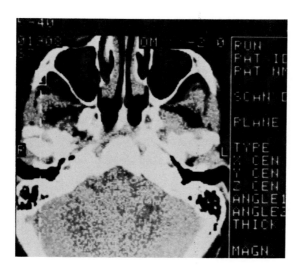

FIG. 12–20. CT scan (blink mode) showing anterior meniscus displacement in a patient with transient locking, a type II internal derangement.

4. Farrar, W. B.: Craniomandibular practice: the state of the art; definition and diagnosis. J. Craniomand. Prac. 1:4, 1983.
5. Bell, W. E.: Understanding temporomandibular biomechanics. J. Craniomand. Prac. 1:28, 1983.

Type III Internal Derangement

Age: Young and middle-aged adults

Sex: Female predilection

Clinical Features: Whereas types I and II manifest pain and clicking of the affected joint(s), type III derangement is characterized by locking with pain. Average jaw opening is 20 mm. The disc is forward and precludes translation of the condyle; therefore, no click can be palpated or auscultated, and the jaw deviates to the affected side. In bilateral involvement, the jaw fails to deviate. Pain

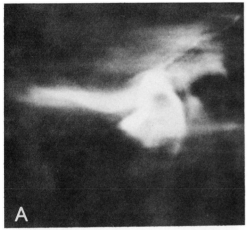

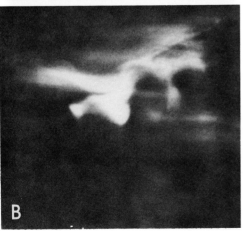

FIG. 12–21. Arthrograms in type III internal derangement. A: Closed with anterior disc displacement. B: Open without reduction, the disc remains forward.

is chronic with a dull ache, that may be exacerbated during masticatory function. Occasionally, the examiner can reduce the disc with manual manipulation of the condyle; however, the patient is unable to do so unassisted. Arthrotomograms will demonstrate anterior dislocation of the disc without reduction. As with the other types of internal derangements, a myogenic pain component may be extant.

Differential Diagnosis: The other types of internal derangements can be excluded from consideration when closed lock is encountered. Other disorders unrelated to TMJ dysfunction must be considered in the differential diagnosis when unilateral locking is encountered. Not all of these conditions are associated with pain symptoms. Post-injection trismus, infections, and tumors of the pterygoid space and lateral pharynx must be considered. These disorders are discussed in detail under the heading *Limited and Deviant Mandibular Opening.*

Treatment: If left untreated, most patients with a type III derangement will progress to degenerative joint disease (localized osteoarthritis). Patients with closed lock should be treated by meniscus reattachment surgery. If myogenic pain is a concomitant, EMG biofeedback with stress management therapeutic modalities are recommended following postoperative recovery. In addition, most patients will develop an immediate posterior open bite on the ipsilateral side. This is usually minimal and self-corrective, yet may require minor orthodontic correction.

References
1. Wilkes, C. H.: Structural and functional alterations of the temporomandibular joint. Northwest Dent. 57:287, 1978.
2. Farrar, W. B. and McCarthy, W. L., Jr.: Inferior joint space arthrography and characteristics of condylar paths in internal derangement of the TMJ. J. Prosthet. Dent. 41:548, 1979.
3. Westesson, P. L., Omnell, K-Å, and Rohlin, M.: Double contrast tomography of the temporomandibular joint: A new technique based on autopsy specimen examinations. Acta Radiol. (Diagn.) 21:777, 1980.
4. Nance, E. P., Jr.: Temporomandibular joint arthrography. J. Craniomand. Prac. 1:36, 1983.
5. Dolwick, M. F.: Surgical treatment of anterior displacement of the TMJ meniscus. Case reports and outlines of selected scientific sessions. 62nd Annual Meeting, AAOMS, 1980, p. 42.

Meniscus Perforation

Age: Young and middle-aged adults

Sex: Female predilection

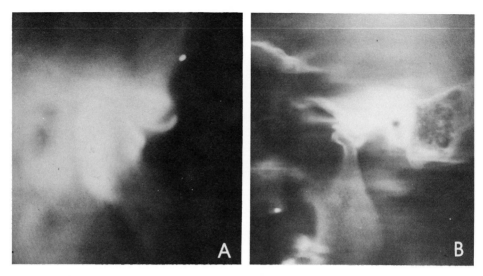

FIG. 12–22. Arthrogram showing contrast media in both upper and lower joint spaces in cases of meniscus perforation. *A:* Closed. *B:* Open.

Clinical Features: Perforation of the meniscus may occur subsequent to chronic anterior displacement, whereby the condylar head articulates with the loose connective tissues of the retrodiscal or bilaminar zone. Alternatively, perforations may occur in the fibrotic intermediate zone or even anterior to the anterior band of the meniscus. In these instances, the condyle has no cushion and may rub directly against the glenoid fossa incline. Characteristically, the patient has a history of clicking and locking and exhibits limited opening. Auscultation reveals crepitus. During arthrographic evaluation with fluoroscopy, contrast media introduced to the lower compartment can be seen to flow into the upper compartment simultaneously. Arthrotomograms also will reveal dye opacity in both joint spaces.

Differential Diagnosis: Similar findings are encountered in degenerative joint disease, which, of course, may coexist with a perforation. Crepitus may also be detected in synovial chondromatosis as well as in other types of chronic arthritis.

Treatment: Surgical correction is the treatment of choice. A simple retrodiscal perforation can be closed primarily. Large perforations with adhesions may require placement of a disc prosthesis. Any condylar osteophytes should be eliminated by arthroplasty.

References

1. Ireland, V. E.: The problem of "the clicking jaw." Proc. Roy. Soc. Med. *44:*191, 1951.
2. Katzberg, R. W., et al.: Arthrotomography of the temporomandibular joint: New technique and preliminary observations. Am. J. Roentgenol. *132:*949, 1979.
3. Helms, C. A., et al.: Arthrotomographic diagnosis of meniscus perforation in the temporomandibular joint. Br. J. Radiol. *53:*283, 1980.

Osteoarthritis (Degenerative Joint Disease)

Age: Middle-aged and elderly adults
Sex: Female predilection

Clinical Features: Generalized osteoarthritis is a degenerative process involving, primarily, weight-bearing joints and metacarpophalangeal joints. The latter may evince nodular excrescences referred to as Heberden's nodes. Limitation of motion and pain are also featured. The TMJ is not often involved in generalized degenerative joint disease, localized TMJ osteoarthritis being more common. Localized arthritis of the TMJ may evolve secondary to trauma; evidence increasingly implicates untreated internal derangements with an anterior meniscus as a precursor to degenerative disease. When the condyle is no longer protected by the meniscus or when the meniscus is loosely attached, perforation may occur, resulting in bone-to-bone contact between the mandibular condylar head and the articular fossa. Erosions, eburnation, and osteophyte formation evolve with resultant chronic pain. The majority of patients with degenerative joint disease will have crepitant joint sounds while opening and closing. Tomograms will reveal flattening of the

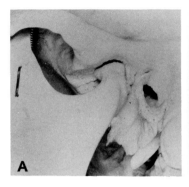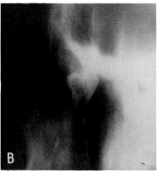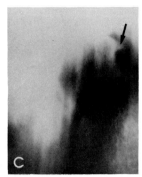

FIG. 12–23. Degenerative joint disease (osteoarthritis). A: Gross skull specimen showing flattened condyle. B: Tomogram showing bulbous condyle with eburnation. C: TMJ tomogram illustrating an anterior osteophyte.

condylar head, eburnation with deformation, erosions, and anterior or superior osteophytic lipping. Similar changes occur on the articular fossa; however, these changes rarely are radiographically demonstrable. In chronic osteoarthritis of long standing, the patient, despite crepitus, may be pain free. Alternatively, ankylosis may develop, but this is unusual.

Differential Diagnosis: A diagnosis of localized TMJ degenerative joint disease is based on the presence of crepitus on auscultation with radiographic confirmation of osseous changes. A history of trauma or of symptoms that indicate a preexistent internal derangement, in conjunction with the aforementioned criteria, provides insight into the possible pathogenesis of the disease. The radiographic changes in TMJ osteoarthritis are similar if not identical to those encountered in rheumatoid arthritis. The latter is a TMJ manifestation of a polyarthritic condition.

Treatment: When the pain is mild, management with analgesics or nonsteroidal prostaglandin inhibitors may be adequate. When pain is moderate and problematic, condylar contouring or condylectomy with placement of a prosthesis may be indicated along with meniscoplasty. Surgical procedures of this nature may alter the occlusion, thus requiring orthodontic or restorative correction.

References

1. Bauer, W. H.: Osteoarthritis of the temporomandibular joint. Am. J. Pathol. *17*:129, 1941.
2. Blackwood, H. J. J.: Arthritis of the mandibular joint. Br. Dent. J. *115*:317, 1963.
3. Toller, P. A.: Osteoarthrosis of the mandibular condyle. Br. Dent. J. *136*:223, 1973.
4. Hecker, R., et al.: Symptomatic osteoarthritis of the temporomandibular joint: report of case. J. Oral Surg. *33*:780, 1975.
5. Ogus, H.: Degenerative disease of the temporomandibular joint in young persons. Br. J. Oral Surg. *17*:17, 1979.
6. Westesson, P-L., and Rohlin, M.: Internal derangement related to osteoarthrosis in temporomandibular joint autopsy specimens. Oral Surg. *57*:17, 1984.

Rheumatoid Arthritis

Age   Young and middle-aged adults
Sex: Female predilection

Clinical Features: Rheumatoid arthritis is a collagen disease associated with poststreptococcal immunopathic tissue changes localized in the joints. This progressive disorder is variable in its regional distribution; however, there is a tendency for symmetrical involvement. The second and third metacarpophalangeal and proximal interphalangeal joints are most frequently involved, followed by the knee, wrist, shoulder, ankle, elbow, and vertebrae. The chief extra-articular manifestation of the disease is anemia. The affected joints are warm to the touch, swollen, and painful. The TMJ is frequently involved; when it is, bilateral pain is accompanied by generalized joint disease. Crepitation with stiffness is more commonly noted than pain. In rheumatic joint disease of childhood onset, involvement of the TMJ may result in retarded development of the mandible and a class II malocclusion with open bite. Condylar destruction and TMJ ankylosis occur in rare instances. Transcranial radiographs or, preferably, TMJ tomograms often disclose pathologic alterations, including irregular condylar articulating surfaces, flattening of the condyle, and osteophyte formation with increased joint space di-

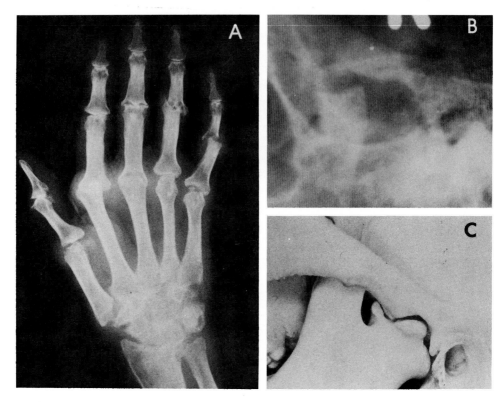

FIG. 12–24.   Rheumatoid Arthritis. *A:* Hand film showing erosions of proximal interphalangeal joints. *B:* Right TMJ radiograph exhibiting condylar erosion and increased joint space. *C:* Skull specimen in rheumatoid ankylosis.

mension. Rheumatoid nodules of the preauricular soft tissues have not been encountered. Rheumatoid factor as assayed by latex agglutination from a serum sample is the primary laboratory finding of diagnostic importance.

Differential Diagnosis: The pain of TMJ rheumatoid arthritis may be confused with that of other arthritides and the myofascial pain dysfunction syndrome. The bilateral nature and association with generalized joint pain and swelling are highly suggestive of rheumatoid arthritis, particularly when rheumatoid nodules are found over extremity joints. The rheumatoid factor is generally positive in the serum.

Treatment: Treatment for TMJ arthritis is not specific. The generalized disease should be managed by a physician and includes the use of steroids or other immunosuppressive drugs along with analgesics. When fibrous ankylosis or severe joint destruction is present, surgical intervention may be indicated.

References

1. Bornstein, L. A., and Ramon, Y.: Bony ankylosis of the temporomandibular joints due to juvenile rheumatoid arthritis. Br. J. Plast. Surg. *16:*95, 1963.
2. Marbach, J. J. and Spiera, H.: Rheumatoid arthritis of the temporomandibular joints. Ann. Rheum. Dis. *26:*538, 1967.
3. Ericson, S. and Lundberg, M.: Alterations in the temporomandibular joint at various stages of rheumatoid arthritis. Acta Rheumatol. Scand. *13:*357, 1967.
4. Ronning, D., Valiaho, M. L., and Laaksonen, A. L.: The involvement of the temporomandibular joint in juvenile arthritis. Scand. J. Rheumatol. *3:*89, 1974.
5. Orgus, H.: Rheumatoid arthritis of the temporomandibular joint. Br. J. Oral Surg. *12:*275, 1975.

Acute Infectious Arthritides

Age: Young adults
Sex: No predilection

Clinical Features: Acute or suppurative TMJ arthritis is usually the result of a bacteremia with pyogenic organisms. Gonococcal, streptococcal, and staphylococcal organisms are seen most frequently in test cultures. The preauricular tissues are swollen and erythematous; they are acutely tender when palpated, both directly and intrameatally. The patient restricts opening; deviation of the mandible toward the affected side is apparent. Aspiration yields an exudate, and a culture should be obtained for specific identification of the infectious agent. Acute arthritis is rare, but chronic granulomatous arthritis, which is usually due to tuberculosis, is even less frequent. In tuberculous arthritis, pain and tenderness are uncommon; however, a preauricular swelling may be present. Acute arthritis causes exudate accumulation in the joint spaces, and tuberculous arthritis causes granulomas; consequently, the joint space dimensions may be enlarged on TMJ tomograms, and a posterior open bite can be seen on the affected side.

Differential Diagnosis: Acute arthritis is unique in that swelling and acute pain coexist with limited opening and deviation. In addition, joint sounds are absent. Aspiration of the periarticular area with evidence of a purulent exudate confirms the initial clinical impression of acute arthritis.

Treatment: Aspiration and drainage should be performed initially, followed by culture and sensitivity testing of the aspirated exudate. An appropriate antibiotic may then be prescribed. Jaw movement exercises during the recovery period will prevent the development of adhesions.

References

1. Winters, S. E.: Staphylococcus infection of the temporomandibular joint. J. Oral Surg. 8:148, 1955.
2. Alexander, W. N. and Nagy, W. W.: Gonococcal arthritis of the temporomandibular joint. Oral Surg. 36:809, 1973.
3. Goodman, W. S.: Infections of the temporomandibular joint. J. Otolaryngol. 8:250, 1979.
4. Wurman, L. H., Flannery, J. V., Jr., and Sack, J. G.: Osteomyelitis of the mandibular condyle secondary to dental extractions. Otolaryngol. Head Neck Surg. 87:190, 1979.

Miscellaneous Arthritides

Age: Adults

Sex: Predilection dependent upon specific disease

Clinical Features: On rare occasions, polyarthritic disease associated with hyperuricemic gout, pyrophosphate arthritis, psoriasis, ankylosing spondylitis, lupus erythematosus, and scleroderma will affect the temporomandibular joint. Most patients with these arthritides do not manifest significant TMJ signs or symptoms. In gout, the synovial tissues are the site of urate crystal formation, which initiates an inflammatory reaction with hyperplasia of the periarticular tissues. With progressive deposition of urates, pain and limitation of motion may be observed along with osseous resorption late in the course of the disease.

A small fraction of psoriasis patients will develop arthritis in the form of monoarticular or oligoarticular symptoms. Ankylosing spondylitis is an asymmetrical oligoarthropathy that primarily affects the spine, particularly the sacroiliac joint, while, in general, sparing small peripheral joints. In systemic lupus erythematosus, fibrinoid necrotic foci may occur in the articular tissue. Dystrophic calcifications and articular erosions may occur in the later stages of systemic sclerosis (scleroderma). In some instances these arthritides affect the TMJ, and the patient may suffer pain, joint swelling, and limited opening. Radiographic evidence of condylar erosions may be identified on tomograms.

Differential Diagnosis: The jaw signs and symptoms appearing in these miscellaneous arthropathies do not differ from those encountered in rheumatoid or degenerative TMJ arthritis. The specific diagnosis is based on distribution of joint symptoms throughout the skeleton in conjunction with other clinical and laboratory findings.

Treatment: In general, conservative therapy is indicated; many other joints are involved, and pain symptoms beyond the craniomandibular articulation tend to be more troublesome. Physical therapy, ultrasound, occlusal splints, and non-narcotic analgesics often alleviate the symptoms. Most of these patients are under the care of a physician, and treatment should be pursued after medical consultation. When unrelenting pain is a feature and is refractory to conservative management, surgical intervention may be indicated.

References

1. Lundberg, M. and Ericson, S.: Changes in the temporomandibular joint in psoriasis arthropathia. Acta Dermatovener (Stockh.) 47:354, 1967.
2. Davison, C., et al.: Temporomandibular joint disease in ankylosing spondylitis. Ann. Rheum. Dis. 34:87, 1975.
3. Pritzker, K. P. H., et al.: Pseudotumor of the temporomandibular joint: destructive calcium pyrophosphate dihydrate arthropathy. J. Rheumatol. 3:70, 1976.
4. Osial, T. A., et al.: Resorption of the mandibular condyles and coronoid processes in progressive systemic sclerosis (scleroderma). Arthritis Rheum. 24:729, 1981.
5. Liebling, M. R. and Gold, R. H.: Erosions of the temporomandibular joint in systemic lupus erythematosus. Arthritis Rheum. 24:948, 1981.

Condylar Fracture

Age: No predilection

Sex: No predilection

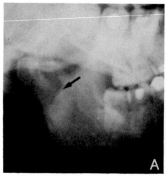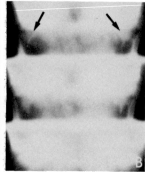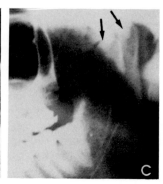

FIG. 12–25. Condylar Fractures. *A:* Lateral jaw showing low subcondylar fracture. *B:* AP tomograms showing bilateral subcondylar fractures with medial displacement. (Courtesy of Dr. William Donlon.) *C:* Double condyle occurring subsequent to nonreducing condylar fracture.

Clinical Features: While trauma to the mandible may occur at any age, condylar neck and symphysis fractures are commonly seen in children. The fracture may be unilateral or bilateral, greenstick, complete, or comminuted. In unilateral subcondylar fractures, the occlusion is altered with a shift of the mandible toward the affected side. Palpation of the preauricular area causes pain, which may be severe; in most cases, swelling is detectable. The jaw deviates on opening, and movement is painful. In bilateral complete fractures, the patient presents with a gagged occlusion that is characterized by retropositioning and an anterior open bite. Towne's, panoramic, ramus lateral jaw, and AP or submental vertex radiographs will disclose the site of fractures. In complete fractures, the condyle is usually anteromedially displaced. Greenstick fractures in children may not show any condylar displacement.

Differential Diagnosis: Restricted or deviant opening due to subcondylar fracture is, of course, preceded by a traumatic blow to the mandible; therefore, the diagnosis is readily suspected and easily confirmed by obtaining radiographs.

Treatment: Most surgeons agree that open reduction is rarely necessary for the treatment of condylar neck fractures. Closed reduction with intermaxillary fixation is the treatment of choice.

References

1. Archer, W. H.: *Oral and Maxillofacial Surgery.* Vol. II, 5th Ed. Philadelphia, W. B. Saunders Co., 1975, pp. 1157–1187.
2. Blevins, C. and Gores, R. J.: Fractures of the mandibular condyloid process: results of conservative treatment in 140 patients. J. Oral Surg. *19:*392, 1961.
3. MacLennan, W. D. and Simpson, W.: Treatment of

fractured mandibular condyle processes in children. Br. J. Plast. Surg. *18:*4–23, 1965.

Synovial Chondromatosis

Age: Middle-aged adults
Sex: Female predilection

Clinical Features: Synovial chondromatosis is a reactive phenomenon that is seldom encoun-

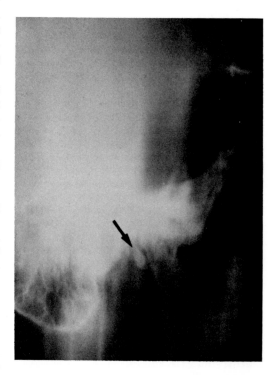

FIG. 12–26. Synovial Chondromatosis. Tomogram showing condylar eburnation in DJD and retrocondylar calcified body. (Courtesy of Dr. Will Forbes.)

tered in the periarticular tissues of the TMJ. Single or multiple ovoid bodies composed of hyaline cartilage form in the subsynovial connective tissue; they enlarge and then become detached, thus forming loose bodies within the joint spaces. Alternatively, it has been suggested that some are generated when osteophytic projections in arthritic joints become detached to form loose bodies. In fact, in some cases, these cartilaginous nodules remain in continuity with the articular tissues, meniscus, or condylar head. They calcify or undergo endochondral ossification and can be visualized as focal radiopacities radiographically. The mandible usually deviates toward the affected side, and the chondroid bodies may cause cross bite or open bite occlusion. Pain, particularly during mastication, is often a complaint. Larger lesions may be palpable over the condyle, and clicking or crepitus can be auscultated. Multiple chondroid bodies may be present with resultant double or triple clicks on opening and closing. Synovial chondromatosis may occur in conjunction with reactive synovial proliferation (villonodular synovitis).

Differential Diagnosis: Internal derangements with meniscus displacement or perforation and arthritic joints manifest similar clinical features. Transcranial and TMJ tomograms will disclose the presence of joint space opacities when calcification is present. It is probable that if contrast media arthrography were used, noncalcified joint bodies would be demonstrable in relief.

Treatment: Surgical removal is the treatment of choice. Meniscus displacement, fibrous adhesions, villonodular synovitis, and arthritic changes may be present; they also require surgical correction.

References

1. Ballard, R. and Weiland, L. H.: Synovial chondromatosis of the temporomandibular joint. Cancer *30*:791, 1972.
2. Tasanen, A., Lamberg, M. A., and Kotilainen, R.: Osteochondromatosis of the temporomandibular joint: report of a case. Oral Surg. *38*:845, 1974.
3. Lomba, J. A., Cabanas, R., and Marrero, I.: Synovial chondrometaplasia of the temporomandibular joint. J. Oral Surg. *35*:675, 1977.
4. Fee, W. E., Jr., et al: Synovial chondromatosis of the temporomandibular joint. Otolaryngol. Head & Neck Surg. *87*:741, 1979.
5. Storeman, D. W., et al: Chondrometaplasia involving the temporomandibular joint. Oral Surg. *49*:556, 1980.

Pigmented Villonodular Synovitis

Age: Middle-aged adults
Sex: No predilection

Clinical Features: Pigmented villonodular synovitis is a reactive proliferation of the synovial lining cells and underlying periarticular connective tissue with a predilection for the knee joint. The lesion is rare in the TMJ. It can be experimentally induced by intra-articular injections of blood and saline, thus suggesting the possibility of traumatic hemarthrosis in its genesis. Microscopically, villous proliferations extend into the joint space, and the supportive fibrovascular tissue contains multinucleated giant cells and hemosiderin pigment deposition. Many of the cases reported in the TMJ have been associated with chondroid metaplasia, thus suggesting the coexistence of synovial condromatosis. In other joints, osseous erosion is uncommon, yet may occur. In the TMJ, radiographic and surgical evidence of condylar erosion may be observed. Clinical findings include pain, swelling, limited opening, and deviation toward the affected side.

Differential Diagnosis: Pigmented villonodular synovitis is diagnosed on the basis of microscopic features. Clinically, the disease may mimic internal derangements, neoplasms, synovial chondromatosis, and arthritis. When condylar erosion is radiographically evident and when a palpable preauricular mass can be detected, surgical intervention with biopsy of the periarticular mass is recommended.

Treatment: Surgical excision and repair of the articular soft tissues is the treatment of choice. Condylar destruction may necessitate placement of a joint prosthesis.

References

1. Jaffe, H. L., Lichtenstein, L., and Sutro, C. J.: Pigmented villonodular synovitis in the temporomandibular joint. A case report. Arch. Pathol. *31*:730, 1941.
2. Barnard, J. D. W.: Pigmented villonodular synovitis in the temporomandibular joint: a case report. Br. J. Oral Surg. *13*:183, 1975.
3. Raibley, S. O.: Villonodular synovitis and synovial chondromatosis. Oral Surg. *44*:279, 1977.
4. Dinerman, W. K. and Myers, E. N.: Pigmented villonodular tenosynovitis of the temporomandibular joint. Trans. Am. Acad. Ophthalmol. Otolaryngol. *84*:132, 1977.
5. Takagi, M. and Ishikawa, G.: Simultaneous villonodular synovitis and synovial chondromatosis of the temporomandibular joint: report of case. J. Oral Surg. *39*:699, 1981.

SIALOGENIC PAIN

Sialolithiasis

Age: Adults

Sex: Male predilection

Clinical Features: Salivary calculi are more common in the submandibular duct than the parotid duct. The pain associated with salivary calculi is experienced during salivation and therefore is notable during meals. Blockage of the main excretory duct causes saliva distention throughout the duct tree, producing a drawing or stinging pain. The submandibular area is often swollen during pain episodes, and the swelling may be tender to palpation. Prolonged blockage may predispose to acute bacterial sialadenitis with constant pain. Occlusal radiographs should be obtained in both anterior and posterior regions. Most stones are located anteriorly; however, some may be found posteriorly underlying the retromylohyoid ductal flexure. A panoramic radiograph or lateral skull film should be ordered when a parotid stone is suspected. When symptoms indicate sialolithiasis yet radiographs fail to uncover a stone, the gland should be milked to evaluate salivary flow. When no flow can be elicited, a sialogram should be ordered to evaluate for the possibility of a noncalcified blockage or focal duct stenosis.

Differential Diagnosis: Pain in the region of the submandibular gland could represent submandibular lymphadenopathy that is secondary to odontogenic infection or is a nonspecific sign of viral infection. The dentition should be evaluated when radiographs are negative for a sialolith.

Treatment: Small stones can occasionally be manipulated digitally and extruded from the duct orifice. Surgery is required in most cases. When duct blockage has persisted for a long time, thus causing sclerosing sialadenitis, sialectomy may be required to prevent multiple recurrent episodes of acute suppurative sialadenitis.

References

1. Harrison, G. R.: Calculi of the salivary glands and ducts. Surg. Gynec. Obstet. *43*:431, 1926.
2. Seldin, H. M., et al.: Conservative surgery for removal of salivary calculi. Oral Surg. 6:579, 1953.
3. Levy, B. M., ReMine, W. H., and DeVine, K. D.: Salivary gland calculi: Pain, swelling associated with eating. J. Am. Med. Assoc. *181*:1115, 1962.

Endemic Parotitis (Mumps)

Age: Children and young adults

Sex: No predilection

Clinical Features: Endemic parotitis is a paramyxovirus infection of the parotid glands causing bilateral parotid swelling and moderate to severe pain. Occasionally, the submandibular glands are enlarged and painful. Pain increases when sour or bitter foods are ingested. Milking the gland often causes exudation at the orifice of Stensen's duct. Constitutional signs and symptoms of infectious disease include malaise, fever, and cervical lymphadenopathy. Orchitis or oophoritis are complications. Serum amylase is elevated. Since development of the mumps vaccine, the disease has become less prevalent.

Differential Diagnosis: The swelling seen in mumps should not be confused with benign lymphoepithelial lesion of Sjögren's syndrome, which is painless. Acute suppurative sialadenitis is encountered in elderly adults. If a bacterial infection is suspected, the duct secretions or exudate can be cultured.

Treatment: Endemic parotitis resolves within 2 weeks. A bland diet, bed rest, and aspirin are

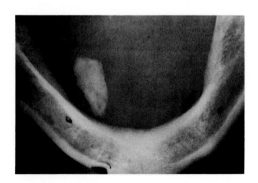

FIG. 12–27. Sialolith in submandibular duct.

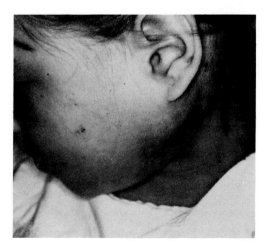

FIG. 12–28. Endemic parotitis.

recommended in conjunction with medical consultation because of possible orchitis, oophoritis, or meningitis.

References

1. Wolman, I. J., et al.: Amylase levels during mumps; the findings in blood and saliva. Am. J. Med. Sci. *213*:477, 1947.
2. Banks, P.: Nonneoplastic parotid swellings: a review. Oral Surg. *25*:732, 1968.

Acute Suppurative Sialadenitis

Age: Middle-aged and elderly adults

Sex: Male predilection

Clinical Features: Acute bacterial sialadenitis is usually caused by streptococcal or staphylococcal microorganisms. Two predisposing factors are associated with nonviral sialadenitis. *Surgical mumps* is uncommon, representing a suppurative bacterial parotitis in elderly patients recovering from surgery (usually abdominal). It has also been reported to occur in xerostomic patients on phenothiazine therapy. The parotids are enlarged and painful, and Stenson's ducts usually have a purulent exudate. *Postobstruction sialadenitis* is a suppurative bacterial infection that develops in an occluded gland. The occlusion may be the consequence of calculus or a focal excretory duct stricture. The involved gland is swollen and painful. If the obstruction is still present and exudate cannot escape, draining cutaneous or oral fistulas may develop. Regardless of the predisposing conditions, fever and malaise are common but not invariable findings.

Differential Diagnosis: Acute suppurative sialadenitis must be differentiated from endemic parotitis and simple, uncomplicated sialolithiasis. Pain and swelling are common to all three diseases. Both an exudate and cultivatable pathogenic organisms are required for the diagnosis.

Treatment: The exudate should be cultured, and penicillin should be prescribed. Pending results of culture and sensitivity, an alternative antibiotic may be necessary, particularly when penicillinase-producing staphylococci are the predominant pathogens.

References

1. Carlson, R. G. and Glas, W. E.: Acute suppurative parotitis; twenty-eight cases at a county hospital. Arch. Surg. *86*:659, 1963.
2. Banning, G. L.: Postoperative suppurative parotitis. Arch. Surg. *89*:653, 1964.

TEMPORAL PAIN

Migraine

Age: Young adults

Sex:;   Female predilection

Clinical Features: Migraine headache has been reported to affect 20 percent of the female population. It is not nearly as prevalent among males. The pain is usually unilateral (hemicrania), yet can be bilateral. The classic form of migraine is characterized by prodromal or concurrent symptoms including nausea, vomiting, flashing lights, scotomas, hemianopia, and/or photophobia. Speech disorders, paresthesias, and confusion are frequently encountered. The pain is moderate to severe, throbbing, and often incapacitating. The episodes may occur 2 or 3 times monthly, and pain may persist for many hours. It is localized around the temporal area and often involves the frontal and retro-orbital regions. The disorder is familial, and emotional problems may precipitate an attack. Evidence supports a vascular source subsequent to vasodilation of the external carotid branches. The superficial temporal vessels are often dilated during an attack; thermograms will show a decrease in facial skin temperature, presumably due to shunting of blood away from the skin. Blood serotonin levels are decreased during attacks.

Differential Diagnosis: The signs and symptoms of migraine are characteristic and usually pathognomonic. Regardless, CNS neoplasms and organic rather than functional vascular disease must be considered in the differential diagnosis, as these conditions may mimic the symptomatology of migraine. Furthermore, migraine may be accompanied by tension headache, with episodic classic attacks being superimposed over constant dull aching pain of the frontalis and temporalis areas.

Treatment: Ergotamine tartrate or caffergot suppositories or sublingual tablets will usually relieve pain. Skin temperature and EMG biofeedback along with stress management have been highly successful.

References

1. Selby, G. and Lance, J. W.: Observations on 500 cases of migraine and allied vascular headache. J. Neurol. Neurosurg. Psychiatr. *23*:23, 1960.
2. Lance, J. W. and Anthony, M.: Some clinical aspects of migraine. Arch. Neurol. *15*:356, 1966.
3. Anthony, M., Hinterberger, H., and Lance, J. W.: Plasma serotonin in migraine and stress. Arch. Neurol. *16*:544, 1967.

4. Lance, J. W. and Anthony, M.: Thermographic studies in vascular headache. Med. J. Aust. 1:240, 1971.

5. Medina, J. L., Diamond, S., and Franklin, M. A.: Biofeedback therapy for migraine. Headache 16:115, 1976.

Myogenic Pain (Tension Headache)

Age: Young and middle-aged adults

Sex: No predilection

Clinical Features: Muscle tension headaches are the most common form of headache. The pain may be referred to the temporomandibular joint; however, diffuse pain over the temporal, frontal, and masseteric regions is more often the chief symptom. Suboccipital, shoulder, and neck pain may occur. Myogenic pain is the result of prolonged and sustained muscle contraction that is related to anxiety or stress. The pain itself is thought to arise subsequent to muscular accumulation of lactic acid. Myogenic facial pain is characterized by a constant dull to moderate ache, which is usually poorly localized. Palpation of the frontalis, temporalis, masseter, pterygoids, sternomastoid, trapezius, and strap muscles of the neck will serve to locate acutely tender foci, referred to as muscle trigger points. Prolonged pressure on a trigger point often causes diffuse referred pain in the areas constituting the chief complaint. Indeed, specific muscles show predictable routes of pain referral. Patients with uncomplicated myogenic facial pain do not manifest clicking or popping joints. Nevertheless, because of muscle spasm and soreness, deviant jaw opening may be a feature.

Differential Diagnosis: A diagnosis of uncomplicated myogenic facial pain is made when no joint sounds are heard and when no palpable clicks are detected in the TMJ. It should be emphasized that myospasm can develop secondarily if other pain disorders are extant. A newly placed high dental restoration or a painful tooth may initiate muscle guarding or splinting to protect against occluding of the tooth in question.

Treatment: Myogenic facial pain is a stress disorder. Treatment is directed toward breaking the myospasm pain cycle. Stress management and electromyographic biofeedback are extremely beneficial in this regard; when bruxism or clenching coexists, an occlusal splint may be employed. Short-term use of muscle relaxants, anxiolytics, and analgesics are initially beneficial, yet should be phased out as the other forms of treatment begin to achieve results. Injection of muscle trigger points with an anesthetic devoid of vasoconstrictor is also beneficial as an adjunctive procedure.

References

1. Travell, J. G.: Temporomandibular joint pain referred from muscles of the head and neck. J. Prosthet. Dent. 10:745, 1960.

2. Travell, J.: Mechanical headache. Headache 7:23, 1967.

3. Travell, J.: Identification of myofascial trigger point syndromes: a case of atypical facial neuralgia. Arch. Phys. Med. Rehabil. 62:100, 1981.

4. Solberg, W. K., Clark, G. T., and Rugh, J. D.: Nocturnal electromyographic evaluation of bruxism patients undergoing short term splint treatment. J. Oral Rehab. 2:215, 1975.

5. Carlsson, S. G. and Gale, E. N.: Biofeedback treatment for muscle pain associated with the temporomandibular joint. J. Behav. Ther. and Exp. Psychiatr. 7:383, 1976.

Giant Cell Arteritis

Age: Elderly adults

Sex: Female predilection

Clinical Features: Giant cell arteritis (GCA), also termed temporal arteritis, is related to polymyalgia rheumatica (PMR), a disorder characterized by shoulder and pelvic girdle pain with muscular weakness, absence of joint disease, and presence of an elevated erythrocyte sedimentation rate. GCA and PMR often coexist. Giant cell arteritis is a granulomatous disease of unknown etiology affecting the muscular-intimal layers of arteries, primarily cranial and facial vessels. The disease is characterized by episodic pain over the temple or temple and maxilla along with palpation tenderness of vessels, fever, anorexia, and eventual blindness. The pain is sharp or shooting with

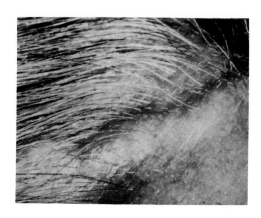

FIG. 12–29. Prominent artery in giant cell (temporal) arteritis. (Courtesy of Drs. G. Arsham and S. Day, Dept. of Ophthalmology, Pacific Medical Center, Series 3390.)

intervening periods of persistent dull ache. The temporal artery may be prominent and visibly tortuous. The overlying skin is often erythematous and hyperalgesic. Involvement is not confined to the temporal artery. Indeed, many vessels supplying the head and neck area may be involved. Cerebral infarction is a complication. Notably, the erythrocyte sedimentation rate and C-reactive protein are elevated.

Differential Diagnosis: The episodic or paroxysmal nature may simulate a true neuralgia. When the patient's age is considered in conjunction with arterial tenderness and elevated sedimentation rate, a preliminary diagnosis of temporal arteritis can be made. Arterial biopsy is then indicated.

Treatment: Prednisone, 20 to 30 mg daily, will usually control the pain associated with temporal arteritis.

References

1. Noshay, W. C. and Roth, R. L.: Giant cell (temporal) arteritis. Henry Ford Hosp. Med. Bull. *10*:455, 1962.
2. Mowat, A. G. and Hazleman, B. L.: Polymyalgia rheumatica. A clinical study with particular reference to arterial disease. J. Rheumatol. *1*:190, 1974.
3. Healy, L. A. and Wilske, K. R.: Manifestations of giant cell arteritis. Med. Clin. North Am. *61*:261, 1977.
4. Malmvall, B. E. and Bengtsson, B. A.: Giant cell arteritis. Clinical features and involvement of different organs. Scand. J. Rheumatol. *7*:154, 1978.
5. Park, J. R., Jones, J. G., and Hazleman, B. L.: Relationship of the erythrocyte sedimentation rate to acute phase proteins in polymyalgia rheumatica and giant cell arteritis. Ann. Rheum. Dis. *40*:493, 1981.

PARESTHESIA

Mental Paresthesia

Age: Adults
Sex: No predilection

Clinical Features: Paresthesia, hypesthesia, or anesthesia of the mental nerve distribution over the lower lip usually represents a complication of third molar extraction subsequent to trauma of the inferior alveolar nerve. Sensitivity to a light touch or a pinprick may be diminished or absent; the ipsilateral mandibular teeth may fail to respond to vitalometer testing. When there is no history of trauma or tooth extraction, metastatic carcinoma to the jaw should be suspected. Periapical and panoramic radiographs will disclose a poorly marginated or moth-eaten radiolucency of the mandibular body. Occasionally, a central or cranial base lesion will compress the third division; when

this occurs, the motor trunk of the fifth nerve is often compressed, resulting in soft palate paresis and/or masticatory muscle weakness.

Differential Diagnosis: With a documented history of trauma or third molar removal, the symptom usually resolves in 6 weeks; however, some patients don't report resolution for 6 months. In some instances of trauma, the paresthesia never resolves, but this is rare. When there is no history of nerve injury, a panoramic radiograph should be ordered; any suspicious radiolucent or mixed radiolucent and radiopaque regions should be biopsied. In the absence of jaw disease, CT scans should be used to evaluate for CNS or cranial base lesions.

Treatment: There is no treatment for post-traumatic mental paresthesia; spontaneous resolution evolves as axis cylinders regenerate. When the sensory deficit persists beyond 6 months, a microsurgical procedure may be successful. Metastatic tumor should be managed by an oncologist.

References

1. Goldstein, N. P., Gibilisco, J. A., and Rushton, J. G.: Trigeminal neuropathy and neuritis: a study of etiology with emphasis on dental causes. J. Am. Med. Assoc. *183*:458, 1963.
2. Moorman, W. C. and Shafer, W. G.: Metastatic carcinoma of the mandible. J. Oral Surg. *12*:205, 1954.

Infraorbital Paresthesia

Age: Adults
Sex: No predilection

Clinical Features: Included under this title of infraorbital paresthesia are other forms of sensory neurologic deficit, including hypesthesia and anesthesia of the infraorbital nerve distribution. In instances of complete anesthesia, light-touch and pinprick testing over the infraorbital skin and usually the ipsilateral palate will not be felt by the patient. In hypesthesia, either a pinprick, a light touch or both may be affected to some degree. In other words, patients may detect these forms of stimulation to a lesser degree than they would on unaffected cutaneous regions. Patients with paresthesias may show a normal response to pinprick and light-touch tests, yet subjectively will describe numbness and tingling of the affected skin. In general, loss of sensation to both a pinprick and a light touch indicates a peripheral nerve lesion, whereas differential loss suggests a central lesion. Antral carcinoma and cranial base tumors are the more common causes of infraorbital sensory deficits when the second division fibers are involved after exit from the skull. Cerebellopontine angle tumors with involvement of the gasserian ganglion are the most prevalent central lesions accounting for these symptoms. Other causes of sensory neuropathy in this area are *multiple sclerosis, Bell's palsy, trauma, vertebrobasilar vascular disease,* and *connective tissue immunopathic disorders. Trigeminal (sensory) neuropathy* is a less frequently encountered disorder in which no organic source can be detected. The sensory deficit is usually temporary with spontaneous resolution. Some of these instances may represent a viral neuritis or a psychological conversion symptom. A few patients with idiopathic atypical facial pain may also experience an attending paresthesia. In all instances of infraorbital paresthesia, hyperthesia, or anesthesia, the remaining cranial nerves should be evaluated for accompanying motor deficits; antral tomograms as well as CT scans should be used to identify a tumor.

Differential Diagnosis: As mentioned previously, loss of both pinprick and light-touch sensation necessitates a search for a central lesion. The presence of ophthalmoplegia or other motor paresis is another sign that suggests a CNS or cranial base tumor. Maxillary or palatal expansion implicates an antral neoplasm.

Treatment: When the cause has been determined and a biopsy diagnosis has been procured, treatment must be planned according to this diagnosis. If an antral source has been ruled out, patients should be referred to a neurologist.

References

1. Thrush, D. C. and Small, M.: How benign a symptom is facial numbness? Lancet 2:851, 1970.
2. Korczyn, A. D.: Sensory deficit in Bell's palsy. N. Engl. J. Med. 282:1493, 1970.
3. Tait, B. and Ashworth, B.: Trigeminal neuropathy in connective tissue disease. Ann. Rheum. Dis. 29:339, 1970.
4. Foley, J. M.: The cranial mononeuropathies. N. Engl. J. Med. 281:905, 1969.
5. Horowitz, S. H.: Isolated facial numbness. Clinical significance and relation to trigeminal neuropathy. Ann. Int. Med. 80:49, 1974.

LOCALIZED MOTOR DEFICITS

Facial Paralysis

Age: Varies according to etiology
Sex: Varies according to etiology

Clinical Features: Seventh nerve paralysis is usually self-limited, and normal function returns within two months. Paralysis of this nature is referred to as Bell's palsy. Notably, the entire dis-

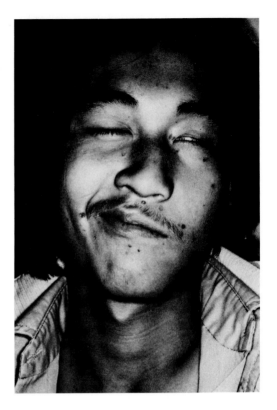

FIG. 12–30. Complete facial nerve paralysis.

tribution of the seventh nerve is involved from the onset; therefore, the patient is unable to raise the eyebrow, close the eye, or smile on the affected side (i.e., complete hemifacial paralysis). Although it has been suggested that Bell's palsy is a herpesvirus neuritis, a variety of other diseases, lesions, and trauma of the temporal region, brain stem, facial canal, middle ear, and infratemporal fossa may produce partial, sequential, or complete seventh nerve palsy. The cortical tracts communicating with the motor nucleus ambiguus of the facial nerve cross over to innervate the lower face musculature, while the upper face fibers are ipsilateral proximal to the nucleus. A cortical lesion will, therefore, cause contralateral lower face palsy; a lesion of the brain stem, main trunk, or peripheral fibers will result in a total hemifacial paralysis. The nervus intermedius carries parasympathetic secretory fibers to the lacrimal and salivary glands. Lesions of the main trunk and facial canal are, therefore, frequently accompanied by ipsilateral xerophthalmia; xerostomia may not be evident due to normal contralateral function. Facial canal and middle ear neoplasms are usually associated with sensorineural hearing loss when seventh nerve palsy is a feature. Tumors of the cranial base, parapharyngeal space, and infratemporal fossa, particularly malignant parotid tumors, often cause seventh nerve palsy and neuropathy of other cranial nerves. CT scans will disclose osseous destructive changes in the temporal bone or a soft tissue mass, depending on the location of the lesion.

Differential Diagnosis: Evaluation of a patient with seventh nerve paralysis must include the following chief factors: precise muscle groups involved, temporal progression of muscle group paresis, middle ear disease, vestibular function, hearing loss, tinnitus, and presence of other cranial nerve deficits. It should also be noted that seventh nerve palsy accompanies cheilitis granulomatosa in the Melkerson-Rosenthal syndrome. Special radiographic and neurologic procedures are required to secure a definitive diagnosis. Referral to an otolaryngologist or neurologist is recommended.

Treatment: Systemic steroids or ACTH injections have been successful in treating Bell's palsy. Even in the absence of treatment, the paralysis generally disappears within 2 months. Lesions arising along the intracranial, temporal bone, and peripheral distributions of the seventh nerve are treated in accordance with the ultimate and definitive diagnosis.

References

1. Boone, P. C.: Bell's palsy. Acta Neurochir. 7:16, 1959.
2. Neely, J. G.: Neoplastic involvement of the facial nerve. Otolaryngol. Clin. North Am. 7:385, 1974.
3. Adour, K. K., Bell, D. N., and Hilsinger, R. L., Jr.: Herpes simplex virus in idiopathic facial paralysis (Bell's palsy). JAMA 233:527, 1975.
4. Seaver, P. R., Jr., and Kuehn, P. G.: Adenoid cystic carcinoma of the salivary glands: a study of ninety-three cases. Am. J. Surg. 137:449, 1979.
5. Gacek, R. R. and Radpour, S.: Fiber orientation of the facial nerve: an experimental study in the cat. Laryngoscope 92:547, 1982.

Horner's Syndrome

Age: Elderly adults

Sex: Male predilection

Clinical Features: Horner's syndrome is a facial sign of a lesion compressing the stellate ganglion, usually bronchogenic carcinoma of the apex of the lung. The sympathetic fibers emerging from the ganglion normally pass into the head and neck regions and innervate the pupil dilator, smooth muscle elevator of the upper eyelid, and perior-

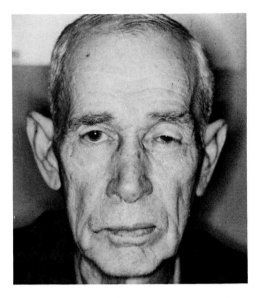

FIG. 12–31. Ptosis and miosis in Horner's syndrome associated with carcinoma of lung apex.

bital sweat glands. Compression of the ganglion leads to miosis or contraction of the pupil, ptosis of the upper eyelid, and anhydrosis of the periorbital and facial skin. In addition to lung cancer, other neoplasms, infections, or aneurysms adjacent to the cervical spine may encroach upon the ganglion or sympathetic fibers arising therefrom.

Differential Diagnosis: The etiology of Horner's syndrome is variable and represents a medical problem. Referral to an internist or neurologist is recommended.

Treatment: The cause must be eliminated. It is important to realize that Horner's syndrome may herald the presence of a serious illness such as cancer or an aneurysm.

References

1. Giles, C. L. and Henderson, J. W.: Horner's syndrome. An analysis of 219 cases. Am. J. Ophthalmol. 46:289, 1958.
2. Jaffee, N. S.: Localization of lesions causing Horner's syndrome. Arch. Ophthalmol. 44:5, 1940.

Ophthalmoplegia

Age: Varies according to disease

Sex: Varies according to disease

Clinical Features: Eye movement paralysis has many complex origins. Lesions may arise in the cerebral motor cortex, the nuclei of nerves III, IV, and VI, or the peripheral nerves may be compressed after they have exited from the brain stem. A lesion of the motor cortex will cause a defect

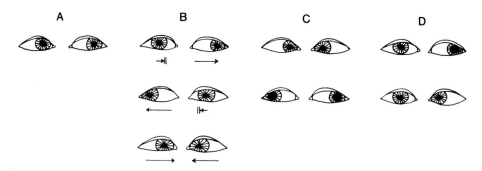

FIG. 12–32. Ophthalmoplegia. *A:* Left cerebral lesion with conjugate gaze. *B:* Medial longitudinal fasciculus lesion with inability to look medially when directed to look left or right, convergence intact. *C:* Bilateral nuclear lesions of abducens (above) and oculomotor (below). *D:* Left unilateral nuclear or peripheral nerve paresis of oculomotor (above) and abducens (below).

in contralateral conjugate gaze. The consequences of a left cerebral lesion will be inability of both eyes to engage in right-sided gaze and a tendency for bilateral left deviation. In other words, the patient "looks toward the lesion." The mechanism involves impairment of neural pathway conduction prior to synapse with the nuclei of III (ipsilateral) and VI (contralateral). Internuclear ophthalmoplegia is characterized by inability to move one eye medially while the opposite eye is directed laterally, despite the fact that the patient is able to converge both eyes. This apparent paradox is reconciled when one realizes that the pathway for convergence is different from the path for lateral conjugate gaze. Multiple sclerosis is usually the underlying disease involving internuclear ophthalmoplegia. Lesions involving each specific nucleus of the three nerves controlling eye movement will manifest specific signs. Bilateral involvement of the abducens nuclei causes convergent gaze due to defective motor supply to the lateral rectus. Divergent gaze is the consequence of a bilateral lesion of the oculomotor nerve. Compression of the peripheral nerves is caused by hemorrhage or tumor. Alternatively, entrapment of ocular muscles may occur in orbital blow-out fractures or in localized orbital lesions. A lesion located in the middle fossa/cavernous sinus region may compress one, two, or all three motor nerves to the eye. Compression of the oculomotor (CN-III) will cause unilateral gaze with pupillary dilation. The cold caloric test will confirm the finding. Involvement of the trochlear nerve (CN-IV) will cause inability to move the affected eye inferolaterally. Unilateral paralysis of the abducens (CN-VI) is characterized by medial gaze of the affected eye.

Differential Diagnosis: Because of the aforementioned clinical signs gleaned from cranial nerve examination of nerves III, IV, and VI, observation of eye position at rest, comparison of pupil size, and use of the cold caloric test, the examiner will have a concept of where the lesion lies. Since the etiology of ophthalmoplegias is so protean, a definitive diagnosis requires a variety of other clinical, radiological, and laboratory tests. A detailed differential diagnosis of ophthalmoplegia is beyond the scope of this book.

Treatment: Patients with eye muscle paresis should be examined and managed by an ophthalmologist or a neurologist when it has been determined that the etiology is not maxillary or orbital fracture.

References

1. Cheek, C. W., et al.: Acquired cranial nerve lesions affecting the ocular system. Am. J. Ophthalmol. 59:13, 1965.
2. Merritt, H. H.: *Textbook of Neurology,* 6th Ed. Philadelphia, Lea & Febiger, 1979, p. 378.
3. Goldberg, S.: *Clinical Neuroanatomy made ridiculously simple.* Miami, MedMaster, Inc. 1979, chap. 5.

Hypoglossal Paralysis

Age: Adults
Sex: No predilection
Clinical Features: The hypoglossal or twelfth nerve supplies motor fibers to the tongue and exits the medulla inferior to the olive. Unilateral injury or a lesion of the nucleus or nerve will cause the affected side of the tongue to undergo atrophy and on protrusion, the tongue will deviate toward the affected side. Attempted movements of the protruded tongue to the normal side are absent or

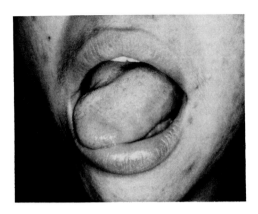

FIG. 12–33. Twelfth nerve paralysis. Tongue deviates toward affected side.

weak. At rest, lying in the floor of the mouth, the tongue deviates slightly toward the healthy side; retrusion of the tongue on the affected side is defective. A lesion may be located within the medulla or along the peripheral course of the nerve. Basilar artery occlusion will cause a lesion of the medulla with ipsilateral tongue paralysis and contralateral arm and leg paralysis. Neoplasms in the vicinity of the occipital condyle frequently compress the hypoglossal nerve with paralysis, dysarthria, and severe pain that is worsened when the neck is flexed. Neoplasms in the lateral neck along the course of the nerve may also cause unilateral paresis or palsy. Bilateral twelfth nerve palsy is rare. Fibrillation of the tongue is seen in syringobulbia, amyotrophic lateral sclerosis, and chronic alcoholism.

Differential Diagnosis: Since unilateral hypoglossal paralysis may be either central or peripheral in origin, complete neurological examination is required to explore other deficits indicative of a lesion within the medulla. CT scans should be obtained to evaluate the possibility of a cranial base primary or metastatic tumor. Palpation of the upper lateral neck for indurated swellings should also be performed.

Treatment: Referral to a neurologist is recommended. Treatment will be determined when the source of the lesion is located and a definitive diagnosis is rendered.

References

1. Merritt, H. H.: *A Textbook of Neurology*, 6th Ed. Philadelphia, Lea & Febiger, 1979, p. 394.
2. Greenburg, H. S., et al.: Metastasis to the base of the skull: Clinical findings in 43 patients. Neurol. *31*:530, 1981.

Soft Palate Paralysis

Age: Varies depending on disease

Sex: No predilection

Clinical Features: The soft palate muscles include the tensor veli palatini, supplied by the motor root of the fifth nerve, and the levator veli palatini, palatoglossus, and palatopharyngeous, all supplied by branches of the tenth nerve from the nucleus ambiguus. Brain stem lesions involving the nucleus or cranial base and parapharyngeal space lesions may cause paralysis with resultant drooping of the palate and loss of the palatal reflex. Bilateral paralysis will result in velopharyngeal insufficiency, thus causing nasal speech and difficulty with velar sounds such as "N" and "NG." Bilateral paralysis is associated with poliomyelitis, diphtheritic polyneuropathy, myasthenia gravis, and brain stem infarction. Unilateral paralysis is characterized by inability of the affected side to elevate when the patient says "ah"; the uvula deviates toward the normal side. An ipsilateral nuclear lesion, cranial base neoplasia, or nasopharyngeal carcinoma may be causative.

Differential Diagnosis: As previously mentioned, a variety of neurologic diseases can cause bilateral palatal paralysis. Unilateral paralysis warrants a thorough nasopharyngeal examination, which should include CT scans of the cranial base to detect the presence of a tumor.

Treatment: Because a variety of neurologic and neoplastic disorders can cause palatal paralysis, referral to a neurologist is recommended.

References

1. Cotton, R. and Nuwayhid, N. S.: The Surgery of Speech. In *Otolaryngology*, 2nd Ed., edited by

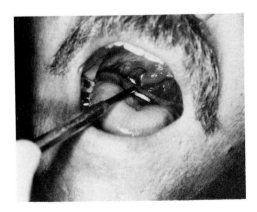

FIG. 12–34. Soft palate paralysis. Uvula deviates toward normal side.

M. M. Paparella and D. A. Shumrick. Philadelphia, W. B. Saunders Co., 1980, p. 2177.

2. Lee, M. C. and Resch, J. A.: Practical clinical neurology for the otolaryngologist. In *Otolaryngology*, 2nd Ed., edited by M. M. Paparella and D. A. Shumrick. Philadelphia, W. B. Saunders Co., 1980, p. 871.

3. Walton, J. N.: *Brain's Diseases of the Nervous System*, 8th Ed. Oxford, Oxford University Press, 1977, p. 208.

LIMITED AND DEVIANT MANDIBULAR OPENING

Muscle Splinting

Age: No predilection
Sex: No predilection

Clinical Features: When patients feel pain, they protect themselves by limiting motion of the associated joint. For instance, wide opening may be painful; thus, the patient may consciously maintain closure or limited opening. The splinting may be unilateral, causing deviation of the mandible on opening. A variety of organic lesions may initiate this protective phenomenon; they include trauma, fracture, pericoronitis, odontogenic infection, salivary gland inflammation, primary TMJ articular disease, and avoidance of a recently placed high dental restoration. Prolonged splinting may actually lead to myospasm, although this is rare. Amelioration of the problem or local anesthesia to the tissues suspected in its etiology will permit the patient to fully depress the mandible.

Differential Diagnosis: Limited opening due to muscle splinting may leave the erroneous impression that the problem is a primary muscle disorder (i. e., myogenic facial pain). Physical evaluation of teeth, occlusion, and periodontium and perioral

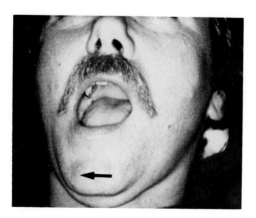

FIG. 12–35.   Deviant jaw opening secondary to muscle splinting.

tissues along with radiographs will disclose the presence of disease. The inflamed or traumatized tissue can be anesthetized so that amelioration of the inability to open can be evaluated.

Treatment: Resolution of the cause will eliminate the effect.

References
1. Bell, W. E.: *Orofacial Pains. Differential Diagnosis.* 2nd Ed. Chicago, Year Book Medical Publishers, 1979, pp. 62–67.

2. Bell, W. E.: Management of Masticatory Pain. In *Facial Pain*, 2nd Ed., edited by Charles C. Alling, III, and Parker E. Mahan. Philadelphia, Lea & Febiger, 1977, chap. 12.

3. Frost, H. M.: Musculoskeletal Pain. In *Facial Pain*, 2nd Ed., edited by Charles C. Alling, III, and Parker E. Mahan. Philadelphia, Lea & Febiger, 1977, chap. 9.

Post-Injection/Post-Infection Trismus

Age: Middle-aged adults
Sex: No predilection

Clinical Features: Limitation in jaw opening may evolve from inferior alveolar nerve block. Occasionally, the patient will complain of pain; however, most patients do not experience pain unless they forcefully attempt full depression of the mandible. The closed-lock phenomenon appears 1 to 6 days following a dental procedure that necessitated inferior nerve block anesthesia. Most patients are unable to open beyond 20 mm. Although the pathogenesis is unknown, the condition probably occurs because a needle has pierced a vessel and caused hematoma followed by organization and scar formation. Occasionally, trismus is encountered in patients with acute pericoronitis or alveolitis sicca. Inflammatory extension into the pterygomandibular space may develop; but in most instances, pain may induce muscle splinting or guarding that prevents a full-range of opening.

Differential Diagnosis: While limited opening may be seen in a variety of disorders, a closed-lock situation due to injection can be readily diagnosed on the basis of history. Inflammation of a pericoronal operculum or extraction site accounting for trismus is also easily recognized on the basis of examination and history.

Treatment: Post-injection trismus will usually resolve after a 3-week course of physiotherapy that includes ultrasound to masticatory muscles, hot packs, and jaw opening exercises 3 times a week. Forced opening under general anesthesia may be required for patients who do not respond to the aforementioned conservative regimen. Rarely, surgical intervention is required to sever a scar band that may form in the pterygoid space. Pericoronitis should be treated with hydrogen peroxide irrigation and antibiotics when fever and malaise are present. With resolution of symptoms, the hyperplastic tissue should be excised with extraction of the associated third molar. A full range of opening should return within a few days.

References

1. Brown, A. E.: Persistent limitation of opening following inferior alveolar nerve block injection. Br. Dent. J. *141*:186, 1976.
2. Campbell, J.: Trismus following inferior dental block anaesthesia: An analysis of a personal experience. Dent. Rec. *74*:180, 1954.
3. Brooke, R. I.: Postinjection trismus due to formation of fibrous band. Oral Surg. *47*:424, 1979.

Conversion Trismus

Age: Young and middle-aged adults
Sex: Female predilection

Clinical Features: Conversion reactions are encountered among patients with hysterical or histrionic personality. The etiology is apparently due to an underlying emotional crisis with which the subject cannot cope, whereby the emotional conflict is converted to a physical sign or symptom. Motor deficits (paralysis), sensory deficits (paresthesia or numbness), and visual loss represent the more common hysterical conversion reactions; notably, the deficits usually do not follow neuroanatomical pathway distributions. Conversion or hysterical trismus is rare and is characterized by inability to open the mouth in the absence of organic disease in the TMJ. Prolonged closure may, however, lead to myospasm with masticatory muscle weakness. The personality profile is important in the diagnosis, and psychometric testing with the Minnesota Multiphasic Personality Inventory (MMPI) will show elevation of the hysteria scale. Patients with histrionic or hysterical personalities exaggerate their symptoms and make multiple unfounded organ-system somatic complaints, yet they maintain an indifferent attitude about their problems (belle indifference). In addition, patients tend to be theatrical with overuse of cosmetics and adornment. The trismus can be reversed with restoration of normal opening while the patient is under general anesthesia or heavy sedation.

Differential Diagnosis: Because many organic disorders result in limited opening or trismus, a thorough workup for joint, muscle, and infectious disease must be pursued. Differentiation from a true closed-lock type III internal derangement is difficult on clinical grounds alone. Psychiatric consultation and MMPI testing should be included in the data base collection. Restoration to normal function following intravenous Valium sedation with manipulation of the mandible will aid in establishing the diagnosis.

Treatment: The immediate problem is easily ameliorated by manipulation of the jaw under general anesthesia or intravenous sedation. Long-term management rests with psychotherapy.

References

1. Marbach, J. J.: Hysterical trismus: a study of six cases. N. Y. State Dent. J. *32*:413, 1966.
2. Salmon, T. N., Tracy, N. H., Jr., and Hiatt, W. R.: Hysterical trismus (conversion reaction). Oral Surg. *34*:187, 1972.

Ankylosis

Age: Children or adults
Sex: No predilection

Clinical Features: Unilateral or bilateral ankylosis of the TMJ is the consequence of trauma, destructive infectious arthritis or rheumatoid arthritis. The ankylosis may be fibrous or bony. When a joint lesion arises during childhood, mandibular retrognathism will occur due to arrest of condylar growth on the affected side(s). The patient may be able to open the jaw only a few millimeters or it may be completely closed. Severe limitation of opening is seen even in unilateral ankylosis, and deviation of the mandible to the affected side is generally not detected because the ankylosed joint often prevents translation of the unaffected condyle. TMJ tomograms will disclose an absent or markedly anomalous-appearing condyle without joint space radiolucency.

Differential Diagnosis: In most of the other disorders showing limitation of opening. the restriction is incomplete. A history of trauma, acute arthritis, or juvenile rheumatoid arthritis and mandibular retrognathia, when considered in conjunction with the radiographic findings, allows for establishment of the diagnosis.

Treatment: A subcondylar through-and-through bony severage may be performed, creating a new focus of articulation. Joint prostheses are usually inadvisable because of the deformation of the glenoid fossa. Postsurgical exercises are mandatory in order to prevent a bony union.

References

1. Blackwood, H. J. J.: Intra-articular fibrous ankylosis of the temporomandibular joint. Oral Surg. *10*:634, 1957.

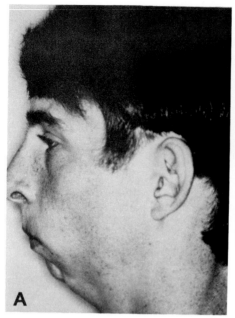
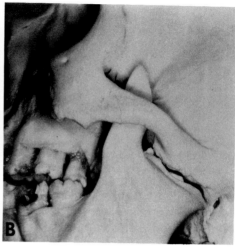

FIG. 12–36. *A:* Retrognathia in bilateral TMJ ankylosis. *B:* Skull specimen in TMJ ankylosis.

2. Hellinger, M. J.: Bony ankylosis of the temporomandibular joint. Oral Surg. *18*:293, 1964.
3. Pizer, M. E.: Ankylosis of the temporomandibular joint treated by subcondylar resection. Oral Surg. *21*:706, 1966.
4. Topazian, R. G.: Etiology of ankylosis of the temporomandibular joint; analysis of 44 cases. J. Oral Surg. *22*:227, 1964.
5. Young, A. H.: A follow-up of 12 cases of ankylosis of the mandibular joint treated by condylectomy. Brit. J. Plast. Surg. *16*:75, 1963.

Hecht-Beals-Wilson Syndrome

Age: Childhood onset
Sex: No predilection

Clinical Features: Inherited as an autosomal dominant trait, the Hecht-Beals-Wilson syndrome is characterized by limited mandibular opening, campylodactyly due to foreshortened flexor tendons of the fingers and wrists, shortened leg and hamstring muscles with consequently short stature, and, occasionally, foot deformities (club foot). The limitation in opening is the result of bilateral abnormal ligaments located within the masseteric region. This fibrotic band can usually be easily palpated bidigitally in the buccal mucosa just anterior and confluent with the masseter.

Differential Diagnosis: This syndrome exhibits classic features allowing for a definitive diagnosis. Limited opening in conjunction with buccal mu-

cosal fibrous bands and flexion of the finger when the wrist is dorsiflexed confirms the diagnosis. Other family members may be affected.

Treatment: The masseteric fibrous bands may be surgically severed. Some surgeons advocate coronoidectomy to free any inhibition of opening as a consequence of temporalis fibrosis, which may be present.

References

1. Hecht, F. and Beals, R. K.: Inability to open the mouth fully: an autosomal dominant phenotype with facultative campylodactyly and short stature. Birth Defects *5*:96, 1969.
2. Wilson, R. V., et al.: Autosomal dominant inheritance of shortening of the flexor profundus muscle-tension unit with limitation of jaw excursion. Birth Defects *5*:99, 1969.
3. deJong, J. G.: A family showing reduced ability to open the mouth and limitation of some movements of the extremities. Humangenetik *13*:210, 1971.
4. Mercuri, L. G.: The Hecht, Beals, and Wilson syndrome: report of case. J. Oral Surg. *39*:53, 1981.

Coronoid Hyperplasia

Age: Children
Sex: Males

Clinical Features: A rare developmental disorder, coronoid hyperplasia is bilateral and causes painless restriction of mandibular opening. Most patients are unable to open beyond 20 mm. The enlarged coronoids impinge upon the posterior aspect of the zygoma, thereby restricting translation of the condyles secondarily. There is no deviation on opening as both coronoids are involved. While some cases are probably sporadic, others have been reported among siblings. The diagnosis must be confirmed radiographically. A lateral skull, high panoramic, or lateral tomograms will disclose enlarged coronoid processes extending high above the zygomatic arch.

Differential Diagnosis: Restricted opening without pain or deviation in a young male should arouse suspicion of coronoid hyperplasia. While the other entities included here must be considered in the differential diagnosis, they are more common in older patients or exhibit restriction of opening with deviation or pain. Radiographs will confirm the diagnosis of condylar hyperplasia.

Treatment: When patients are not bothered by their inability to open and they are able to function adequately, no treatment is necessary. With severe limitation, bilateral coronoidectomy is the treatment of choice.

References

1. Rowe, N. L.: Bilateral developmental hyperplasia of the mandibular coronoid process. A report of two cases. Br. J. Oral Surg. *1*:90, 1963.
2. Van Hoof, R. J. and Besling, W. T.: Coronoid process enlargement. Br. J. Oral Surg. *10*:339, 1973.
3. Hecker, R. and Corwin, J. O.: Bilateral coronoid hyperplasia: review of the literature and report of case. J. Oral Surg. *38*:606, 1980.

Condylar Hyperplasia

Age: Children and young adults
Sex: Female predilection

Clinical Features: Unilateral hyperplasia of the mandibular condyle is of unknown etiology yet is considered to be a developmental defect. Clini-cally, facial asymmetry is seen and the patient will exhibit either an open bite on the affected side or a crossbite with open bite. The face is elongated on the affected side, and restricted opening may or may not be observed. Similarly, deviation toward the affected side is a variable finding. TMJ tomograms will disclose a markedly thickened condyle, which may represent a two- or threefold increase in dimension when compared radiographically with the normal condyle.

Differential Diagnosis: Condylar hyperplasia is easily differentiated from the other disorders included here with restricted or deviant mandibular movement. The facial asymmetry, open bite or crossbite, and radiographic evidence of an enlarged condyle confirm the diagnosis of condylar hyperplasia. Condylar hypoplasia is rare yet must be considered in the differential diagnosis because the normal side may be mistaken for hyperplasia.

Treatment: Surgical correction with subcondylar osteotomy is the treatment of choice. The case should be planned with models and radiographs because bilateral procedures may be required to obtain optimal results. Orthodontic consultation should be obtained; most patients will require combined orthodontic and surgical therapy.

References

1. Gruca, A. and Meisels, E.: Asymmetry of mandible from unilateral hypertrophy. Ann. Surg. *83*:755, 1926.
2. Bruce, R. A. and Hayward, J. R.: Condylar hyperplasia and mandibular asymmetry: a review. J. Oral Surg. *26*:281, 1968.
3. Wang-Norderud, R. and Ragab, R. R.: Unilateral condylar hyperplasia and the associated deformity of facial asymmetry. Case Report. Scand. J. Plast. Reconstr. Surg. *11*:91, 1977.
4. Ferguson, M. W. J. and Whitlock, R. I. H.: An un-

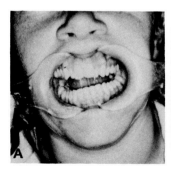
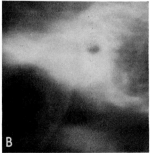
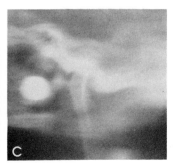

FIG. 12–37. Condylar Hyperplasia. *A:* Asymmetry with unilateral open bite on affected side. *B:* Hyperplastic condyle. *C:* Normal condyle for comparison. (Courtesy of Dr. John Ditmer.)

usual case of acquired unilateral condylar hypoplasia. Br. J. Oral Surg. *16*:156, 1978.

5. Jouck, L. M.: Condylar hyperplasia. A case for early treatment. Int. J. Oral Surg. *10*:154, 1981.

TMJ Region Neoplasms

Age:; Variable

Sex: Variable

Clinical Features: Most so-called neoplasms of the temporomandibular joint region are, in actuality, represented by hyperplastic or reactive processes including synovial chondromatosis and villonodular tenosynovitis. These reactive lesions involve the joint space or synovium and rarely distort or erode the condylar bone. Nevertheless, true benign and malignant neoplasms, while extremely rare, do arise in the region of the TMJ. The most common benign tumor is osteochondroma. The lesion arises from the cortex as an exostotic projection with a narrow neck. Actually, most osteochondromas arise from the coronoid process. Limitation of opening with deviation toward the affected side is a common sign; pain usually is not a complaint, although it certainly can be. Radiographs will disclose a radiopaque nodular projection emanating from either the condyle or coronoid; the projection is usually oriented medially or superiorly. Other benign neoplasms including osteomas, hemangiomas, and nerve sheath neoplasms may arise within articular tissues and cause restricted opening. Sarcomas are extremely rare, whereas parotid adenocarcinomas are not uncommon. These malignancies may proliferate within the infratemporal space and cause limited opening, cranial nerve deficits, and condylar or coronoid erosion as evidenced radiographically. In these instances, a parapharyngeal mass is usually palpable with deflection of the tonsilar region or soft palate.

Differential Diagnosis: Submental vertex, TMJ tomograms, and/or CT scans should be obtained when patients present with unilateral restricted opening and jaw deviation. Soft tissue opacification; irregular foci of resorption, particularly below the articular cortex; and soft tissue swelling over the joint or in the parapharyngeal region should arouse suspicion of neoplasia and a biopsy should be obtained.

Treatment: Treatment is usually surgical, and the extent of surgical removal will depend on the microscopic diagnosis.

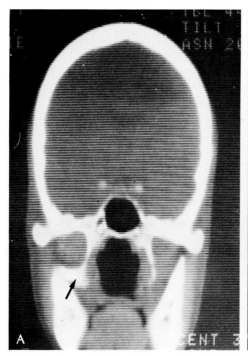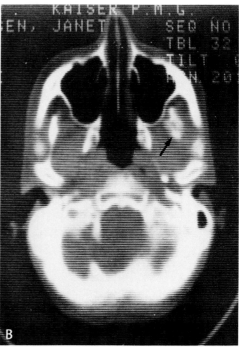

FIG. 12–38. Osteochondroma of the coronoid with fusion to the pterygoid plates. *A:* AP CT scan. *B:* Coronal CT scan.

References

1. Thoma, K. H.: Tumors of the condyle and tempo-romandibular joint. Oral Surg. 7:1091, 1954.
2. Gingrass, R. P.: Chondrosarcoma of the mandibular joint. J. Oral Surg. 12:61, 1954.
3. Goodsell, J. O. and Hubinger, H. L.: Benign chondroblastoma of the mandibular condyle. J. Oral Surg. 22:355, 1964.
4. Uotila, E. and Westerholm, N.: Hemangioma of the temporomandibular joint. Odont. T. 74:202, 1966.
5. James, R. B., Alexander, R. W., and Traver, J. G.: Osteochondroma of the mandibular coronoid process. Report of a case. Oral Surg. 37:189, 1974.
6. Simon, G. T., Kendrick, R. W., and Whitlock, R. I. H.: Osteochondroma of the mandibular condyle. Case report and its management. Oral Surg. 43:18, 1977.

Scleroderma

Age: Adults
Sex: Female predilection

Clinical Features: Scleroderma or progressive systemic sclerosis is grouped with the collagen diseases; while the etiology is unknown, evidence suggests an immunopathic or autoimmune mechanism. Although the onset is early adult life, many years evolve before severe symptoms develop. Progressive fibrosis of the skin, lungs,and esophagus is the end result with expressionless facies, board-like skin, sclerodactyly, and dysphagia. The CREST syndrome is a variant and is characterized by soft tissue calcinosis, Raynaud's phenomenon, esophageal stricture, sclerodactyly, and telangiectasia of the skin. Microstomia with restricted opening occurs late in the course of the disease. The major cause is fibrosis of the perioral tissues including the buccal mucosa. The fibrous induration is palpable and may restrict opening severely. In addition, some patients manifest temporomandibular joint symptoms, usually crepitus, and radiographs occasionally exhibit arthritic erosive changes.

Differential Diagnosis: Since scleroderma is a systemic disease with multisystem involvement, the diagnosis in a patient with restricted mandibular opening is usually straightforward. Board-hard facial skin, microstomia, widened periodontal ligament spaces, loss of attached gingiva with foci of stripping, and xerostomia are all head and neck manifestations of the disease.

Treatment: There is no effective therapy for the restricted opening observed in scleroderma. Plasmaphoresis has been beneficial for the other manifestations of the disease.

References

1. Seiffert, M. H., Steigerwald, J. C., and Cliff, M. M.: Bone resorption of the mandible in progressive systemic sclerosis. Arthritis Rheum. 18:507, 1975.
2. Weisman, R. A. and Calcaterra, T. C.: Head and neck manifestations of scleroderma. Ann. Otol. 87:332, 1978.
3. Marmary, Y., Glaiss, R., and Pisanty, S.: Scleroderma: oral manifestations. Oral Surg. 52:32, 1981.
4. Eversole, L. R., Jacobsen, P. L., and Stone, C. E.: Oral and gingival changes in systemic sclerosis (scleroderma). J. Periodontol. 55:175, 1984.

Tetanus

Age: No predilection
Sex: No predilection

Clinical Features: Tetany represents sustained tonic muscular contraction and is seen in *Clostridium tetani* infection and in *hypoparathyroidism* secondary to hypocalcemia. Infectious tetanus occurs primarily as a result of accidental injury from fomites on which *C. tetani* spores reside. The organism secretes the tetanus toxin that is transported to the central nervous system and acts upon autonomic nerves, end plates, the spinal cord, and the brain, where it binds to gangliosides. Headache is a prodromal sign followed by generalized muscle rigidity. During the early stages of the disease, masticatory muscle trismus occurs along with facial muscle spasms, producing a distorted demoniacal grin referred to as *risus sardonicus*. The myotonic spasm becomes progressively generalized with dysphasia, laryngospasm, and autonomic effects including hypertension, cardiac arrythmias, elevated pulse rate, and profuse perspiration. Hyperflexia is also featured. Death may result from asphyxia. In hypoparathyroidism, low serum calcium initiates neuromuscular electrolyte disturbances with appearance of convulsions and tetanus. Jaw trismus is rarely seen alone or as the chief presenting sign. Carpopedal spasm is the predominant finding. Latent tetany is evaluated by trapping the preauricular skin over the facial nerve that is followed by facial muscle contraction (Chvostek's sign) and by producing carpal spasm by reducing blood flow to the arm by means of a blood pressure cuff (Trousseau's sign). In addition, lowered-threshold electrical excitability of nerves is observed (Erb's sign). In addition to tetany and convulsions, other features of the disease include basal ganglia calcifications, dry skin with alopecia and atrophic nails, and cataracts. The serum calcium may dip to 5 mg/100 ml with acalciuria; serum phosphate is elevated.

Differential Diagnosis: Unlike most of the

other disorders with limited opening, tetanus is a systemic disorder involving numerous other muscle groups. The diagnosis is made on the basis of the aforementioned signs, symptoms, and laboratory findings.

Treatment: Infectious tetanus is treated by administration of tetanus antitoxin. Hypoparathyroid tetany is treated by management of the etiology of parathyroid dysfunction and restitution of electrolyte balance by administration of calcium and dihydrotachysterol. These patients should be managed by a physician.

References

1. Moersch, F. and Woltman, H.: Progressive fluctuating muscular rigidity and spasm (stiff-man syndrome). Proc. Staff Meet. Mayo Clinic. *31*:421, 1956.
2. Patel, J. and Mehta, B.: Tetanus: A study of 2007 cases. Indian J. M. Sci. *17*:791, 1963.
3. Nusynowitz, M. L., Frame, B., and Kolb, P. O.: The spectrum of hypoparathyroid states. Medicine *53*:127, 1974.
4. Smith, M. J. A. and Myall, R. W. T.: Tetanus: review of the literature and report of a case. Oral Surg. *41*:451, 1976.

GENERALIZED MOTOR FUNCTION DISORDERS

Auriculotemporal Syndrome

Age: No predilection
Sex: No predilection

Clinical Features: A complication of conservative parotid surgery, the auriculotemporal syndrome may also develop as a consequence of trauma or infection of the parotid or preauricular tissues. The syndrome, also termed *gustatory sweating*, is characterized by preauricular sweating, flushing, and sometimes pain following ingestion of food or visual stimulation by foods that initiate salivation. These symptoms emerge after severance of the auriculotemporal nerve, which, in addition to its sensory function, supplies parasympathetic fibers to the parotid. The fibers regenerate, become misdirected, and follow the course of sympathetic fibers to the skin and sweat glands. Parasympathetic fibers that would ordinarily induce salivation inadvertently stimulate the preauricular dermal sweat glands and arterioles, causing hydrosis and vasodilation. A similar disorder may accompany facial nerve palsy of surgical or traumatic origin in which parasympathetic fibers are misdirected into the lacrimal gland, causing gustatory lacrimation (crocodile tears).

Differential Diagnosis: Not applicable.

Treatment: Control of gustatory sweating may be maintained for up to 3 days by topical application to the affected skin of 1 percent glycopyrrolate lotion or cream.

References

1. Gardner, W. J. and McCubbin, J. W.: Auriculotemporal syndrome; gustatory sweating due to misdirection of regenerating nerve fibers. J. Am. Med. Assoc. *160*:272, 1956.
2. Hemenway, W. G.: Gustatory sweating and flushing; the auriculo-temporal syndrome—Frey's syndrome. Laryngoscope *70*:84, 1960.
3. Scouteris, C. A., et al.: Frey's syndrome. Report of a case. Oral Surg. *52*:368, 1981.
4. Hays, L. L., Novack, A. J., and Worsham, J. C.: The Frey Syndrome: A simple, effective treatment. Otolaryngol. Head Neck Surg. *90*:419, 1982.

Jaw-Winking Syndrome

Age: Childhood or congenital
Sex: Slight male predilection

Clinical Features: The jaw-winking syndrome is a misnomer in that this bizarre neuromuscular disorder is characterized by exaggerated opening of the eye upon moving of the mandible in a contralateral direction. The involved eye shows ptosis at rest. The pupils of both eyes show normal reflexes without miosis of the ptotic eye. Half of the affected patients manifest exaggerated opening by simply abducting the jaw, while the other half show this change only when the jaw is depressed with lateral movement to the opposite direction of the ptotic eye. The etiology and pathogenesis are unknown. It has been theorized that neural fiber crossovers occur between the pterygoid innervation and innervation to the upper lid. Supranuclear involvement has been suggested as responsible.

Differential Diagnosis: Unilateral ptosis as seen in the jaw-winking syndrome may be confused with Horner's syndrome. In the former, miosis with anhydrosis is lacking; conversely, the upper lid fails to open upon depression of the mandible in Horner's syndrome.

Treatment: No treatment is available. The defect is annoying to the patient yet is of no consequence with regard to association with a serious or life-threatening neurologic lesion.

References

1. Haynes, P. R.: A quantitative investigation of the Marcus Gunn phenomenon. Am. J. Optom. *32*:621, 1955.
2. Smith, E. E. and Gans, M. E.: Jaw-winking (Marcus Gunn phenomenon). J. Pediatr. *50*:52, 1957.

Motor System Disease

Age: Varies according to subtype
Sex: Male predilection

Clinical Features: The motor system diseases include *progressive muscular atrophy,* which begins in childhood and involves the extremities, *amyotrophic lateral sclerosis,* and *progressive bulbar palsy.* The motor system diseases result from degeneration of the corticospinal and anterior horn cells. The latter two variants begin in adulthood and result in bulbar signs. These two disorders may show a familial pattern or may develop after a neurotropic infection. In amyotrophic lateral scerosis (ALS) patients show ambulatory difficulties and weakness of the oropharyngeal musculature evidenced by difficulty with swallowing and speech. In progressive bulbar palsy, deglutition and articulation defects are present in conjunction with atrophy of masticatory and facial muscles. Fasciculation of the tongue is often present in both forms with bulbar manifestations.

Differential Diagnosis: Difficulty with swallowing and articulation, cardinal signs of bulbar degenerative motor system disorders, may also be seen in organic disease such as cancer of the larynx or base of the tongue. For this reason a thorough physical examination is required when these symptoms emerge. Bulbar lesions subsequent to cerebrovascular accident may cause similar signs and symptoms.

Treatment: No known treatment exists. The motor system diseases are progressive, eventually resulting in death.

References

1. Koerner, D. R.: Amyotrophic lateral sclerosis on Guam; a clinical study and review of the literature. Ann. Intern. Med. *37*:1204, 1952.
2. Roe, P. F.: Familial motor neuron disease. J. Neurol. Neurosurg. Psychiatry *27*:140, 1964.
3. Roller, N. W., et al.: Amyotrophic lateral sclerosis. Oral Surg. *37*:46, 1974.
4. Horton, W. A., Eldridge, R., and Brody, J. A.: Familial motor neuron disease. Neurology *26*:460, 1976.

Multiple Sclerosis

Age: Young adults
Sex: Slight female predilection

Clinical Features: Multiple sclerosis is a demyelinating disease, probably of either viral or autoimmune origin, that involves the central nervous system without demyelinization of peripheral nerves. The disease is chronic with periods of remission and exacerbation. A variety of neurologic signs and symptoms are observed, depending upon anatomical location and severity of lesions. These signs and symptoms can be extremely diverse; the more common include spasticity, hyperreflexia, Babinski's sign, absent abdominal reflexes, intention tremor, nystagmus, sensory deficits, paresthesias, muscle weakness, ocular disturbance, urinary disturbance, and ataxia. Facially, the more prevalent or noteworthy manifestations are ocular (diplopia, blurring of vision, visual field defects, and scotoma), sensory (trigeminal paresthesia or neuralgia), and motor (seventh nerve paresis and dysarthria). The more significant laboratory abnormalities include elevated CSF immunoglobulin G and white cells. Cortical-evoked responses from visual, auditory, and sensorimotor stimulation have been shown to be of value in early diagnosis. CT scans will often disclose ventricular enlargement, cortical atrophy, and periventricular plaques.

Differential Diagnosis: Myelinoclastic infectious diseases are easily confused with multiple sclerosis because the signs and symptoms can be identical. Neurologic lesions in other diseases including lupus erythematosus, polyarteritis nodosa, vascular malformations and gliomas of the brain stem, syringomyelia, and lymphoma may exhibit features similar to those enumerated for multiple sclerosis. Patients with unexplained facial weakness, paresthesia, or trigeminal neuralgia should be evaluated for the disease.

Treatment: Referral to a neurologist is recommended. The disease may be quite mild or may remain in long-term remission. Alternatively, in some instances it is a progressive disease that leaves the patient severely disabled.

References

1. Poser, C. M.: Diseases of the myelin sheath. In *A Textbook of Neurology,* 6th Ed., edited by H. H. Merritt. Philadelphia, Lea & Febiger, 1979, pp. 768–798.
2. Poser, C., et al.: Clinical characteristics of autopsy-proved multiple sclerosis. Neurol. *16*:791, 1966.
3. Mackay, R. and Hirano, A.: Forms of benign multiple sclerosis. Arch. Neurol. *17*:588, 1967.

Muscular Dystrophies

Age: Childhood onset
Sex: Male predilection

Clinical Features: Muscular dystrophy of Duchenne is a generalized progressive disease of muscle with an X-linked recessive mode of inheritance, occurring in males. A restricted form, fascioscapulohumeral dystrophy, shows no sex predilection, and the disorder is restricted to muscles of the face, neck, and shoulder. In all forms of muscular dystrophy, the primary defect lies in the muscle fiber; neural function and reflexes are not affected. In the generalized form, which is more common, early childhood onset is characterized by inability to ambulate, with pseudohypertrophy of the limb muscles. The increase in muscle bulk is the result of fatty infiltration so that weakness and poor function are encountered. The muscles eventually become atrophic. Masticatory, facial, and strap muscles are involved late in the course of the disease, with difficulty chewing, swallowing and articulating. Serum creatinine phosphokinase is elevated early in the course of the disease. Fascioscapulohumeral dystrophy spares the lower limbs and does not show pseudohypertrophic enlargement. Onset may be later in life and is characterized by profound weakness of the arms, inability to close the eyes, drooping of the facies and inability to purse the lips (which are protuberant). Cardiac failure is a common complication.

Differential Diagnosis: The two forms of muscular dystrophy may be differentiated on the basis of age and distribution of muscle involvement. Both may show myopathic facies, which occur in the myotonias, and myasthenia gravis. A muscle biopsy may be helpful in determining whether the patient suffers from muscular dystrophy. Muscle fibers show variation in size with infiltration of adipose tissue, and enzyme histochemical stains are useful.

Treatment: No treatment is presently effective. In Duchenne's muscular dystrophy, survival beyond the second decade is rare. Fascioscapulohumeral muscular dystrophy is compatible with life; however, many patients develop cardiac failure.

References

1. Pearson, C. M.: Muscular dystrophy. Am. J. Med. *35:*632, 1963.
2. Zundel, W. S. and Tyler, F. H.: The muscular dystrophies. N. Engl. J. Med. *273:*537, 1965.
3. Hanson, P. and Rowland, L. P.: Möbius syndrome and fascioscapulo-humeral muscular dystrophy. Arch. Neurol. *24:*31, 1971.
4. Black, J. T., et al.: Diagnostic accuracy of clinical data, quantitative electromyography and histochemistry in neuromuscular disease. J. Neurol. Sci. *21:*59, 1974.

Myotonias

Age: Children and young adults
Sex: No predilection

Clinical Features: The myotonias are characterized by failure of muscle relaxation following contraction. Two major forms exist: dystrophic and congenital myotonias. Myotonic contractions may also be acquired after trismus, with spread of infection to muscle. This form is most common, and in the head and neck area, myositis of the masticatory muscles generally develops as a complication of odontogenic infection or pericoronitis. Dystrophic myotonia develops in late childhood as an autosomal dominant trait. In addition to sustained contractions after voluntary neuromuscular activity, atrophy of the masticatory and strap muscles occurs to yield the so-called myopathic facies. Testicular atrophy is often present. Congenital myotonia, a familial disorder, commences early in life and affects virtually all skeletal muscles. The myotonic contractions are severe but painless. The affected individuals manifest marked generalized muscular hypertrophy so that they appear to be muscle-bound.

Differential Diagnosis: Dystrophic myotonia may resemble late muscular dystrophy and myasthenia gravis, as muscular atrophy with a myopathic facies may be seen in all three of these muscular disorders. Characteristic myotonic contractions are seen only in myotonia. The muscle hypertrophy of congenital myotonia is also accompanied by myotonic contraction, aiding in differentiating this disorder from pseudohypertrophic muscular dystrophy.

Treatment: No treatment is available for the familial myotonias. The dystrophic form is ultimately fatal, whereas the congenital form carries a favorable prognosis. Acquired myotonia may be treated by removing the source of infection and employing antibiotics.

References

1. Adams, R. S., Denny-Brown, D., and Pearson, C. M.: *Diseases of Muscle. A Study in Pathology,* 2nd Ed. New York, Harper and Row, 1962.
2. Thayer, H. H. and Crenshaw, J.: Oral manifestations of myotonic muscular dystrophy, report of a case. J. Am. Dent. Assoc. *72:*1405, 1966.
3. Becker, P. E.: Genetic approaches to the nosology of muscular disease: Myotonias and similar diseases. Birth Defects *7:*52, 1971.
4. Dyken, P. R. and Harper, P. S.: Congenital dystrophia myotonia. Neurology *23:*465, 1973.

Congenital Facial Diplegia

Age: Congenital
Sex: No predilection

Clinical Features: The Möbius syndrome is a nonfamilial congenital primary myopathy of the facial muscles with secondary degeneration of the abducens and facial nerves. In utero necrosis of brain stem nuclei has been reported and may have been due to an episode of anoxia. The paralysis is bilateral with expressionless facies and inability to close the eyes. The muscles of mastication may also be affected, with difficulty in chewing and swallowing. Drooling is often uncontrollable. Patients also show a variety of other congenital defects including deafness, epilepsy, and club foot.

Differential Diagnosis: Congenital facial diplegia shows myopathic facies seen in other myopathies; however, onset at birth and restriction to the facial musculature allow for differentiation from these other disorders.

Treatment: No treatment is effective. The disease is not fatal.

References

1. McDougal, J. J.: Möbius syndrome: A congenital facial diplegia syndrome. J. Conn. State Dent. Assoc. *34:*21, 1960.
2. Pitner, S. E., Edwards, J. E., and McCormick, W. F.: Observations on the pathology of the Moebius syndrome. J. Neurol. Neurosurg. & Psychiatr. *28:*362, 1965.
3. Thakkar, N., et al.: Möbius syndrome due to brainstem tegmental necrosis. Arch. Neurol. *34:*124, 1977.

Hemifacial Atrophy

Age: Teenagers
Sex: Female predilection

Clinical Features: Unilateral progressive atrophy of the face, known as Romberg's syndrome, is an uncommon disorder of unknown origin. It begins during the second decade with slowly progressive atrophy of the skin, muscle, and often even the maxilla and mandible on one side of the face. The disease progresses for 3 or 4 years and ultimately becomes static. The teeth on the affected side may be smaller than normal, and eruption may be somewhat retarded. Contralateral epilepsy and trigeminal neuralgia may accompany the atrophic changes.

Differential Diagnosis: The marked facial asymmetry with atrophy on one side may be confused with hemifacial hypertrophy. Close observation will of course show that the larger side of the face is normal, the smaller side atrophic. Unilateral TMJ ankylosis may show features similar to Romberg's syndrome; however, in the former only the mandible is atrophic, whereas in the latter the entire hemiface is involved.

Treatment: Elective plastic surgery may be performed once the atrophic process has stabilized.

References

1. Crikelair, G. F., et al.: Facial hemiatrophy. Plast. Reconstr. Surg. *29:*5, 1962.
2. Glass, D.: Hemifacial atrophy. Br. J. Oral Surg. *1:*194, 1964.
3. Stringer, D. E., et al.: Correction of hemifacial microsomia. J. Oral Surg. *39:*35, 1981.

Myasthenia Gravis

Age: Middle-aged adults
Sex: Female predilection

Clinical Features: Myasthenia gravis is characterized by generalized muscular weakness involving only voluntary muscle, the heart being spared. Often the facial and masticatory muscles are the first to show fatigue after limited movement. As the disease progresses, ptosis with an expressionless myopathic facies develops. In advanced cases, the jaw and head droop; eventually, the respiratory muscles become fatigued. The cause for this condition is unknown but has been linked to immunopathologic mechanisms operating at the level of the neuromuscular junction with interference in the release-binding of acetylcholine. Thymic hyperplasia or thymoma is found in most patients with myasthenia gravis.

Differential Diagnosis: The myopathic facies with generalized muscular weakness is seen in muscular dystrophy, myotonias and Möbius syndrome. The onset during midlife, predilection for females, lack of myotonic contraction, and lack of muscle hypertrophy favor a diagnosis of myasthenia. A muscle biopsy may be helpful in that perivascular lymphoid aggregates appear between muscle bundles in this disorder, but are not featured in the aforementioned disorders. A classic diagnostic finding is the ability of intramuscular injection of physostigmine to restore normal functions.

Treatment: Myasthenia gravis is treated with anticholinesterases such as neostigmine or related drugs and should be managed by an internist or neurologist.

References

1. Keeling, C. W.: Myasthenia gravis. J. Oral Surg. *9:*224, 1951.
2. Garvin, J. S.: Differential diagnosis of muscle weakness in myasthenia gravis, polymyositis, and muscular dystrophy. Med. Clin. North Am. *49:*189, 1965.
3. Kornfeld, O. and Genkins, G.: Current concepts in myasthenia gravis. J. Med. Soc. N. J. *71:*562, 1974.
4. Gallagher, D. M., Erickson, K. L., and Genkins, G.: Current concepts in the surgical treatment of patients with myasthenia gravis. J. Oral Surg. *39:*30, 1981.

Appendices

APPENDIX I. CLASSIFICATION OF CERTAIN ORAL CYSTS, REACTIVE PROLIFERATIONS, AND NEOPLASMS

I. **Odontogenic Cysts**
   Dental lamina cyst
   Gingival cyst
   Primordial cyst
   Lateral periodontal cyst
   Dentigerous (follicular) cyst
   Eruption cyst
   Apical periodontal cyst
   Calcifying epithelial odontogenic cyst
   Odontogenic keratocyst

II. **Developmental and Nonodontogenic Cysts**
   A. Intraosseous Cysts
      Incisive canal (nasopalatine) cyst
      Globulomaxillary cyst
      Surgical ciliated cyst of the maxilla
   B. Soft Tissue Cysts
      Epidermoid cyst
      Dermoid cyst
      Lymphoepithelial (branchial cleft) cyst
      Benign cystic lymph node
      Lingual gastric cyst
      Thyroglossal duct cyst
      Nasoalveolar (Kledstadt) cyst
      Cyst of incisive papilla
      True mucous cyst
   C. Pseudocysts
      Mucous retention phenomenon (mucocele)
      Ranula (mucocele)
      Traumatic (hemorrhagic) cyst

III. **Benign Odontogenic Neoplasms and Hamartomas**
   A. Epithelial Group
      Ameloblastoma
      Calcifying epithelial odontogenic tumor
      Odontogenic adenomatoid tumor
      Epithelial odontogenic hamartoma
      Squamous odontogenic tumor
   B. Mixed Group
      Ameloblastic fibroma
      Ameloblastic fibrodentinoma
      Ameloblastic fibro-odontoma

        Odontoma
        Odontoameloblastoma
   C. Mesenchymal Group
        Odontogenic fibroma
        Odontogenic myxoma
        Periapical cemental dysplasia (cementoma)
        Benign cementoblastoma
        Cementifying fibroma
   D. Malignant Odontogenic Neoplasms
        Malignant ameloblastoma
        Ameloblastic carcinoma
        Intraosseous squamous cell carcinoma
        Ameloblastic fibrosarcoma

IV.   Salivary Neoplasms
   A. Benign
        Pleomorphic adenoma (mixed tumor)
        Monomorphic adenoma
        Canalicular (basal cell) adenoma
        Papillary cystadenoma lymphomatosum
        Oxyphilic adenoma (oncocytoma)
        Ductal papilloma
        Sebaceous lymphadenoma
        Glycogen-rich adenoma
   B. Malignant
        Adenoid cystic carcinoma (cylindroma)
        Mucoepidermoid carcinoma
        Malignant mixed tumor
        Ductal epidermoid carcinoma
        Oat cell adenocarcinoma
        Acinic cell carcinoma
        Epithelial-myoepithelial carcinoma of intercalated duct
        Adenocarcinoma (not otherwise specified)

V.   Oral Epithelial Neoplasms
   A. Benign
        Papilloma
        Verruca vulgaris
        Condyloma acuminatum
        Keratoacanthoma
   B. Malignant
        Epidermoid (squamous cell) carcinoma
        Verrucous carcinoma
        Adenoacanthoma (pseudoglandular squamous cell carcinoma)
        Spindle cell carcinoma

VI.   Neuroectodermal Hamartomas and Neoplasms
   Ephilis
   Nevocellular nevi
   Melanocytic nevi (blue nevus)
   Spindle cell nevus
   Melanotic neuroectodermal tumor of infancy

Hutchinson's freckle (superficial spreading melanoma)
Malignant melanoma

VII. Mesenchymal Neoplasms of Soft Tissue

A. Benign
Fibroma
Giant cell fibroma
Lipoma
Leiomyoma
Rhabdomyoma
Granular sheath cell lesion (myoblastoma)
Neurofibroma
Neurilemmoma (schwannoma)
Osseous and cartilaginous choristoma
Fibrous histiocytoma
Hemangioma
Lymphangioma and cystic hygroma

B. Aggressive
Hemangioendothelioma
Hemangiopericytoma

C. Malignant
Fibrosarcoma
Liposarcoma
Leiomyosarcoma
Rhabdomyosarcoma
Alveolar soft part sarcoma
Neurogenic sarcoma
Malignant fibrous histiocytoma
Synovial sarcoma
Angiosarcoma
Kaposi's sarcoma
Malignant lymphoma (Hodgkin's and non-Hodgkin's types)

VIII. Reactive Proliferations

Pyogenic granuloma
Traumatic fibroma
Inflammatory fibrous hyperplasia (epulis fissuratum)
Papillomatosis
Peripheral ossifying fibroma
Peripheral giant cell granuloma
Pseudosarcomatous fasciitis
Myositis ossificans
Proliferative myositis

IX. Central Nonodontogenic Bone Tumors of the Jaws

A. Benign
Desmoplastic fibroma
Hemangioma and arteriovenous malformation
Neurofibroma
Neurilemmoma
Central ossifying fibroma
Osteoma

B. Malignant
Osteogenic sarcoma
Chondrosarcoma
Fibrosarcoma
Neurogenic sarcoma
Ewing's sarcoma
Angiosarcoma
Non-Hodgkin's lymphoma
Burkitt's lymphoma
Multiple myeloma

APPENDIX II. CLASSIFICATION OF BENIGN FIBRO-OSSEOUS LESIONS

I. **Giant Cell Group**
Central giant cell granuloma
Hyperparathyroid brown tumor
Aneurysmal bone cyst
Cherubism (familial fibrous dysplasia)

II. **Nongiant Cell Group (Pure Fibro-Osseous)**
Fibrous dysplasia
Osteitis deformans
Ossifying and cementifying fibroma
Periapical cemental dysplasia (cementoma)
Focal sclerosing osteomyelitis
Diffuse sclerosing osteomyelitis (florid cemento-osseous dysplasia)
Garre's proliferative periostitis

APPENDIX III. CLINICAL LABORATORY PARAMETERS

The following diseases, which are associated with elevated or depressed values, are by no means all inclusive. Rather, they represent the more common disease states showing alterations in laboratory values.

I. **Hemogram**
A. Red Blood Cell Count, Hemoglobin, and Hematocrit

1. *Elevated*
Fluid loss
Polycythemia vera
Secondary polycythemia

2. *Depressed*
Iron deficiency anemia
Pernicious anemia
Malaria
Hemorrhage
Thalassemia
Sickle-cell anemia
Hemolytic anemias
Leukemia
Metastatic cancer
Osteopetrosis
Multiple myeloma
Pancytopenia
Erythroblastosis fetalis
Renal disease

B. White Blood Cell Count
   1. *Elevated*
      Infections
      Leukemia

   2. *Depressed*
      Certain viral infections
      Leukemia (leukopenic phase)
      Agranulocytosis
      Cyclic neutropenia
      Hemorrhage
      Pancytopenia
      Typhoid fever

C. Differential White Count
   1. *Neutrophilic Leukocytosis*
      a. Pyogenic infections
      b. Myelogenous leukemia
   2. *Lymphocytic Leukocytosis*
      a. Viral infections
      b. Typhoid fever
      c. Lymphocytic leukemia
      d. Infectious mononucleosis
   3. *Eosinophilic Leukocytosis*
      a. Allergy
      b. Parasitic infections, particularly helminths
   4. *Neutrophilic Leukopenia*
      a. Agranulocytosis
      b. Cyclic neutropenia
      c. Leukemia
D. Thrombocytes
   1. *Depressed Count*
      Thrombocytopenic purpura
      Secondary thrombocytopenia
      Pancytopenia
      Leukemia
      Metastatic cancer
      Multiple myeloma
      Consumptive coagulopathy (DIC)
      Postinfections
   2. *Delayed Aggregation*
      Thrombocytopathic purpura
      von Willebrand's disease
      Salicylates and other drugs

II. **Coagulation Panel**
   A. Prothrombin Time Prolonged
      Alcoholic cirrhosis
      Biliary cirrhosis
      Hepatitis
      Idiopathic steatorrhea
      Hypovitaminosis K
      Coumadin therapy
      Afibrinogenemia
      Hypoprothrombinemia

   B. Partial Thromboplastin Time Prolonged
      Hemophilia
      Christmas disease
      von Willebrand's disease
      Hageman deficiency
      All disorders manifesting prolonged prothrombin time
   C. Fibrin Split Products
      Disseminated intravascular coagulation

III. **Serology (Elevated or Positive Tests)**
   A. VDRL, TPI, FTA—Syphilis
   B. Monospot, Heterophil Antibody—Infectious Mononucleosis
   C. Antistreptolysin-O—Scarlet Fever, Rheumatic Fever, Erysipelas, Streptococcal
      Sore Throat
   D. RA Factor—Rheumatoid Arthritis
   E. Antinuclear Antibodies and Anti-DNA Antibodies—Lupus Erythematosus,
      Miscellaneous Collagen Diseases
   F. Antimitotic Spindle Antibody—Scleroderma
   G. Coombs' Test—Erythroblastosis Fetalis and Other Immune Hemolytic Anemias
   H. HBS-AB—Immunity to Hepatitis B
   I. HBS-AG, Hepatitis Core AG—Active or Carrier Status for Hepatitis B

IV. **Immunofluorescence/Immunoperoxidase**
   A. Antibasal Lamina Antibodies (Smooth)—Bullous Pemphigoid, Benign Mucous
      Membrane Pemphigoid
   B. Antibasal Lamina Antibodies (Granular)—Lupus Erythematosus
   C. Anti-Intercellular Cement Antibodies—Pemphigus Vulgaris
   D. Antibasal Lamina Fibrinogen—Lichen Planus
   E. Submucosal Papillae IgA Antibodies—Dermatitis Herpetiformis
   F. Antiductal Salivary Antibodies—Sjögren's Syndrome

V. **Clinical Laboratory**

Test	Elevated Values	Depressed Values
A. Glucose 70–110 mg/100 ml	Diabetes mellitus Acute pancreatitis Cushing's syndrome Pheochromocytoma Acromegaly Anabolic hormones Hemochromatosis	Insulinoma Addison's disease Liver disease Early diabetes Glycogenosis Renal glycosuria
B. Total Bilirubin 0.1–1.0 mg/100 ml	Biliary obstruction Liver diseases Hemolytic anemias Hepatitis Postextravasation Dubin-Johnson syndrome Gilbert's disease Crigler-Najjar syndrome Rotor's syndrome Malnutrition	

C. Cholesterol
150–300 mg/100 ml

Atherosclerosis	Liver disease
Diabetes mellitus	Malnutrition
Nephrotic syndrome	Anemia
Hypothyroidism	
Hyperlipoproteinemia	
Gout	
Myeloma	
Biliary obstruction	

D. Uric Acid
2.5–8.0 mg/100 ml

Gout	Cirrhosis
Malignancy	Renal tubular disease
Infectious mononucleosis	Various drugs
Renal disease	Wilson's disease
Tissue necrosis	
Anemias	

E. Creatinine
.05–1.5 mg/100 ml

Muscle necrosis	
Renal disease	

F. Total Protein
6–8 gm/100 ml

Liver disease	Renal disease
Collagen disease	Debilitating disease
Chronic infection	Malnutrition
Myeloma	Burns
Cryoglobulinemia	Hypogammaglobulinemia

G. Albumin
3.5–5 gm/100 ml

	Liver disease
	Nephrotic syndrome
	Malnutrition
	Burns

H. Calcium
8.5–10.5 mg/100 ml

Hyperparathyroidism	Renal disease
Milk-alkali syndrome	Malnutrition
Malignancy	Acute pancreatitis
Sarcoidosis	Hypoparathyroidism
Hypothyroidism	Vitamin D refractory
Addison's disease	rickets
Hypophosphatasia	

I. Phosphorus
2.5–4.5 mg/100 ml

Malignancy in bone	Hyperparathyroidism
Renal disease	Malnutrition
Hypoparathyroidism	Osteomalacia
Milk-alkali syndrome	Renal tubular disease
Sarcoidosis	Vitamin D refractory
Addison's disease	rickets
	Hypophosphatasia

J. Alkaline
    Phosphatase   Bone metastasis   Hypophosphatasia
    1.5–5 Bodansky   Hepatobiliary disease   Malnutrition
    U/ml   Renal disease
    5–10 King-   Paget's disease
    Armstrong U/ml   Bone fractures
                               Fibrous dysplasia
                               Ulcerative colitis
                               Hyperthyroidism
                               Pancreatitis
                               Sarcoidosis
                               Rickets
                               Amyloidosis

K. SGOT
    10–40 U/ml   Acute myocardial
                                 infarction
                               Liver disease
                               Skeletal muscle disease
                               Congestive heart failure
                               Renal infarction
                               Pulmonary infarction
                               Malignancy
                               Burns
                               Certain anemias
                               Eclampsia
                               Trauma

L. LDH
    100–225 U/ml   Myocardial infarction
                               Liver disease
                               Skeletal muscle disease
                               Renal infarction
                               Pulmonary infarction
                               Cerebral vascular accident
                               Collagen vascular diseases
                               Acute pancreatitis
                               Trauma

APPENDIX IV. PRESCRIPTIONS USEFUL IN THE MANAGEMENT OF ORAL DISEASES

I. Antibiotics (Endocarditis Prophylaxis)

Regimen A (Adults/Oral)

Penicillin V 500 mg
Dsp #12
Sig: 4 caps 1 hour prior to procedure, then 1 cap q6h for 8 doses
Use: Patients with rheumatic or congenital heart defects *excluding* prosthetic valves

Erythromycin 500 mg
Dsp #10
Sig: 2 caps 1½ hours prior to procedure, then 1 cap q6h for 8 doses

Use: Penicillin allergic patients with rheumatic or congenital heart defects excluding prosthetic valves

Regimen A (Children/Oral)
Penicillin V 250 mg
Dsp #12
Sig: 4 caps 1 hour prior to procedure, then 1 cap q6h for 8 doses
Use: Child patients under 60 lbs with rheumatic or congenital heart defects excluding prosthetic valves

Erythromycin
20 mg/kg initial oral dose $1\frac{1}{2}$ hours prior to procedure
10 mg/kg dose q6h for 8 doses
Use: Child patients allergic to penicillin with rheumatic or congenital heart disease

Regimen B (Adults)
Aqueous crystalline penicillin G 1,000,000 U
Penicillin G procaine, 600,000 U
Streptomycin 1 gm
Intramuscular injection $\frac{1}{2}$–1 hour prior to procedure, then
Penicillin V 500 mg orally q6h for 8 doses
Use: Patients with prosthetic valves

Vancomycin 1 gm intravenously over $\frac{1}{2}$–1 hour prior to procedure, then
Erythromycin 500 mg orally q6h for 8 doses
Use: Patients allergic to penicillin with prosthetic valves

Regimen B (Children)
Aqueous crystalline penicillin G 30,000 U/kg
Penicillin G procaine 600,000 U
Streptomycin 20 mg/kg
Intramuscular injection $\frac{1}{2}$–1 hour prior to procedure, then
Penicillin V 500 mg or 250 mg q6h for 8 doses
Use: Children over 60 lbs (500 mg q6h) and children under 60 lbs (250 mg q6h) with prosthetic valves

II.   **Antibiotics (Infections)**
Penicillin VK 500 mg
Dsp #40
Sig: 1 cap q6h
Use: Odontogenic infections (i.e., abscess cellulitis), acute necrotizing ulcerative gingivitis with fever, oral gonorrhea

Erythromycin stearate 500 mg
Dsp #40
Sig: 1 cap q6h
Use: Odontogenic infections in the patient allergic to penicillin

Dicloxacillin 150 mg
Dsp #40
Sig: 2 caps q6h
Use: Possible drug of choice when penicillin is ineffective in 48 hours. Effective for staphylococci or penicillinase secreting organisms.

Clindamycin 150 mg
Dsp #40
Sig: 2 caps q6h
Use: Most effective against bacteroides infections.
        Caution, may cause clostridia pseudomembranous ulcerative colitis.

Cephalexin 250 mg
Dsp #40
Sig: 1 cap q6h
Use: Possible drug of choice when penicillin is ineffective in 48 hours. Often
        ineffective for penicillinase secreting organisms.

Tetracycline oral suspension 250 mg/tsp
Dsp 4 oz
Sig: 1 tsp q.i.d., rinse orally for 5 minutes and swallow
Use: Minor and major aphthous stomatitis

Mycostatin oral suspension 500,000 U/tsp
Dsp 4 oz
Sig: 1 tsp q6h; rinse orally for 5 minutes then swallow (7 days)
Use: Oral candidiasis

Mycostatin vaginal tablets 100,000 U
Dsp #56
Sig: 2 tabs q6h; use orally as lozenge
Use: Oral candidiasis

Nizoral 200 mg
Dsp #10
Sig: 1 tab per day
Use: Oral candidiasis

III. Antihistamines and Topical Anesthetics
Benadryl 50 mg
Dsp #20
Sig: 1 cap t.i.d.
Use: Allergic stomatitis of the immediate type, erythema multiforme

Phenergan 12.5 mg
Dsp #20
Sig: 1 cap t.i.d.
Use: Allergic stomatitis of the immediate type, erythema multiforme

Benadryl elixir 12.5 mg/tsp 50:50 with Kaopectate
Dsp 6 oz
Sig: 2 tsp as oral rinse t.i.d.
Use: Palliation of painful vesiculoulcerative lesions

Phenergan syrup 6.25 mg/tsp 50:50 with Kaopectate
Dsp 6 oz
Sig: 2 tsp as oral rinse t.i.d.
Use: Palliation of painful vesiculoulcerative lesions

2% Xylocaine viscous
Dsp 4 oz

Sig: 3 drops with fingertip to oral sores p.r.n. for pain
Use: Palliation of painful vesiculoulcerative lesions
Caution: Instruct patient not to swallow medication to avoid anesthetizing gag reflex

IV. Steroid Anti-Inflammatory Preparations

0.1% Triamcinolone in Orabase
Dsp 5-gm tube
Sig: Apply to oral sores q.i.d.
Use: Erosive lichen planus, bullous pemphigoid, oral lesions of pemphigus vulgaris, contact (delayed) allergic stomatitis

.05% Lidex ointment 50:50 with Orabase
Dsp 10 gm
Sig: Apply to oral lesions 6 times daily
Use: Erosive lichen planus, bullous pemphigoid, pemphigus vulgaris, contact (delayed) allergic stomatitis

Dapsone 25 mg
Dsp #30
Sig: 1 tab daily for 3 days, then 2 tabs daily for 3 days, then 3 tabs daily for 3 days, followed by 2 tabs b.i.d. for 3 days
Use: Benign mucous membrane pemphigoid. Maintenance dose after accelerated schedule is between 100 and 150 mg daily.
Caution: Dapsone may cause hemolysis; red cell counts, hemoglobin, and hematocrit should be obtained regularly.

Prednisone 5 mg or dexamethasone 0.75 mg
Dsp #40
Sig: 1 tab q6h for 7 days, followed by 1 tab q12h for 4 days, followed by ½ tab q12h for 3 days
Use: Severe erosive lichen planus, major aphthous stomatitis, benign mucous membrane pemphigoid, erythema multiforme
Caution: Do not prescribe for patients with existing infectious disease or diabetes mellitus

1% Hydrocortisone with polymyxin B, bacitracin, neomycin cream 50:50 with 5% lidocaine ointment
Dsp 5 gm
Sig: Apply to lip sores t.i.d.
Use: Recurrent herpes labialis
Caution: Do not apply during early active stages. Use 4 days following onset of vesicular eruption, after vesicles have ruptured

V. Antiviral Topicals

5% Zovirax ointment
Dsp 15 gm
Sig: Apply to lip sores 6 times daily
Use: Herpes labialis. Recommend application during onset of prodromal paresthesia if possible; otherwise apply directly over vesicles.

VI. Muscle Relaxants

Paraflex 250 mg
Dsp #100
Sig: 2 tabs q.i.d.

Use: Myogenic facial pain, tension headache

Parafon Forte 500 mg
Dsp #100
Sig: 2 tabs q.i.d.
Use: Myogenic facial pain, tension headache

Lioresal 10 mg
Dsp #60
Sig: ½ tab t.i.d. for 3 days, then 1 tab t.i.d. for 3 days, then 1½ tab t.i.d.
Use: Myogenic facial pain, tension headache

VII. Anxiolytics

Valium 5 mg
Dsp #20
Sig: 1–2 tabs daily
Use: Tension reduction prior to appointments, myogenic facial pain

Ativan 1 mg
Dsp #20
Sig: 1 tab daily
Use: Tension reduction prior to appointments, myogenic facial pain

VIII. Antidepressants

Sinequan 25 mg
Dsp #45
Sig: 1 cap each evening for 5 days, then 2 caps each evening for 5 days, then 4
       caps each evening for 7 days
Use: Atypical facial pain of psychogenic origin, most effective in depressed patients
       with anxiety. Dexamethasone suppression test advisable initially. Maintenance
       dose varies from 100–200 mg daily.

Desyrel 50 mg
Dsp #70
Sig: 2 tabs each evening for 5 days, then 3 tabs each evening for 5 days, then 3
       tabs b.i.d. for 7 days
Use: Atypical facial pain of psychogenic origin, most effective in depressed patients.
       Dexamethasone suppression test advisable initially. Maintenance dose is
       250–350 mg/day in divided doses.

IX. Analgesics

Aspirin 325 mg or Tylenol
Dsp: OTC
Sig: 2 tabs q6h, p.r.n. pain
Use: Mild pain

Motrin 600 mg
Dsp #20
Sig: 1 tab q.i.d., p.r.n. pain
Use: Mild pain

ASA #2 (Codeine 15 mg)
       #3 (Codeine 30 mg)
       #4 (Codeine 60 mg)
Dsp #20

Sig: 1 tab q4h, p.r.n. pain
Use: Mild to moderate pain

Percodan or Percocet
Dsp #20
Sig: 1 tab q4h, p.r.n. pain
Use: Moderate pain

Demerol 50 mg
Dsp #12
Sig: 1 tab q4h, p.r.n. pain
Use: Severe pain

Dilaudid 2 mg
Dsp #12
Sig: 1 tab q4h, p.r.n. pain
Use: Severe pain

Cafergot suppositories
Dsp #10
Sig: Place 1 tab rectally at onset of pain attack
Use: Migraine headache, midface cluster headache, not to exceed 5 per week.
Caution: Contraindicated in gravid women; use cautiously in hypertensive
patients.

Tegretol 100 mg
Dsp #40
Sig: 1 tab b.i.d. for 2 days, then 1 tab q.i.d.
Use: Trigeminal and glossopharyngeal neuralgias. Most patients can be maintained
on 400–800 mg per day. Caution: While escalating, complete blood counts
should be monitored regularly as Tegretol will induce a dose-related marrow
suppression.

Index